Dictionary of Medical Acronyms & Abbreviations

Fourth Edition

Compiled and edited by
Stanley Jablonski

HANLEY & BELFUS, INC. / *Philadelphia*

Publisher: HANLEY & BELFUS, INC.
                Medical Publishers
                210 South 13th Street
                Philadelphia, PA 19107
                (215) 546-7293; 800-962-1892
                FAX (215) 790-9330
                Web site: http://www.hanleyandbelfus.com

Library of Congress Cataloging-in-Publication Data

Dictionary of medical acronyms and abbreviations / Stanley Jablonski—4th ed.
     p. cm.
   ISBN 1-56053-460-5 (alk. paper)
     1. Medicine—Abbreviations—Dictionaries. 2. Medicine—Acronyms—Dictionaries.
Jablonski, Stanley.

   R123.J24 2001
   610'.1'48—dc21   2001016717

**Dictionary of Medical Acronyms
& Abbreviations, 4th edition**   ISBN 1-56053-460-5

Last digit is the print number: 9   8   7   6   5   4   3   2

Preface to the First Edition

Acronyms and abbreviations are used extensively in medicine, science and technology for good reason—they are more essential in such fields. It would be difficult to imagine how one could write down chemical and mathematical formulas and equations without using abbreviations or symbols. In medicine, they are used as a convenient shorthand in writing medical records, instructions, and prescriptions, and as space-saving devices in printed literature. It is easier and more economical to write down the acronyms HETE and RAAS than their full names 12-L-hydroxy-5,8,10,14-eicosatetraenoic acid and renin-angiotensin-aldosterone system, respectively.

The main reason for abbreviations is said to be economy. Some actually save space in print, such as acronyms for the names of institutions and organizational units, as well as being convenient to use. Many are used for other reasons, as for instance, when trying to be delicate, we may euphemistically refer to bowel movement as BM, an unprincipled individual as SOB, and body odor as BO. Also, it is sometimes difficult to fathom the reasoning of bureaucratic acronym makers, who have created some tongue-twisting monstrosities, such as ADCOMSUBORDCOMPHIBSPAC (for Administrative Command, Amphibious Forces, Pacific Fleet, Subordinate Command).

Abbreviations and acronyms used in medicine can be grouped into two broad categories. The first consists of official abbreviations and symbols used in chemistry, mathematics, and other sciences, and those designating weights and measures, whose exact form, capitalization, and punctuation have been determined by official governing bodies In this category, they mean only one thing (e.g., kg is the symbol for kilogram and Hz for hertz), and their form, capitalization, and punctuation have been established by the International System of Units (Système International d'Unités). Abbreviations in the second group, on the other hand, may appear in a variety of forms, the same abbreviation having a different number of letters, sometimes capitalized, at other times not, with or without punctuation. Moreover, they may also have numerous meanings. The abbreviation AP may mean alkaline phosphatase, acid phosphatase, action potential, angina pectoris, and many other things.

Editors of individual scientific publications make an effort to standardize the form of abbreviations and symbols in their journals and books, but they generally vary from one publication to another.

This dictionary lists acronyms and abbreviations occurring with a reasonable frequency in the medical literature that were identified by a systematic scanning of collections of books and periodicals at the National Library of Medicine. Except as they take the form of Greek letters, pure geometric symbols are not included. Although we have attempted to be as inclusive as possible, a book such as this one can never be complete, in spite of the most diligent effort, and it is expected that some abbreviations and acronyms may have escaped detection and others may have been introduced since completion of the manuscript.

Stanley Jablonski

Preface to the Second Edition

It is a reality of medicine and science that the number of acronyms and abbreviations is increasing dramatically. Despite the efforts of teachers and editors to contain them, clinicians and researchers constantly introduce new ones, as perusal of any current journal demonstrates. This growth attests to the fact that acronyms and abbreviations are necessary and useful in medical writing and speaking, conserving space and preventing needless repetition.

This edition, like its predecessor, is a selective collection of the most frequently used acronyms and abbreviations. Over 2,000 entries have been added. We trust you will find it to be a handy reference to be kept within easy reach.

Stanley Jablonski

Preface to the Third Edition

The purpose of this edition, like that of the previous two editions, is to provide a compact, useful, and affordable collection of the most frequently used acronyms and abbreviations in medicine and the health care professions. As in previous editions, the goal was not to be comprehensive but rather to focus on acronyms and abbreviations that occur with reasonable frequency in the health care literature.

Approximately 5,000 entries have been added to reflect new material related to burgeoning fields such as health care management, long-term care, outcomes research, medical informatics, molecular biology, and outpatient care, to name just a few. The symbol section in the front of the book has also been expanded and now includes genetic symbols as well as the Greek alphabet.

We welcome feedback and suggestions from readers, which can be sent to me in care of the publisher, Hanley & Belfus in Philadelphia. I hope you find this new edition user friendly and helpful.

Stanley Jablonski

Preface to the Fourth Edition

There has been a veritable explosion in the number of acronyms over the past few years, especially in the fields of medical informatics, computer technology, cardiology, and molecular biology, to name just a few. As in previous editions, the goal of this book is not to be exhaustive in coverage but rather to focus on medical acronyms and abbreviations that are encountered with reasonable frequency by health care professionals or those in other professions that use medical or health care terminology.

This edition boasts an amazing 10,000 new entries that cover recent advances in medicine. This enormous growth attests to the usefulness of acronyms and abbreviations in avoiding needless repetition and in providing a mechanism for coping with the unwieldy, lengthy descriptions related to new clinical trials and new technologies.

Acronyms and abbreviations are being created at such a rapid pace that a book such as this can never contain every last one, but new entries were included up to the very day this book went to press. I invite readers to send or email suggestions to the publisher. I hope you find this 4th edition to be a valuable, convenient, easy-to-use resource.

Stanley Jablonski

Acknowledgments

The author would like to thank Christopher Peterson, MD, PhD, from Rio de Janeiro, Brazil, for supplying several hundred entries for this edition. The work of Tsung O. Cheng, MD, from Washington, DC, was extremely useful for verifying acronyms for cardiology trials and is gratefully acknowledged: Cheng TO: Acronyms of clinical trials in cardiology—1998. American Heart Journal 137:726–765, 1999.

Symbols

°	degree
′	foot
″	inch
/	per
%	per cent
:	ratio
∞	infinity
+	positive
−	negative
±	positive or negative
#	number; fracture; pound
÷	divided by
×	multiplied by; magnification
=	equals
≠	does not equal
~	approximate
↓	decreased
↑	increased
→	to (in direction of)
∅	normal
∨	systolic blood pressure
∧	diastolic blood pressure
∠	angle
∠	angle of entry
∡	angle of exit
⌞	right lower quadrant
⌐	right upper quadrant
⌐	left upper quadrant
⌟	left lower quadrant
>	greater than
<	less than
Δ	change
√	root; square root
χ^2	chi square (test)
σ	1/1000 of a second standard deviation
Σ	sum of
π	3.1415—ratio of circumference of a circle to its diameter

τ	life (time)
τ½	half-life (time)
λ	wavelength
@	at
ā	before
c̄	with
√c̄	check with
p̄	after
s̄	without
24°	24 hours
Δt	time interval
2d	second
1°	primary
2°	secondary to
♀	female
♂	male
ℨ	dram
℥	ounce
−ve	negative
+ve	positive
D_x	diagnosis
R_x	treatment or therapy
†	deceased
◊	lozenge; sex unknown or unspecified
Ⓐ , ⓐₓ	axilla (temperature)
Ⓗ , ⓗ	hypodermically
Ⓜ	intramuscularly
Ⓥ	intravenously
Ⓛ	left
Ⓜ	murmur
ⓜ	by mouth, murmur
Ⓞ	by mouth, orally
Ⓡ	rectally, registered trademark, right
Ⓧ	end of anesthesia, end of operation

Genetic Symbols

□	male
○	female
◇	sex unspecified
□─○	mating or marriage
□═○	consanguinity
□┬○	illegitimate offspring
□─╫─○	divorce
□─○─□	multiple marriage
⌃ (□ ○)	dizygotic twins
⌃ (□ ○)	monozygotic twins
4 ③	number of children of sex indicated

(□)(○)	adopted
□──//──○	half siblings
□ ○ ◇	stillbirth or abortion
□┬○	no offspring
■ ●	affected offspring
■ ●	proband, propositus, or index case
◧ ◐	heterozygotes for autosomal recessive
⊙	carrier of sex-linked recessive
⊘ Ø	death

Greek Alphabet and Symbols

α	A	alpha	ω	Ω	omega
β	B	beta	o	O	omicron
χ	X	chi	φ	Φ	phi
δ	Δ	delta (diagnosis; change)	π	Π	pi
ε	E	epsilon	ψ	Ψ	psi
η	H	eta	ρ	P	rho
γ	Γ	gamma	σ	Σ	sigma
ι	I	iota	τ	T	tau
κ	K	kappa	θ	Θ	theta
λ	Λ	lambda	υ	Y	upsilon
μ	M	mu	ξ	Ξ	xi
ν	N	nu	ζ	Z	zeta

A abnormal; abortion; absolute temperature; absorbance; acceptor; accommodation; acetone; acetum; achondroplasia; acid; acidophil, acidophilic; acromion; actin; *Actinomyces*; activity [radiation]; adenine; adenoma; adenosine; admittance; adrenalin; adriamycin; adult; age; akinetic; alanine; albino [guinea pig]; albumin; allergologist, allergy; alpha [cell]; alveolar gas; ambulation; ampere; amphetamine; ampicillin; anaphylaxis; androsterone; anesthetic; angstrom, Ångström unit; anode; *Anopheles*; antagonism; anterior; antibody; antrectomy; apical; aqueous; area; argon; artery [Lat. *arteria*]; atomic weight; atrium; atropine; auricle; auscultation; axial; axilla, axillary; before [Lat. *ante*] blood group A; ear [Lat. *auris*]; mass number; subspinale; total acidity; water [Lat. *aqua*]; year [Lat. *annum*]

A [band] the dark-staining zone of a striated muscle

Å Ångström unit

Ā cumulated activity; antinuclear antibody

A₁ aortic first sound

A₂ aortic second sound

A₂₋ₒₛ aortic second sound, opening snap

A₂ P₂ aortic second sound; pulmonary second sound

AI, AII, AIII angiotensin I, II, III

a absorptivity; acceleration; accommodation; acidity; activated; ampere; anode; ante [before]; anterior; area; arterial blood; arterial; artery [Lat. *arteria*]; atto-; thermodynamic activity; total acidity; water [Lat. *aqua*]

ā before [Lat. *ante*]

A see *alpha*

α see *alpha*

AA abdominal aorta; acetic acid; achievement age; active alcoholic; active assistive [range of motion]; active avoidance; acupuncture analgesia; adenine arabinoside; adenylic acid; adjuvant arthritis; adrenal androgen; agranulocytic angina; Alcoholics Anonymous; allergic alveolitis; alopecia areata; alveolo-arterial; amino acid; aminoacyl; amyloid A; anticipatory avoidance; antigen aerosol; aortic arch; aplastic anemia; arachidonic acid; arteries; ascending aorta; atlanto-axial; atomic absorption; Australia antigen; autoanalyzer; automobile accident; axonal arborization

2AA 2-aminoanthracene

A-a alveolar-arterial; alveolar-atrial

aa arteries [Lat. *arteriae*]

A&A aid and attendance; awake and aware

aA abampere

AAA abdominal aortic aneurysm/aneurysmectomy; acne-associated arthritis; acquired aplastic anemia; acute anxiety attack; alacrimia-achalasia-addisonianism [syndrome]; American Academy of Addictionology; American Academy of Allergy; American Association of Anatomists; androgenic anabolic agent; aneurysm of ascending aorta; angiography of abdominal aorta; Area Agency on Aging; aromatic amino acid; arrest after arrival

AAAD aromatic amino acid decarboxylase

AA/AD alcohol abuse/alcohol dependence

AAAE amino acid activating enzyme

AAAHC Accreditation Association for Ambulatory Health Care

AAAHE American Association for the Advancement of Health Education

AAAI American Academy of Allergy and Immunology; American Association of Artificial Intelligence

AAALAC American Association for Accreditation of Laboratory Animal Care

AAAM Association for the Advancement of Automotive Medicine

AAAS American Association for the Advancement of Science

AAASPS African-American Antiplatelet Stroke Prevention Study

AAB American Association of Bioanalysts; aminoazobenzene

AABB American Association of Blood Banks; axis-aligned bounding boxes

AABCC alertness (consciousness), airway, breathing, circulation, cervical spine

AABS automobile accident, broadside

AAC antibiotic-associated [pseudomembranous] colitis; antimicrobial agent-induced colitis; augmentative and alternative communication

AACA acylaminocephalosporanic acid

6'AAC-2"APH 6'-acetyltransferase-2"-phosphotransferase

AACC American Association for Clinical Chemistry

AACCN American Association of Critical Care Nurses

AACD aging-associated cognitive decline

AACE acute acquired comitant esotropia

AACEM Association of Academic Chairs in Emergency Medicine

AACG acute angle closure glaucoma

AACHP American Association for Comprehensive Health Planning

AACIA American Association for Clinical Immunology and Allergy

AACN American Association of Colleges of Nursing; American Association of Critical-Care Nurses

AACOM American Association of Colleges of Osteopathic Medicine

AACP American Academy of Cerebral Palsy; American Association of Colleges of Pharmacy

AACPDM American Academy for Cerebral Palsy and Developmental Medicine

AACS American Academy of Cosmetic Surgery

AACSH adrenal androgen corticotropic stimulating hormone

AACT American Academy of Clinical Toxicology

AACVPR American Association of Cardiovascular and Pulmonary Rehabilitation

AAD acute agitated delirium; acute aortic dissection; alloxazine adenine dinucleotide; alpha-1-antitrypsin deficiency; American Academy of Dermatology; antibiotic-associated diarrhea; aromatic acid decarboxylase

7-AAD 7-amino-actinomycin D

AADC amino acid decarboxylase

AADE American Association of Dental Editors; American Association of Dental Examiners

AADGP American Academy of Dental Group Practice

AADH alopecia-anosmia-deafness-hypogonadism [syndrome]

$(A-a)D_{N2}$ alveolo-arterial nitrogen tension difference

AAD_{O2}, $(a-A) D_{O2}$ arterio-alveolar oxygen tension difference

AADP American Academy of Denture Prosthetics; amyloid A-degrading protease

AADPA American Academy of Dental Practice Administration

AADR American Academy of Dental Radiology

AADS American Academy of Dental Schools

AAE active assistive exercise; acute allergic encephalitis; American Association of Endodontists; annuloaortic ectasia

AAEE American Association of Electromyography and Electrodiagnosis

AAEM American Academy of Emergency Medicine; American Academy of Environmental Medicine; American Association of Electrodiagnostic Medicine

AA ex active assistive exercise

AAF acetylaminofluorene; aortic arch flush; ascorbic acid factor

AAFP American Academy of Family Physicians; American Academy of Family Practice

AAFPRS American Academy of Facial Plastic and Reconstructive Surgery

AAG 3-alkaladenine deoxyribonucleic acid glycosylase; allergic angiitis and granulomatosis; alpha-1-acid glycoprotein; alveolar arterial gradient; autoantigen

AAGL American Academy of Gynecologic Laparoscopists

AAGP American Academy of General Practice; American Association for Geriatric Psychiatry

AAH Academy of Architecture for Health

AAHA American Academy of Hospital Attorneys; American Association of Homes for the Aging

AAHC American Academy of Healthcare Consultants; American Accreditation HealthCare Commission; Association of Academic Health Centers

AAHD American Association of Hospital Dentists

AAHE Association for the Advancement of Health Education

AAHP American Association of Health Plans

AAHPER American Association for Health, Physical Education, and Recreation

AAHS American Association for Hand Surgery

AAHSL Association of Academic Health Sciences Libraries

AAHSLD Association of Academic Health Sciences Library Directors

AAI acute alveolar injury; Adolescent Alienation Index; American Association of Immunologists; atrial inhibited [pacemaker]

AAIB alpha-1-aminoisobutyrate

AAID American Academy of Implant Dentures

AAIN American Association of Industrial Nurses

AAK allo-activated killer

AAL anterior axillary line

AALAC American Association for Laboratory Animal Care

AALAS American Association of Laboratory Animal Science

AALib amino acid library

AALL American Association for Labor Legislation

AALNC American Association of Legal Nurse Consultants

AAm acrylamide

AAM acute aseptic meningitis; American Academy of Microbiology; amino acid mixture

AAMA American Academy of Medical Administrators; American Association of Medical Assistants

AAMC American Association of Medical Clinics; Association of American Medical Colleges

AAMD American Academy of Medical Directors; American Association of Mental Deficiency

AAME acetylarginine methyl ester

AAMFT American Association for Marriage and Family Therapy

AAMI Association for the Advancement of Medical Instrumentation

AAMIH American Association for Maternal and Infant Health

AAMMC American Association of Medical Milk Commissioners

AAMP American Academy of Maxillofacial Prosthetics; American Academy of Medical Prevention

AAMR American Academy of Mental Retardation

AAMRL American Association of Medical Record Librarians

AAMRS automated ambulatory medical record system

AAMS acute aseptic meningitis syndrome

AAMSI American Association for Medical Systems and Informatics

AAMT American Association for Medical Transcription

AAN AIDS-associated nephropathy; alpha-amino nitrogen; American Academy of Neurology; American Academy of Nursing; American Academy of Nutrition; American Association of Neuropathologists; amino acid nitrogen; analgesic-associated nephropathy; attending's admission notes

AANA American Association of Nurse Anesthetists

AANE American Association of Nurse Executives

AANM American Association of Nurse-Midwives

AANPI American Association of Nurses Practicing Independently

AAO American Academy of Ophthalmology; American Academy of Optometry; American Academy of Osteopathy; American Academy of Otolaryngology; American Association of Ophthalmologists; American Association of Orthodontists; amino acid oxidase; ascending aorta; awake, alert, and oriented

AAo ascending aorta

A-a O$_2$ alveolar-arterial oxygen gradient; alveolo-arterial oxygen tension

AAOC antacid of choice

AAofA Ambulance Association of America

AAOHN American Association of Occupational Health Nurses

AAOM American Academy of Oral Medicine

AAOMS American Association of Oral and Maxillofacial Surgery

AAOO American Academy of Ophthalmology and Otolaryngology

AAOP American Academy of Oral Pathology

AAOPP American Association of Osteopathic Postgraduate Physicians

AAOS American Academy of Orthopedic Surgeons; American Association of Osteopathic Specialists

AAP acute abdominal pain; air at atmospheric pressure; American Academy of Pediatrics; American Academy of Pedodontics; American Academy of Periodontology; American Academy of Psychoanalysts; American Academy of Psychotherapists; American Association of Pathologists; Association for the Advancement of Psychoanalysis; Association for the Advancement of Psychotherapy; Association of Academic Physiatrists; Association of American Physicians

AAPA American Academy of Physician Assistants; American Association of Pathologist Assistants

AAPB American Association of Pathologists and Bacteriologists

AAPC antibiotic-associated pseudomembranous colitis; average annual percent change

AAPCC adjusted annual per capita cost; adjusted average per capita costs; American Association of Poison Control Centers

AaP$_{CO2}$, (A-a)P$_{CO2}$ alveolo-arterial carbon dioxide tension difference

AAPF anti-arteriosclerosis polysaccharide factor

AAPH azobis amidino propane hydrochloride

AAPHD American Association of Public Health Dentists

AAPHP American Association of Public Health Physicians

AAPL American Academy of Psychiatry and the Law

AAPM American Association of Physicists in Medicine

AAPMC antibiotic-associated pseudomembranous colitis

AAPM&R American Academy of Physical Medicine and Rehabilitation

AaP$_{O2}$, (A-a) P$_{O2}$ alveolo-arterial oxygen tension difference

AAPP American Academy on Physician and Patient

AAPPO American Association of Preferred Provider Organizations

AAPS American Association of Pharmaceutical Scientists; American Association of Plastic Surgeons; Arizona Articulation Proficiency Scale; Association of American Physicians and Surgeons

AAPT Adolescent Alcohol Prevention Trial

AAR active avoidance reaction; acute articular rheumatism; antigen-antiglobulin reaction

aar against all risks

AARE automobile accident, rear end

AARNet Australian Academic and Research Network

AAROM active assertive range of motion; active-assisted range of motion

AARP American Association of Retired Persons

AART American Association for Rehabilitation Therapy; American Association for Respiratory Therapy

AAS Aarskog-Scott [syndrome]; acid aspiration syndrome; alcoholic abstinence syndrome; American Academy of Sanitarians; American Analgesia Society; aneurysm of atrial septum; anthrax antiserum; aortic arch syndrome; atomic absorption spectrophotometry

AASD American Academy of Stress Disorders

aa seq amino acid sequence

AASH adrenal androgen stimulating hormone; American Association for the Study of Headache

AASK African American Study of Kidney Disease and Hypertension Pilot Study

AASP acute atrophic spinal paralysis; American Association of Senior Physicians; ascending aorta synchronized pulsation

AASS American Association for Social Security

AAST American Association for the Surgery of Trauma

AAT Aachen Aphasia Test; academic aptitude test; Accolate Asthma Trial; alanine aminotransferase; alkylating agent therapy; alpha-1-antitrypsin; atrial triggered [pacemaker]; auditory apperception test; automatic atrial tachycardia

α_1AT alpha-1-antitrypsin

AATS American Association for Thoracic Surgery

AAU acute anterior uveitis

AAV adeno-associated virus

AAVMC Association of American Veterinary Medical Colleges

AAVP American Association of Veterinary Parasitologists

AAW anterior aortic wall

AB abdominal; abnormal; abortion; Ace bandage; active bilaterally; aid to the blind; airbag; alcian blue; alertness behavior; antibiotic; antibody; antigen binding; apex beat; asbestos body; asthmatic bronchitis; axiobuccal; Bachelor of Arts [Lat. *Artium Baccalaureus*]; blood group AB

A/B acid-base ratio

A&B apnea and bradycardia

A>B air greater than bone [conduction]

Ab abortion; antibiotic; antibody; antivenom

aB azure B

ab abortion; antibody; from [Lat.]

3AD 3-aminobenzamide

ABA abscissic acid; allergic bronchopulmonary aspergillosis; American Board of Anesthesiologists; American Burn Association; antibacterial activity; arrest before arrival

ABACAS Adjunctive Balloon Angioplasty Following Coronary Arthrectomy Study

ABAT American Board of Applied Toxicology

ABB Albright-Butler-Bloomberg [syndrome]; American Board of Bioanalysis

ABBI advanced breast biopsy instrument

ABBQ AIDS Beliefs and Behavior Questionnaire

abbr abbreviation, abbreviated

ABC abacavir; absolute basophil count; absolute bone conduction; acalculous biliary colic; acid balance control; aconite-belladonna-chloroform; airway, breathing, and circulation; alignment, blue, calcium [synovial fluid pearls in gout and pseudogout]; Alpha Beta Canadian [trial]; alternative birth center; alum, blood, and charcoal [purification and deodorizing method]; alum, blood, and clay [sludge deodorizing method]; American Blood Commission; aneurysmal bone cyst; antigen-binding capacity; apnea, bradycardia, cyanosis;

aspiration biopsy cytology; assessment of basic competency; atomic, biological, and chemical [warfare]; axiobuccocervical; autism behavior checklist

A&BC air and bone conduction

ABCC Atomic Bomb Casualty Commission

ABCD airway, breathing, circulation, differential diagnosis (or defibrillate) [in cardiopulmonary resuscitation]; appropriate blood pressure control in diabetes; asymmetry, borders are irregular, color variegated, diameter > 6 mm [biopsy in melanoma]

ABCDE airway, breathing, circulation, disability, exposure [in trauma patients]; botulism toxin pentavalent

ABCDES abnormal alignment, bones-periarticular osteoporosis, cartilage—joint space loss, deformities, marginal erosions, soft tissue swelling [x-ray features in rheumatoid arthritis]; adjust medication, bacterial prophylaxis, cervical spine disease, deep vein thrombosis prophylaxis, evaluate extent and activity of disease, stress-dose steroid coverage [preoperative evaluation in rheumatoid diseases]; alignment, bone mineralization, calcifications, distribution of joints, erosions, soft tissue and nails [x-ray features in arthritis]; ankylosis, bone osteoporosis, cartilage destruction, deformity of joints, erosions, swelling of soft tissues [x-ray features of septic arthritis]

ABCIC airway, breathing, circulation, intravenous crystalloid

ABCIL antibody-mediated cell-dependent immunolympholysis

ABCN American Board of Clinical Neuropsychology

ABD abdomen; aged, blind, and disabled; aggressive behavioral disturbance; automatic border detection; average body dose

Abd, abd abdomen, abdominal; abduct, abduction, abductor

abdom abdomen, abdominal

ABDPH American Board of Dental Public Health

ABE acute bacterial endocarditis; American Board of Endodontics; botulism equine trivalent antitoxin

ABEM American Board of Emergency Medicine

ABEPP American Board of Examiners in Professional Psychology

ABER auditory brainstem evoked response

aber aberrant

A-β amyloid beta-peptide

ABF aortic blood flow; aortobifemoral

ABG arterial blood gas; axiobucco-gingival

ABI ankle/brachial index; atherothrombotic brain infarct

ABIC Adaptive Behavior Inventory for Children

ABIM American Board of Internal Medicine

ABIMCE American Board of Internal Medicine certifying examination

ABIT assertive behavior inventory tool

ABK aphakic bullous keratopathy

ABL abetalipoproteinemia; acceptable blood loss; African Burkitt lymphoma; Albright-Butler-Lightwood [syndrome]; angioblastic lymphadenopathy; antigen-binding lymphocyte; Army Biological Laboratory; automated biological laboratory; axiobuccolingual

ABLB alternate binaural loudness balance

ABM adjusted body mass; alveolar basement membrane; autologous bone marrow

ABMG American Board of Medical Genetics

ABMI autologous bone marrow transplantation

AbMLV Abelson murine leukemia virus

ABMM American Board of Medical Management

ABMS American Board of Medical Specialties

ABMT American Board of Medical Toxicology; autologous bone marrow transplantation

AbN antibody nitrogen

Abn, abn abnormal; abnormality(ies)

ABNMP alpha-benzyl-N-methyl phenethylamine

ABNO anatomic abnormality [UMLS]

abnor abnormal

ABO abortion; absent bed occupancy; American Board of Orthodontists; blood group system consisting of groups A, AB, B, and O

ABOHN American Board for Occupational Health Nurses

ABOMS American Board of Oral and Maxillofacial Surgery

ABOP American Board of Oral Pathology

Abor, abor abortion

ABOS American Board of Orthopaedic Surgery

ABOVE Acute Bleeding Oesophageal Variceal Episodes [study]

ABP actin-binding protein; ambulatory blood pressure; American Board of Pedodontics; American Board of Periodontology; American Board of Prosthodontists; antigen-binding protein; androgen-binding protein; arterial blood pressure; automatic systolic blood pressure measurement; avidin-biotin peroxidase

aBP arterial blood pressure

ABPA actin-binding protein, autosomal form; allergic bronchopulmonary aspergillosis

ABPC antibody-producing cell

ABPE acute bovine pulmonary edema

ABPM ambulatory blood pressure monitoring

ABPM&R American Board of Physical Medicine and Rehabilitation

ABPS American Board of Plastic Surgery

ABR abortus Bang ring [test]; absolute bed rest; arterial baroreflex; auditory brainstem response

ABr agglutination test for brucellosis

Abr, Abras abrasion

ABS abdominal surgery; acute brain syndrome; Adaptive Behavior Scale; admitting blood sugar; adult bovine serum; aging brain syndrome; alkylbenzene sulfonate; aloin, belladonna, strychnine; American Board of Surgery; amniotic band sequence; amniotic band syndrome; anti-B serum; Antley-Bixler syndrome; arterial blood sample; at bed side; Australian Bureau of Statistics

Abs absorption

abs absent; absolute

AB-SAAP autologous blood selective aortic arch perfusion

absc abscess; abscissa

abs conf absolute configuration

ABSe ascending bladder septum

abs feb while fever is absent

ABSITE American Board of Surgery In-Training Examination

absorp absorption

AbSR abnormal skin reflex

abst, abstr abstract
ABT autologous blood transfusion
abt about
ABU asymptomatic bacteriuria
ABV actinomycin D–bleomycin–vincristine; arthropod-borne virus
ABVD Adriamycin, bleomycin, vinblastine, and dacarbazine
ABW average body weight
ABX abciximab; antibiotics
ABY acid bismuth yeast [medium]
AC abdominal circumference; abdominal compression; ablation catheter; abrupt closure; absorption coefficient; abuse case; acetate; acetylcholine; acidified complement; *Acinetobacter calcoaceticus;* acromioclavicular; activated charcoal; acupuncture clinic; acute; acute cholecystitis; adenocarcinoma; adenylate cyclase; adherent cell; adrenal cortex; adrenocorticoid; adriamycin/cyclophosphamide; air chamber; air conditioning; air conduction; alcoholic cirrhosis; alternating current; alveolar crest; ambulatory care; anesthesia circuit; angiocellular; anodal closure; antecubital; anterior chamber; anterior column; anterior commissure; antibiotic concentrate; anticholinergic; anticoagulant; anticomplement; antiphlogistic corticoid; aortic closure; aortic compliance; aortocoronary; arm circumference; ascending colon; atriocarotid; axiocervical
A-C acromioclavicular; adult-versus-child; aortocoronary bypass
A/C albumin/coagulin [ratio]; anterior chamber of eye; assist control [ventilation]
A2C apical two-chamber [view]
A4C apical four-chamber [view]
Ac accelerator [globulin]; acetate; acetyl; actinium; aortic closure; arabinosyl cytosine
aC abcoulomb; arabinsyl cytosine
ac acceleration; acetyl; acid; acromioclavicular; acute; alternating current; antecubital; anterior chamber; atrial contraction; axiocervical
5-AC azacitidine
ACA abnormal coronary artery; acrodermatitis chronica atrophicans; acute cerebellar ataxia; adenocarcinoma; adult child of an alcoholic; American Chiropractic Association; American College of Allergists; American College of Anesthesiologists;

American College of Angiology; American College of Apothecaries; American Council on Alcoholism; aminocephalosporanic acid; ammonia, copper, and acetate; amyotrophic choreo-acanthocytosis; anterior cerebral artery; anterior communicating aneurysm [or artery]; anticapsulary antibody; anticardiolipin antibody; anticentromere antibody; anticollagen antibody; anticomplement activity; anticytoplasmic antibody; arrhythmic cardiac arrest; Automatic Clinical Analyzer
AC/A accommodative convergence/accommodation [ratio]
ACAAI American College of Allergy, Asthma and Immunology
ACAC acetyl-coenzyme A cocarboxylase; activated charcoal artificial cell
ACACN American Council of Applied Clinical Nutrition
ACACT acyl-coenzyme A:cholesterol acyl transferase
ACAD asymptomatic coronary artery disease; Azithromycin in Coronary Artery Disease [study]
Acad academy
ACADEMIC Azithromycin in Coronary Artery Disease Elimination of Myocardial Infection with Chlamydia [study]
A-CAH autoimmune chronic active hepatitis
ACAO acyl coenzyme A oxidase
ACAT acetocoenzyme A acetyltransferase; automated computerized axial tomography
ACB antibody-coated bacteria; aortocoronary bypass; arterialized capillary blood; asymptomatic carotid bruit
ACBaE air contrast barium enema
ACBC aminocyclobutanecarboxylic acid
AC/BC air conduction/bone conduction [time ratio]
ACBE air contrast barium enema
ACBG aortocoronary bypass graft
ACBS Asymptomatic Cervical Bruit Study
ACC accommodation; acetyl coenzyme A carboxylase; acinic cell carcinoma; acute care center; adenoid cystic carcinoma; administrative control center; adrenocortical carcinoma; agenesis of corpus callosum; alveolar cell carcinoma; ambulatory care center; American College of Cardiology;

anodal closure contraction; anterior cingulate cortex; antitoxin-containing cell; aplasia cutis congenita; articular chondrocalcinosis; automated cell count; automated cell counter

Acc adenoid cystic carcinoma; acceleration

acc acceleration, accelerator; accident; accommodation

ACCA Advisory Committee on Casualty Assessment [Canada]; American College of Cardiovascular Administrators

ACC/AHA American College of Cardiology/American Hospital Association [Task Force]

ACCE American College of Clinical Engineering

ACCEPT Accupril Canadian Clinical Evaluation and Patient Teaching; American College of Cardiology Electrocardiogram Proficiency Test; American College of Cardiology Evaluation of Preventive Therapies [study]

ACCESS A Comparison of Percutaneous Entry Sites for Coronary Angioplasty; Acute Candesartan Cilexetil Evaluation in Stroke Survivors; Ambulatory Care Clinic Effectiveness Systems Study; Atorvastatin Comparative Cholesterol Efficacy and Safety Study; automated cervical cell screening system

ACCH Association for the Care of Children's Health

AcCh acetylcholine

AcChR acetylcholine receptor

AcCHS acetylcholinesterase

accid accident, accidental

acc insuff accommodation insufficiency

ACCL, Accl anodal closure clonus

ACCME Accreditation Council for Continuing Medical Education

AcCoA acetyl coenzyme A

accom accommodation

ACCP American College of Chest Physicians; American College of Clinical Pharmacology; American College of Clinical Pharmacy

ACCR amylase-creatinine clearance ratio

ACCS American-Canadian Cooperative Study

ACCT Amlodipine Cardiovascular Community Trial

accum accumulation

accur accurately [lat. *accuratissime*]

ACD absolute cardiac dullness; absolute claudication distance; acid-citrate-dextrose [solution]; actinomycin D; active compression-decompression; adult celiac disease; advanced care directive; allergic contact dermatitis; alopecia-contractures-dwarfism [syndrome]; American College of Dentists; ammonium citrate dextrose; angiokeratoma corporis diffusum; anterior chamber depth; anterior chest diameter; anticoagulant citrate dextrose; area of cardiac dullness

AC-DC, ac/dc alternating current or direct current

ACD-CPR active compression-decompression cardiopulmonary resuscitation

ACD-PCR active compression-decompression post-compression remodeling

ACE acetonitrile; acetylcholine esterase; acute cerebral encephalopathy; acute coronary event; adrenocortical extract; Adverse Childhood Experience [study]; alcohol, chloroform, and ether; angiotensin-converting enzyme; Aspirin and Carotid Endarterectomy [trial]

ace acentric; acetone

ACED anhydrotic congenital ectodermal dysplasia

ACEDS angiotensin-converting enzyme dysfunction syndrome

ACEH acid cholesterol ester hydrolase

ACEI angiotensin-converting enzyme inhibitor

ACEP American College of Emergency Physicians

ACES Alternans Cardiac Electrical Safety [study]; Azithromycin and Coronary Events Study

AcEst acetyl esterase

ACET Advisory Committee for the Elimination of Tuberculosis; Azmacort Cost Effectiveness Trial

ACET, acet acetone; vinegar [*Lat.* acetum]

acetab acetabular, acetabulum

acetyl-CoA acetyl coenzyme A

ACF accessory clinical findings; acute care facility; anterior cervical fusion; area correction factor; asymmetric crying facies; autocorrelation function

ACFAO American College of Foot and Ankle Orthopedics and Medicine

ACFAS American College of Foot and Ankle Surgeons

ACET Advisory Committee for the Elimination of Tuberculosis

ACG accelerator globulin; alternative care grant; ambulatory care group; American College of Gastroenterology; angiocardiography, angiocardiogram; aortocoronary graft; apexcardiogram

AC-G, AcG, ac-g accelerator globulin

ACGIH American Conference of Governmental Industrial Hygienists

ACGME Accreditation Council for Graduate Medical Education

ACGP American College of General Practitioners

ACGPOMS American College of General Practitioners in Osteopathic Medicine and Surgery

ACGT antibody-coated grid technique

ACH acetylcholine; achalasia; active chronic hepatitis; adrenocortical hormone; amyotrophic cerebellar hypoplasia; arm girth, chest depth, and hip width [nutritional index]

ACh acetylcholine

ACHA American College Health Association; American College of Hospital Administrators

AChA anterior choroidal artery

ACHE American College of Healthcare Executives; American Council for Headache Education

AChE acetylcholinesterase

ACHIEVE Accupril Congestive Heart Failure Investigation and Economic Variable Evaluation

ACHOO autosomal dominant compelling helio-ophthalmic outburst [syndrome]

ACHPER Australian Council for Health, Physical Education and Recreation [survey]

ACHPR Agency for Health Care Policy and Research

AChR acetylcholine receptor

AChRAb acetylcholine receptor antibody

AChRP acetylcholine receptor protein

ACI acceleration index; acoustic comfort index; acute cardiac ischemia; acute coronary infarction; acute coronary insufficiency; adenylate cyclase inhibitor; adrenocortical insufficiency; anticlonus index

ACID Arithmetic, Coding, Information, and Digit Span; automatic implantable cardioverter defibrillator

ACIF acute care index of functions; anti-complement immunofluorescence

AcINH acid labile isonicotinic acid hydrazide

ACIP acute canine idiopathic polyneuropathy; Advisory Committee on Immunization Practices [CDC]; ambulatory care incentive payment; Asymptomatic Cardiac Ischemia Pilot Study

ACIR Automotive Crash Injury Research; Australian Clinical Immunisation Register

ACIS ambulatory care information system; automated clinical information system

ACIT Asymptomatic Cardiac Ischemia Trial

ACI-TIPI acute cardiac ischemia-time insensitive predictive instrument

AcK francium [actinium K]

ACKD acquired cystic kidney disease

ACL access control list; Achievement Check List; acromegaloid features, cutis verticis gyrata, corneal leukoma [syndrome]; anterior chamber lens; anterior cruciate ligament

ACl aspiryl chloride

aCL anticardiolipin [antibody]

ACLA American Clinical Laboratory Association

ACLC Assessment of Children's Language Comprehension

ACLD Association for Children with Learning Disabilities

ACLE acute cutaneous lupus erythematosus

ACLF adult congregate living facility

ACLI American Council on Life Insurance

ACLM American College of Legal Medicine

ACLPS Academy of Clinical Laboratory Physicians and Scientists

ACLR anterior capsulolabral reconstruction

ACLS acrocallosal syndrome; advanced cardiac life support; Assessment of Children's Language Comprehension

AcLV avian acute leukemia virus

ACM acetaminophen; acute cerebrospinal meningitis; adaptive fuzzy c-means algorithm; Adriamycin, cyclophosphamide, methotrexate; albumin-calcium-magnesium;

alveolar capillary membrane; anticardiac myosin; Arnold-Chiari malformation

ACMA American Occupational Medical Association

ACMC Association of Canadian Medical Colleges

ACMD associate chief medical director

ACME Advisory Council on Medical Education; Angioplasty Compared to Medicine [study]; assessing changes in medical education; Automated Classification of Medical Entities

ACMF arachnoid cyst of the middle fossa

ACMG American College of Medical Genetics

ACMI age-consistent memory impairment; American College of Medical Informatics

ACML atypical chronic myeloid leukemia

AcMNPV *Autographa californica* multicapsid nuclear polyhedrosis virus

ACMP alveolar-capillary membrane permeability

ACMR Advisory Committee on Medical Research

ACMS American Chinese Medical Society

ACMT artificial circus movement tachycardia

ACMV assist-controlled mechanical ventilation

ACN acute conditioned neurosis; Ambulatory Care Network; American College of Neuropsychiatrists; American College of Nutrition

ACNM American College of Nuclear Medicine; American College of Nurse-Midwives

ACNP acute care nurse practitioner; American College of Nuclear Physicians

ACO acute coronary occlusion; alert, cooperative, and oriented; anodal closure odor

ACOA adult children of alcoholics

ACoA anterior communicating artery

ACODENIC Advisory Committee on Dental Electronic Nomenclature, Indexing and Classification

ACOEM American College of Occupational and Environmental Medicine

ACOEP American College of Osteopathic Emergency Physicians

ACOG American College of Obstetricians and Gynecologists

ACOHA American College of Osteopathic Hospital Administrators

ACO-HNS American Council of Otolaryngology-Head and Neck Surgery

ACOI American College of Osteopathic Internists

ACOM American College of Occupational Medicine; anterior communicating [artery]

AComA anterior communicating artery

ACOMS American College of Oral and Maxillofacial Surgeons

ACOOG American College of Osteopathic Obstetricians and Gynecologists

ACOP American College of Osteopathic Pediatricians; approved code of practice

ACORDE A Corsortium on Restorative Dentistry Education

ACOS American College of Osteopathic Surgeons; associate chief of staff

ACOS/AC associate chief of staff for ambulatory care

Acous acoustics, acoustic

ACP accessory conduction pathway; acid phosphatase; acyl carrier protein; American College of Pathologists; American College of Pharmacists; American College of Physicians; American College of Prosthodontists; American College of Psychiatrists; Animal Care Panel; anodal closure picture; aspirin-caffeine-phenacetin; Association for Child Psychiatrists; Association of Clinical Pathologists; Association of Correctional Psychologists; Asymptomatic Cardiac Ischemia Pilot Study

ACPA American Cleft Palate Association

AcPase acid phosphatase

ACPC aminocyclopentane carboxylic [acid]

ACPE American College of Physician Executives

AC-PH, ac phos acid phosphatase

ACPM American College of Preventive Medicine

ACPP adrenocortical polypeptide; prostate-specific acid phosphatase

ACPS acrocephalopolysyndactyly

ACQUIP Ambulatory Care Quality Improvement Project

ACR abnormally contracting region; absolute catabolic rate; acriflavine; adenomatosis of colon and rectum; adjusted community rate; ambulance call report;

American College of Radiology; American College of Rheumatology; anticonstipation regimen; axillary count rate

Acr acrylic

ACRE Appropriateness of Coronary Revascularization [study]

ACRF acute-on-chronic respiratory failure; ambulatory care research facility

ACRM American Congress of Rehabilitation Medicine

ACR/NEMA American College of Radiology/National Electrical Manufacturers' Association [standard for transferring radiologic images]

ACS acrocallosal syndrome; acrocephalosyndactyly; acute chest syndrome; acute confusional state; acute coronary syndrome; Alcon Closure System; American Cancer Society; American Chemical Society; American College of Surgeons; anodal closure sound; antireticular cytotoxic serum; aperture current setting; Association of Clinical Scientists; automatic corneal shaper

ACSA adenylate cyclase-stimulating activity

ACS AO ascending aorta

ACSCEPT Assessment for Carotid Stenosis: Correlation with Endarterectomy Specimen Trial

ACS CPS American Cancer Society Cancer Prevention Studies

ACSE association control service element

aCSF artificial cerebrospinal fluid

ACSF artificial cerebrospinal fluid

ACSM American College of Sports Medicine

AC/SIUG ambulatory care special-interest user group

ACSP adenylate cyclase-stimulating protein

ACST Asymptomatic Carotid Surgery Trial

ACSV aortocoronary saphenous vein

ACSVBG aortocoronary saphenous vein bypass graft

ACT abdominal computed tomography; ablation catheter tip; achievement through counseling and treatment; actin; actinomycin; activated clotting time; adaptive current tomography; advanced coronary treatment; Angioplasty Compliance Trial; anterocolic transposition; antichymotrypsin;

anticoagulant therapy; anxiety control training; Association of Cytogenetic Technologists; asthma care training; atropine coma therapy; Attacking Claudication with Ticlopidine [study]; Australian Capital Territory [heroin trial]

AcT acceleration time

act actinomycin; activity, active

ACTA American Cardiology Technologists Association; automatic computerized transverse axial [scanning]

Act-C actinomycin C

ACTC alpha-actin, cardiac muscle

Act-D actinomycin D

ACT/DB Adaptable Clinical Trials Database

ACTe anodal closure tetanus

ACTG AIDS Clinical Trial Group [study]

ACTH adrenocorticotropic hormone

ACTH-LI adrenocorticotropin-like immunoreactivity

ACTHR adrenocorticotropic hormone receptor

ACTHR/MC-2 adrenocorticotropin receptor/melanocortin receptor 2

ACTH-RF adrenocorticotropic hormone releasing factor

ACTION A Coronary Disease Trial Investigating Outcome with Nifedipine GITS

ACTIS AIDS Clinical Trials Information Service

activ active, activity

ACTN adrenocorticotropin

ACTOBAT Australasian Clinical Trial of Betamethasone and Thyroid-Releasing Hormone

ACTP adrenocorticotropic polypeptide

ACT/PD actual nursing hours per patient/day

ACTS acute cervical traumatic sprain or syndrome; advanced communication technology satellite; advanced computational testing and simulation [toolkit]; American-Canadian Thrombosis Study; American College Testing Services; Auditory Comprehension Test for Sentences

ACTUR Automated Central Tumor Registry

ACTV activity [UMLS]

ACU acquired cold urticaria; acute care unit; agar colony-forming unit; ambulatory care unit

ACURP American College of Utilization Review Physicians

ACUTE Analysis of Coronary Ultrasound Thrombolysis Endpoints; Assessment of Cardioversion Utilizing Transesophageal Echocardiography [pilot study]

ACV acute cardiovascular [disease]; acyclovir; assisted controlled ventilation; atrial/carotid/ventricular; autonomic conduction velocity

ACVB aortocoronary venous bypass

ACVD acute cardiovascular disease, atherosclerotic cardiovascular disease

ACx anomalous circumflex [coronary artery]

AD accident dispensary; accidental death; acetate dialysis; active disease; active domain; acute dermatomyositis; addict, addiction; adenoid degeneration [agent]; adjuvant disease; admitting diagnosis; adrenodoxin; adrenostenedione; adult disease; advanced directive; aerosol deposition; affective disorder; after discharge; alcohol dehydrogenase; Aleutian disease; alveolar diffusion; alveolar duct; Alzheimer dementia; Alzheimer disease; analgesic dose; anodal duration; anterior division; antigenic determinant; appropriate disability; arthritic dose; associate degree; atopic dermatitis; attentional disturbance; Aujeszky disease; autistic disorder; autonomic dysreflexia; autosomal dominant; average deviation; axiodistal; axis deviation; right ear [Lat. *auris dextra*]

A/D analog-to-digital

A&D admission and discharge; ascending and descending

Ad adenovirus; adrenal; anisotropic disk

ad add [Lat. *adde*] let there be added [up to a specified amount] [Lat. *addetur*]; axiodistal; right ear [Lat. *auris dextra*]

AD1 Alzheimer disease type I

ADA adenosine deaminase; American Dental Association; American Dermatological Association; American Diabetes Association; American Dietetic Association; Americans with Disabilities Act; anterior descending artery; antideoxyribonucleic acid antibody; approved dietary allowance

ADAA American Dental Assistants Association

ADAM adhesion, mutilation [syndrome]; amniotic deformity, Amsterdam Duration of Antiretroviral Medication [study]

ADAMHA Alcohol, Drug Abuse, and Mental Health Administration

ADAP American Dental Assistant's Program; Assistant Director of Army Psychiatry

ADAPT American Disabled for Attendant Programs Today [organization]

ADAPTS acute directional atherectomy prior to stenting

ADAS Alzheimer disease assessment scale

ADAS-COG cognitive portion of the Alzheimer's Disease Assessment Scale

AdASDiM Adaptive Advisory System for Diabetic Management

ADase adenosine deaminase

ADAU adolescent drug abuse unit

ADB accidental death benefit

ADC adenylate cyclase; adult day care [facility]; affective disorders clinic; Aid to [Families with] Dependent Children; AIDS-dementia complex; albumin, dextrose, and catalase [medium]; ambulance design criteria; analog-to-digital converter; anodal duration contraction; apparent diffusion coefficient; average daily census; axiodistocervical

AdC adenylate cyclase; adrenal cortex

ADCA autosomal dominant cerebellar ataxia

ADCC acute disorder of cerebral circulation; antibody-dependent cell-mediated cytotoxicity

ADCH autosomal dominant cyclic hematopoiesis

AD-CHF acutely decompensated congestive heart failure

ADCMC antibody-dependent complement-mediated cytotoxicity

AdCMVHSV-TK adenovirus carrying the gene for herpes simplex thymidine kinase

ADCP adenosine deaminase complexing protein

ADCS Argonz del Castillo syndrome

ADCY adenyl cyclase

ADD acceptable daily dose; adduction; adenosine deaminase; Anti-Epileptic Drug Development [program]; attention deficit disorder; auditory discrimination in depth; average daily dose

add addition; adductor, adduction; let there be added [Lat. *addatur*]

ADDH attention deficit disorder with hyperactivity

ADD/HA attention deficit disorder/hyperactivity

addict addiction, addictive

add poll adductor pollicis

ADDS American Digestive Disease Society

ADDU alcohol and drug dependence unit

ADE acute disseminated encephalitis; advanced large scale integrated computational environment [ALICE] differencing engine; adverse drug event; antibody-dependent enhancement; apparent digestible energy

Ade adenine

ADEAR Alzheimer Disease Education and Referral [center]

AdeCbl adenosyl cobalamine

ADEE age-dependent epileptic encephalopathy

ADEG Antiarrhythmic Drug Evaluation Group [trial]

ADEM academic department of emergency medicine; acute disseminated encephalomyelitis

AdenCa adenocarcinoma

ADEP Atherosclerotic Disease Evolution by Picotamide [study]

adeq adequate

ADF administrative determination of fault; average duration of failures

ADFN albinism-deafness [syndrome]; albinism-deafness syndrome

ADFR activate, depress, free, repeat [coherence therapy]

ADFS alternative delivery and financing system

AD-FSP autosomal dominant familial spastic paraplegia

ADG ambulatory diagnostic group; atrial diastolic gallop; axiodistogingival

ADH Academy of Dentistry for the Handicapped; adhesion; alcohol dehydrogenase; antidiuretic hormone; arginine dihydrolase; atypical ductal hyperplasia

adh adhesion, adhesive; antidiuretic hormone

ADHA American Dental Hygienists Association

ADHD attention deficit-hyperactivity disorder

ADHDP action-dependent dual heuristic programming

ADI Academy of Dentistry International; acceptable daily intake; AIDS-defining illness; allowable daily intake; alternating directions implicit [method]; artificial diverticulum of the ileum; atlas-dens interval; autism diagnostic interview; average daily intake; axiodistoincisal

adj adjacent; adjoining; adjuvant

ADK adenosine kinase

ADKC atopic dermatitis with keratoconjunctivitis

ADL active digital library; activities of daily living; Amsterdam Depression List; annual dose limit

ADLAR advanced design linear accelerator radiosurgery

ADLC antibody-dependent lymphocyte-mediated cytotoxicity

ad lib as desired [Lat. *ad libitum*]

ADLS Activities of Daily Living Survey

ADM abductor digiti minimi; add-drop multiplexer; administrative medicine; admission; Adriamycin; Alcohol, Drug Abuse and Mental Health [grant of US Department of Health and Human Services]

AdM adrenal medulla

adm administration; admission; apply [Lat. *admove*]

Adm Dr admitting doctor

ADME [drug] absorption, distribution, metabolism, and excretion

Admin administration

ADMIRE AMP 579 Delivery for Myocardial Infarction Reduction

ADMIT Arterial Disease Multiple Intervention Trial

Adm Ph admitting physician

ADMR average daily metabolic rate

ADMS analysis of disorders of masticatory system

ADMX adrenal medullectomy

ADN antideoxyribonuclease; aortic depressor nerve; associate degree in nursing

ad naus to the point of producing nausea [Lat. *ad nauseam*]

ADN-B antideoxyribonuclease B

ADO adolescent medicine; allele dropout; axiodisto-occlusal

Ado adenosine
ADOA autosomal dominant ocular albinism
AdoCbl 5′-adenosylcobalamin
ADOD arthrodentosteodysplasia
AdoDABA adenosyldiaminobutyric acid
AdoHcy S-adenosylhomocysteine
adol adolescence, adolescent
AdoMet S-adenosylmethionine
ADOPT Accupril Decision on Pharmacotherapy [trial]
ADOS autism diagnostic observation scale; autosomal dominant Opitz syndrome
ADOTS affective disorder outpatient telephone screening
Adox oxidized adenosine
ADP adenopathy; adenosine diphosphate; administrative psychiatry; approved drug product; approximate dynamic programming; area diastolic pressure; automatic data processing
AdP adductor pollicis
ADPase adenosine diphosphatase
ADPK autosomal dominant polycystic kidney [disease]
ADPKD autosomal dominant polycystic kidney disease
ADPL average daily patient load
ADPR adenosine diphosphate ribose
ADPRT adenosine diphosphate ribosyltransferase
ADQ abductor digiti quinti; adolescent drinking questionnaire
ADR activation, depression, repetition [in bone remodeling]; adrenalin; adrenergic receptor; adrenodoxin reductase; Adriamycin; adverse drug reaction; airway dilation reflex; alternative dispute resolution; arrested development of righting response; ataxia-deafness-retardation [syndrome]
Adr adrenalin; Adriamycin
adr adrenal, adrenalectomy
ADRA1A alpha-1A-adrenergic receptor
ADRA1B beta-1B-adrenergic receptor
ADRA1C alpha-1C-adrenergic receptor
ADRA2C alpha-2C-adrenergic receptor
ADRAR alpha-2-adrenergic receptor
ADRBK beta-1-adrenergic receptor kinase
ADRBR adrenergic beta-receptor
ADRC Alzheimer Disease Research Center
ADRDA Alzheimer Disease and Related Disorders Association

ADRP adipose differentiation-related protein; autosomal dominant retinitis pigmentosa
ADS acute death syndrome; acute diarrheal syndrome; Alcohol Dependence Scale; alternative delivery system; anatomical dead space; anonymous donor's sperm; antibody deficiency syndrome; antidiuretic substance; Army Dental Service
ADSD adductor spasmodic dysphonia
ADSL adenylsuccinate lyase; asymmetrical digital single line
ADSP analog devices digital signal processor
ADSS adenylsuccinate synthetase
ADSTGD Stargardt-like muscular dystrophy
ADT Accepted Dental Therapeutics; adenosine triphosphate; admission, discharge, and transfer; agar-gel diffusion test; alternate day therapy; any, what you desire, thing (a placebo); Alzheimer-type dementia; asphyxiating thoracic dystrophy; Auditory Discrimination Test
ADTA American Dental Trade Association
ADTe anodal duration tetanus
ADU alkaline deoxyribonucleic acid unwinding
AD&U acid dissociation and ultrafiltration
ADV adenovirus; adventitia; Aleutian disease virus; Aujeszky disease virus
Adv adenovirus
adv advanced; against [Lat. *adversum*]
ADVENT antithrombin for deep venous thrombosis
ADVIRC autosomal dominant vitreoretinochoroidopathy
ADVS activities of daily vision survey
ADW assault with deadly weapon
A5D5W alcohol 5%, dextrose 5%, in water
ADX adrenalectomized; adrenodoxin
AE above-elbow [amputation]; acrodermatitis enteropathica; activation energy; adult erythrocyte; adverse event; aftereffect; agarose electrophoresis; air embolism; air entry; alcoholic embryopathy; anion exchange; anoxic encephalopathy; autiepileptic; antitoxic unit [Ger. *Antitoxineinheit*]; apoenzyme; aryepiglottic; atherosclerotic encephalopathy; atrial ectopic [heart beat]; avian encephalomyelitis

A&E accident and emergency [department]

A+E accident and emergency [department]; analysis and evaluation

A/E above elbow [amputation]

AEA alcohol, ether, and acetone [solution]; apocrine membrane antigen

AEB acute erythroblastopenia; avian erythroblastosis

AEC ankyloblepharon, ectodermal defects, and cleft lip [syndrome]; at earliest convenience; Atomic Energy Commission

AECB acute exacerbation of chronic bronchitis

AECD allergic eczematous contact dermatitis

AECE-6-AZUMP 5-{2-(aminoethyl) carbamyl}-6-azauridine-5'monophosphate

AECS acute exacerbation of chronic sinusitis

AED academic emergency department; antiepileptic drug; antihidrotic ectodermal dysplasia; automated external defibrillator

AEDP automated external defibrillator pacemaker

AEE atomic energy establishment

AEF allogenic effect factor; amyloid enhancing factor; aorto-enteric fistula

A$_{EFF}$ effective area

AEG air encephalography, air encephalogram; atrial electrogram

AEGIS Aid for the Elderly in Government Institutions

AEI arbitrary evolution index; atrial emptying index

AEL acute erythroleukemia

AEM Academic Emergency Medicine [journal]; analytical electron microscopy; ambulatory electrocardiographic monitoring; ataxia episodica with myokymia; avian encephalomyelitis

AEMIS Aerospace and Environmental Medicine Information System

AEMK ataxia episodica with myokymia

A-EMT advanced emergency medical technician

AEN anal epithelial neoplasia; aseptic epiphyseal necrosis

AEP acute edematous pancreatitis; artificial endocrine pancreas; auditory evoked potential; average evoked potential

AEq age equivalent

AER abduction/external rotation; acoustic evoked response; acute exertional rhabdomyolysis; agranular endoplasmic reticulum; albumin excretion rate; aldosterone excretion rate; apical ectodermal ridge; auditory evoked response; average electroencephalic response; average evoked response

AERE Atomic Energy Research Establishment

Aero Aerobacter

AERP antegrade effective refractory period; atrial effective refractory period

AERPAP antegrade effective refractory period accessory pathway

AERS acute equine respiratory syndrome

AES acetone-extracted serum; ambulatory encounter system; American Electroencephalographic Society; American Encephalographic Society; American Endocrine Society; American Endodontic Society; American Epidemiological Society; American Equilibration Society; anterior esophageal sensor; anti-embolic stockings; antral ethmoidal sphenoidectomy; aortic ejection sound; Auger's electron spectroscopy; auto-erythrocyte sensitization

AEs adverse events

AEST aeromedical evacuation support team

AET absorption-equivalent thickness;S-(2-aminoethyl) isothiuronium

AEV avian erythroblastosis virus

AEZ acrodermatitis enteropathica, zinc deficient

AF abnormal frequency; acid-fast; active force; adult female; afebrile; affected female; aflatoxin; albumin-free; albumose-free; aldehyde fuchsin; amaurosis fugax; aminofluorine; aminophylline; amniotic fluid; angiogenesis factor; anteflexion; anterior fontanelle; antibody-forming; anti-fog; aortic flow; Arthritis Foundation; artificial feeding; ascitic fluid; atrial fibrillation; atrial flutter; atrial fusion; attenuation factor; attributable fraction; audio frequency

aF abfarad

af audio frequency

AFA acromegaloid facial appearance [syndrome]; advanced first aid; alcohol-formaldehyde-acetic [fixative]

AFAFP amniotic fluid alpha-fetoprotein

AFAR American Foundation for Aging Research

AFASAK Atrial Fibrillation, Aspirin, Anticoagulation [trial]

AFB acid-fast bacillus; aflatoxin B; air fluidized bed; aortofemoral bypass

AFBAC affected family-based control test

AFBG aortofemoral bypass graft

AFC adult foster care; alternative forced choice; amplitude frequency characteristics; antibody-forming cell

AFCAPS Air Force Coronary Atherosclerosis Prevention Study

AFCI acute focal cerebral ischemia

AFCR American Federation for Clinical Research

AFD accelerated freeze drying; acrofacial dysostosis

AFDC Aid to Families with Dependent Children

AFDH American Fund for Dental Health

AFDW ash-free dry weight

AFE amniotic fluid embolism

afeb afebrile

AFEDI Association Francophone Europeenne des Infirmiers [Canada]

AFF atrial fibrillation; atrial filling fraction; atrial flutter

aff afferent

AFFIRM Atrial Fibrillation Follow-Up Investigation of Rhythm Management

AFFN acrofrontofacionasal [dysostosis]

AFG aflatoxin G; amniotic fluid glucose; arbitrary function generator

aFGF acidic fibroblast growth factor

AFH angiofollicular hyperplasia; anterior facial height

AFI amaurotic familial idiocy; Atrial Fibrillation Investigators [1993 pooled study]

AFib atrial fibrillation

AFIB Atrial Fibrillation Investigation with Bidisomide [trial]

AFIP Armed Forces Institute of Pathology

AFIPS American Federation of Information Processing Societies

AFIRME antagonist of the fibrinogen receptor after myocardial events

AFIS amniotic fluid infection syndrome

AFL antifibrinolysin; artificial limb; atrial flutter

AFLNH angiofollicular lymph node hyperplasia

AFLP acute fatty liver of pregnancy

AFM aflatoxin M; after fatty meal; American Federation of Musicians; atomic force microscopy

AFMA automated fabrication of modality aids

AFN afunctional neutrophil

AFNC Air Force Nurse Corps

AFND acute febrile neutrophilic dermatosis

AFO ankle/foot orthotic [brace or cast]; ankle-foot orthosis

AFORMED alternating failure of response, mechanical, [to] electrical depolarization

AFP acute flaccid paralysis; alpha-fetoprotein; anterior faucial pillar; atypical facial pain

AFPP acute fibropurulent pneumonia

AFQ aflatoxin Q

AFR aqueous flare response; ascorbic free radical

AFRAX autism-fragile X [syndrome]

AFRD acute febrile respiratory disease

AFRI acute febrile respiratory illness

AFROC Association for Freestanding Radiation Oncology Centers

AFS acquired or adult Fanconi syndrome; alternative financing system; American Fertility Society; antifibroblast serum

AFSAM Air Force School of Aviation Medicine

AFSCME American Federation of State, County and Municipal Employees

AFSM adaptive Fourier series modeling

AFSP acute fibrinoserous pneumonia

AFT aflatoxin; agglutination-flocculation test

AFTA American Family Therapy Association

AFTER Antistreplase Following Thrombolysis Effect on Reocclusion [study]; Aspirin/Anticoagulants Following Thrombolysis with Eminase in Recurrent Infarction [study]; Aspirin/Anticoagulants Following Thrombolysis with Eminase Results [study]

AFTN autonomously functioning thyroid nodule

AFV amniotic fluid volume; aortic flow velocity

AFX atypical fibroxanthoma

AG abdominal girth; agarose; aminoglutethimide; analytical grade; anion gap;

antigen; antigenomic; antiglobulin; anti-gravity; atrial gallop; attached gingiva; axiogingival; azurophilic granule

AG, A/G albumin-globulin [ratio]

Ag antigen; silver [Lat. *argentum*]

ag androgenetic; antigen

AGA accelerated growth area; allergic granulomatosis and angiitis; American Gastroenterological Association; American Genetic Association; American Geriatrics Association; American Goiter Association; anti-IgG autoantibody; antiglomerular antibody; appropriate for gestational age [birthweight]; aspartylglucosaminidase

Ag-Ab antigen-antibody complex

AGAG acidic glycosaminoglycans

AGAR Australian Group on Antimicrobial Resistance [study]

AGBAD Alexander Graham Bell Association for the Deaf

AGC absolute granulocyte count; atypical glandular cell; automatic gain control

AGC-FN atypical glandular cell—favor neoplasia

AGC-FR atypical glandular cell—favor reactive

AGCT antiglobulin consumption test; Army General Classification Test

AGC-U atypical glandular cell— unqualified

AGD agar gel diffusion; agarose diffusion; alpha-ketoglutarate dehydrogenase

AGDD agar gel double diffusion

AGE acrylamide gel; acute gastroenteritis; advanced glycosylation end-product; agarose gel electrophoresis; angle of greatest extension; arterial gas embolism

AGED automated general experimental device

AGEG age group

AGEPC acetyl glyceryl ether phosphorylcholine

AGES age grade extension size [thyroid tumor]

AGF adrenal growth factor; angle of greatest flexion

AGG agammaglobulinemia

agg agglutination; aggravation; aggregation

aggl, agglut agglutination

aggrav aggravated, aggravation

aggreg aggregated, aggregation

AGGS anti-gas gangrene serum

AGI adjusted gross income

agit agitated, agitation

AGL acute granulocytic leukemia; agglutination; aminoglutethimide

AGM absorbent gelling material

AGMK African green monkey kidney [cell]

AGMkK African green monkey kidney [cell]

AGN acute glomerulonephritis; agnosia

VIII$_{AGN}$ factor VIII antigen

agn agnosia

AGNB aerobic gram-negative bacillus

AgNOR silver-staining nucleolar organizer region

AGOS American Gynecological and Obstetrical Society

AGP acid glycoprotein; agar gel precipitation; azurophil granule protein; ambulatory glucose profile

AGPA American Group Practice Association; American Group Psychotherapy Association

AGPI agar gel precipitin inhibition

AGPT agar-gel precipitation test

AGR aniridia–ambiguous genitalia–mental retardation [syndrome]; anticipatory goal response

agri agriculture

AGS adrenogenital syndrome; Alagille syndrome; American Geriatrics Society; audiogenic seizures

AGSP Australian Gonococcal Surveillance Programme

AGT abnormal glucose tolerance; activity group therapy; acute generalized tuberculosis; alkylguanine deoxyribonucleic acid alkyltransferase; angiotensin; aniline/glyoxylate aminotransferase; antiglobulin test

agt agent

AGTH adrenoglomerulotropic hormone

AGTr adrenoglomerulotropin

AGTT abnormal glucose tolerance test

AGU aspartylglucosaminuria

AGUS atypia of gland cells of undetermined significance

AGV aniline gentian violet

AH abdominal hysterectomy; absorptive hypercalciuria; accidental hypothermia; acetohexamide; acid hydrolysis; acute hepatitis; adrenal hypoplasia; after hyperpolarization; agnathia-holoprosencephaly;

alcoholic hepatitis; amenorrhea and hirsutism; aminohippurate; anterior heel; anterior hypothalamus; antihyaluronidase; arcuate hypothalamus; Army Hospital; arterial hypertension; artificial heart; ascites hepatoma; assisted hatching; astigmatic hypermetropia; ataxic hemiparesis; autoimmune hepatitis; autonomic hyperreflexia; axillary hair

A/H amenorrhea-hyperprolactinemia

A + H accident & health [policy]

A·h ampere hour

aH abhenry

ah hyperopic astigmatism

AHA acetohydroxamic acid; acquired hemolytic anemia; acute hemolytic anemia; American Heart Association; American Hospital Association; anterior hypothalamic area; anti-heart antibody; antihistone antibody; area health authority; arthritis-hives-angioedema [syndrome]; aspartylhydroxamic acid; autoimmune hemolytic anemia

AHA/ACC American Heart Association/American College of Cardiology [Task Force]

AHB alpha-hydroxybutyric acid

AHC academic health care; academic health center; acute hemorrhagic conjunctivitis; acute hemorrhagic cystitis; adrenal hypoplasia congenita; antihemophilic factor C

AHCA Agency for Health Care Administration; American Health Care Association

AHCD acquired hepatocellular degeneration

AHC/HHG adrenal hypoplasia congenita-hypogonadopic hypogonadism [syndrome]

AHCN American Housecall Network [consumer health information]

AHCP Allied health care professional

AHCPR Agency for Health Care Policy and Research (see **AHRQ**)

AHCy adenosyl homocysteine

AHD acquired hepatocerebral degeneration; acute heart disease; antihyaluronidase; antihypertensive drug; arterio-hepatic dysplasia; arteriosclerotic heart disease; atherosclerotic heart disease; autoimmune hemolytic disease

AHDMS automated hospital data management system

AHDP azacycloheptane diphosphonate

AHDS Allan-Herndon-Dudley syndrome

AHE acute hazardous events [database]; acute hemorrhagic encephalomyelitis

AHEA area health education activity

AHEC area health education center

AHES artificial heart energy system

AHF acute heart failure; American Health Foundation; American Hepatic Foundation; American Hospital Formulary; antihemolytic factor; antihemophilic factor; Argentinian hemorrhagic fever; Associated Health Foundation

AHFS American Hospital Formulary Service

AHF SCENE Advanced Heart Failure Shared Clinical Experience Network

AHG aggregated human globulin; antihemophilic globulin; antihuman globulin

AHGG antihuman gammaglobulin; aggregated human gammaglobulin

AHGS acute herpetic gingival stomatitis

AHH alpha-hydrazine analog of histidine; anosmia and hypogonadotropic hypogonadism [syndrome]; arylhydrocarbon hydroxylase; Association for Holistic Health

AHI active hostility index; Animal Health Institute; apnea-plus-hypopnea index

AHIMA American Health Information Management Association

AHIP assisted health insurance plan

AHIS automated hospital information system

AHJ artificial hip joint

AHL apparent half-life

AHLE acute hemorrhagic leukoencephalitis

AHLG antihuman lymphocyte globulin

AHLS antihuman lymphocyte serum

AHM Allied health manpower; ambulatory Holter monitor

AHMA American Holistic Medicine Association; antiheart muscle autoantibody

AHMC Association of Hospital Management Committees

AHMC Association of Hospital Management Committees

AHN Army Head Nurse; assistant head nurse

AHO Albright hereditary osteodystrophy

AHP accountable health plan or partnership; acute hemorrhagic pancreatitis; after hyperpolarization; air at high pressure; aminohydroxyphenylalanine; analytic hierarchy process; approved health plan; Assistant House Physician

AHPA American Health Planning Association

AHPO anterior hypothalamic preoptic [area]

AHR antihyaluronidase reaction; Association for Health Records; atrial heart rate

AHRA American Hospital Radiology Administration

AHRF acute hypoxemic respiratory failure; American Hearing Research Foundation

AHRQ Agency for Healthcare Research and Quality [formerly Agency for Health Care Policy and Research]

AHS Academy of Health Sciences; Adventist Health Study; African horse sickness; alveolar hypoventilation syndrome; American Hearing Society; American Hospital Society; area health service; assistant house surgeon

AHSA American Health Security Act

AHSDF area health service development fund

AHSG alpha-2HS-glycoprotein

AHSN Assembly of Hospital Schools of Nursing

AHSP AIDS Health Services Program [of the Robert Wood Johnson Foundation]

AHSR Association for Health Services Research

AHT aggregation half time; antihyaluronidase titer; augmented histamine test; autogenous hamster tumor

AHTG antihuman thymocyte globulin

AHTP antihuman thymocyte plasma

AHTS antihuman thymus serum

AHU acute hemolytic uremic [syndrome]; arginine, hypoxanthine, and uracil

AHuG aggregated human IgG

AHV avian herpes virus

AI accidental injury; accidentally incurred; adiposity index; aggregation index; allergy and immunology; amylogenesis imperfecta; anaphylatoxin inactivator; angiogenesis inhibitor; angiotensin I; anxiety index; aortic incompetence; aortic insufficiency; apical impulse; articulation index; artificial insemination; artificial intelligence; atherogenic index; atrial insufficiency; autoimmune, autoimmunity; avidity index; axio-incisal; first meiotic anaphase

A&I allergy and immunology

aI active ingredient

AIA allylisopropylacetamide; amylase inhibitor activity; anti-immunoglobulin antibody; anti-insulin antibody; aspirin-induced asthma; automated image analysis

AIB aminoisobutyrate; avian infectious bronchitis

AIBA aminoisobutyric acid

AIBS American Institute of Biological Sciences

AIC Akaike information criterion [a goodness-of-fit measure]; aminoimidazole carboxamide; Association des Infirmières Canadiennes

A-IC average integrated concentration

AICA anterior inferior cerebellar artery; anterior inferior communicating artery

AI-CAH autoimmune-type chronic active hepatitis

AICAR aminoimidazole carboxamide ribonucleotide

AICD automatic implantable cardioverter defibrillator

AICE angiotensin I converting enzyme

AICF adaptive impulse correlated filtering; autoimmune complement fixation

AI/COAG artificial intelligence hemostasis consultant system

AID acquired immunodeficiency disease; acute infectious disease; acute ionization detector; Agency for International Development; argon ionization detector; artificial insemination by donor; autoimmune deficiency; autoimmune disease; automatic implantable defibrillator; average interocular difference

AIDA automatic interpretation for diagnostic assistance; automatic interpretation of data analysis

AIDCI angle independent Doppler color imaging

AIDP acute idiopathic demyelinating polyneuropathy

AIDS acquired immune deficiency syndrome

AIDSDRUGS Clinical Trials of AIDS drugs [National Library of Medicine (NLM) database]

AIDS-KS acquired immune deficiency syndrome with Kaposi's sarcoma

AIDSLINE on-line information on acquired immunodeficiency syndrome [MEDLARS data base]

AIDSPIT Artificial Insulin Delivery System Pancreas and Islet Transplantation [study]

AIDSTRIALS clinical trials of acquired immunodeficiency syndrome drugs [MEDLARS data base]

AIE acute inclusion-body encephalitis; acute infectious encephalitis; acute infective endocarditis

AIEP amount of insulin extractable from pancreas

AIF anemia-inducing factor; anti-inflammatory; anti-invasion factor

AIFD acute intrapartum fetal distress

AIG anti-immunoglobulin

AIgE anti-immunoglobulin E antibody

AIH amelogenesis imperfecta, hypomaturation type; American Institute of Homeopathy; artificial insemination, homologous; artificial insemination by husband

AIHA American Industrial Hygiene Association; American International Health Alliance; autoimmune hemolytic anemia

AIHC American Industrial Health Conference

AIHD acquired immune hemolytic disease

AII acute intestinal infection; second meiotic anaphase; angiotensin II

AIIS anterior inferior iliac spine

AIIT amiodarone-iodine-induced thyrotoxicosis

AIL acute infectious lymphocytosis; angiocentric immunoproliferative lesion; angioimmunoblastic lymphadenopathy

AILD alveolar interstitial lung disease; angioimmunoblastic lymphadenopathy

AIM Abridged Index Medicus; acquisition interface module; acuity index method; acute transverse myelopathy; advanced informatics and medicine; all in medicine; area of interest magnification; artificial intelligence in medicine; atypical immature squamous metaplasia

AIMBE American Institute for Medical and Biological Engineering

AIMD abnormal involuntary movement disorder

AIMS abnormal involuntary movement scale; Acylated Plasminogen-Streptokinase Activator Complex [APSAC] Intervention Mortality Study; aid for the impaired medical student; arthritis impact measurement scale

AIN acute interstitial nephritis; American Institute of Nutrition; anterior interosseous nerve

AINA automated immunonephelometric assay

AINS anterior interosseous nerve syndrome; anti-inflammatory nonsteroidal

AION anterior ischemic optic neuropathy

AIOS acute illness observation scale

AIP acute idiopathic pericarditis; acute infectious polyneuritis; acute intermittent porphyria; aldosterone-induced protein; automated immunoprecipitation; average intravascular pressure; integral anatuberculin, Petragnani

AIPE acute interstitial pulmonary emphysema; alcoholism intervention performance evaluation

AIPFP acute idiopathic peripheral facial nerve palsy

AIPRI ACE Inhibition in Progressive Renal Insufficiency [study]

AIPS American Institute of Pathologic Science

AIR amino-imidazole ribonucleotide; automated image registration; average impairment rating

AIRA anti-insulin receptor antibody

AIRE Acute Infarction Ramipril Efficacy [study]; Acute Infarction Ramipril Efficacy [trial]; Acute Infarction Reperfusion Efficacy [study]

AIREX Acute Infarction Ramipril Efficacy Extension [study]

AIRF alterations in respiratory function

AI/RHEUM artificial intelligence rheumatology consultant system

AIRS Amphetamine Interview Rating Scale

AIS Abbreviated Injury Scale; absolute increase in survival; acute ischemic stroke; acute ischemic syndrome; adenocarcinoma in situ; administrative information system; aggregate injury score; amniotic infection syndrome; analyzer of interrated sequences [model of a beating ventricle]; androgen insensitivity syndrome; anterior interosseous nerve syndrome; anti-insulin serum; automatic information system; automotive injury score

AISA acquired idiopathic sideroblastic anemia

AIS/MR Alternative Intermediate Services for the Mentally Retarded

AIT acute intensive treatment

AITIA aspirin in transient ischemic attacks

AITIAIS Aspirin in Transient Ischemic Attacks Italian Study

AITP autoimmune idiopathic thrombocytopenic purpura

AITT arginine insulin tolerance test; augmented insulin tolerance test

AIU absolute iodine uptake; antigen-inducing unit

AIUM American Institute of Ultrasound in Medicine

AIVC Australian Influenza Vaccine Committee

AIVR accelerated idioventricular rhythm

AIVV anterior informal vertebral vein

AJ adherens junction

AJ, A/J ankle jerk

AJCC American Joint Commission for Cancer

AJCCS American Joint Committee on Cancer Staging

AJDL arteriojugular venous lactate content difference

AJDO₂ arteriojugular venous oxygen content difference

AJR abdominojugular reflux maneuver

AJS acute joint syndrome

AK above knee; acetate kinase; actinic keratosis; adenosine kinase; adenylate kinase; artificial kidney

A/K, ak above knee [amputation]

A→K ankle to knee

AKA above-knee amputation; alcoholic ketoacidosis; also known as; antikeratin antibody

aka also known as

AK amp above-knee amputation

AKE acrokeratoelastoidosis

A/kg amperes per kilogram

AKP alkaline phosphatase

AKS alcoholic Korsakoff syndrome; auditory and kinesthetic sensation

AKU alkaptonuria

AL absolute latency; acinar lumen; acute leukemia; adaptation level; albumin; alcoholism [and other drug dependence services]; alignment; amyloid L; amyloidosis; analyzer and loader; anatomic location, anatomical localizer; anterior leaflet; antihuman lymphocytic [globulin]; avian leukosis; axial length; axillary loop; axiolingual; left ear [Lat. *auris laeva*]

A_L angiographic area of lateral projection

Al allantoic; allergic, allergy; aluminum

al left ear [Lat. *auris laeva*]

ALA amebic liver abscess; American Laryngological Association; American Lung Association; aminolevulinic acid; axiolabial

ALa axiolabial

Ala alanine

AL-Ab antilymphocyte antibody

ALAD abnormal left axis deviation

ALAD, ALA-D aminolevulinic acid dehydrase

ALADH delta-aminolevulinate dehydratase

ALADP aminolevulinic acid dehydrogenase deficiency porphyria

ALAG, ALaG axiolabiogingival

A-LAK adherent lymphokine-activated killer [cell]

ALAL, ALaL axiolabiolingual

A_LAO angiographic area of left anterior oblique projection

AlaP, ala-P alafosfalin

ALARA as low as reasonably achievable [radiation exposure]

ALARM adjustable leg and ankle repositioning mechanism

ALARP as low as reasonably possible

ALAS delta-aminolevulinate synthase

ALASH delta-aminolevulinate synthase, housekeeping type

ALAT alanine aminotransferase

ALB albumin; avian lymphoblastosis

alb albumin; white [Lat. *albus*]

ALBC albumin clearance

ALB/GLOB albumin/globulin [ratio]

ALC absolute lymphocyte count; acute lethal catatonia; aided living center; Alternative Lifestyle Checklist; approximate lethal concentration; avian leukosis complex; axiolinguocervical

alc alcohol, alcoholism, alcoholic

ALCA anomalous left coronary artery

ALCAPA anomalous origin of left coronary artery from pulmonary artery

ALCAR acetyl-L-carnitine

ALCEQ Adolescent Life Change Event Questionnaire

alcoh alcohol, alcoholic, alcoholism

AlcR, alcR alcohol rub

AlCr aluminum crown

ALD adrenoleukodystrophy; alcoholic liver disease; aldolase; anterior latissimus dorsi; Appraisal of Language Disturbance; assistive listening device

Ald aldolase

ALDA aldolase A

ALDB aldolase B

ALDC aldolase C

ALDF American Lyme Disease Foundation

ALDH aldehyde dehydrogenase

Aldo, ALDOST aldosterone

ALDOA aldolase A

ALDOC aldolase C

ALDP adrenoleukodystrophy protein

ALDR aldose reductase

ALDS albinism-deafness syndrome

ALDUSA aspirin low dosage in unstable angina

ALE active life expectancy; adaptive line enhancer; allowable limits of error; amputated lower extremity

ALEC artificial lung-expanding compound

ALEP atypical lymphoepithelioid cell proliferation

ALERT Amiodarone vs Lidocaine Inpatient Emergency Resuscitation Trial

ALF acute liver failure; American Liver Foundation; assisted living facilities; automated laser fluorescence

ALFT abnormal liver function test

ALG antilymphocytic globulin; axiolinguogingival

alg allergy

ALGOL algorithmic oriented language

ALH angiolymphoid hyperplasia; anterior lobe hormone; anterior lobe of hypophysis

ALHE angiolymphoid hyperplasia with eosinophilia

ALI acute lung injury; annual limit of intake; average lobe index

ALICE advanced large-scale integrated computational environment

ALIF anterior lumbar interbody fusion

ALIP abnormal localized immature myeloid precursor

ALIVE Adenosine Lidocaine Infarct Zone Viability Enhancement [trial]; Amiodarone vs Lidocaine in Prehospital Refractory Ventricular Fibrillation [study]; Azimilide Postinfarction Survival Evaluation [trial]

ALK automated lamellar keratoplasty

ALK, alk alkaline; alkylating

ALK-P alkaline phosphatase

ALL acute lymphoblastic leukemia; acute lymphocytic leukemia; Antihypertensive and Lipid-Lowering [study]

all allergy, allergic

ALLHAT Antihypertensive and Lipid-Lowering Treatment to Prevent Heart Attack Trial

ALLA acute lymphocytic leukemia antigen

ALLO atypical *Legionella*-like organism

ALM aerial lentiginous melanoma; alveolar living material

ALME acetyl-lysine methyl ester

ALMI anterior lateral myocardial infarct

ALMV anterior leaflet of the mitral valve

ALN allylnitrile; anterior lymph node

ALO average lymphocyte output; axiolinguo-occlusal

ALOS average length of stay

ALOSH Appalachian Laboratory for Occupational Safety and Health

ALOX aluminum oxide

ALP acute leukemia protocol; acute lupus pericarditis; alkaline phosphatase; alveolar proteinosis; anterior lobe of pituitary; antileukoproteinase; antilymphocytic plasma; argon laser photocoagulation; automated linkage preprocessor

AlPase alkaline phosphatase

ALPG alkaline phosphatase, germ-cell

α Greek letter alpha; angular acceleration; first [carbon atom next to the carbon atom bearing the active group in organic compounds]; optical rotation; probability of type I error; solubility coefficient

α_1-**AT** alpha$_1$-antitrypsin

alpha$_2$-AP alpha 2-antiplasmin

alpha-GLUC alpha-glucosidase

alpha$_2$M alpha$_2$-macroglobulin

ALPL alkaline phosphatase, liver

ALPP alkaline phosphatase, placental

ALPPL alkaline phosphatase-like, placental

ALPS angiolymphoproliferative syndrome; Aphasia Language Performance Scale; attitudinal listening profile system

ALR aldehyde reductase

ALRI anterolateral rotatory instability

ALROS American Laryngological, Rhinological, and Otological Society

ALS acute lateral sclerosis; advanced life support; afferent loop syndrome; alkali-labile site; amyotrophic lateral sclerosis; angiotensin-like substance; anterolateral sclerosis; anticipated life span; antilymphocyte serum

ALSD Alzheimer-like senile dementia

ALSPAC Avon Longitudinal Study of Pregnancy and Childhood

ALS-PD amyotrophic lateral sclerosis-parkinsonism-dementia [complex]

AL-SV avian leukosis sarcoma virus

ALT alanine aminotransferase; argon laser trabeculoplasty; avian laryngotracheitis

Alt, alt aluminum tartrate; alternate; altitude

AlT aluminum tartrate

ALTB acute laryngotracheobronchitis

ALTE apparent life threatening event

ALTEE acetyl-*L*-tyrosine ethyl ester

ALTS acute lumbar traumatic sprain [or syndrome]

ALU arithmetic and logic unit

ALV Abelson leukemia virus; adeno-like virus; alveolar, alveolus; ascending lumbar vein; avian leukosis virus

Alv alveolus, alveolar

ALVAD abdominal left ventricular assist device

ALVF acute left ventricular failure

ALV M alveolar mucosa

ALVT aortic and left ventricular tunnel

alv vent alveolar ventilation

ALVX alveolectomy

ALW arch-loop whorl

ALWMI anterolateral wall myocardial infarct

AM Academic Medicine [journal]; actomyosin; acute myelofibrosis; adult male; adult monocyte; aerospace medicine; affected male; akinetic mutism; alveolar macrophage; alveolar mucosa; amacrine cell; ambulatory; amethopterin; ametropia; ammeter; amperemeter; ampicillin; amplitude modulation; amyl; anovular menstruation; arithmetic mean; arousal mechanism; articular manipulation; aviation medicine; axiomesial; meter angle; myopic astigmatism

Am americium; amnion; amyl

A/m amperes per meter

A-m² ampere-square meter

am ametropia; amyl; amplitude; meter angle; myopic astigmatism

AMA against medical advice; alkaline membrane assay; American Management Association; American Medical Association; antimitochondrial antibody; antimyosin antibody; antithyroid microsomal antibody; arm muscle area; Australian Medical Association

AMA-DE American Medical Association Drug Evaluation

AMAL Aero-Medical Acceleration Laboratory

AMANET, AMA/Net American Medical Association Network

AMAP American Medical Accreditation Program; as much as possible

A-MAT amorphous material

AMB avian myeloblastosis; amphotericin B; anomalous muscle bundle

Amb ambulance; ambulatory, ambulation

amb ambient; ambiguous; ambulance; ambulatory

AMBER advanced multiple-beam equalization radiography; assisted model building with energy refinement

ambig ambiguous

AMBL acute megakaryoblastic leukemia

AMbL acute myeloblastic leukemia

AMBRE atraumatic multidirectional bilateral rehabilitation [shoulder]

ambul ambulatory

AMC academic medical center; acetylmethyl carbinol; Animal Medical Center; antibody-mediated cytotoxicity; antimalaria campaign; arm muscle circumference; Army Medical Corps; arthrogryposis multiplex congenita; ataxia-microcephaly-retardation [syndrome]; automated mixture control; axiomesiocervical

AMCAS American Medical College Application Service

AMCHA aminomethylcyclohexane-carboxylic acid

AMCN anteromedial caudate nucleus

AMCRA American Managed Care and Review Association

AMD acid maltase deficiency; acromandibular dysplasia; actinomycin D; adrenomyelodystrophy; age-related macular degeneration; Aleutian mink disease; alpha-methyldopa; Association for Macular Diseases; axiomesiodistal; S-adenosylmethionine decarboxylase

AMDA American Medical Directors Association

AMDGF alveolar macrophage-derived growth factor

AMDS Association of Military Dental Surgeons

AME amphotericin methyl ester; apparent minerallocorticoid excess; aseptic meningoencephalitis

AMEA American Medical Electroencephalographic Association

AMEAE acute monophasic experimental autoimmune encephalomyelitis

AMEDS Army Medical Service

AMEGL, AMegL acute megakaryoblastic leukemia

AMEND aiding mothers and fathers experiencing neonatal death

AMES age metastasis extension size

AMet adenosyl-*L*-methionine

AMETHIST Ambroxol Efficacy and Tolerability on Hypersecretion, Italian Study

AMF antimuscle factor

AMFAR American Foundation for AIDS Research

AMG amyloglucosidase; antimacrophage globulin; axiomesiogingival

A₂MG alpha-2-macroglobulin

AMH Accreditation Manual for Hospitals; anti-müllerian hormone; automated medical history

Amh mixed astigmatism with myopia predominating

AMHA Association of Mental Health Administrators

AMHIS Alberta Mental Health Information System

AMHT automated multiphasic health testing

AMI acquired monosaccharide intolerance; acute myocardial infarct; amitriptyline; anterior myocardial infarction; Argatroban in Myocardial Infarction [study]; Association

of Medical Illustrators; Athletic Motivation Inventory; axiomesioincisal

AMIA American Medical Informatics Association

AMIABLE Acute Myocardial Infarction Angioplasty Bolus Lysis Evaluation

AMICUS Austrian Multicenter Isradipine cum Spirapril Study

AMIS Ambulatory Medical Information System; Aspirin in Myocardial Infarction Study; Automated Management Information System

AMISTAD Acute Myocardial Infarction Study of Adenosine

AMKL acute megakaryoblastic leukemia

AML acute monocytic leukemia; acute mucosal lesion; acute myeloblastic leukemia; acute myelocytic leukemia; acute myelogenous leukemia; anatomic medullary locking; angiomyolipoma; anterior mitral leaflet; automated multitest laboratory

AMLB alternate monoaural loudness balance

AMLC adherent macrophage-like cell; autologous mixed lymphocyte culture

AMLR autologous mixed lymphocyte reaction

AMLS antimouse lymphocyte serum

AMLSGA acute myeloblastic leukemia surface glycoprotein antigen

AMM agnogenic myeloid metaplasia; ammonia; antibody to murine cardiac myosin; World Medical Association [Fr. *Association Médicale Mondiale*]

amm, ammonia

AMML acute myelomonocytic leukemia

AMMoL acute myelomonocytic or myelomonoblastic leukemia

ammon ammonia

AMN adrenomyeloneuropathy; alloxazine mononucleotide; aminonucleoside; anterior median nucleus

AMNS aminonucleoside

AMO assistant medical officer; axiomesio-occlusal

AmO alarm object

A-mode amplitude mode; amplitude modulation

AMOG adhesion molecule on glia

AMOL, AMoL acute monocytic or monoblastic leukemia

amo, amor amorphous

AMP accelerated mental processes; acid mucopolysaccharide; adenosine monophosphate; amphetamine; ampicillin; ampule; amputation; average mean pressure

amp ampere; amplification; amplitude; ampule; amputation, amputee

AMPA alpha-amino-3-hydroxy-5-methyl-4-isoxazolepropionate; American Medical Publishers Association; aminoisopropyl propionic acid

AMPAC American Medical Political Action Committee

AMP-c cyclic adenosine monophosphate

AMPH, amphet amphetamine

amp-hr ampere-hour

AMPI Aspac in Acute Myocardial Infarction Placebo Controlled Investigation

ampl large [Lat. *amplus*]

AMPLE allergies, medications, past medical history, last meal, events preceding present condition

A-M pr Austin-Moore prosthesis

AMPS abnormal mucopolysacchariduria; acid mucopolysacch…

AMPT alpha-methylparatyrosine

ampul ampule

AMR acoustic muscle reflex; activity metabolic rate; acute mitral stenosis; alopecia-mental retardation [syndrome]; alternate motion rate; alternating motion reflex; ambulatory medical record

AMRA American Medical Record Association

AMRF American Medical Resources Foundation

AMRI anteromedial rotatory instability

AMRL Aerospace Medical Research Laboratories

AMRNL Army Medical Research and Nutrition Laboratory

AMRO Amsterdam-Rotterdam Trial Comparing Excimer Laser and Percutaneous Transluminal Coronary Angioplasty

AMRS automated medical record system

AMS ablepharon-microstomia syndrome; acute mountain sickness; adenosylmethionine synthetase; advanced large scale integrated computational environment [ALICE] memory snooper; advanced medical systems [fetal monitor]; aggravated in military service; altered mental status; American Microscopical Society; amount of substance;

amylase; antimacrophage serum; Army Medical Service; aseptic meningitis syndrome; Association of Military Surgeons; auditory memory span; automated multiphasic screening

ams amount of a substance

AMSA acridinylamine methanesulfon-m-anisidide; American Medical Society on Alcoholism; American Medical Students Association; amsacrine

AMSAODD American Medical Society on Alcoholism and Other Drug Dependencies

AMSC Army Medical Specialist Corps

AMSP Association of Medical School Pharmacology

AMSRDC Army Medical Service Research and Development Command

AMSU ambulatory minor surgery unit

AMT acute miliary tuberculosis; Adenosine Scan Multicenter Trial; alpha-methyltyrosine; American Medical Technologists; amethopterin; amitriptyline; amphetamine; anxiety management training

amt amount

AMU Army Medical Unit

amu atomic mass unit

AmuLV Abelson murine leukemia virus; amphotrophic murine leukemia virus

AMV assisted mechanical ventilation; avian myeloblastosis virus

AMVF additive multiattribute value function

AMVI acute mesenteric vascular insufficiency

aMVL anterior mitral valve leaflet

AMWA American Medical Women's Association; American Medical Writers' Association

AMX advanced multiprocessor extension; amoxicillin

AMY, amy amylase

AN acanthosis nigricans; acne neonatorum; acoustic neuroma; adult, normal; ala nasi; amyl nitrate; aneurysm; anisometropia; anode; anorexia nervosa; antenatal; anterior; antineuraminidase; aseptic necrosis; atmosphere normal; atrionodal; autonomic neuropathy; avascular necrosis

A/N antenatal; as needed

An actinon; anisometropia; anode, anodal; atmosphere normal

A$_n$ atmosphere normal

A1-NA A1 area of the nucleus ambiguus

ANA acetylneuraminic acid; American Narcolepsy Association; American Neurological Association; American Nurses Association; anesthesia [*anaesthesia*]; antibody to nuclear antigens; antinuclear antibody; aspartyl naphthylamide

Ana anaplastic

ANAD anorexia nervosa with associated disorders

ANAE alpha-naphthyl acetate esterase

anal analgesia, analgesic; analysis, analytic

ANAG acute narrow angle glaucoma

ANAL, anal analgesia, analgesic; analysis, analytic

ANAM automated neuropsychological assessment metrics

ANAP agglutination negative, absorption positive [reaction]

ANAS anastomosis; auditory nerve activating substance

ANASCD American Nurses Association Steering Committee on Databases

anast anastomosis

ANAT anatomic structure [UMLS]

Anat, anat anatomy, anatomist

ANB avascular necrosis of bone

ANBP Australian National Blood Pressure [trial]

ANC absolute neutrophil count; acid neutralization capacity; adult neuronal ceroid [lipofuscinosis]; antigen-neutralizing capacity; Army Nurse Corps

ANCA antineutrophilic cytoplasmic antibody

ANCC, AnCC anodal closure contraction

ANCHR Access to National Claims History Repository [Medicare database]

ANCL adult neuronal ceroid lipofuscinosis

ANCOVA analysis of covariance

ANCR Association of the Nordic Cancer Registries

AND algoneurodystrophy; anterior nasal discharge

ANDA Abbreviated New Drug Application

ANDRO, andro androsterone

ANDTE, AnDTe anodal duration tetanus

anes, anesth anesthesia, anesthetic

ANESR apparent norepinephrine secretion rate

AnEx, an ex anodal excitation

ANF alpha-naphthoflavone; American Nurses' Foundation; antineuritic factor; antinuclear factor; atrial natriuretic factor

ANG angiogenin; angiogram, angiography; angiotensin

Ang II angiotensin II

ang angiogram; angiography, angle, angular

ANGFA antinerve growth factor antibody

Ang GR angiotensin generation rate

Angio angiography, angiogram, angiographic

ang pect angina pectoris

ANH academic nursing home

anh anhydrous

ANI acute nerve irritation

ANIA automated nephelometric immunoassay

ANIM animal [UMLS]

ANIMAL automatic nonlinear image matching and anatomical labeling

ANIR Advanced Networking Infrastructure and Research [National Science Foundation]

ANIS Anorexia Nervosa Inventory for Self-rating

aniso anisocytosis

ANIT alpha-naphthyl-isothiocyanate

ANK, Ank ankyrin

ank ankle

ANL acute nonlymphoblastic leukemia

ANLI antibody-negative with latent infection

ANLL acute nonlymphocytic leukemia

ANN artificial neural network

Ann annual

ann fib annulus fibrosus

ANOC, AnOC anodal opening contraction

ANOCL anodal opening clonus

ANOCOVA analysis of covariance

ANOP anophthalmia

ANOV, ANOVA analysis of variance

ANP acute necrotizing pancreatitis; adult nurse practitioner; advanced nurse practitioner; ancillary nursing personnel; A-norprogesterone; atrial natriuretic peptide

ANP-A atrial natriuretic peptide A

ANP-B atrial natriuretic peptide B

ANP-C atrial natriuretic peptide C

A-NPP absorbed normal pooled plasma

ANRC American National Red Cross

ANRL antihypertensive neutral renomedullary lipid

ANS acanthion; American Nimodipine Study; American Nutrition Society; 8-anilino-1-naphthalene-sulfonic acid; anterior nasal spine; antineutrophilic serum; antirat neutrophil serum; Army Nursing Service; arterionephrosclerosis; Associate in Nursing Science; autonomic nervous system

ANSCII American National Standard Code for Information Interchange

ANSI American National Standards Institute

ANSWER Agency for Toxic Substances and Disease Registry/National Library of Medicine's Workstation for Emergency Response

ANT acoustic noise test; adenine nucleotide translocator; aminonitrothiazole; anterior

ant anterior; antimycin

ANT3Y adenine nucleotide translocator 3 Y

AntA antimycin A

antag antagonist

ANTENOX [Switch to oral] Anticoagulant from Enoxaparin [In treatment of acute deep venous thrombosis]

Anth-Gly anthraquinone-glycine [conjugate]

Anth-IDA anthraquinone-iminodiacetate [conjugate]

anti-HB$_c$ antibody to hepatitis B core antigen

anti-HB$_e$ antibody to hepatitis B early antigen

anti-HB$_s$ antibody to hepatitis B surface antigen

anti-PNM Ab anti-peripheral nerve myelin antibody

ANTR apparent net transfer rate

ANTU alpha-naphthylthiourea

ANU artificial neural unit

ANuA antinuclear antibody

ANUG acute necrotizing ulcerative gingivitis

ANV avian nephritis virus

ANX annexin

anx anxiety

ANZ Australia and New Zealand [heart failure collaborative study]

AO abdominal aorta; achievement orientation; acid output; acridine orange; age of onset; ankle orthosis; anodal opening; anterior oblique; antisense oligonucleotide; aorta; aortic opening; arthro-ophthalmopathy; assessment-object; atelosteogenesis; atomic orbital; atrioventricular valve opening; average optical [density]; axio-occlusal

Ao aorta

A$_o$ orifice area

A/O atlanto-occipital

A&O, A/O alert and oriented

AOA Administration on Aging; Alpha Omega Alpha Honor Society; American Optometric Association; American Orthopedic Association; American Orthopsychiatric Association; American Osteopathic Association; ascending aorta

AoA age of acquisition

AOAA amino-oxyacetic acid

AOAC Association of Official Agricultural Chemists

AOAP as often as possible

AoArE aortic arch epinephrine

AOAS American Osteopathic Academy of Sclerotherapy

AOB accessory olfactory bulb; alcohol on breath

AOBEM American Osteopathic Board of Emergency Medicine

AOBS acute organic brain syndrome

AOC abridged ocular chart; allyloxycarbonyl; amyloxycarbonyl; anodal opening contraction; area of concern

AOCA American Osteopathic College of Anesthesiologists

AOCD American Osteopathic College of Dermatology

AOCl anodal opening clonus

AOCN advanced oncology certified nurse

AOCPA American Osteopathic College of Pathologists

AOCPR American Osteopathic College of Proctology

AOCR American Osteopathic College of Radiology; American Osteopathic College of Rheumatology

AOD Academy of Operative Dentistry; Academy of Oral Dynamics; adult onset diabetes; anesthesiologist-on-duty; arterial oxygen desaturation; arteriosclerotic occlusive disease; auriculo-osteodysplasia

AODM adult onset diabetes mellitus

AODME Academy of Osteopathic Directors of Medical Education

AODP alcohol and other drug problems

AOE admission order entry

AoE aortic epinephrine

AOHA American Osteopathic Hospital Association

AOI apnea of infancy

AOIVM angiographically occult intracranial vascular malformation

AOL acro-osteolysis

AOM acute otitis media; alternatives of management; arthroophthalmopathy; azoxymethane

AOMA American Occupational Medical Association

AOMP, AoMP aortic mean pressure

AONE American Organization of Nurse Executives

AOO anodal opening odor; atrial asynchronous (competitive, fixed-rate) [pacemaker]

AOP anodal opening picture; aortic pressure

AoP aortic pressure

AOPA American Orthotics and Prosthetics Association

AOPC adult outpatient psychotherapy clinic

AOPW, AoPW aortic posterior wall

AOR adjusted odds ratio; Alvarado Orthopedic Research [instruments]; auditory oculogyric reflex

AORN Association of Operating Room Nurses

AOS American Ophthalmological Society; American Otological Society; anodal opening sound; anterior [o]esophageal sensor

AOSF adaptive order statistic filter

AOSSM American Orthopedic Society for Sports Medicine

AOT accessory optic tract; acute occlusive thrombus or thrombosis; Anderson Olsson table; anodal opening tetanus; Association of Occupational Therapists

AOTA American Occupational Therapy Association

AOTe anodal opening tetanus

AOTF American Occupational Therapy Foundation

AOU apparent oxygen utilization

AOV, AoV aortic valve

AP abdominal pain; accessory pathway; accounts payable; acid phosphatase; acinar parenchyma; action plan; action potential; activator protein; active pepsin; active pressure; acute pancreatitis; acute phase; acute pneumonia; acute proliferative; adenomatous polyposis; adolescent psychiatry; agno protein; alkaline phosphatase; alum precipitated; aminopeptidase; aminopurine; amyloid P-component; amyloid peptide; anatomic profile; angina pectoris; antepartal [Lat. *ante partum*]; anterior pituitary; anteroposterior; antidromic potential; antipyrine; antral peristalsis; aortic pressure; aortopulmonary; apical pulse; apothecary; appendectomy; appendicitis; appendix; apurinic acid; apurinic/apyrimidinic [site in DNA]; area postrema; arithmetic progression; arterial pressure; artificial pneumothorax; aspiration pneumonia; assessment and plans; association period; atherosclerotic plaque; atrial pacing; atrioventricular pathway; axiopulpal; before parturition [Lat. *ante partum*]

A-P anteroposterior

A/P abdominal/perineal; antepartum; ascites/plasma [ratio]

A&P anterior and posterior; assessment and plans; auscultation and percussion

Ap apex

aP acellular pertussis [vaccine]

ap anteroposterior; attachment point

APA action potential amplitude; aldosterone-producing adenoma; Ambulatory Pediatric Association; American Pancreatic Association; American Pharmaceutic Association; American Physiotherapy Association; American Podiatric Association; American Psychiatric Association; American Psychoanalytic Association; American Psychological Association; American Psychopathological Association; American Psychotherapy Association; aminopenicillanic acid; anterior margin of pulmonary artery; antipernicious anemia [factor]; antiphospholipid antibody; antiproliferative antibody; arcuate premotor area; azidophenacyl

ApA adenylyl (3'-5') adenosine; azidophenacyl

APAAP alkaline phosphatase-antialkaline phosphatase [labeling]

APAB antiphospholipid antibody; azidophenacyl bromide

APACHE Acute Physiology, Age, and Chronic Health Evaluation

APAF antipernicious anemia factor

APAMI Asian Pacific Association of Medical Informatics

APAN Asian-Pacific Advanced Network

APAP acetaminophen; adaptive positive airway pressure

APASS Antiphospholipid Antibodies in Stroke Studies

APB abductor pollicis brevis; atrial premature beat

APBD adult polyglucosan body disease

APC acetylsalicylic acid, phenacetin, and caffeine; activated protein C; adenoidalpharyngeal-conjunctival [agent]; adenomatous polyposis coli; allophyocyanin; all-purpose capsule; angiotensin presenting cell; antigen-presenting cell; antiphlogistic corticoid; aortopulmonary collateral artery; aperture current; apneustic center; argon plasma coagulation; aspirin-phenacetin-caffeine; atrial premature contraction

aPC activated protein C

APCC aspirin-phenacetin-caffeine-codeine

APCD acquired prothrombin complex deficiency [syndrome]; adult polycystic kidney disease

APCF acute pharyngoconjunctival fever

APCG apex cardiogram

Ap4CH apical four-chamber plane

APCKD adult-type polycystic kidney disease

APD action potential duration; acute polycystic disease; advanced physical diagnosis; anteroposterior diameter; antipsychotic drug; articulation-phonological disorders; atrial premature depolarization; autoimmune progesterone dermatitis; automated peritoneal dialysis

APD$_{80}$ action potential duration at 80% repolarization

A-PD anteroposterior diameter

APDF amplitude probability density function

APDI Adult Personal Data Inventory

APDIM Association of Program Directors in Internal Medicine

AP-DRG all patients–diagnosis-related group

APE acetone powder extract; acute polioencephalitis; acute psychotic episode; acute pulmonary edema; airway pressure excursion; aminophylline, phenobarbital, and ephedrine; anterior pituitary extract; asthma of physical effort; avian pneumoencephalitis

APECED autoimmune polyendocrinopathy-candidosis-ectodermal dystrophy

APF acidulated phosphofluoride; adaptive pattern filtering; American Psychological Foundation; anabolism-promoting factor; animal protein factor; antiperinuclear factor

APG acid-precipitated globulin; air plethysmography; ambulatory patient group; animal pituitary gonadotropin; antegrade pyelography

APGAR American Pediatric Gross Assessment Record

APGL alkaline phosphatase activity of granular leukocytes

APGO Association of Professors of Gynecology and Obstetrics

APH alcohol-positive history; alternative pathway hemolysis; aminoglycoside phosphotransferase; antepartum hemorrhage; anterior pituitary hormone; Association of Private Hospitals

Aph aphasia

APHA American Protestant Hospital Association; American Public Health Association

APhA American Pharmaceutical Association

APHEA Air Pollution in Health, European Approach

APHIS Animal and Plant Health Inspection Service

APHL Association of Public Health Laboratories

APHP anti-Pseudomonas human plasma

API alkaline protease inhibitor; Analytical Profile Index; applications programming interface; arterial pressure index; atmospheric pressure ionization; Autonomy Preference Index

APIC Acenocoumarin vs Pentoxifylline in Intermittent Claudication [trial]; Association for Practitioners in Infection Control

APIE assessment, plan, implementation, and evaluation

APIM Association Professionnelle Internationale des Médecins

APIP additional personal injury protection

APIS Antihypertensive Patch, Italian Study

APIVR artificial pacemaker-induced ventricular rhythm

APKD adult-onset polycystic kidney disease

APL abductor pollicis longus; accelerated painless labor; acute promyelocytic leukemia; animal placenta lactogen; anterior pituitary-like; anterior pulmonary leaflet

aPL antiphospholipid

A-P&L anteroposterior and lateral

APLA, aPLA antiphospholipid antibody

APLAUD Antiplatelet Useful Dose [trial]

APLAUSE Antiplatelet Treatment After Intravascular Ultrasound Guided Optimal Stent Expansion [trial]

APLP amyloid precursor-like protein

APLS advanced pediatric life support

APM Academy of Parapsychology and Medicine; Academy of Physical Medicine; Academy of Psychosomatic Medicine; acid precipitable material; admission pattern monitoring; affected pedigree member; alternating pressure mattress; anteroposterior movement; aspartame; Association of Professors of Medicine

APML acute promyelocytic leukemia

APMOMS Advisory Panel on the Mission and Organization of Medical Schools

APMR Association for Physical and Mental Retardation

APN acute pyelonephritis; advanced practice nurse; average peak noise

APNH antiporter sodium-hydrogen ion

APO abductor pollicis obliguus; acquired pendular oscillation; adriamycin, prednisone, vincristine; adverse patient occurrence; aphoxide; apolipoprotein; apomorphine; apoprotein

Apo, apo apolipoprotein

APOA, apoA apolipoprotein A

APOB, apoB apolipoprotein B

APOC, apoC apolipoprotein C

APOE, apoE apolipoprotein E

APOJ, apoJ apolipoprotein J

APORF acute postoperative renal failure

apoth apothecary

APP acute phase protein; alum-precipitated pyridine; aminopyrazolopyrimidine; amyloid peptide precursor; amyloid precursor protein; antiplatelet plasma; aqueous procaine penicillin; automated physiologic profile; avian pancreatic polypeptide

App, app appendix

APPA American Psychopathological Association

appar apparatus

APPC application or advanced program-to-program communication

APPCR, AP-PCR arbitrarily primed polymerase chain reaction

APPG aqueous procaine penicillin G

APPI Active Persantine in Postischemic Injury [study]

appl appliance; application, applied

APPROACH Alberta Provincial Project for Outcomes Assessment in Coronary Heart Disease

approp appropriate

approx approximate

APPS amyloid precursor protein secretase

appt appointment

appx appendix

appy appendectomy

APR abdominoperineal resection; absolute proximal reabsorption; acute phase reaction or reactant; amebic prevalence rate; anatomic porous replacement; anterior pituitary reaction; average payment rate

APRAIS Acute Phase Reactions and Ischemic Coronary Syndromes

APRAISE Antisense to Prevent Restenosis After Intervention, Stent Evaluation

aprax apraxia

APRICOT Antithrombotics in the Prevention of Reocclusion in Coronary Thrombolysis [trial]; Aspirin vs. Coumadin Trial; Aspirin vs. Coumadin in the Prevention of Reocclusion and Recurrent Ischemia after Successful Thrombolysis Trial

APRL American Prosthetic Research Laboratory

AProL acute promyelocytic leukemia

APRP acidic proline-rich protein; acute phase reactant protein

APRT adenine phosphoribosyl transferase

APRV airway pressure release ventilation

APS acute physiology score; adenosine phosphosulfate; advanced photon source; American Pain Society; American Pediatric Society; American Physiological Society; American Proctologic Society; American Prosthodontic Society; American Psychological Society; American Psychosomatic Society; aminopropylsilane; ammonium persulfate; analog processing stage; annual person summary [Medicare data file]; antiphospholipid antibody syndrome; attending physician's statement; autoimmune polyglandular syndrome; automated patent system; prostate-specific antigen

APSAC acylated plasminogen-streptokinase activator complex; anisoylated plasminogen streptokinase activator complex

APSD aorticopulmonary septal defect

APSGN acute poststreptococcal glomerulonephritis

APSIS Angina Prognosis Study in Stockholm; Angina Prognosis Study with Isoptin and Seloken [trial]

APSP assisted peak systolic pressure

APSQ Abbreviated Parent Symptom Questionnaire

APSS Association for the Psychophysiological Study of Sleep

APSU Australian Paediatric Surveillance Unit

APT Ablate and Pace Trial; alum-precipitated toxoid; aminophenylthioether; antiplatelet trials; applied potential tomography

APTA American Physical Therapy Association

APTD Aid to Permanently and Totally Disabled

APTF American Physical Therapy Foundation

APTH ambulatory blood pressure monitoring and treatment of hypertension

APTI airway pressure time index

APTT, aPTT activated partial thromboplastin time

APUD amine precursor uptake and decarboxylation

APV abnormal posterior vector

aPV acellular pertussis vaccine

APVC anomalous pulmonary venous connection

APW alkaline peptone water

APWS attending physician work station

AQ achievement quotient; any quantity; aphasia quotient

aq aqueous; water [Lat. *aqua*]

AQAB acquired abnormality [UMLS]

AQCESS Automated Quality of Care Evaluation Support System

AQL acceptable quality level

AQLQ Asthma Quality of Life Questionnaire

AQP aquaporin

AQS additional qualifying symptoms

aqu aqueous

AR absolute risk; accounts receivable; achievement ratio; actinic reticuloid [syndrome]; active resistance; acute rejection; adherence ratio; admission rate; admitting room; adrenodoxin reductase; airway resistance; alarm reaction; alcohol related; alkali reserve; allergic rhinitis; alloy restoration; ambulance report; amphiregulin; amplitude ratio; analytical reagent; androgen receptor; anterior root; aortic regurgitation; apical-radial; Argyll Robertson [pupil]; aromatase; arsphenamine; articulare; artificial respiration; ascorbate reductase; assisted respiration; at risk; atrial rate; atrial reversal; atrophic rhinitis; augmented reality [computer graphics]; autoradiography; autoregressive; autosomal recessive

Ar argon; articulare

ar aromatic

A/R apical/radial

A&R advised and released

ARA Academy of Rehabilitative Audiometry; acetylene reduction activity, American Rheumatism Association; anorectal agenesis; antireticulin antibody; aortic root angiogram; arabinose; Associate of the Royal Academy

ara arabinose

ara-A adenine arabinoside

Ara-C arabinosylcytidine

ara-C acytosine arabinose; cytosine arabinoside

ARAL adjustment reaction to adult life

ARAM antigen recognition activation motif

ARAMIS American Rheumatism Association Medical Information System

A$_{RAO}$ angiographic area of right anterior oblique projection

ARAS ascending reticular activating system

ara-U arabinosyluracil

ARB adrenergic receptor binder; angiotensin receptor blocker

arb arbitrary unit

ARBD alcohol-related birth defects

ARC accelerating rate calorimetry; Accreditation Review Council; acquired immunodeficiency syndrome-related complex; active renin concentration; AIDS-related complex; American Red Cross; anomalous retinal correspondence; antigen reactive cell; arcuate; Arthritis Rehabilitation Center; arthrogryposis-renal dysfunction-cholestasis [syndrome]; Association for Retarded Children; atypical reparative changes

ARCA acquired red cell aplasia

ARCH Amiodarone Reduces Coronary Artery Bypass Grafting Hospitalization [trial]; automated record for child health

ARCI Addiction Research Center Inventory

ARCOS Auckland Region Coronary or Stroke [study]

ARCS Associate of the Royal College of Science; Atherosclerosis Risk in Communities Study

ARC-ST Accreditation Review Council for Educational Programs in Surgical Technology

ARD absolute reaction of degeneration; acute radiation disease; acute respiratory disease; adult respiratory distress; allergic respiratory disease; ancillary report display; anorectal dressing; arthritis and rheumatic diseases; atopic respiratory disease

AR-DLMD autosomal recessive Duchenne-like muscular dystrophy

ARDMS American Registry of Diagnostic Medical Sonographers

ARDS acute respiratory distress syndrome; adult respiratory distress syndrome

ARE active-resistive exercises; AIDS-related encephalitis

AREDS Age-Related Eye Disease Study

AREDYLD acrorenal field defect, ectodermal dysplasia, lipoatrophic diabetes [syndrome]

AREPA acetazolamide-responsive familial paroxysmal ataxia

ARES antireticulo-endothelial serum

AREV Advanced Revelations [platform for database distribution]

ARF acute renal failure; acute respiratory failure; acute rheumatic fever; Addiction Research Foundation; ambulance report form; area resource file

ARFC active rosette-forming T-cell; autologous rosette-forming cell

ARFD acrorenal field defect

AR-FSP autosomal recessive familial spastic paraplegia

ARG, Arg arginine

arg arginine; silver [Lat. *argentum*]

ARGAMI Argatroban Compared with Heparin in Myocardial Infarction Treated with Recombinant Tissue Plasminogen Activator

ARGS antitrypsin-related gene sequence

ARI absolute risk increase; acute respiratory illness; airway reactivity index; anxiety reaction, intense

ARIA acetylcholine receptor-inducing activity; automated radioimmunoassay

ARIC Atherosclerosis Risk in Communities [study]

ARIMA autoregressive integrated moving average

ARIS Andrology Research Information System; Anturan Reinfarction Italian Study; auto-regulated inspiratory support

Ar Kr argon-krypton [laser]

ARL Association of Research Libraries; average remaining lifetime

ARLD alcohol related liver disease

AR-LGMD autosomal recessive limb muscular dystrophy

ARM adrenergic receptor material; aerosol rebreathing method; ambulatory renal monitor; anorectal manometry; anxiety reaction, mild; Armenian [hamster]; artificial rupture of membranes; atomic resolution microscopy

ARMA autoregressive moving average

ARMD age-related muscle degeneration

ARMS access by radial artery multilink stent; adverse reaction monitoring system; amplification refractory mutation system

ArMV arabis mosaic virus

ARN acute renal necrosis; acute retinal necrosis; arcuate nucleus; Association of Rehabilitation Nurses

ARNMD Association for Research in Nervous and Mental Diseases

ARNP Advanced Registered Nurse Practitioner

ARNSHL autosomal recessive non-syndromic hearing loss

ARO Associate for Research in Ophthalmology

AROA autosomal recessive ocular albinism

AROM active range of motion; artificial rupture of membranes

arom aromatic

ARP absolute refractory period; American Registry of Pathologists; anticipated recovery path; apolipoprotein regulatory protein; assay reference plasma; assimilation regulatory protein; at risk period; automaticity recovery phase

ARPA Advanced Research Projects Agency

ARPANET Advanced Research Projects Agency Network

ARPC Akaike relative power contribution

ARPD autosomal recessive polycystic disease

ARPES angular resolved photoelectron spectroscopy

ARPKD autosomal recessive polycystic kidney disease

ARPT American Registry of Physical Therapists

ARR absolute risk reduction; aortic root replacement

arr arrest, arrested

ARRC Associate of the Royal Red Cross

ARREST Amiodarone in Out-of-Hospital Resuscitation of Refractory Sustained Ventricular Tachyarrhythmia, Amsterdam Resuscitation Study

ARRP autosomal recessive retinitis pigmentosa

ARRS American Roentgen Ray Society

ARRT American Registry of Radiologic Technologists

ARS acquiescence response scale; acute radiation syndrome or sickness; adult Reye's syndrome; alcohol-related seizures; alizarin red S; American Radium Society; American Rhinologic Society; antirabies serum; arsphenamine; arylsulfatase; Atherogenic Risk Study; autonomously replicating sequence

Ars arsphenamine

ARSA American Reye's Syndrome Association; arylsulfatase A

ARSACS autosomal recessive spastic ataxia of Charlevoix-Saguenay

ARSB arylsulfatase B

ARSC arylsulfatase C; Associate of the Royal Society of Chemistry

ARSM acute respiratory system malfunction

ARSPH Associate of the Royal Society for the Promotion of Health

ART absolute retention time; Accredited Record Technician; Achilles reflex time; acoustic reflex test; adaptive resonance theory; algebraic reconstruction technique; algebraic reconstructive technique; artery; Angiojet Rapid Thrombectomy Catheter Study; antiretroviral therapy; assisted reproductive technique; automated reagin test; automaticity recovery time

art artery, arterial; articulation; artificial

arth arthritis

artic articulation, articulated

artif artificial

ARTISTIC Angiorad Radiation Technology for In-Stent Restenosis Trial in Coronaries

ARTMAP adaptive resonance theory mapping

Art O$_2$ arterial oxygen flow

ARTS Arterial Revascularization Therapies Study

ARU arthritis rehabilitation unit

ARV acquired immunodeficiency syndrome-related virus; anterior right ventricle; avian reovirus

ARVD arrhythmogenic right ventricular dysplasia

ARVP arginine-vasopressin

ARX autoregressive with exogenous input [model]

AS acetylstrophanthidin; acidified serum; acoustic schwannoma; acoustic stimulation; active sarcoidosis; active sleep; Adams-Stokes [disease]; allele-specific; Alport syndrome; alveolar sac; amyloid substance; anal sphincter; androsterone sulfate; Angelman syndrome; ankylosing spondylitis; anovulatory syndrome; antiserum; antisocial; antistreptolysin; antral spasm; anxiety state; aortic sound; aortic stenosis; approaching significance [statistical]; aqueous solution; aqueous suspension; area of stenosis; arteriosclerosis; artificial sweetener; aseptic meningitis; asparagine synthetase; assisted suicide; astigmatism; asymmetric; atherosclerosis; atrial septum; atrial stenosis; atropine sulfate; audiogenic seizure; Auto-Suture; left ear [Lat. *auris sinistra*]

As arsenic; astigmatism; asymptomatic

A(s) asplenia syndrome

A·s ampere second

A x s ampere per second

aS absiemens

as left ear [Lat. *auris sinistra*]

ASA acetylsalicylic acid; active systemic anaphylaxis; acute severe asthma; Adams-Stokes attack; ambulatory services architecture; American Society of Anesthesiologists; American Standards Association; American Surgical Association; aminosalicylic acid; anterior spinal artery; antibody to surface antigen; argininosuccinic acid; arylsulfatase-A; aspirin-sensitive asthma; asthmanasal polyps-aspirin intolerance [triad]

ASAAC Acetylsalicylic Acid Aorto-Coronary Bypass Surgery; Acetylsalicylic Acid vs. Anticoagulants [study]

ASAAD American Society for the Advancement of Anesthesia in Dentistry

ASAC acidified serum-acidified complement

ASAH antibiotic sterilized aortic valve homograft

ASAHP American Society of Allied Health Professions

ASAIO American Society for Artificial Internal Organs

ASAL arginosuccinic acid lyase

ASAP Academic Strategic Alliance Program; acetylsalicylic acid persantine [study]; American Society for Adolescent Psychology; arbitrary signatures from amplification profiles; Areawide Stroke Awareness Program; as soon as possible; Azimilide Supraventricular Arrhythmia Program [trial]

ASAS argininosuccinate synthetase

ASAT aspartate aminotransferase

ASB American Society of Bacteriologists; anencephaly–spina bifida [syndrome]; anesthesia standby; Anxiety Scale for the Blind; asymptomatic bacteriuria

ASBS American Society for Bariatric Surgery

ASBV avocado sunblotch viroid

ASC acetylsulfanilyl chloride; altered state of consciousness; ambulatory surgical center; American Society of Cytology; antibody-secreting cell; antigen-sensitive cell; ascorbate, ascorbic acid; asthma symptom checklist

asc ascending; anterior subcapsular

ASCAD atherosclerotic coronary artery disease

ASCAo ascending aorta

ASCB Asymptomatic Cervical Bruit [study]

ASCH American Society of Clinical Hypnosis

ASCI Accelerated Strategic Computing Initiative; acute spinal cord injury; American Society for Clinical Investigation

ASCII American Standard Code for Information Interchange

ASCLT American Society of Clinical Laboratory Technicians

ASCMS American Society of Contemporary Medicine and Surgery

ASCN American Society for Clinical Nutrition

ASCO American Society of Clinical Oncology; American Society of Contemporary Ophthalmology

ASCOT Anglo-Scandinavian Cardiac Outcomes Trial; a severity characterization of trauma

ASCOTA American Student Committee of the Occupational Therapy Association

ASCP American Society of Clinical Pathologists; American Society of Consulting Pharmacists

ASCR American Society of Chiropodical Roentgenology

ASCS admissions scheduling system

ASCT autologous stem cell transplantation

ASCUS atypia of squamous cells of undetermined significance

ASCVD arteriosclerotic cardiovascular disease; atherosclerotic cardiovascular disease

ASD adaptive seating device; aldosterone secretion defect; Alzheimer senile dementia; antisiphon device; arthritis syphilitica deformans; arthroscopic subacromial decompression; atrial septal defect

A-SDC anomaly-symptomatic deformity complex

ASDC American Society of Dentistry for Children; Association of Sleep Disorders Centers

ASDE Accelerated Strategic Computing Initiative [ASCI] Simulation Development Environment

ASDH acute subdural hemorrhage or hematoma

ASDOS Atrial Septal Defect Occlusion System [study]

ASDP anal sphincter dysplasia

ASDS American Society for Dermatological Surgery

ASE acute stress erosion; American Society of Electrocardiography; application service element; axilla, shoulder, and elbow

ASF African swine fever; aniline-sulfur-formaldehyde [resin]

ASFR age-specific fertility rate

ASG advanced cell group; American Society for Genetics; Army Surgeon General; aspermiogenesis

ASGBI Association of Surgeons of Great Britain and Ireland

ASGE American Society for Gastrointestinal Endoscopy

ASGP asialoglycoprotein

AS/GP antiserum, guinea pig

ASGR asialoglycoprotein receptor

ASH Action on Smoking and Health; aldosterone-stimulating hormone; alkylosing spinal hyperostosis; American Society of Hematology; antistreptococcal hyaluronidase; asymmetric septal hypertrophy

AsH astigmatism, hypermetropic

A&Sh arm and shoulder

ASHA American School Health Association; American Social Health Association; American Speech and Hearing Association

ASHAC acquired immunodeficiency syndrome self-help and care

ASHBEAMS American Society of Hospital-Based Emergency Aeromedical Services

ASHBM Associate Scottish Hospital Bureau of Management

ASHCRM American Society of Health Care Risk Managers

ASHCSP American Society for Hospital Central Service Personnel [of AHA]

ASHCVD atherosclerotic hypertensive cardiovascular disease

ASHD arteriosclerotic heart disease; atrioseptal heart disease

ASHE American Society for Hospital Engineering

ASHET American Society for Health Manpower Education and Training

ASHFSA American Society for Hospital Food Service Administrators

ASHG American Society for Human Genetics

ASHI Association for the Study of Human Infertility

ASHM Australasian Society for Human Immunodeficiency Virus Medicine

ASHN acute sclerosing hyaline necrosis

AS/Ho antiserum, horse

ASHP American Society for Hospital Planning; American Society of Hospital Pharmacists

ASHPA American Society for Hospital Personnel Administration

ASHT American Society of Hand Therapists

ASI addiction severity index; anxiety state inventory; anxiety status inventory; arthroscopic screw installation

ASIA American Spinal Injury Association

ASIC application-specific integrated circuit

ASIF Association for Study of Internal Fixation

ASII American Science Information Institute

ASIM American Society of Internal Medicine

ASIR age-standardized incidence rate

ASIS American Society for Information Science; American Study of Infarct Survival; Angina and Silent Ischemia Study; average severity of index score; anterior superior iliac spine

ASIST Atenolol Silent Ischemia Trial

ASK antistreptokinase; Australian Streptokinase [trial in stroke]

ASL antistreptolysin; argininosuccinate lyase

ASLIB Association of Special Libraries and Information Bureau

ASLM American Society of Law and Medicine

ASLN Alport syndrome-like hereditary nephritis

ASLO antistreptolysin O

ASLT antistreptolysin test

ASM acid sphingomyelinase; age-specific mortality; airway smooth muscle; American Society for Microbiology; angular second moment; anterior scalenus muscle

AsM astigmatism, myopic

asm age-specific mortality

ASMA antismooth muscle antibody

ASMC arterial smooth muscle cell

ASMD anterior segment mesenchymal dysgenesis; atonic sclerotic muscle dystrophy

ASME Association for the Study of Medical Education

ASMI anteroseptal myocardial infarct

As/Mk antiserum, monkey

ASMPA Armed Services Medical Procurement Agency

ASMR age-standardized mortality ratio

ASMT acetylserotonin methyltransferase; American Society for Medical Technology

ASMTY acetylserotonin methyltransferase Y

ASN abstract syntax notation; alkali-soluble nitrogen; American Society of Nephrology; American Society of Neurochemistry; arteriosclerotic nephritis; asparagine; Associate in Nursing

Asn asparagine

ASO administrative services only; AIDS service organization; allele-specific oligonucleoside; antistreptolysin O; arteriosclerosis obliterans

ASOD anterior segmental ocular dysgenesis

ASOS American Society of Oral Surgeons

ASOT antistreptolysin-O test

ASP abnormal spinal posture; active server page; acute symmetric polyarthritis; affected sibling pair; African swine pox; aged substrate plasma; alkali-stable pepsin; American Society of Parasitology; ankylosing spondylitis; anorectal malformation, sacral bony abnormality, presacral mass [association]; antibody-specific prediction; antisocial personality; aortic systolic pressure; area systolic pressure; asparaginase; aspartic acid

Asp aspartic acid; asparaginase

asp aspartate, aspartic acid; aspiration

ASPA American Society of Physician Analysts; American Society of Podiatric Assistants; aspartoacylase

ASPAC Asia-Pacific [regional study]

ASPAT antistreptococcal polysaccharide test

ASPCR, AS-PCR allele-specific polymerase chain reaction

ASPD antisocial personality disorder

ASPDM American Society of Psychosomatic Dentistry and Medicine

ASPECT Anticoagulants in Secondary Prevention of Events in Coronary Thrombosis; approach to systematic planning and evaluation of clinical trials

ASPEN American Society for Parenteral and Enteral Nutrition

ASPG antispleen globulin

ASPIRE action on secondary prevention by intervention to reduce events

ASPM American Society of Paramedics

ASPO American Society for Psychoprophylaxis in Obstetrics

ASPP Association for Sane Psychiatric Practices

ASPREN Australian Sentinel Practice Research Network

ASPRS American Society of Plastic and Reconstructive Surgeons

ASPS advanced sleep phase syndrome; Australian Swedish Pindolol Study

ASPSOM adaptive structure probabilistic self-organizing map

ASPVD atherosclerotic peripheral vascular disease

ASQ Abbreviated Symptom Questionnaire; Anxiety Scale Questionnaire

ASR age-standardized rate; aldosterone secretion rate; antistreptolysin reaction; automated speech recognition

AS/Rab antiserum, rabbit

ASRT American Society of Radiologic Technologists

ASS Aarskog-Scott syndrome; acute serum sickness; acute spinal stenosis; acute stroke study; anterior superior spine; argininosuccinate synthetase; Auckland Stroke Study

ASSA, ASSAS aminopterin-like syndrome sine aminopterin

ASSC acute splenic sequestration crisis

AS-SCORE age, stage of disease, physiological system involved, complications, response to therapy

ASSENT Assessment of the Safety and Efficacy of a New Thrombolytic Agent

ASSERT [improving] Alcohol and Substance Abuse Services and Educating Providers to Refer Patients to Treatment

ASSET Anglo-Scandinavian Study of Early Thrombolysis; Atorvastatin Simvastatin Safety and Efficacy Trial

ASSH American Society for Surgery of the Hand

ASSI Accurate Surgical and Scientific Instruments

assim assiimilate, assimilation

ASSIST American Stop Smoking Intervention Study

ASSO American Society for the Study of Orthodontics

Assoc association, associate

ASSP argininosuccinate synthetase pseudogene

ASSR adult situation stress reaction

ASSURE A Stent vs Stent Ultrasound Remodeling Evaluation

ASSX argininosuccinate synthetase pseudogene

AST allele-specific transcript; allergy serum transfer; angiotensin sensitivity test; anterior spinothalamic tract; antimicrobial susceptibility test; antistreptolysin test; aspartate aminotransferase (SGOT); Association of Surgical Technologists; astigmatism; atrial overdrive stimulation rate; audiometry sweep test; Australian Streptokinase Trial

Ast astigmatism

ASTA anti alpha-staphylolysin

ASTAM American Society for Testing and Materials

ASTECS Antenatal Steroid Therapy in Elective Cesarean Section [study]

ASTH, Asth asthenopia

ASTHO Association of State and Territorial Health Officers

ASTI antispasticity index

ASTM American Society for Testing and Materials; asynchronous transfer protocol

ASTMH American Society of Tropical Medicine and Hygiene

ASTO antistreptolysin O

as tol as tolerated

ASTRO American Society for Therapeutic Radiology and Oncology

ASTZ antistreptozyme

ASUB active substance [UMLS]

ASV anodic stripping voltammetry; antisiphon valve; antisnake venom; autologous saphenous vein; avian sarcoma virus

ASVO American Society of Veterinary Ophthalmology

ASVPP American Society of Veterinary Physiologists and Pharmacologists

ASW artificial sweetener

Asx amino acid that gives aspartic acid after hydrolysis; asymptomatic

asym asymmetry, asymmetric

AT abdominal thrusts; achievement test; Achilles tendon; Achard-Thiers [syndrome]; adaptive thermogenesis; adenine-thymine; adenine-thyronine; adipose tissue; adjunctive therapy; adnexal torsion; air temperature; allergy treatment; aminotransferase; amitriptyline; anaerobic threshold; anaphylotoxin; angiotensin; anterior tibia; antithrombin; antitrypsin; antral transplantation; applanation tonometry; ataxia-telangiectasia; atmosphere; atraumatic; atresia, tricuspid; atrial tachycardia; atropine; attenuate, attenuation; axonal terminal; old tuberculin [Gr. *alt Tuberkulin*]

A-T ataxia telangiectasia

At angiotensin; antithrombin

AT$_1$ angiotensin II type 1

AT$_{10}$ dihydrotachysterol

AT I angiotensin I

AT II angiotensin II

AT III angiotensin III; antithrombin III

At acidity, total; astatine; atrium, atrial

at air tight; atom, atomic

ATA alimentary toxic aleukia; American Telemedicine Association; American Thyroid Association; aminotriazole; antithymic activity; antithyroglobulin antibody; anti-Toxoplasma antibody; atmosphere absolute; aurintricarboxylic acid

ATACS Antithrombotic Therapy in Acute Coronary Syndromes [trial]

ATB at the time of the bomb [A-bomb in Japan]; atrial tachycardia with block

Atb antibiotic

ATBC Alpha-Tocopherol/Beta Carotene [cancer prevention study]

ATC activated thymus cell; anaplastic thyroid carcinoma; anatomical therapeutic chemical; around the clock; certified athletic trainer

ATCase aspartate transcarbomoylase

ATCC American Type Culture Collection

ATCL adult T-cell leukemia or lymphoma

ATCS anterior tibial compartment syndrome

ATD Alzheimer-type dementia; androstatrienedione; anthropomorphic test dummy; antithyroid drug; aqueous tear deficiency; asphyxiating thoracic dystrophy

ATDC Association of Thalidomide Damaged Children

ATDNet Advanced Technology Demonstration Network

ATDP attitude toward disabled persons [scale]

ATE acute toxic encephalopathy; adipose tissue extract; autologous tumor extract

ATEE N-acetyl-1-tyrosyl-ethyl ester

ATEM analytic transmission electron microscopy

Aten atenolol

ATEST Atenolol and Streptokinase Trial

ATF activating transcription factor; anterior talofibular [ligament]; ascites tumor fluid

At fib atrial fibrillation

ATG adenine-thymidine-guanine antihuman thymocyte globulin; antithrombocyte globulin; antithymocyte globulin; antithyroglobulin

ATGAM antithymocyte gamma-globulin

AT/GC adenine-thymine/guanine-cytosine [ratio]

ATH acetyl-tyrosine hydrazide

ATh Associate in Therapy

Athsc atherosclerosis

ATI abdominal trauma index; attitude-treatment interaction

ATIAIS Anturane Transient Ischemic Attack Italian Study

ATIME Accupril Titration Intervention Management Interval Management Evaluation [trial]

ATL Achilles tendon lengthening; acute T-cell leukemia; adult T-cell leukemia; anterior tricuspid leaflet; antitension line; atypical lymphocyte

ATLA adult T-cell leukemia virus-associated antigen; alternatives to laboratory animals

ATLANTIC Angina Treatment, Lasers and Normal Therapy in Comparison [trial]

ATLANTIS Alteplase Thrombolysis for Acute Noninterventional Therapy in Ischemic Stroke

ATLAS Adolescents Training and Learning to Avoid Steroids; Aspirin and Ticlid vs Anticoagulants for Stents [study]; Assessment of Treatment with Lisinopril and Survival [trial]

ATLAST Antiplatelet Therapy vs Lovenox Plus Antiplatelet Therapy for Patients with Increased Risk of Stent Thrombosis; Aspirin/Ticlopidine vs Low-Molecular-Weight Heparin/Aspirin/Ticlopidine Stent Trial

ATLL adult T-cell leukemia/lymphoma

ATLS acute tumor lysis syndrome; advanced trauma life support

ATLV adult T-cell leukemia virus

ATM abnormal tubular myelin; acute transverse myelopathy; adaptive template moderated; Arizona Asynchronous Transfer Mode [network]; asynchronous transfer mode; ataxia-telangiectasia-mutated [protein]; atmosphere; average time of maintenance

atm standard atmosphere

ATMA Amiodarone Trials Meta Analysis; antithyroid plasma membrane antibody

atmos atmospheric

ATN acute tubular necrosis; augmented transition network

ATNC atraumatic normocephalic

at no atomic number

ATNR asymmetric tonic neck reflex

A-to-D analog-to-digital

ATP adenosine triphosphate; ambient temperature and pressure; Arizona Telemedicine Program; autoimmune thrombocytopenic purpura

A-TP adsorbed test plasma

AT-P antitrypsin-Pittsburgh

AtP attending physician

ATPA 2-amino-3-(hydroxy-5-*tert*-butyl-isoxazol-4-yl) propanoic acid

AT-PAS aldehyde-thionine-periodic acid Schiff [test]

ATPase adenosine triphosphatase

ATPD dried at ambient temperature and pressure

ATP-2Na adenosine triphosphate disodium

ATPS ambient temperature and pressure, saturated

ATR Achilles tendon reflex; alpha-thalassemia-mental retardation [syndrome]; ataxia-telangiectasia and rad-related [protein]; attenuated total reflectance; axial trunk rotation

atr atrophy

ATR1 alpha-thalassemia mental retardation [syndrome] type 1

ATR2 alpha-thalassemia mental retardation [syndrome] type 2

ATRA all-*trans*retinoic acid

ATRAMI Autonomic Tone and Reflexes After Myocardial Infarction [trial]

ATRAS Adrenal Test Retrieval and Analysis System

Atr fib atrial fibrillation

ATRX, ATR-X X-linked alpha-thalassemia mental retardation [syndrome]

ATS Achard-Thiers syndrome; acid test solution; alpha-D-tocopherol acid succinate; American Thoracic Society; American Trudeau Society; American Trauma Society; antirat thymocyte serum; antitetanus serum; antithymocyte serum; anxiety tension state; arteriosclerosis; autologous transfusion system

ATSDR Agency for Toxic Substances and Disease Registry

ATT arginine tolerance test; aspirin tolerance time

att attending

ATTMH Australian Therapeutic Trial of Mild Hypertension

ATV Abelson virus transformed; avian tumor virus

at vol atomic volume

at wt atomic weight

ATx adult thymectomy

atyp atypical

ATZ acetazolamide; atypical transformation zone

AU allergenic unit; Ångström unit; antitoxin unit; arbitrary unit; Australia antigen; azauridine

Au Australia [antigen]; authorization

AUA American Urological Association; asymptomatic urinary abnormalities

Au Ag Australia antigen

AUB abnormal uterine bleeding

AUC area under the curve

AUD arthritis of unknown diagnosis

aud auditory

AUDEX automated urologic diagnostic expert [ultrasonographic imaging]

AUDIT alcohol use disorders identification test

AUDIT-C alcohol use disorders identification test–alcohol consumption questions

aud-vis audiovisual

AUG acute ulcerative gingivitis; adenosine-uracil-guanine

AUGH acute upper gastrointestinal hemorrhage

AuHAA Australia hepatitis-associated antigen

AUI Alcohol Use Inventory

AUL acute undifferentiated leukemia

AUO amyloid of unknown origin

AuP Australian antigen protein

AUPHA Association of University Programs in Health Administration

aur, auric auricle, auricular

AUS acute urethral syndrome

AuS Australia serum hepatitis

aus, ausc auscultation

AuSH Australia serum hepatitis

AUST Australian Urokinase Stroke Trial

Auto-PEEP self-controlled positive end-expiratory pressure

AUV anterior urethral valve

aux auxiliary

AV adenovirus; Adriamycin and vincristine; air velocity; allergic vasculitis; anteroventral; anteversion; anticipatory vomiting; antivirin; aortic valve; arteriovenous; artificial ventilation; assisted ventilation; atrioventricular; audiovisual; augmented vector; average; aviation medicine; avoirdupois

A-V arteriovenous; atrioventricular

A/V ampere/volt; arteriovenous

Av average; avoirdupois

aV abvolt

av air velocity; average; avulsion

AVA activity vector analysis; antiviral antibody; aortic valve annulus; aortic valve area; aortic valve atresia; arteriovenous anastomosis

AV/AF anteverted, anteflexed

AVB atrioventricular block

AVC aberrant ventricular conduction; Academy of Veterinary Cardiology; aortic valve closure; arteriovenous communication; associative visual cortex; Association of Vitamin Chemists; associative visual cortex; atrioventricular canal; automatic volume control

AVCN anteroventral cochlear nucleus

AVCO₂R arteriovenous carbon dioxide removal

AVCS atrioventricular conduction system

AVCx atrioventricular circumflex branch

AVD aortic valvular disease; apparent volume of distribution; Army Veterinary Department; atrioventricular dissociation

AVDO₂ arteriovenous oxygen saturation difference

AVDO₂B arteriovenous oxygen saturation difference, basal

AVDP average diastolic pressure

avdp avoirdupois

AVE aortic valve echocardiogram

ave, aver average

AVED ataxia with vitamin E deficiency

AVERT Atorvastatin vs Revascularization Treatment [trial]

AVEU AIDS Vaccine Evaluation [group]

AVF antiviral factor; arteriovenous fistula

aVF automated volt foot

aV$_F$ unipolar limb lead on the left leg in electrocardiography

AVG ambulatory visit group

avg average

AVH acute viral hepatitis

AVHD acquired valvular heart disease

AVHS acquired valvular heart syndrome

AVI air velocity index; Association of Veterinary Inspectors

AVID Amiodarone vs Implantable Defibrillators [trial]; Angiography vs Intravascular Ultrasound Directed Coronary Stent Placement [trial]; Antiarrhythmics vs Implantable Defibrillators [study]

AVIR aortic valve replacement

AVJ atrioventricular junction

AVJR atrioventricular junction rhythm

AVJRe atrioventricular junctional reentrant

AVL automatic vehicle locator

aVL automated volt left

aV$_L$ unipolar limb lead on the left arm in electrocardiography

AVLINE Audiovisuals Online [NLM database]

AVM arteriovenous malformation; atrioventricular malformation; aviation medicine

AVMA American Veterinary Medical Association

AVN acute vasomotor nephropathy; atrioventricular nodal [conduction]; atrioventricular node; avascular necrosis

AVND atrioventricular node dysfunction

AVNFH avascular necrosis of the femoral head

AVNFRP atrioventricular node functional refractory period

AVNR atrioventricular nodal reentry

AVNRT atrioventricular node reentry tachycardia

AVO aortic valve opening; aortic valve orifice; atrioventricular opening

AVO$_2$ arteriovenous oxygen ratio

AVP abnormal vasopressin; actinomycin-vincristine-Platinol; ambulatory venous pressure; antiviral protein; aqueous vasopressin; arginine–vasopressin; arteriovenous passage time

AVPU alert, verbal, painful, unresponsive [neurologic test]

AVR accelerated ventricular rhythm; antiviral regulator; aortic valve replacement

aVR automated volt right

aV$_R$ unipolar limb lead on the right arm in electrocardiography

AVRI acute viral respiratory infection

AVRP atrioventricular refractory period

AVRR antiviral repressor regulator

AVRT atrioventricular reentrant tachycardia; atrioventricular reciprocating tachycardia

AVS aortic valve stenosis; arteriovenous shunt; auditory vocal sequencing

AVSD atrioventricular septal defect

AVSV aortic valve stroke volume

AVT Allen vision test; arginine vasotocin; Aviation Medicine Technician

AVV atrioventricular valve

Av3V anteroventral third ventricle

AVZ avascular zone

AW able to work; above waist; abrupt withdrawal; alcohol withdrawal; alveolar wall; anterior wall; atomic warfare; atomic weight

A&W alive and well

aw airway; water activity

AWAR anterior wall of aortic root

AWBM alveolar wall basement membrane

AWESOME Angina with Extremely Serious Operative Mortality Evaluation

AWFM adaptive Walsh function modeling

AWG American Wire Gauge

AWI anterior wall infarction

AWL active waiting list

AWM abnormal wall motion

AWMI anterior wall myocardial infarction

AWMV amplitude-weighted mean velocity

AWO airway obstruction

AWOL absent without official leave

AWP airway pressure; any willing provider; average of the wholesale prices; average wholesale price

AWR absolute weighted residual; airway restriction

AWRS anti-whole rabbit serum

AWRU active wrist rotation unit
AWS Alagille-Watson syndrome; alcohol withdrawal syndrome
AWTA aniridia-Wilms tumor association
awu atomic weight unit
ax axillary; axis, axial
AXD axillary dissection
AXF advanced x-ray facility
AXG adult xanthogranuloma
AXL anexelekto [oncogene]; axillary lymphoscintigraphy
AXR abdominal x-ray [examination]
AXT alternating exotropia
AYA acute yellow atrophy
AYF antiyeast factor
AYP autolyzed yeast protein
AYV aster yellow virus
AZ Aschheim-Zondek [test]; 5-azacytidine; azathioprine
Az nitrogen [Fr. *azote*]
AZA azathioprine
AzC azacytosine

AZF azospermia factor
AzG; azg azaguanine
AZGP zinc-alpha-2-glycoprotein
AZO [indicates presence of the group –N:N–]
AZOA azaorotic acid
AZQ diaziquone
AZR alizarin
AZT Aschheim-Zondek test; azidothymidine; 3'-azido-3'-deoxythymidine; zidovudine (azidothymidine)
AZTEC amplitude zone time epoch coding [in ECG]
AZTMP azidothymidine monophosphate
AZT-R azidothymidine-resistant
AZT-S azidothymidine-susceptible or sensitive
AZTTP azidothymidine trithiophosphate
AZT-TP 3'azido-3'-dexythymidine triphosphate
AZU azauracil; azurodicin
AzUr 6-azauridine

B bacillus; bands; barometric; base; basophil, basophilic; bath [Lat. *balneum*]; Baumé scale; behavior; bel; Benoist scale; benzoate; beta; biscuspid; black; blood, bloody; blue; body; boils at; Bolton point; bone marrow-derived [cell or lymphocyte]; born; boron; bound; bovine; break; bregma; bronchial, bronchus; brother; *Brucella*; bruit; buccal; Bucky [film in cassette in Potter-Bucky diaphragm]; Bucky factor; bursa cells; bypass; byte; magnetic induction; minimal detectable blurring; supramentale [point]

b barn; base; boils at; born; brain; branched; [chromosome] break; supramentale [point]; twice [Lat. *bis*]

b⁺ positron emission

b⁻ beta emission

B₀ constant magnetic field in nuclear magnetic resonance

B₁ induced field in magnetic resonance imaging; radiofrequency magnetic field in nuclear magnetic resonance; thiamine

B₂ riboflavin

B₆ pyridoxine

B₇ biotin

B₈ adenosine phosphate

B₁₂ cyanocobalamin

β see beta

BA Bachelor of Arts; backache; bacterial agglutination; barbituric acid; basion; benzyladenine; best amplitude; beta adrenergic; betamethasone acetate; bilateral asymmetrical; bile acid; biliary atresia; biological activity; blocking antibody; blood agar; blood alcohol; bone age; boric acid; bovine albumin; brachial artery; breathing apparatus; bronchial asthma; buccoaxial; buffered acetone

Ba barium; barium enema; basion

ba basion

BAA benzoylarginine amide; branched amino acid

BAATAF Boston Area Anticoagulation Trial for Atrial Fibrillation

BAB blood agar base

Bab Babinski's reflex; baboon

BabK baboon kidney

BAC baclofen; bacterial adherent colony; bacterial antigen complex; bacterial artificial chromosome; blood alcohol concentration; British Association of Chemists; bronchoalveolar carcinoma; bronchoalveolar cells; buccoaxiocervical

Bac, bac *Bacillus*, bacillary

BACT bacterium [UMLS]

Bact, bact *Bacterium*; bacterium, bacteria

BACUS Balloon Angioplasty Compliance Ultrasound Study

BAD biological aerosol detection; British Association of Dermatologists

BADE [Thoracic] Bioimpedance as an Adjunct to Dobutamine Echocardiography [study]

BADS black locks-albinism-deafness syndrome

BAE bovine aortic endothelium; bronchial artery embolization

BaE barium enema

BAEC bovine aortic endothelial cell

BAEDP balloon aortic end-diastolic pressure

BAEE benzoylarginine ethyl ester

BaEn barium enema

BAEP brainstem auditory evoked potential

BAER brainstem auditory evoked response

BaEV baboon endogenous virus

BaFBr:Eu europium-activated barium fluorohalide

BAG buccoaxiogingival

BAGG buffered azide glucose glycerol

BAHAMA Baragwanath Hypertension Ambulatory Blood Pressure Monitoring Multiarm

BA/HPCC biomedical application of high performance computing and communication

BAHS Boston Area Health Study; butoctamide hydrogen succinate

BAI beta-aminoisobutyrate

BAIB beta-aminoisobutyric [acid]

BAIF bile acid independent flow

BAIT bacterial automated identification technique

BAL blood alcohol level; British anti-lewisite; bronchoalveolar lavage

bal balance; balsam

BALB binaural alternate loudness balance

BALF broncho-alveolar lavage fluid

bals balsam

BALT broncho-alveolar lavage fluid; bronchus-associated lymphoid tissue

BAM basilar artery migraine; bilateral augmentation mammoplasty; brachial artery mean [pressure]

BaM barium meal

Bam benzamide

BAME benzoylarginine methyl ester

BAN British Approved Name; British Association of Neurologists

BANS back, arms, neck, and scalp

BANTER Bayesian Network Tutoring and Explanation

BAO basal acid output; brachial artery output

BAO-MAO basal acid output to maximal acid output [ratio]

BAP bacterial alkaline phosphatase; Behavior Activity Profile; beta-amyloid peptide; blood-agar plate; bovine albumin in phosphate buffer; brachial artery pressure

BAPhysMed British Association of Physical Medicine

BAPI barley alkaline protease inhibitor

BAPN beta-aminoproprionitrile fumarate

BAPP beta amyloid precursor protein

BAPS biomechanical ankle platform system; bovine albumin phosphate saline; British Association of Paediatric Surgeons; British Association of Plastic Surgeons

BAPT British Association of Physical Training

BAPTA 1,2-bis (aminophenoxy) ethane-N,N,N',N'-tetraacetic acid

BAPV bovine alimentary papilloma virus

BAQ brain-age quotient

BAR bariatrics; barometer, barometric; beta-adrenergic receptor

bar barometric

BARASTER Balloon Angioplasty vs Rotational Atherectomy for Stent Restenosis

Barb, barb barbiturate, barbituric

BARI Bypass Angioplasty Revascularization Investigation [trial]

BARK beta-adrenergic receptor kinase

BARN bilateral acute retinal necrosis; Body Awareness Resource Network

BAROCCO Balloon Angioplasty vs Rotacs for Total Chronic Coronary Occlusion [trial]

BARS behaviorally anchored rating scale

BART blood-activated recalcification time

BAS balloon atrial septostomy; benzyl anti-serotinin; beta-adrenergic stimulation; boric acid solution; Bronx Longitudinal Aging Study

BaS barium swallow

bas basilar; basophil, basophilic

BASA Boston Assessment of Severe Aphasia

BASC Blood Pressure in Acute Stroke Collaboration

BASE B27-arthritis-sacroiliitis-extra-articular features [syndrome]

BASH body acceleration synchronous with heart rate

BASIC Beginner's All-Purpose Symbolic Introduction Code

BASIS Basel Antiarrhythmic Study of Infarct Survival

baso basophil

BAT basic aid training; best available technology; blunt abdominal trauma; bright acuity test; brown adipose tissue

BAUP Bovie-assisted uvulopalatoplasty

BAUS British Association of Urological Surgeons

BAV bicuspid aortic valve

BAVCP bilateral abductor vocal cord paralysis

BAVFO bradycardia after arteriovenous fistula occlusion

BAW bronchoalveolar washing

BB bad breath; bed bath; beta blockade, beta blocker; BioBreeding [rat]; blanket bath; blood bank; blood buffer; blow bottle; blue bloaters [emphysema]; bombesin; borderline; both bones; breakthrough bleeding; breast biopsy; brush border; buffer base; bundle branch; isoenzyme of creatine kinase containing two B subunits

bb Bolton point; both bones

BBA born before arrival

BBB blood-brain barrier; blood buffer base; bundle-branch block

BBBB bilateral bundle-branch block

BBBD blood brain barrier disruption

BBC bromobenzycyanide; buccal bifurcation cyst

BBD benign breast disease

BBE *Bacteroides* bile esculin [agar]

BBEP brush border endopeptidase

BBF bronchial blood flow

BBI Biomedical Business International; Bowman-Birk soybean inhibitor

BBM brush border membrane

BBMV brush border membrane vesicle

BBN broad band noise

BBPP Beta-Blocker Pooling Project

BBRS Burks' Behavior Rating Scale

BBS Barolet-Biedl syndrome; bashful bladder syndrome; benign breast syndrome; bilateral breath sounds; bombesin; borate-buffered saline; brown bowel syndrome; bulletin board system

BBT basal body temperature

BBTD baby bottle tooth decay

BB/W BioBreeding/Worcester [rat]

BC Bachelor of Surgery [Lat. *Baccalaureus Chirurgiae*]; back care; bactericidal concentration; basal cell; basket cell; battle casualty; bicarbonate; biliary colic; bipolar cell; birth control; blastic crisis; blood count; blood culture; Blue Cross [plan]; board certified; bone conduction; brachiocephalic; brain contour; breast cancer; bronchial carcinoma; buccal cartilage; buccocervical; buffy coat

B&C biopsy and curettage

b/c benefit/cost [ratio]

BCA balloon catheter angioplasty; bicinchoninic acid; blood color analyzer; Blue Cross Association; branchial cleft anomaly; Breast Cancer Action; breast cancer antigen

BCAA branched chain amino acid

BCAPS Beta-Blocker Cholesterol-Lowering Asymptomatic Plaque Study

BCAT brachiocephalic arterial trunk

BCB blood-cerebrospinal fluid barrier; brilliant cresyl blue

BCBR bilateral carotid body resection

BC/BS Blue Cross/Blue Shield [plan]

BCBSA Blue Cross and Blue Shield Association

BCC basal-cell carcinoma; bedside communication controller; biliary cholesterol concentration; birth control clinic; business card computer

bcc body-centered-cubic

BC-CFC blast cell colony-forming cell

BCCG British Cooperative Clinical Group

BCCP biotin carboxyl carrier protein

BCD binary-coded decimal; bleomycin, cyclophosphamide, dactinomycin

BCDDP Breast Cancer Detection Demonstration Project

BCDF B-cell differentiation factor

BCDL Brachmann-Cornelia de Lange [syndrome]

BCDRS brief Carroll depression rating scale

BCDS bulimia cognitive distortions scale

BCDSP Boston Collaborative Drug Surveillance Program

BCE basal cell epithelioma; benign childhood epilepsy; bubble chamber equipment

BCEI breast cancer estrogen-inducible

BCF basic conditioning factor; basophil chemotactic factor; bioconcentration factor; breast cyst fluid

BCFP breast cyst fluid protein

BCG bacille Calmette-Guérin [vaccine]; ballistocardiography, ballistocardiogram; bicolor guaiac test; bromcresol green

BCGF B-cell growth factor

BCGM bi-conjugate gradient method

BCH basal cell hyperplasia

BCh Bachelor of Surgery [Lat. *Baccalaureus Chirurgiae*]

BChD Bachelor of Dental Surgery

BCHE butyrylcholinesterase

BChir Bachelor of Surgery [Lat. *Baccalaureus Chirurgiae*]

Bchl, bChl bacterial chlorophyll

BCHS Bureau of Community Health Services

BCI behavioral cues index; brain-computer interface

BCIA Biomedical Clinical Instrumentation Association

BCIP 5-bromo-4-chloro-3-inodolyl phosphate

BCIS British Cardiovascular Intervention Society

BCKA branched-chain keto acid

BCKD branched-chain alpha-keto acid dehydrogenase

BCL basic cycle length; B-cell leukemia/lymphoma

BCLL B-cell chronic lymphocytic leukemia

BCLM below critical length material

BCLP bilateral cleft of lip and palate

BCLS basic cardiac life support

BCM B-cell maturation; birth control medication; blood-clotting mechanism; body cell mass; body control and movement
BCME bis-chloromethyl ether
BCMF B-cell maturation factor
BCMS Bioethic Citation Maintenance System
BCN basal cell nevus; bilateral cortical necrosis
BCNS basal cell nevus syndrome
BCNU 1,3-bis-(2-chloroethyl)-1-nitrosourea; bleomycin and camustine
BCO biliary cholesterol output
BCOC bowel care of choice
BCP basic calcium phosphate; birth control pill; blue cone pigment; Blue Cross Plan; bromcresol purple
BCPD bromcresol purple deoxylate
BCPR bystander cardiopulmonary resuscitation
BCPT breast cancer prevention trial
BCPV bovine cutaneous papilloma virus
BCQ breast cancer questionnaire
BCR B-cell reactivity; birth control regimen; breakpoint cluster region; bromocriptine; bulbocavernous reflex
bcr break point cluster region
BCRS brief cognitive rating scale
BCRx birth control drug
BCS battered child syndrome; blood cell separator; breast cancer screening; British Cardiac Society; Budd-Chiari syndrome
BCSI breast cancer screening indicator
BCSP Bavarian Cholesterol Screening Project
BCT brachiocephalic trunk; branched-chain amino acid transferase; breast conservation therapy
BCTF Breast Cancer Task Force
BCtg bovine chymotrypsinogen
BCtr bovine chymotrypsin
BCV between class variance
BCVA best corrected visual acuity
BCW biological and chemical warfare
BCYE buffered charcoal-yeast extract [agar]
BD barbital-dependent; barbiturate dependence; base deficit; base of prism down; basophilic degeneration; Batten disease; behavioral disorder; Behçet disease; belladonna; Bessel distribution; bicarbonate dialysis; bile duct; binocular deprivation; birth date; black death; bladder drainage; block design [test]; blood donor; blue diaper [syndrome]; borderline dull; bound; brain damage; brain dead, brain death; Briquet disorder; bronchodilation, bronchodilator; buccodistal; Byler disease
B-D Becton-Dickinson
Bd board; buoyant density
bd band; bundle
BDA balloon dilation angioplasty; British Dental Association
BDAC Bureau of Drug Abuse Control
BDAE Boston Diagnostic Aphasia Examination
BDC Bazex-Dupré-Christol [syndrome]; burn-dressing change
BDE bile duct examination
BDentSci Bachelor of Dental Science
BDG buccal developmental groove; buffered desoxycholate glucose
BDHI Buss Durkee hostility inventory
BDI Beck depression inventory
BDIP biomedical digital image processing
BDIS Becton-Dickinson immunocytometry system; Birth Defects Information Service
BDL behaviors of daily living; below detectable limits; bile duct ligation
BDLS Brachmann-de Lange syndrome
BDM Becker's muscular dystrophy
BDMS Bureau of Data Management Strategy [Health Care Financing Administration (HCFA)]
bDNA branched deoxyribonucleic acid [DNA]
BDNF brain-derived neurotrophic factor
BDP beclomethasone dipropionate; benzodiazepine; bilateral diaphragmatic paralysis; bronchopulmonary dysplasia
BDR background diabetic retinopathy
BDRS Blessed Dementia Rating Scale
BDS Bachelor of Dental Surgery; biological detection system; Blessed Dementia Scale
BDSc Bachelor of Dental Science
BDUR bromodeoxyuridine
BDW biphasic defibrillation waveform; buffered distilled water
BE bacillary emulsion; bacterial endocarditis; barium enema; Barrett's esophagus; base excess; below-elbow; bile-esculin [test]; bovine enteritis; brain edema; bread equivalent; breast examination; bronchoesophagology

B/E below-elbow

B&E brisk and equal

Be beryllium

Bé Baumé scale

BEA below-elbow amputation; bioelectrical activity; bromoethylamine

BEAM brain electrical activity monitoring

BEAP bronchiectasis, eosinophilia, asthma, pneumonia

BEAR biological effects of atomic radiation

BEB Biomedical Engineering Branch [of US Army]

BEC bacterial endocarditis; behavioral emergency committee; blood ethyl alcohol; bromo-ergocryptine

BECAIT Bezafibrate Coronary Atherosclerosis Intervention Trial

BECF blood extracellular fluid

BED binge eating disorder

BEE basal energy expenditure

beg begin, beginning

BEH benign exertional headache

beh behavior, behavioral

BEHA behavior [UMLS]

BEI back-scattered electron imaging; biological exposure indexes; butanol-extractable iodine

BEIR biological effects of ionizing radiation

BEK bovine embryonic kidney [cells]

BEL blood ethanol level; bovine embryonic lung

BELIR beta-endorphin-like immunoreactivity

BEM boundary element method

BEMS Bioelectromagnetics Society

BENAR blood eosinophilic non-allergic rhinitis

BENEDICT Bergamo Nephrologic Diabetes Complications Trial

BENESTENT Belgian-Netherlands Stent [study]

Benz, benz benzene; benzidine; benzoate

BEP brain evoked potential; basic element of performance

B-EP β-endorphin

BEPS Belgian Eminase Prehospital Study

BER base encoding rule; base excision repair; basic electrical rhythm

BERA brainstem evoked response audiometry

BERNWARD building essential concept representations in well-arranged restricted domains

BERT Beneficiary Enrollment Retrieval System [Medicare]; Beta Energy Restenosis Trial

BES balanced electrolyte solution; Baltimore Eye Study

BESM bovine embryonic skeletal muscle

BESMART Bestent in Small Arteries Study

BESP bovine embryonic spleen [cells]

BESS Berlin Pacemaker Study on Syncope; Part B Extract and Summary System [Medicare]

BESSAMI Berlin Stent Study in Acute Myocardial Infarction

BEST Beta-blocker Evaluation of Survival Trial; Beta-blocker Stroke Trial; Beta-Cath System Trial; Bolus Dose Escalation Study of Tissue-Type Plasminogen Activator; Bucindolol Evaluation of Survival Trial; Medtronic Bestent Coronary Stent vs Palmz-Schatz Coronary Stent

BET benign epithelial tumor; bleeding esophageal varix; Brunauer-Emmet-Teller [method]

BETA Biomedical Electronics Technicians Association

β [Greek letter beta] an anomer of a carbohydrate; buffer capacity; carbon separated from a carboxyl by one other carbon in aliphatic compounds; a constituent of a plasma protein fraction; probability of Type II error; a substituent group of a steroid that projects above the plane of the ring

1–β power of statistical test

β₂m beta$_2$-microglobulin

BEV baboon endogenous virus; beam's eye view; bovine enterovirus

BeV, Bev billion electron volts

bev beverage

BF Barmah Forest [virus]; bentonite flocculation; bile flow; black female; blastogenic factor; blister fluid; blood flow; body fat; bouillon filtrate [tuberculin] [Fr. *bouillon filtré*]; brain factor; breakfast fed; breast feeding; buffered; burning feet [syndrome]; butter fat

bf black female; bouillon filtrate [tuberculin]

B3F band 3 cytoplasmic fragment

B/F black female; bound/free [antigen ratio]

BFB biological feedback; bronchial foreign body

BFDI bronchodilation following deep inspiration

BFEC benign focal epilepsy of childhood

BFC benign febrile convulsion

BFE blood flow energy

bFGF basic fibroblast growth factor

BFH benign familial hematuria

BFHD Beukes familial hip dysplasia

BFHR basal fetal heart rate

BFL bird fancier's lung; Börjeson-Forssman-Lehman [syndrome]

BFLS Börjeson-Forssman-Lehmann syndrome

BFM benign familial megalocephaly or macrocephaly

BFO balanced forearm orthosis; ball-bearing forearm orthosis; blood-forming organ

BFOD binary frames of discernment

BFP biologic false-positive

BFPR biologic false-positive reaction

BFPSTS biologic false-positive serological test for syphilis

BFR biologic false reaction; blood flow rate; bone formation rate; buffered Ringer [solution]

BFS blood fasting sugar

BFT bentonite flocculation test; biofeedback training

BFU burst-forming unit

BFU-E burst-forming unit, erythrocytes

BFU-ME burst-forming unit, myeloid/erythroid

BFU-Meg burst-forming unit-megakaryocyte

BFV bovine feces virus

BG basal ganglion; basic gastrin; Bender Gestalt [test]; beta-galactosidase; beta-glucuronidase; bicolor guaiac [test]; Birbeck granule; blood glucose; bone graft; brilliant green; buccogingival

B-G Bordet-Gengou [agar, bacillus, phenomenon]

BGA blue-green algae

BGAg blood group antigen

BGAV blue-green algae virus

BGC basal ganglion calcification; blood group class

BGCA bronchogenic carcinoma

BGD blood group degradation

BGE butyl glycidyl ether

BGG bovine gamma-globulin

bGH bovine growth hormone

Bg^J beige [mouse]

BGLB brilliant green lactose broth

BGlu blood glucose

BGM bedside glucose monitoring

BGMR basal ganglion disorder-mental retardation [syndrome]

BGMV bean golden mosaic virus

BGO bismuth germanium oxide

BGP beta-glycerophosphatase

BGPS Belgian General Practitioners' Study

BGS balance, gait, and station; Baller-Gerold syndrome; blood group substance; British Geriatrics Society

BGSA blood granulocyte-specific activity

BGTT borderline glucose tolerance test

BH base hospital; benzalkonium and heparin; bill of health; birth history; Bishop-Harman [instruments]; boarding home; board of health; Bolton-Hunter [reagent]; borderline hypertensive; both hands; brain hormone; Braxton-Hicks contractions; breathholding; bronchial hyperreactivity; Bryan high titer; bundle of His

BH$_4$ tetrahydrobiopterin

BHA bound hepatitis antibody; butylated hydroxyanisole

BHAT Beta Blocker Heart Attack Trial

BHB beta-hydroxybutyrate

bHb bovine hemoglobin

BHBA beta-hydroxybutyric acid

BHC benzene hexachloride

BHCDA Bureau of Health Care Delivery and Assistance

β-hCG beta human chorionic gonadotropin

BHF Bolivian hemorrhagic fever; British Heart Foundation

BHFS Benzapril Heart Failure Study

BHI biosynthetic human insulin; brain-heart infusion [broth]; British Humanities Index; Bureau of Health Insurance

BHIA brain-heart infusion agar

BHIBA brain-heart infusion blood agar

BHIRS brain-heart infusion and rabbit serum

BHIS beef heart infusion supplemented [broth]

BHK baby hamster kidney [cells]; type-B Hong Kong [influenza virus]

BHL bilateral hilar lymphadenopathy; biological half-life

bHLH basic helix-loop-helix

bHLH-ZIP basic helix-loop-helix-leucine zipper

BHM Bureau of Health Manpower

BHN bephenium hydroxynaphthoate; Brinell hardness number

BHP basic health profile

BHPr Bureau of Health Professions

BHR basal heart rate; benign hypertrophic prostatitis; borderline hypertensive rat; bronchial hyperreactivity

BHS Bachelor of Health Science; Beck Hopelessness Scale; beta-hemolytic streptococcus; Bogalusa Heart Study; breath-holding spell; Brisighella Heart Study

BHT beta-hydroxytheophylline; breath hydrogen test; bronchial hygiene therapy; butylated hydroxytoluene

BHTE bioheat transfer equation

BHU basic health unit

BHV bovine herpes virus

BH/VH body hematocrit-venous hematocrit [ratio]

BHyg Bachelor of Hygiene

BI background interval; bacterial or bactericidal index; base-in [prism]; basilar impression; Billroth I [operation]; biological indicator; biotehnology infomatics; bodily injury; bone injury; bowel impaction; brain injury; burn index

Bi bismuth

BIA biolectric impedance analysis; bioimmunoassay; biomechanical impedance analyses

BIAC Bioinstrumentation Advisory Council

BIAD blind insertion airway device

BIB bibliography; biliointestinal bypass; brought in by

bib, biblio bibliography

BIBRA British Industrial Biological Research Association

BIBRA British Industrial Biological Research Association

B-IBS B-immunoblastic sarcoma

BIC Bayes information criterion; bicoherence; blood isotope clearance; brain imaging center

Bic biceps

BICAO bilateral internal carotid artery occlusion

bicarb bicarbonate

BiCAT bilateral carotid artery traction

BICC Biomedical Information Communications Center

Bicnu 1,3-bis-(2-chloroethyl)-1-nitrosourea

BICS Brigham Integrated Computing System

BICST biceps skin tone

BID bibliographic information and documentation; brought in dead

BIDLB block in posteroinferior division of left branch

BIDS brittle hair, intellectual impairment, decreased fertility, and short stature [syndrome]

BIE Bayes inference engine; bullous ichthyosiform erythroderma

BIG bone injection gun

BIG 6 analysis of 6 serum components

BIGGY bismuth glycine glucose yeast

BIGMAC Beaumont Interventional Group-Mevacor, ACE Inhibitor, Colchicine Restenosis [trial]; Bidirectional Gantry Multiarray Coil [study]

BIGPRO Biguanides and the Prevention of the Risk of Obesity [study]

BIH benign intracranial hypertension; Beth Israel Hospital

BII beat inclusion index; Billroth II [operation]; butanol-insoluble iodine

BIL basal insulin level; bilirubin

Bil bilirubin

bil bilateral

BILAG British Isles Lupus Assessment Group [Index]

BIL/ALB bilirubin/albumin [rate]

bilat bilateral

bili bilirubin

bili-c conjugated bilirubin

bilirub bilirubin

bili T&D bilirubin total and direct

BIMA bilateral internal mammary artery

BIN butylisonitrile

biochem biochemistry, biochemical

BIOD bony intraorbital distance

bioeng bioengineering

BIOETHICSLINE Bioethical Information Online

BIOF biologic function [UMLS]

biol biology, biological

bioLH bioassay of luteinizing hormone

biophys biophysics, biophysical

BIOSIS BioScience Information Service

biotyping biochemical typing

BIP bacterial intravenous protein; Bezafibrate Infarction Prevention [study]; biparietal; bismuth iodoform paraffin; Blue Cross interim payment; brief infertility period

Bip binding protein

BIPAP biphasic positive airway pressure

BIPLED bilateral, independent, periodic, lateralized epileptiform discharge

BIPM International Bureau of Weights and Measures [Fr. *Bureau International des Poids et Mesures*]

BIPP bismuth iodoform paraffin paste

BIR basic incidence rate; British Institute of Radiology

BIRADS Breast Imaging Reporting and Data System

BIRD Bolus vs Infusion Rescupase Development

BIRLS Beneficiary Identification and Record Locator Subsystem [Veterans Benefit Administration]

BIRNH Belgian Interuniversity Research on Nutrition and Health [study]

BIS bioimpedance spectroscopy; bispectral index; bone cement implantation syndrome; Brain Information Service; British Infection Society; building illness syndrome

B-ISDN broadband-integrated services digital network

BiSP between ischial spines

hisp hispinous [diameter]

BIT binary digit; bitrochanteric

bit binary digit

BITE Bulimic Investigatory Test

BITNET Because It's Time Network [mail-only electronic network]

BIU barrier isolation unit

BIVAS body image visual analogue scale

BJ Bence Jones [protein, proteinuria]; biceps jerk; Bielschowsky-Jansky [syndrome]; bones and joints

B&J bones and joints

BJE bones, joints, and examination

BJM bones, joints, and muscles

BJP Bence Jones protein or proteinuria

BK below the knee; bovine kidney [cells]; bradykinin

B-K initials of two patients after whom a multiple cutaneous nevus [mole] was named

B/K below knee [amputation]

Bk berkelium

bk back

BKA below-knee amputation

BK-A basophil kallikrein of anaphylaxis

BK amp below-knee amputation

BKAT Basic Knowledge Assessment Tool for Critical Care

bkf breakfast

Bkg background

BKS beekeeper serum

BKTT below knee to toe

BKWP below knee walking plaster

BL Barré-Lieou [syndrome]; basal lamina; baseline; Bessey-Lowry [unit]; black light; bladder; bleeding; blind loop; blood loss; bone marrow lymphocyte; borderline lepromatous; bronchial lavage; buccolingual; buffered lidocaine; Burkitt lymphoma

Bl black

B-l bursa-equivalent lymphocyte

bl black; blood, bleeding; blue

BLA Biologics License Application

BLAD borderline left axis deviation

blad bladder

BLAS Bronx Longitudinal Aging Study

BLASP Barbados Low-Dose Aspirin Study in Pregnancy

BLAT Blind Learning Aptitute Test

BLB Baker-Lima-Baker [mask]; Bessey-Lowry-Brock [method or unit]; black light bulb; Boothby-Lovelace-Bulbulian [oxygen mask]; bulb [syringe]

BL=BS bilateral equal breath sounds

BlC blood culture

BLCL Burkitt lymphoma cell line

B-LCL B-lymphocyte cell line

bl cult blood culture

BLD basal liquefactive degeneration; benign lymphoepithelial disease

bld blood

Bld Bnk blood bank

BLE both lower extremities; buffered lidocaine with epinephrine

BLEL benign lympho-epithelial lesion

BLEO bleomycin

bleph blepharitis

BLFD buccolinguofacial dyskinesia

BLG beta-lactoglobulin

blH biologically active luteinizing hormone

BLI bombesin-like immunoreactivity

blk black

BLL below lower limit

BLLD British Library Lending Division

BLM basolateral membrane; bilayer lipid membrane; bimolecular liquid membrane; bleomycin; Bloom syndrome; buccolinguomasticatory

BLN bronchial lymph node

BLOB binary large object

BLOBS bladder obstruction

BLOC body location [UMLS]

BLOT Bimodality Lung Oncology Trial; British Library of Tape

BLP beta-lipoprotein

BlP blood pressure

B-LPH beta-lipoprotein hormone

B-LPN beta-lipotropin

bl pr blood pressure

BLQ both lower quadrants

BLRC Biomedical Library Review Committee

BLROA British Laryngological, Rhinological, and Otological Association

BLS bare lymphocyte syndrome; basic life support; blind loop syndrome; blood and lymphatic system; blood sugar; Bloom syndrome; Bureau of Labor Statistics

BlS blood sugar

BLSA Baltimore Longitudinal Study of Aging; basic life support ambulance

BLSD bovine lumpy skin disease

BLS-D basic life support–defibrillation; Blessed scale-dementia

BLT bleeding time; blood-clot lysis time; blood test

BlT bleeding time; blood test; blood type, blood typing

BLU Bessey-Lowry unit

BLV blood volume; bovine leukemia virus

BlV blood viscosity; blood volume

BLVR biliverdin reductase

Blx bleeding time

BM Bachelor of Medicine; barium meal; basal medium; basal metabolism; basement membrane; basilar membrane; betamethasone; biomedical; black male; blood monitoring; body mass; Bohr magneton; bone marrow; bowel movement; breast milk; buccal mass; buccomesial

B/M black male

bm black male

B2M beta-2-microglobulin

BMA biological movement artifacts; bone marrow arrest; bone mineral area; British Medical Association

BmA Brugia malayi adult antigen

BMAD Medicare Part B Annual Data [file]

BMAP bone marrow acid phosphatase

B-MAST short Michigan Alcoholism Screening Test

B$_{max}$ maximum binding capacity

BMB biomedical belt; bone marrow biopsy

BMBL benign monoclonal B cell lymphocytosis

BMBMA bulk motion biological movement artifacts

BMC blood mononuclear cell; bone marrow cell; bone mineral content

BMCC beta-methylcrotonyl coenzyme A carboxylase

BMCHRD Bureau of Maternal and Child Health and Resources Development

BMD Becker muscular dystrophy; Boehringer Mannheim Diagnostics; bone marrow depression; bone mineral density; bovine mucosal disease

BMDC Biomedical Documentation Center

BMDP biomedical [computer] program

BMDW Bone Marrow Donor Worldwide

BME basal medium Eagle; biundulant meningoencephalitis; brief maximal effort

BMed Bachelor of Medicine

BMedBiol Bachelor of Medical Biology

BMedSci Bachelor of Medical Science

BMET biomedical equipment technician

BMF bone marrow failure

BMG benign monoclonal gammopathy

BMI body mass index; brief motivational intervention

BMic Bachelor of Microbiology

BMIPP beta-methylidophenylpentadecanoic acid

BMJ bones, muscles, joints

bmk birthmark

BML biomedical library; bone marrow lymphocytosis

BMLS billowing mitral leaflet syndrome

BMM bone marrow-derived macrophages

BMMP benign mucous membrane pemphigoid

BMN bone marrow necrosis

BMNC blood mononuclear cell

BMOC Brinster's medium for ovum culture

Bmod behavior modification

B-mode brightness modulation

BMP bone morphogenetic protein
bmp bone morphogenetic protein
BMPI bronchial mucous proteinase inhibitor
BMPP benign mucous membrane pemphigus; beta-methyliodophenylpentadecanoic acid
BMQA Board of Medical Quality Assurance
BMR basal metabolic rate
BMRC British Medical Research Council
BMS Bachelor of Medical Science; Belfast Metoprolol Study; betamethasone; biomedical monitoring system; biomedical science; bleomycin sulfate; broadcast message server; Bureau of Medical Services; Bureau of Medicine and Surgery; burning mouth syndrome
BMSA British Medical Students Association
BMSP biomedical sciences program
BMST Bruce maximum stress test
BMT Bachelor of Medical Technology; basement membrane thickening; benign mesenchymal tumor; bone marrow transplant; bone marrow transplantation
BMTU bone marrow transplantation unit
BMU basic metabolic unit; basic multicellular unit
BMZ basement membrane zone
BN bladder neck; branchial neuritis; bronchial node; brown Norway [rat]; bulimia nervosa
BNA Basle Nomina Anatomica
BNCT boron neutron capture therapy
BND barely noticeable difference
BNDD Bureau of Narcotics and Dangerous Drugs
BNEd Bachelor of Nursing Education
BNF British National Formulary
BNG Bayesian Network Generation [system]
BNIST National Bureau of Scientific Information [Fr. *Bureau National d'Information Scientifique*]
BNML brown Norway rat myelocytic leukemia
BNO bladder neck obstruction; bowels not opened
bNOS brain nitric oxide synthase
BNP brain natriuretic peptide
BNPA binasal pharyngeal airway

BN/RN baccalaurate registered nurse
BNS Belfast Nifedipine Study; benign nephrosclerosis
BNSc Bachelor of Nursing Science
BNT Boston Naming Test; brain neurotransmitter
BNYVV beet necrotic yellow vein virus
BO Bachelor of Osteopathy; base of prism out; behavior objective; belladonna and opium; body odor; bowel obstruction; bowels opened; bronchiolitis obliterans; bucco-occlusal
Bo Bolton point
bo bowels
B$_o$ constant magnetic field in a magnetic resonance scanner
B&O belladonna and opium
BOA born on arrival; British Orthopaedic Association
BOAS Bank of America Study [of retiree population]
BOAT back pain outcome assessment team; Balloon vs Optimal Atherectomy Trial
BOB biorthogonal basis
BOBA beta-oxybutyric acid
BOC blood oxygen capacity; Bureau of Census; butyloxycarbonyl
BOCC biomedical occupation [UMLS]
BOD biochemical oxygen demand; brachymorphism-onychodysplasia-dysphalangism [syndrome]
Bod Bodansky [unit]
BOE benign occipital epilepsy
BOEA ethyl biscoumacetate
BOF branchio-oculofacial [syndrome]
BOFS branchio-oculofacial syndrome
BOH board of health
BOILER Balloon Occlusive Intravascular Lysis Enhanced Recanalization Strategy
BOLD bleomycin, Oncovin, lomustin, dacarbazine; blood oxygenation level dependent
BOM bilateral otitis media
BOMA bilateral otitis media, acute
BOOP bronchiolitis obliterans-organizing pneumonia
BOP buffalo orphan prototype [virus]
BOR basal optic root; before time of operation; bowels open regularly; branchio-oto-renal [syndrome]
BORR blood oxygen release rate

BORSA borderline resistant *Staphylococcus aureus*
BOS Bioethics Online Service
BOSC Board of Scientific Counselors
BoSM Bolivian squirrel monkey
BOSS Balloon Optimization vs Stent Study
BOT botulinum toxin
bot bottle
BOU branchio-oto-ureteral [syndrome]
BOW bag of waters
BP Bachelor of Pharmacy; back pressure; barometric pressure; basic protein; bathroom privileges; bed pan; before present; behavior pattern; Bell palsy; benzpyrene; beta-protein; binding protein; biotic potential; biparietal; biphenyl; bipolar; birth place; bisphosphonate; blood pressure; body plethysmography; boiling point; Bolton point; borderline personality; breech presentation; British Pharmacopoeia; bronchopleural; buccopulpal; bullous pemphigus; bypass
B/P blood pressure
bp base pair; bed pan; boiling point
BP II bipolar type II disorder
BPA blood pressure assembly; bovine plasma albumin; British Paediatric Association; bronchopulmonary aspergillosis; burst-promoting activity
BPAEC bovine pulmonary artery endothelial cell
BPAG bullous pemphigoid antigen
BPAR body part [UMLS]
BPB bromphenol blue; biliopancreatic bypass
BPC Behavior Problem Checklist; bile phospholipid concentration; blood pressure cuff; British Pharmaceutical Codex
BPCS back pain classification scale
BPD biparental disomy; biparietal diameter; blood pressure decrease; borderline personality disorder; bronchopulmonary dysplasia
BPDE benzo(α)pyrene-diol-epoxide
BPE bacterial phosphatidylethanolamine
BPEC benign partial epilepsy of childhood; bipolar electrocardiogram
BPEG British Pacing and Electrophysiology Group [study]
BPEI blepharophimosis, ptosis, epicanthus inversus
BPES blepharophimosis-ptosis-epicanthus inversus syndrome

BPF bradykinin-potentiating factor; bronchopulmonary fistula; burst-promoting factor
BPG benzathine penicillin G; D-2,3-bisphosphoglycerate; blood pressure gauge; bypass graft
BPGM bisphosphoglyceromutase
BPH Bachelor of Public Health; benign prostatic hypertrophy
BPh British Pharmacopoeia; buccopharyngeal
Bph bacteriopheophytin
BPharm Bachelor of Pharmacy
BPHEng Bachelor of Public Health Engineering
BPheo bacteriopheophytin
BPHN Bachelor of Public Health Nursing
BPI bactericidal/permeability increasing [protein]; Basic Personality Inventory; beef-pork insulin; bipolar type I; blood pressure increase; blood pressure index; brief pain inventory
BPL Beneficiary Program Liability [data file]; benign proliferative lesion; benzyl penicilloyl-polylysine; beta-propiolactone
BPLA blood pressure, left arm
BPM beats per minute; biperidyl mustard; body protein monitor; bone morphogenetic protein; breaths per minute; brompheniramine maleate
bpm beats per minute
BPMF British Postgraduate Medical Federation
BPMS blood plasma measuring system
BPN bacitracin, polymyxin B, neomycin sulfate; brachial plexus neuropathy
BPO basal pepsin output; benzyl penicilloyl
BPP biophysical profile; bovine pancreatic polypeptide; bradykinin potentiating peptide
BP&P blood pressure and pulse
BPPN benign paroxysmal positioning nystagmus
BPPV benign paroxysmal positional vertigo; bovine paragenital papilloma virus
BPQ Berne pain questionnaire
BPR blood pressure recorder; blood production rate
BPRA blood pressure, right arm
BPROP backpropagation neural network
BPRS brief psychiatric rating scale; brief psychiatric reacting scale

BPS Basel Prospective Study; beats per second; Behavioral Pharmacological Society; biophysical profile score; bits per second; bovine papular stomatitis; brain protein solvent; breaths per second; bytes per second; systolic blood pressure

Bps, bps bits per second; bytes per second

BPSA bronchopulmonary segmental artery

BPSMC Blood Pressure Study in Mexican Children

BPsTh Bachelor of Psychotherapy

BPSU British Paediatric Surveillance Unit

BPT benign paroxysmal torticollis

BPTI basic pancreatic trypsin inhibitor; basic polyvalent trypsin inhibitor; bovine pancreatic trypsin inhibitor

BPV bat paramyxovirus; benign paroxysmal vertigo; benign positional vertigo; bioprosthetic valve; bovine papilloma virus

BP(Vet) British Pharmacopoeia (Veterinary)

Bq becquerel

BQA Bureau of Quality Assurance

BR baroreflex; barrier reared [experimental animals]; baseline recovery; bathroom; bed rest; bedside rounds; bilirubin; biologic response; branchial; breathing rate; breathing training; bronchial, bronchitis, bronchus; *Brucella*, brucellosis

Br brain; breech; bregma; bridge; bromine; bronchitis; brown, *Brucella*; brucellosis

bR bacteriorhodopsin

br boiling range; brachial; branch; branchial; breath; brother

BRA bilateral renal agenesis; bone-resorbing activity; brain-reactive antibody; brainstem auditory [response]

BRAC basic rest-activity cycle

Brach brachial

Brady, brady bradycardia

BRAFE brachial, radial and femoral [approach for elective coronary stent implantation]

BRAGS Bioelectric Repair and Growth Society

BRAINS Biochemical Research and Information Study; Brain Research, Analysis of Images, Networks, and Systems

BRAMS Bech-Rafaelson melancholia scale

BRAO branch retinal artery occlusion

BRAP burst of rapid atrial pacing

BrAP brachial artery pressure

BRAT Baylor rapid autologous transfusion [system]

BRATT bananas, rice, applesauce, tea and toast

BRAVE biosense revascularization approach for viable endocardium

BRB bright red blood

BRBC bovine red blood cell

BRBN blue rubber bleb nevus

BRBNS blue rubber bleb nevus syndrome

BRBPR bright red blood per rectum

BRbx breast biopsy

BRC brain reserve capacity

Brc bromocriptine

BRCA breast cancer

BRCA1, BRCA2 breast cancer susceptibility genes

BRCD breast cancer, ductal

BRCM below right costal margin

BRCS British Red Cross Society

BRCT Brain Resuscitation Clinical Trial

BRD bladder retraining drill; bovine respiratory disease

BrdU bromodeoxyuridine

BrdUrd bromodeoxyuridine

BREASTS bronchopulmonary aspergillosis, radiotherapy, extrinsic allergic alveolitis, ankylosing spondylitis, sarcoidosis, tuberculosis, silicosis [x-ray findings in fibrotic pulmonary changes]

BRESEK brain anomalies–retardation of mentality–ectodermal dysplasia–kidney dysplasia/hypoplasia [syndrome]

BRESHECK brain anomalies–retardation of mentality and growth–ectodermal hypoplasia–Hirschsprung disease–ear deformity and deafness–eye hypoplasia–cleft palate–cryptorchidism–kidney dysplasia/hypoplasia [syndrome]

BRESUS British Hospital Resuscitation Study

BRF bone-resorbing factor

BRFSS Behavioral Risk Factor Surveillance System

BRH benign recurrent hematuria; British Regional Heart [study]; Bureau of Radiological Health

BRHS British Regional Heart Study

BRIC benign recurrent intrahepatic cholestasis

BRIC benign recurrent intrahepatic cholestasis

BRILLIANT Blood Pressure, Renal Effects, Insulin Control, Lipids, Lisinopril and Nifedipine Trial
BRIME brief repetitive isometric maximal exercise
Brkf breakfast
BRM biological response modifier; biuret reactive material
BRMS Bannayan-Riley-Myhre-Smith [syndrome]; Bech-Rafaelsen melancholia scale
BRN Board of Registered Nursing
brn brown
BRO bronchiolitis obliterans; bronchoscopy
bro brother
brom bromide
Bron, Bronch bronchi, bronchial; bronchoscopy
Broncho bronchoscopy
BRP bathroom privileges; bilirubin production; bronchophony
Brph bronchophony
BRR Bannayan-Riley-Ruvalcaba [syndrome]; baroreceptor reflex response; breathing reserve ratio
BRS baroreflex sensitivity; behavior rating scale; battered root syndrome; Bibliographic Retrieval Services; British Roentgen Society
BrSM Brazilian squirrel monkey
BRT Brook reaction test
brth breath
5-BrU 5-bromouracil
BRU bone remodeling unit
BrU bromouracil
Bruc Brucella
BRVO branch retinal vein occlusion
BRW Brown-Robert-Wells [stereotactic system]
BS Bachelor of Science; Bachelor of Surgery; *Bacillus subtilis*; Bartter syndrome; base strap; bedside; before sleep; Behçet syndrome; bilateral symmetrical; bile salt; Binet-Simon [test]; bismuth sulfite; blood sugar; Bloom syndrome; Blue Shield [plan]; body system; borderline schizophrenia; bowel sound; breaking strength; breath sound; British Standard; buffered saline; Bureau of Standards
B-S Bjork-Shiley [valve]
B&S Brown and Sharp [sutures]
B/s, b/s bytes per second
bs bedside; bowel sound; breath sound

b x s brother x sister inbreeding
BSA benzenesulfonic acid; Biofeedback Society of America; bismuth-sulfite agar; bis-trimethylsilyl-acetamide; Blind Service Association; Blue Shield Association; body surface area; bovine serum albumin; bowel sounds active
bsa bovine serum albumin
BSAG Bristol Social Adjustment Guides
BSAM basic sequential access method
BSAP brief short-action potential; brief, small, abundant potentials
BSB body surface burned
BS=BL breath sounds equal bilaterally
BSC bedside commode; bedside care; bench scale calorimeter; best supportive care; bile salt concentration; Biological Stain Commission; Biomedical Science Corps
BSc Bachelor of Science
BSC-1, BS-C-1 *Cercopithecus* monkey kidney cells
BSCC Björk-Shiley convexo-concave [heart valve]; British Society for Clinical Cytology
BSCP bovine spinal cord protein
BSD bedside drainage
BSDLB block in anterosuperior division of left branch
BSE behavior summarized evaluation; bilateral intranasal sphenoethmoidectomy; bilateral symmetrical and equal; bovine spongiform encephalopathy; breast self-examination; bystander effect [ability of genetically modified cells to survive cytotoxic effects]
BSEP brain stem evoked potential
BSER brain stem evoked response [audiometry]
BSF back scatter factor; B-cell stimulatory factor; benign senescent forgetfulness; busulfan
BSG basigin; biotin-streptavidin-gold; branchio-skeleto-genital [syndrome]
BSG-DNA biotin-streptavidin-gold-deoxyribonucleic acid [DNA]
BSH benign sexual headache
BSI behavior status inventory; blood stream infection; body substance isolation; borderline syndrome index; bound serum iron; brainstem injury; brief symptom inventory; British Standards Institution
BSID Bayley scale of infant development
BSIF bile salt independent fraction

BSL benign symmetric lipomatosis; biosafety level; blood sugar level

BSM Bachelor of Science in Medicine; body surface mapping

BSMC bronchial smooth muscle cell

BSN baccalaureate of science in nursing; Bachelor of Science in Nursing; bowel sounds normal

BSNA bowel sounds normal and active

BSO bilateral sagittal osteotomy; bilateral salpingo-oophorectomy; butathione sulfoximine

BSOFP blood spotted on filter paper

BSOP blood spot on filter paper

BSP bromosulphthalein

BSp bronchospasm

BSPA body space [UMLS]

BSPh bachelor of science in pharmacy

BSPM body surface potential mapping

BSQ behavior style questionnaire

BSR basal skin resistance; blood sedimentation rate; bowel sounds regular; brain stimulation reinforcement; burst suppression ratio; Buschke selective reminding [test]

BSS Bachelor of Sanitary Science; balanced salt solution; Bernard-Soulier syndrome; black silk suture; buffered salt solution; buffered single substrate

B-SS Bernard-Soulier syndrome

BSSE bile salt-stimulated esterase

BSSG sitogluside

BSSL bile salt-stimulated lipase

BST bacteriuria screening test; bed nucleus of the striae terminalis; blood serologic test; brief stimulus therapy

BSTFA bis-trimethylsilyltrifluoroacetamide

BSU Bartholin, Skene, urethral [glands]; basic structural unit; British standard unit

BSUB body substance [UMLS]

BSV binocular single vision

BT base of tongue; bedtime; bitemporal; bitrochanteric; bladder tumor; Blalock-Taussig [shunt]; bleeding time; blood type, blood typing; blue tetrazolium; blue tongue; body temperature; borderline tuberculoid; bovine turbinate [cells]; brain tumor; breast tumor

BTA Blood Transfusion Association

BTB breakthrough bleeding; bromthymol blue

BTBL bromothymol blue lactose

BTC basal temperature chart; body temperature chart; butylcholinesterase

BTCG Brain Tumor Cooperative Group

BTD biliary tract disease

BTDG Biological Therapeutics Development Group

BTDS benzoylthiamine disulfide

BTE behind the ear [hearing aid]; biphasic truncated exponential; bovine thymus extract

BTFS breast tumor frozen section

BTG beta-thromboglobulin

BTg bovine trypsinogen

BThU British thermal unit

Btk Bruton's tyrosine kinase

BTL bilateral tubal ligation

BTLS basic trauma life support

BTM benign tertian malaria; blood temperature monitor; body temperature monitor

BTMSA bis-trimethylsilacetylene

BTP biliary tract pain; biological treatment planning; broad terminal phalanges

BTPABA N-benzoyl-L-tyrosyl-p-amino-benzoic acid

BTPS at body temperature and ambient pressure, and saturated with water vapor [gas]

BTR Bezold-type reflex; biceps tendon reflex

BTr bovine trypsin

BTRID binomial transform reduced interference distribution

BTRS Belgian Ticlodipine Retinopathy Study

BTS Batten syndrome; blood transfusion service; blue toe syndrome; bradycardia-tachycardia syndrome

BTSG Brain Tumor Study Group

bTSH bovine thyroid-stimulating hormone

BTU British thermal unit

BTV blue tongue virus

BTWC Biological and Toxin Weapons Convention

BTX botulinum toxin; brevetoxin; bungarotoxin

BTx blood transfusion

BTX-B brevetoxin-B

BTZ benzothiazepine

BU base of prism up; Bethesda unit; blood urea; Bodansky unit; bromouracil; burn unit

Bu butyl
bu bushel
BUA blood uric acid; broadband ultrasonic attenuation
Buc, Bucc buccal
BUB budding uninhibited by benzimidazole
BUDR bromodeoxyuridine
BUDS bilateral upper dorsal sympathectomy
BUE both upper extremities
BUF buffalo [rat]
BUFUL bumetanide and furosemide on lipid [profile]
BUG buccal ganglion
BUGT bilirubin-uridine diphosphate glucuronysyltransferase
BUI brain uptake index
BULIT bulimia test
BULL buccal or upper lingual of lower
BuMed Bureau of Medicine and Surgery
BUMP behavioral regression or upset in hospitalized medical patients [scale]
BUN blood urea nitrogen
bun br bundle branch
BUN/CR blood urea nitrogen/creatine ratio
BUO bleeding of undetermined origin, bruising of undetermined origin
BUQ both upper quadrants
BUR bilateral ureteral occlusion
Burd Burdick suction
BUS Bartholin, urethral, and Skene glands; busulfan
But, but butyrate, butyric
BV bacitracin V; bacterial vaginosis; balloon valvuloplasty; biologic value; blood vessel; blood volume; bronchovesicular
BVA Blind Veterans Association; British Veterinary Association
BVAD biventricular assist device
BVC British Veterinary Codex
BVD bovine viral diarrhea
BVDT brief vestibular disorientation test
BVDU bromovinyldeoxyuridine
BVDV bovine virus diarrhea virus
BVE binocular visual efficiency; blood vessel endothelium; blood volume expander
BVH biventricular hypertrophy
BVI blood vessel invasion
BVL bilateral vas ligation

BVM bag-valve-mask; bronchovascular markings; Bureau of Veterinary Medicine
BVMGT Bender Visual-Motor Gestalt Test
BVMOT Bender Visual-Motor Gestalt Test
BVMS Bachelor of Veterinary Medicine and Science
BVO branch vein occlusion
BVP blood vessel prosthesis; blood volume pulse; burst of ventricular pacing
BVR baboon virus replication; Balloon Valvuloplasty Registry
BVS biventricular support; blanked ventricular sense
BVSc Bachelor of Veterinary Science
BVU bromoisovalerylurea
BVV bovine vaginitis virus
BW bacteriological warfare; Beckwith-Wiedeman [syndrome]; bed wetting; below waist; biological warfare; biological weapon; birth weight; bladder washout; blood Wasserman [reaction]; body water; body weight
B&W black and white [milk of magnesia and cascara extract]
bw body weight
BWC bladder wash cytology
BWD bacillary white diarrhea
BWFCM bladder wash flow cytometry
BWFI bacteriostatic water for injection
BWIS Baltimore-Washington Infant Study
BWS battered woman (or wife) syndrome; Beckwith-Wiedemann syndrome
BWST black widow spider toxin
BWSV black widow spider venom
BWt birth weight
Bwt body weight
BWYV beet western yellow virus
BX, bx bacitracin X; biopsy
Bx biopsy
BXO balanitis xerotica obliterans
ByCPR bystander cardiac pulmonary resuscitation
BYDV barley yellow dwarf virus
BYE Barila-Yaguchi-Eveland [medium]
BZ benzodiazepine
Bz, Bzl benzoyl
BZD benzodiazepine
BZQ benzquinamide
BZRP benzodiazepine receptor peripheral [type]
BZS Bannayan-Zonana syndrome

C about [Lat. *circa*]; ascorbic acid; bruised [Lat. *contusus*]; calcitonin-forming [cell]; calculus; calorie [large]; Campylobacter; Candida; canine tooth; capability [list]; capacitance; carbohydrate; carbon; cardiac; cardiovascular disease; carrier; cast; cathode; Caucasian; cell; Celsius; centigrade; central; central electrode placement in electroencephalography; centromeric or constitutive heterochromatic chromosome [banding]; cerebrospinal; certified; cervical; cesarean [section]; chest (precordial) lead in electrocardiography; chicken; *Chlamydia;* chloramphenicol; cholesterol; class; clearance; clonus; *Clostridium;* closure; clubbing; coarse [bacterial colonies]; cocaine; coefficient; color sense; colored [guinea pig]; complement; complex; compliance; component; compound [Lat. *compositus*]; concentration; conditioned, conditioning; condyle; constant; consultation; contraction; control; conventionally reared [experimental animal]; convergence; correct; cortex; coulomb, count; criteria; *Cryptococcus;* cubic; cubitus; curie; cyanosis; cylinder; cysteine; cytidine; cytochrome; cytosine; gallon [Lat. *congius*]; horn [Lat. *cornu*]; hundred [Lat. *centum*]; large calorie; molar heat capacity; rib [Lat. *costa*]; total capacitance; velocity of light; with [Lat. *cum*]

C1 first cervical nerve; first cervical vertebra; first component of complement

C₁ first rib

C̄1 activated first component of complement

C1 INH inhibitor of first component of complement

CI first cranial nerve

2C 2-component

C2 second cervical nerve; second cervical vertebra; second component of complement

C₂ second rib

C̄2 activated second component of complement

CII second cranial nerve

3C 3-component; cranio-cerebello-cardiac syndrome

C3 third cervical nerve; third cervical vertebra; third component of complement

C₃ Collins' solution; third rib

C̄3 activated third component of complement

CIII third cranial nerve

C4 controlled collapse chip connection; fourth cervical nerve; fourth cervical vertebra; fourth component of complement

C̄4 activated fourth component of complement

CIV fourth cranial nerve

C5 fifth cervical nerve; fifth cervical vertebra; fifth component of complement

C̄5 activated fifth component of complement

CV fifth cranial nerve

C6 sixth cervical nerve; sixth cervical vertebra; sixth component of complement

C̄6 activated sixth component of complement

CVI sixth cranial nerve

C7 seventh cervical nerve; seventh cervical vertebra; seventh component of complement

C̄7 activated seventh component of complement

CVII seventh cranial nerve

C8 eighth component of complement

C̄8 activated eighth component of complement

CVIII eighth cranial nerve

C9 ninth component of complement

C̄9 activated ninth component of complement

CIX-CXII ninth to twelfth cranial nerves

°C degree Celsius

C' complement

c about [Lat. *circa*]; calorie [small]; candle; canine tooth; capacity; carat; centi-; complementary [strand]; concentration; contact; cup; curie; cyclic; meal [Lat. *cibus*]; specific heat capacity; with [Lat. *cum*]

c' coefficient of portage

CA anterior commissure [Lat. *commissura anterior*]; calcium antagonist; California [rabbit]; cancer; *Candida albicans;* caproic acid; carbonic anhydrase; carcinoma; cardiac angiography; cardiac arrest; cardiac arrhythmia; carotid artery; cast; catecholamine, catecholaminergic; cathode; Caucasian adult; cell automation; celiac axis; cerebral aqueduct; cerebral atrophy; cervicoaxial; Chemical Abstracts; chemotactic activity; child abuse; chloroamphetamine; cholic acid; chromosomal aberration; chronic anovulation; chronological age; citric acid; clotting assay; coagglutination; coarctation of the aorta; Cocaine Anonymous; coefficient of absorption; cold agglutinin; colloid antigen; common antigen; compressed air; conceptional age; coracoacromial; coronary artery; corpora alata; corpora amylacea; corpus albicans; corrected [echo] area; cortisone acetate; cricoarytenoid; cricoid arch; croup-associated [virus]; cytosine arabinoside; cytotoxic antibody

Ca calcium; cancer, carcinoma; *Candida albicans;* cathode

ca about [Lat. *circa*]; candle; carcinoma

C&A Clinitest and Acetest

CA1 carbonic anhydrase I

CA-2 second colloid antigen

Ca²⁺-blocker calcium channel blocker

CAA carotid audiofrequency analysis; cerebral amyloid angiopathy; circulating anodic antigen; Clean Air Act; computer-assisted assessment; constitutional aplastic anemia; coronary artery aneurysm; crystalline amino acids

CAAH chronic active autoimmune hepatitis

CAAS cardiovascular angiographic analysis system; Commission on Accreditation of Ambulance Services

CAASET Canadian Amlodipine and Atenolol Stress Echo [trial]

CAAT computer-assisted axial tomography

CAAX [box] protein segment in which C is cysteine, A is usually but not always an aliphatic amino acid, and X is methionine or serine

CAB captive air bubble; cellulose acetate butyrate; coronary artery bypass

CABADAS [prevention of] Coronary Artery Bypass Graft Occlusion by Aspirin, Dipyridamole and Acenocoumarol Study

CABF coronary artery blood flow

CABG coronary artery bypass grafting

CABGS coronary artery bypass graft surgery

CaBI calcium bone index

CABM Center for Advanced Biotechnology and Medicine

CABMET Colorado Association of Biomedical Engineering Technicians

CaBP calcium-binding protein

CABRI Coronary Angioplasty versus Bypass Revascularization Investigation; Coronary Artery Bypass Revascularization Investigation

CABS citric acid-buffered saline [solution]; continuous ambulatory blood sampler; coronary artery bypass surgery

CAC Carcinogeneity Assessment Committee [FDA]; cardiac-accelerator center; cardiac arrest code; children's asthma center; circulating anticoagulant; clinical application coordinator

CaCC cathodal closure contraction

CAC/CIC chronic active/inactive cirrhosis

CACCN Canadian Association of Critical Care Nurses

CACHET Comparison of Abciximab Complications with Hirulog for Ischemic Events Trial

CACP cisplatin

CaCTe cathodal closure tetanus

CACTIS Comparison of Aspirin with Clopidogrel or Ticlopidine in Stents [trial]

CaCV calicivirus

CaCX cancer of cervix

CACY calcyclin

CAD cadaver, cadaveric; coenzyme A dehydrogenase; cold agglutinin disease; collisionally activated dissociation; compressed air disease; computer-aided design; computer-aided dispatch; computer-assisted design; computer-assisted diagnosis; congenital abduction deficiency; coronary artery disease; coronoradiographic documentation

Cad cadaver, cadaveric

CADA Council on Alcohol and Drug Abuse

CADASIL cerebral autosomal dominant arteriopathy with subcortical infarcts and leukoencephalopathy

CAD/CAM computer-aided design/computer-aided manufacturing

CADD computer-aided drug design

CADHYP Coronary Artery Disease in Hypertension [study]

CADI coronary artery disease index

CADILLAC Controlled Abciximab and Device Investigation to Lower Late Angioplasty Complications [study]

CADL Communicative Abilities in Daily Living

CADMIO computer-assisted design for medical information objectives

cADPR cyclic adenosinephosphate-ribose

CADR coronary artery descriptors and restenosis

CADRES Coronary Artery Descriptors and Restenosis [project]

CADS Captopril and Digoxin Study

CaDTe cathodal-duration tetanus

CADx computer-aided diagnosis

CAE caprine arthritis-encephalitis; cellulose acetate electrophoresis; contingent after-effects; coronary artery embolism

CaE calcium excretion

CaEDTA calcium disodium ethylene-diaminetetraacetate

CAEP Canadian Association of Emergency Physicians; cortical auditory evoked potential

CAESAR Canada, Australia, Europe and South Africa Republic [trial]; Computer-Assisted Evaluation of Stenosis and Restenosis [system]

CAEV caprine arthritis-encephalitis virus

CAF cell adhesion factor; citric acid fermentation

Caf caffeine

CAFA Canadian Atrial Fibrillation Anticoagulation [study]

CAFE Coronary Artery Flow Evaluation

CAFS Canadian Atrial Fibrillation Study

CAG cholangiogram, cholangiography; chronic atrophic gastritis; coronary angiography

CAGA calgranulin A

CAGB calgranulin B

CAGE capillary affinity gell electrophoresis; *c*ut down, *a*nnoyed by criticism, *g*uilty about drinking, *e*ye-opener drinks (a test for alcoholism)

CAH chronic active hepatitis; chronic aggressive hepatitis; combined atrial hypertrophy; congenital adrenal hyperplasia; cyanacetic acid hydrazide

CAHD coronary arteriosclerotic heart disease

CAHEA Committee on Allied Health Education and Accreditation

CAHMR cataract-hypertrichosis-mental retardation [syndrome]

CAHPS Consumer Assessment of Health Plans Study

CAHS central alveolar hypoventilation syndrome

CAHV central alveolar hypoventilation

CAI cellular adaptive immunotherapy; complete androgen insensitivity; computer-assisted instruction; computer-assisted interview

CAIS complete androgen insensitivity syndrome

CAIUS Carotid Atherosclerosis Italian Ultrasound Study

C(a-jb)O$_2$ arterial-jugular bulb venous oxygen ratio

CAK cyclin-dependent kinase-activating kinase

CAL café au lait; calcium test; calculated average life; calories; chronic airflow limitation; computer-assisted learning; coracoacromial ligament

Cal caliber; large calorie

cal small calorie

C$_{alb}$ albumin clearance

Calc calcium

CALC calcitonin

calc calculation

calcif calcification

CALCR calcitonin receptor

CALD chronic active liver disease

CALGB cancer and leukemia group B

CALH chronic active lupoid hepatitis

cALL common null cell acute lymphocytic leukemia

CALLA, cALLA common acute lymphoblastic leukemia antigen

CALM café-au-lait macules

CALP congenital absence of left pericardium

CALS café-au-lait spots

CALYPSO Cylexin as an Adjunct to Lytic Therapy to Prevent Superoxide Reflow Injury

CAM calf aortic microsome; cell adhesion molecule; cell-associating molecule; chorioallantoic membrane; complementary and alternative medicine(s); computer assisted myelography; confusion assessment method [rating for delirium]; contralateral axillary metastasis; cystic adenomatoid malformation

CaM calmodulin

C$_{am}$ amylase clearance

CAMAC computer automated measurement and control

CAMAK cataract-microcephaly-arthrogryposis-kyphosis [syndrome]

CAMAT Canadian Amiodarone Myocardial Infarction Arrhythmia Trial

CAMCAM Center for Assessment and Management of Changes in Academic Medicine

CAMCAT Canadian Multicenter Clentiazem Angina Trial

CAMCOG Cambridge cognitive capacity scale

CAMD computer-aided molecular design

CAMDEX Cambridge mental disorders of the elderly examination

CAMF cyclophosphamide, Adriamycin, methotrexate, fluorouracil

CAMFAK cataract–microcephaly–failure to thrive–kyphoscoliosis [syndrome]

CAMI Canadian Assessment of Myocardial Infarction [study]

CAMIAT Canadian Amiodarone Myocardial Infarction Arrhythmia Trial; Canadian Myocardial Infarction Amiodarone Trial

CAMIS Center for Applied Medical Information Systems Research

CAMK calmodulin-dependent protein kinase

CaMK calcium-mediated kinase

CAML cystic adenomatoid malformation of the lung

CAMP Christie-Atkins-Munch-Petersen [test]; computer-assisted management protocol; computer-assisted menu planning; concentration of adenosine monophosphate; cyclic adenosine monophosphote; cyclophosphamide, Adriamycin, methotrexate, and procarbazine

cAMP cyclic adenosine monophosphate

CAMS computer-assisted monitoring system

CAMTS Commission for Accreditation of Medical Transport Services

CaMV cauliflower mosaic virus

CAMVA chorioallantoic membrane vascular assay

CAN cardiac autonomic neuropathy

Can cancer; Candida; *Cannabis*

CA/N child abuse and neglect

CANA circulating antineuronal antibody

CaNaEDTA calcium-disodium ethylenediamine tetraacetic acid

CANAHOP Canadian Ambulatory, Home and Office Pressure Study

canc cancelled

C-ANCA cytoplasmic anti-neutrophilic cytoplasmic antibody

CANCERLIT Cancer Literature [NLM database]

CANCERPROJ Cancer Research Projects

CANDA computer-assisted new drug application

CANDELA computer-assisted notification of drug effects on laboratory animals [test]

CANDY Communication Aids Negating Disabilities of Youth [laboratory]

CA*Net Canada's High Performance Network

CANP calcium-activated neutral protease

CANS central auditory nervous system

CAN'T LEAP cyclosporine, alcohol, nicotinic acid, thiazides, lasix, ethambutanol, aspirin, pyrazinamide [substances causing hyperuricemia]

CANX calnexin

CAO chronic airway obstruction; coronary artery obstruction

CAO$_2$ arterial oxygen content

C$_a$O$_2$ arterial oxygen content

CaOC cathodal opening contraction

CaOCL cathodal opening clonus

CAOD coronary artery occlusive disease

CAOHC Council for Accreditation of Occupational Hearing Conservation

CAOM chronic adhesive otitis media

CAOT Canadian Association of Occupational Therapy

CaOTe cathodal opening tetanus

CAP camptodactyly-arthropathy-pericarditis [syndrome]; Canada Assistance Plan; capsule; captopril; catabolite gene activator protein; cell attachment protein; cellular acetate propionate; cellulose acetate phthalate; central apical part; chloramphenicol; chronic alcoholic pancreatitis; clinical access program; College of American Pathologists;

community-acquired pneumonia; complement-activated plasma; compound action potential; coupled atrial pacing; cyclosphosphamide, Adriamycin, and Platino [cisplatin]; cystine aminopeptidase

C_{AP} cationic antimicrobial protein; circumference of apex

CaP carcinoma of the prostate

cap capacity; capsule

CAPA cancer-associated polypeptide antigen

CAPARES Coronary Angioplasty Amlodipine in Restenosis Trial

CAPAS Cutting Balloon Angioplasty vs Plain Old Balloon Angioplasty Randomized Study

CAPCC Canadian Association of Poison Control Centers

CAPD continuous ambulatory peritoneal dialysis

CAPE Circadian Anti-Ischemia Program in Europe; Clifton assessment procedures for the elderly; computer-assisted patient emulator

CAPERS Computer Assisted Psychiatric Evaluation and Review System

CAPHIS Consumer and Patient Health Information Section [American Library Association]

CAPI cryptographic applications programming interface

CAPITOL Captopril Postinfarction Tolerance [trial]

CAPM continuous airway pressure monitoring

CAPP Captopril Prevention Project [study]; Concerted Action Polyp Prevention

CAPPHY Captopril Primary Prevention in Hypertension [study]

CAPPP Captopril Prevention Project

CAPPS Current and Past Psychopathology Scale

CAPRCA chronic, acquired, pure red cell aplasia

CAPRI Cardiopulmonary Research Institute

CAPRICORN Carvedilol Postinfarct Survival Controlled Evaluation

CAPRIE Clopidogrel vs Aspirin in Patients at Risk of Ischemic Events

CAPS Cardiac Arrhythmia Pilot Study; care profile system; community adjustment profile system; computer-aided prototyping system

caps capsule

CAPTIN Captopril Before Reperfusion in Acute Myocardial Infarction; Captopril Plus Tissue Plasminogen Activator Following Acute Myocardial Infarction

CAPTISM Captopril Insulin Sensitivity Multicenter [study]

CAPTURE Chimeric 7E3 Antiplatelet Therapy in Unstable Refractory Angina [trial]

CAR Canadian Association of Radiologists; cancer-associated retinopathy; Cardiac Ablation Registry; cardiac ambulation routine; carvedilol; cell adhesion regulator; chronic articular rheumatism; computer-assisted radiology; computer-assisted research; conditioned avoidance response

car carotid

CARA chronic aspecific respiratory ailment

CARAF Canadian Registry of Atrial Fibrillation

CARAFE Cocktail Attenuation of Rotational Ablation Flow Effects [study]

CAR AMP carotid pulse amplitude

CARAT Coronary Angioplasty and Rotablator Atherectomy Trial; coronary artery risk assessment and treatment

CARB carbohydrate; coronary artery bypass graft

carb carbohydrate; carbonate

carbo carbohydrate

CARD cardiac automatic resuscitative device

card cardiac

CARDIA Coronary Artery Risk Development in Young Adults [study]

CARDIAC Cardiovascular Disease and Alimentary Comparison [study]

card insuff cardiac insufficiency

cardiol cardiology

CARD PORT Cardiac Arrhythmia and Risk of Death Patient Outcome Research Team

CARE calcium antagonist in reperfusion; cardiac arrhythmias research and education; Carvedilol Arthrectomy Restenosis [trial]; Cholesterol and Recurrent Events [study]; comprehensive assessment and referral evaluation; computerized adult and records evaluation [system]; computerized clinical assessment, research and education; cyclic adenosine monophosphate response element

CAREC Caribbean Epidemiology Centre

CARES cancer rehabilitation evaluation system

CARET Beta-Carotene and Retinol Efficacy Trial

CARF Commission on Accreditation and Rehabilitation Facilities

CARG coronary artery bypass grafting

CAR$_{hd}$ high-dose carvedilol

CARMEN Carvedilol Angiotensin Converting Enzyme Inhibitors Remodelling Mild Heart Failure Evaluation

CARP carbonic anhydrase-related polypeptide

CARPORT Coronary Artery Restenosis Prevention on Repeated Thromboxane A$_2$-Receptor Antagonism Study

CARS Childhood Autism Rating Scale; Children's Affective Rating Scale; Coronary Artery Regression Study; Coumadin Aspirin Reinfarction Study; cysteinyltransfer ribonucleic acid synthetase

CART classification and regression tree; Colchicine Angioplasty Restenosis Trial; computer-assisted radiotherapy

cart cartilage

CAS calcarine sulcus; calcific aortic stenosis; Cancer Attitude Survey; carbohydrate-active steroid; cardiac adjustment scale; cardiac surgery; Celite-activated normal serum; Center for Alcohol Studies; central anticholinergic syndrome; cerebral atherosclerosis; Chemical Abstract Service; clinical application suite; clinical assessment score; clinical asthma score; cognitive assessment scale; cold agglutinin syndrome; computer-assisted surgery; congenital alcoholic syndrome; control adjustment strap; coronary artery spasm; Council of Academic Societies

Cas casualty

cas castration, castrated

CASA center for addiction and substance abuse; computer-assisted self assessment

CASANOVA Coronary Artery Stenosis with Asymptomatic Narrowing: Operation vs Aspirin [study]

CASCADE Cardiac Arrest in Seattle: Conventional vs Amiodarone Drug Evaluation; Conventional Arrhythmic vs Amiodarone in Survivors of Cardiac Arrest Drug Evaluation

CASCO Calcium Sensitization in Congestive Heart Failure

CASE Community, Attachment, Structures and Epidemic [study]; computer-aided systems engineering

CASET Carotid Artery Stenting vs Endarterectomy Trial

CASH Cardiac Arrest Study, Hamburg; Caring About Seniors' Health [study]; Commission for Administrative Services in Hospitals; Consensus Action on Salt and Hypertension; corticoadrenal stimulating hormone; cruciform anterior spinal hyperextension

CASHD coronary arteriosclerotic heart disease

CASI cognitive abilities screening instrument

CASIS Canadian Amlodipine/Atenolol in Silent Ischemia Study; Coronary Artery Stent Implantation Study

CASMD congenital atonic sclerotic muscular dystrophy

CASPER computer-assisted pericardial puncture; computer-assisted pericardial surgery

CASQ calsequestrin

CASR calcium-sensing receptor

CAS-REGN Chemical Abstracts Service Registry Number

CAS-REGN Chemical Abstracts Service Registry Number

CASRT corrected adjusted sinus node recovery time

CASS cataract-alopecia-sclerodactyly syndrome; Coronary Artery Surgery Study

CASSIS Classification and Search Support Information System [Patent Office]; Czech and Slovak Spirapril Intervention Study

CAST calpastatin; Cardiac Arrhythmia Suppression Trial; Carotid Artery Stenting Trial; Children of Alcoholism Screening Test; Chinese Acute Stroke Trial

CASTEL Cardiovascular Study in the Elderly

CASTOR Coronary Angioscopic Study of Restenosis

CAT California Achievement Test; cancer after transplantation; capillary agglutination test; Cardiomyopathy Trial; care support terminal; catalase; cataract; catecholamine; Children's Apperception Test; Chinese Angiotensin Converting Enzyme Inhibitor in Acute Myocardial Infarction Trial; chloramphenicol acetyltransferase; chlormerodrin accumulation test; choline acetyltransferase; chronic abdominal tympany; Cognitive Abilities Test; Columbia Center for Advanced Technology; computed abdominal tomography; computed axial tomography; computer-assisted tomography; computer of average transients; coronary angioplasty trial; critically appraised topic

cat catalysis, catalyst; cataract

CAT'ase catalase

CATB catalase B

CATCEC Computer-Supported Assessment and Treatment Consultation for Emotional Crises

CATCH Child and Adolescent Trial for Cardiovascular Health; Community Action to Control High Blood Pressure

CATCH 22 cardiac defects–abnormal facies–thymic hypoplasia–cleft palate–hypocalcemia [syndrome]

Cath cathartic; catheter, catheterize

cath catheterization

CATLINE Catalog Online [NLM database]

CATPO computer-aided therapy planning in pediatric oncology

CATS Canadian American Ticlopidine Study; Captopril and Thrombolysis Study

CAT-S Children's Apperception Test, Supplemental

CAT scan computed axial tomography scan

CATSIM computer case simulation

CATT calcium tolerance test

Cauc Caucasian

caud caudal

caut cauterization

CAV congenital absence of vagina; congenital adrenal virilism; constant angular velocity; croup-associated virus

cav cavity

CAVA Coronary Atherectomy vs Angioplasty [study]

CAVATAS Carotid and Vertebral Artery Transluminal Angioplasty Study

CAVB complete atrioventricular block

CAVD complete atrioventricular dissociation; completion, arithmetic problems, vocabulary, following directions [test]; congenital aplasia of vas deferens

CAVE cerebroacrovisceral–early lethality [phenotype]

CAVEAT Coronary Angioplasty vs Excisional Atherectomy Trial

CAVEAT-I Comparison of Directional Atherectomy vs Coronary Angioplasty Trial

CAVEAT-II Coronary Angioplasty vs Directional Atherectomy for Patients with Saphenous Vein Bypass Graft Lesions [trial]

CAVG coronary artery vein graft

CAVH continuous arteriovenous hemofiltration

CAVHD continuous arteriovenous hemodialysis

CAVHDF continuous arteriovenous hemodiafiltration

CAVLT Children's Auditory Verbal Learning Test

CAVO common atrioventricular orifice

$C(a-v)_{O_2}$ arterio-venous oxygen tension difference

CAVR continuous arteriovenous rewarming

CAVS Conformance Assessment to Voluntary Standards

CAVU continuous arteriovenous ultrafiltration

CAW central airways

C_{AW} airway conductance

CB Bachelor of Surgery [Lat. *Chirurgiae Baccalaureus*]; calcium blocker; carbenicillin; carotid body; chocolate blood [agar]; chromatin body; chronic bronchitis; circumflex branch; code blue; color blind; compensated base; conus branch; Coomassie blue; coprocessor board; coracobrachial

8CB octylcyanobiphenyl

Cb cerebellum; niobium [columbium]

CBA chronic bronchitis and asthma; Columbia blood agar [test]; cost-benefit analysis

CBAB complement-binding antibody

CBADAA Certifying Board of the American Dental Assistants Association

CBAVD congenital bilateral absence of vas deferens

CBBEST cutting balloon before stent

CBBM color blindness, blue mono-cone-monochromatic type

CBC capillary blood gases; carbenicillin; child behavior characteristics; compensatory base change; complete blood cell count

cbc complete blood cell count

CBCL Child Behavior Checklist

CBCL/2-3 Child Behavior Checklist for ages 2-3

CBCN carbenicillin

CbCtx cerebellar cortex

CBD carotid body denervation; closed bladder drainage; color blindness, deutan type; common bile duct; Convention on Biological Diversity

CBDC chronic bullous disease of children

CBDE common bile duct exploration

CBDPR computer-based dental patient record

CBDMP California Birth Defects Monitoring Program

CBE clinical breast examination

CBER Center for Biologic Evaluation and Research

CBET certified biomedical equipment technician

CBF capillary blood flow; cerebral blood flow; ciliary beat frequency; collagen-binding factor; core-binding factor; coronary blood flow; cortical blood flow

CBFB core binding factor, beta

CBFb beta subunit of core-binding factor

CBG capillary blood gases; coronary bypass graft; corticosteroid-binding globulin; cortisol-binding globulin

CBGv corticosteroid-binding globulin variant

CBH chronic benign hepatitis; cutaneous basophilic hypersensitivity

CBI children's behavior inventory; continuous bladder irrigation

CBIC Certification Board in Infection Control

CBL circulating blood lymphocytes; chronic blood loss; cord blood leukocytes

Cbl cobalamin

CBM capillary basement membrane

CBMMP chronic benign mucous membrane pemphigus

CBN cannabinol; central benign neoplasm; Commission on Biological Nomenclature

CBO community-based organization; Congressional Budget Office

CBOC completion bed occupancy care

CBP calcium-binding protein; cAMP-binding protein; carbohydrate-binding protein; cardiopulmonary bypass; chlorobiphenyl; cobalamin-binding protein; color blindness, protan type; cruciform binding protein

C4BP complement 4 binding protein

CBPA competitive protein-binding assay

CBPR computer-based patient record

CBPS congenital bilateral perisylvian syndrome

CBR carbonyl reductase; case-based reasoning; chemical, biological, and radiological [warfare]; chemically-bound residue; chronic bed rest; complete bed rest; crude birth rate

CBRL contextual Bayesian relaxation labeling technique

CB3S Coxsackie B3 virus susceptibility

CBS cervicobrachial syndrome; chronic brain syndrome; clinical behavioral science; conjugated bile salts; culture-bound syndrome; cystathionine beta-synthase

CBT carotid body tumor; code blue team; cognitive behavioral treatment/therapy; computed body tomography; computer-based training instruction

CBV capillary blood cell velocity; catheter balloon valvuloplasty; central blood volume; cerebral blood volume; circulating blood volume; cortical blood volume; corrected blood volume; Coxsackie B virus

CBVD cerebrovascular disease

CBVI computer-based video instruction

CBW chemical and biological warfare

CBX computer-based examination

CBZ carbamazepine

CC calcaneal-cuboid; calcium cyclamate; cardiac catheterization; cardiac center; cardiac contusion; cardiac cycle; cardiovascular clinic; cell culture; central compartment; cerebral commissure; cerebral cortex; cervical cancer; chest circumference; chief complaint; cholecalciferol; choledochocholedochostomy; chondrocalcinosis; choriocarcinoma; chronic complainer; circulatory collapse; classical conditioning; clean catch [of urine]; Clinical Center [NIH]; clinical course; clomiphene citrate; closed cup; closing capacity; coefficient of consistency; collagenous colitis; colony count; colorectal cancer; columnar cells; commission certified; common cold; complicating condition; complications and co-morbidity; compound cathartic; computation constant; computer calculated; computer center; concordance; congenital cardiopathy; congenital cataract; consumptive coagulopathy; contrast cystogram; conversion complete; coracoclavicular; cord compression; coronary care; corpus callosum; correlation coefficient; costochondral; Coulter counter; craniocaudal; craniocervical; creatinine clearance; critical care; critical condition; Crohn colitis; Cronkhite-Canada [syndrome]; cross correlation; crus cerebri; cubic centimeter; current complaint; Current Contents

C-C convexo-concave

C&C cold and clammy

Cc concave

cc clean catch [urine]; concave; corrected; cubic centimeter

CCA canonical correlation; cephalin cholesterol antigen; chick cell agglutination; chimpanzee coryza agent; choriocarcinoma; circulating cathodic antigen; circumflex coronary artery; common carotid artery; congenital contractural arachnodactyly; constitutional chromosome abnormality

CCABOT Cornell Coronary Artery Bypass Outcomes Trial

CCAg corpus callosum agenesis

CCAIT Canadian Coronary Atherosclerosis Intervention Trial

CCAT Canadian Coronary Atherectomy Trial; chick cell agglutination test; conglutinating complement absorption test

CCB calcium channel blocker

CCBV central circulating blood volume

CCC Canadian Cardiovascular Coalition [study]; care-cure coordination; cathodal closure contraction; child care center; children communication checklist; chronic calculus cholecystitis; chronic catarrhal colitis; comprehensive cancer center; comprehensive care clinic; concentration, clustering and continuity; concurrent care concern; consecutive case conference; continuous curvilinear capsulotomy; craniocerebello-cardiac [dysplasia or syndrome];

critical care complex; council on clinical classification; cylindrical confronting cisternae

CC&C colony count and culture

CCCC centrifugal countercurrent chromatography

CCCCP Comprehensive Cardiovascular Community Control Program

cccDNA covalently closed circular deoxyribonucleic acid

CCCE cross-cultural cognitive examination

CCCl cathodal closure clonus

CCCN community care coordination network

CCCP carbonyl cyanide m-chloro-phenyl-hydrazone

CCCR closed chest cardiac resuscitation

CCCS condom catheter collecting system; critical care computer system

CCCT closed craniocerebral trauma

CCCU comprehensive cardiac care unit

CCD calibration curve data; charge-coupled device; childhood core disease; childhood celiac disease; cleidocranial dysplasia; clinical cardiovascular disease; cortical collecting duct; countercurrent distribution; cumulative cardiotoxic dose

CCDC Canadian Communicable Disease Center; consultant in communicable disease control

CCDN Central Council for District Nursing

ccDNA closed circle deoxyribonucleic acid

CCDS case cart delivery system

CCE carboline carboxylic acid ester; chamois contagious ecthyma; clear-cell endothelioma; clubbing, cyanosis, and edema; countercurrent electrophoresis; cruciform cutting endonuclease

CCEHRP Committee to Coordinate Environmental Health and Related Programs

CCEI Crown-Crisp Experimental Index

CCF cancer coagulation factor; cardiolipin complement fixation; carotid-cavernous fistula; centrifuged culture fluid; cephalin-cholesterol flocculation; compound comminuted fracture; congestive heart failure; cross-correlation function; crystal-induced chemotactic factor

CCFA cefotoxin-cycloserine fructose agar

CCFAS compact colony-forming active substance

CCFE cyclophosphamide, cisplatin, fluorouracil, and extramustine

CCFMG Cooperating Committee on Foreign Medical Graduates

CCG Children's Cancer Study Group; cholecystogram, cholecystography; clinically coherent group

CCGC capillary column gas chromotography

CCGS cell cycle G and S

CCH C-cell hyperplasia; central clinical hospital; chronic chloride hemagglutination; chronic cholestatic hepatitis; cross-correlation histogram

CCHA Canadian Council on Hospital Accreditation

CCHAT Canadian Cozaar, Hyzaar and Amlodipine Trial

CCHD Caephilly Collaborative Heart Disease [study]; cyanotic congenital heart disease

CCHE Central Council for Health Education

CCHF Crimean-Congo hemorrhagic fever

CCHFA Canadian Council on Health Facilities Accreditation

CCHMS Central Committee for Hospital Medical Services

CCHP Consumer Choice Health Plan; Corpus Christi Heart Project

CCHS congenital central hypoventilation syndrome; Copenhagen City Heart Study

CCI Canadian Classification of Health Interventions; Cancer Care International; Cardiovascular Credentialing International; cholesterol crystallization inhibitor; chronic coronary insufficiency; common client interface; component communication interface; corrected count increment; crowded cell index

CC-IMED California Consortium of Information in Medical Education and Development

CCK cholecystokinin

CCK-8 cholecystokinin octapeptide

CCKLI cholecystokinin-like immunoreactivity

CCK-OP cholecystokinin octapeptide

CCK-PZ cholecystokinin-pancreozymin

CCKRB cholecystokinin receptor B

CCL carcinoma cell line; certified cell line; Charcot-Leyden crystal; continuing care level; continuous cell line; critical carbohydrate level

CCLE chronic cutaneous lupus erythematosus

CCLI composite clinical and laboratory index

CCM cerebrocostomandibular [syndrome]; chemical cleavage of mismatch; congestive cardiomyopathy; craniocervical malformation; critical care medicine

c cm cubic centimeter

CCMC Committee on the Costs of Medical Care

CCMDS Core Community Minimum Data Set [Scotland]

CCME Coordinating Council on Medical Education

CCML Comprehensive Core Medical Library

CCMS cerebrocostomandibular syndrome; clean catch midstream [urine]; clinical care management system

CCMSU clean catch midstream urine

CCMT catechol methyltransferase

CCMU critical care medical unit

CCN cancer center network; caudal central nucleus; community care network; coronary care nursing; critical care nursing

CCNHP community college nursing home project

CCNU N-(2-chloroethyl)-N'-cyclo-hexyl-N-nitrosourea

CCO cytochrome C oxidase

CcO$_2$ capillary oxygen content

CCORP Cornell-China-Oxford Research Project

CCOT cervical compression overloading test

CCP Canadian Classification of Diagnostic, Therapeutic, and Surgical Interventions; cephalin-cholesterol flocculation; chronic calcifying pancreatitis; ciliocytophthoria; community care plan; comprehensive care plan; cooperative cardiovascular project; coordinated care program; critical control point [food safety]; cytidine cyclic phosphate

CCPD continuous cycling (cyclical) peritoneal dialysis

CCPDS Centralized Cancer Patient Data System

CCPR closed-chest cardiopulmonary resuscitation; crypt cell production rate

CCPT Chinese Cancer Prevention Project

CCR Canadian Cancer Registry; complete continuous remission; complex chromosome rearrangement; consistency and concurrency reporting

C-CR Computing-Communications Research Division [National Science Foundation (NSF)]

CCRC comprehensive care retirement community; continuing care retirement community

Ccr, C$_{cr}$ creatinine clearance

CCRG Cooperative Cataract Research Group

CCRIS Chemical Carcinogenesis Research Information System [NLM database]

CCRN Critical Care Registered Nurse

CCRS Chemical Carcinogenesis Research Information System

CCRT Cardiac Catheter Reuse Trial; computer-controlled radiation therapy

CCS Canadian Cardiovascular Society; casualty clearing station; cell cycle specific; Chinese Cardiac Study; cholecystosonography; chronic cerebellar stimulation; chronic compartment syndrome; clear cell sarcoma; cloudy cornea syndrome; composite cultured skin; concentration camp syndrome; costoclavicular syndrome; crippled children's service

CCSCS central cervical spinal cord syndrome

CCSE Cognitive Capacity Screening Examination

CCSG Canadian Cooperative Study Group; Children's Cancer Study Group

CCSK clear cell sarcoma of the kidney

CCSP Clara cell-specific protein

CCSRG Cochrane Collaboration Stroke Review Group

CCT carotid compression tomography; central conduction time; cerebrocranial trauma; Chinese Captopril Trial; chocolate-coated tablet; coated compressed tablet; combined cortical thickness; composite cyclic therapy; computerized cranial tomography; contrast-enhanced computed tomography; controlled cord traction; coronary care team; cranial computed tomography; critical care technician; cyclocarbothiamine

CCTe cathodal closure tetanus

CC-TGA congenitally corrected transposition of great vessels

CC-TOE continuum of care trauma outcome evaluation

CCTP coronary care training program

CCTV closed circuit television

CCU cardiac care unit; Cherry-Crandall unit; coronary care unit; critical care unit

ccua clean catch urinalysis

CCUP colpocystourethropexy

CCV channel catfish virus; conductivity cell volume

CCVD chronic cerebrovascular disease

CCVM congenital cardiovascular malformation

CCW critical care workstation; counterclockwise

CCX cycloxygenase

CD cadaver donor; caldesmon; canine distemper; canine dose; carbohydrate dehydratase; carbon dioxide; cardiac disease; cardiac dullness; cardiac dysrhythmia; cardiovascular disease; Carrel-Dakin [fluid]; Castleman disease; cation-dependent; caudad, caudal; celiac disease; cell dissociation; cervicodorsal; cesarean delivery; chemical dependency; circular dichroism; cluster of differentiation [antigens]; color Doppler; combination drug; common [bile] duct; communicable disease; compact disk; completely denatured; conduct disorder; conduction disorder; conjugata diagonalis; consanguineous donor; contact dermatitis; contagious disease; contrast-detail [imaging]; control diet; controlled drug; conventional dialysis; convulsive disorder; convulsive dose; corneal dystrophy; Cotrel-Dubousset [rod]; Crohn disease; crossed diagonal; curative dose; cutdown; cystic duct

C/D cigarettes per day; cup to disc ratio

C&D cystoscopy and dilatation

Cd cadmium; caudal; coccygeal; condylion

cd candela; caudal

c/d cigarettes per day

CD4 HIV helper cell count

CD8 HIV suppressor cell count

CD$_{50}$ median curative dose

CDA Canadian Dental Association; Certified Dental Assistant; chenodeoxycholic acid; ciliary dyskinesia activity; complement-dependent antibody; completely denatured alcohol; compound document architecture; computer diagnostic assistant; congenital dyserythropoietic anemia

CdA chlorodeoxyadenosine

CDAC Clinical Data Abstraction Center

CDAI Crohn disease activity index

CDAL clinical data analysis laboratory

CDAP continuous distending airway pressure

C&DB cough and deep breath

CDC calculated date of confinement; cancer diagnosis center; capillary diffusion capacity; cell division control; cell division cycle; Centers for Disease Control and Prevention; chenodeoxycholate; children's diagnostic classification; Communicable Disease Center; complement-dependent cytotoxicity

CD-C controlled drinker-control

CDCA chenodeoxycholic acid

CDC-BRFS Centers for Disease Control Behavioral Risk Factor Survey

cDCIS comedo-type ductal carcinoma in situ

CDC NAC Centers for Disease Control and Prevention of AIDS Clearinghouse

CDD certificate of disability for discharge; choledochoduodenostomy; chronic degenerative disease; chronic disabling dermatosis; congenital diaphragmatic defect; contrast-detail-dose [imaging]; craniodiaphyseal dysplasia; current disease descriptions

CDDP cis-diaminedichloroplatinum

CDE canine distemper encephalitis; chlordiazepoxide; color Doppler energy [imaging]; common duct exploration

CDEC Comprehensive Developmental Evaluation Chart

CDER Center for Drug Evaluation and Research; chronic granulomatous disease

CDF chondrodystrophia foetalis; clinical data field; common data format

CDG carbohydrate-deficient glycoprotein syndrome; central developmental groove

CDGE constant denaturant gel electrophoresis

CDGG corneal dystrophy Groenouw type, granular

CDGS carbohydrate-deficient glycoprotein syndrome

cDGS complete form of DiGeorge syndrome

CDH ceramide dihexoside; congenital diaphragmatic hernia; congenital dislocation of hip; congenital dysplasia of hip

CDI cell-directed inhibitor; central or chronic diabetes insipidus; Children's Depression Inventory; clinical data interchange; color Doppler imaging; communicable disease intelligence; cranial diabetes insipidus; cyclin-dependent kinase interactor

CDILD chronic diffuse interstitial lung disease

CDK caldesmon kinase; cell division kinase; climatic droplet keratopathy; cyclin-dependent kinase

CDL chlordeoxylincomycin; Cornelia de Lange [syndrome]

CDLE chronic discoid lupus erythematosus

CDLS Cornelia de Lange syndrome

CDM chemically-defined medium; clinical decision making; common data model

CDMMS chorioretinal dysplasia–microcephaly–mental retardation syndrome

CDMNS clinical decision making in nursing scale

CD-MPR cation-dependent mannose-6-phosphate receptor

cDNA circular deoxyribonucleic acid; complementary deoxyribonucleic acid

CDNANZ Communicable Disease Network of Australia and New Zealand

CDNB 1-chloro-2,4-dinitrobenzene

CDP chondrodysplasia punctata; chronic destructive periodontitis; collagenase-digestible protein; continuous distending pressure; coronary drug project; Council on Dental Practice; cytidine diphosphate; cytosine diphosphate

CDPAS Coronary Disease Prevention with Aspirin Study; Coronary Drug Project Aspirin Study

CDPC cytidine diphosphate choline

CDPR chondrodysplasia punctata, rhizomelic

CDPS calcium-dependent protease small subunit

CDPX X-linked chondrodysplasia punctata

CDR calcium-dependent regulator; clinical data repository; clinical dementia rating; computerized digital radiography; cup/disk ratio

CDRH Center for Devices and Radiological Health

CD-ROM compact disk-read only memory

CDRP clinical database research program

CDRS Children's Depression Rating Scale

CDS cardiovascular surgery; catechol-3, 5-disulfonate; caudal dysplasia syndrome; Chemical Data System; children's diagnostic scale; Christian Dental Society; clinical decision-support; cumulative duration of survival

CDSA common data security architecture

CDSC Communicable Diseases Surveillance Centre [UK]

CDSM Committee on Dental and Surgical Materials

CDSR Cochrane Database of Systematic Reviews

cd-sr candela-steradian

CDSRF chronic disease and sociodemographic risk factors

CDSS clinical decision support system

CDT carbohydrate-deficient transferrin; carbon dioxide therapy; Certified Dental Technician; children's day treatment; *Clostridium difficile* toxin; color discrimination test; combined diphtheria-tetanus [vaccine]

CDTe cathode duration tetanus

CDU cardiac diagnostic unit; clinical decision unit; color Doppler ultrasound

CDV canine distemper virus; clinical diagnostic validity

cDVH cumulative dose-volume histogram

Cdyn, C$_{dyn}$ dynamic compliance

Cdyn, rs dynamic compliance of the respiratory system

CDYS cell dysfunction [UMLS]

CDZ chlordiazepoxide; conduction delay zone

CE California encephalitis; capillary electrophoresis; carboxylesterase; cardiac enlargement; cardioesophageal; carotid endarterectomy; catamenial epilepsy; cataract extraction; cell extract; center-edge [angle]; central episiotomy; chemical energy; chick embryo; chloroform ether; cholesterol esters; chorioepithelioma; chromatoelectrophoresis; ciliated epithelium; cloning efficiency; coded element; coefficient of error; columnar epithelium; conical elevation; conjugated estrogens; constant error; continuing education; contractile element; contrast-enhancement [imaging]; converting enzyme; cornified epithelium; crude extract; cytoplasmic extract; cytopathic effect

Ce cerium

C-E chloroform-ether

CEA carcinoembryonic antigen; carotid endarterectomy; cholesterol-esterifying activity; cost-effectiveness analysis; cranial epidural abscess; crystalline egg albumin; cultured epithelial autograft

CEAC clinical education and assessment center

CEAL carcinoembryonic antigen-like [protein]

CEAP Clinical Efficacy Assessment Project

CEARP Continuing Education Approval and Recognition Program

CEASE Collaborative European Anti-Smoking Evaluation

CEAT chronic ectopic atrial tachycardia

CEB calcium entry blocker

cEBV chronic Epstein-Barr virus [infection]

CEC central echo complex; ciliated epithelial cell; Commission of the European Community

CECCC confidential enquiry into cardiac catheterization complications

CECR cat eye syndrome chromosome region

CECT contrast-enhanced computed tomography

CED chondroectodermal dysplasia

CEDARS Comprehensive Evaluation of Defibrillators and Resuscitative Shock Study

CEE Central European encephalitis; chick embryo extract

CEEA curved end-to-end anastomosis [stapler]

CEEF clinical evaluation encounter form

CEEG computer-analyzed electroencephalography

CEES chloroethyl ethyl sulfide

CEET chicken enucleated eye test

CEEV Central European encephalitis virus

CEF centrifugation extractable fluid; chick embryo fibroblast; constant electric field

CEFA continuous epidural fentanyl anesthesia

CEFMG Council on Education for Foreign Medical Graduates

CEG chronic erosive gastritis

CEH cholesterol ester hydrolase

CEHC calf embryonic heart cell; cost-effective healthcare

CEHO Chief Environmental Health Officer [UK]

CEI character education inquiry; converting enzyme inhibitor

CEI-AMI converting enzyme inhibitor [CEI] in the treatment of acute myocardial infarction [AMI]

CEID crossed electroimmunodiffusion

CEJ cement-enamel junction

CEJA Council on Ethical and Judicial Affairs [American Medical Association]

CEK chick embryo kidney

CEL carboxyl-ester lipase

CELDIC Commission on Emotional and Learning Disorders in Children

CELL Cost Effectiveness of Lipid Lowering [study]

Cell celluloid

CELO chick embryonal lethal orphan [virus]

CELP code excited linear prediction [ECG]

Cels Celsius

CEM care environment management; computerized electroencephalographic map; conventional transmission electron microscope

CEMIA Center for Engineering and Medical Image Analysis

CEMIS community-based environmental management information system

CEN Certificate for Emergency Nursing; Clinical Experience Network [study]; Comité European de Normalisation (standards); continuous enteral nutrition

cen centromere; central

CENMR capillary electrophoresis nuclear magnetic resonance

CENOG computerized electro-neuro-ophthalmography

CENP centromere protein

CENPA centromeric protein A

CENPB centromeric protein B

CENPC centromeric protein C

CENPD centromeric protein D

CENPE centromeric protein E

CENT Committee for European Normalisation

cent centigrade; central

CEO chick embryo origin; Chief Executive Officer

CEOEECP Clinical Evaluation of Enhanced External Counterpulsation

CEOT calcifying epithelial odontogenic tumor

CEP chronic eosinophilic pneumonia; chronic erythropoietic porphyria; congenital erythropoietic porphyria; continuing education program; cortical evoked potential; counter-electrophoresis

CEPA chloroethane phosphoric acid

CEPH cephalic; cephalosporin; Council on Education for Public Health

ceph cephalin

CEPH FLOC cephalin flocculation

CEQ Council on Environmental Quality

CER capital expenditure review; ceramide; conditioned emotional response; control electrical rhythm; cortical evoked response

CERAD Consortium to Establish a Registry for Alzheimer disease

CERCLA The Comprehensive Environmental Response, Compensation, and Liability Act

CERD chronic end-stage renal disease

CERP complex event-related potential; Continuing Education Recognition Program

CERT Cardiovascular Event Reduction Trial; computer emergency response team

Cert, cert certified

cerv cervix, cervical

CES carboxylesterase; cauda equina syndrome; cat's eye syndrome; central excitatory state; chronic electrophysiological study; clinical engineering services; conditioned escape response

CESAR Centralised European Studies in Angina Research

CESARZ Clinical European Studies in Angina and Revascularization

CES-D Center for Epidemiological Studies of Depression [scale]

CESD cholesterol ester storage disease

CESG Cerebral Embolism Study Group [trial]

CESNA Comparative Efficacy and Safety of Nisolpidine and Amlopidine [in hypertension]

CESNA II Comparative Efficacy and Safety of Nisolipidine and Amlopidine [in hypertension with ischemic heart disease]

CESS Cooperative Ewings Sarcoma Study
CET capital expenditure threshold; cholesterol-ester transfer; Collaborative Eclampsia Trial; congenital eyelid tetrad
CETE Central European tick-borne encephalitis
CETP cholesteryl ester transfer protein
CEU congenital ectropion uveae; continuing education unit
CEV California encephalitis virus; *Citrus exocortis* viroid
CEX clinical evaluation exercise
CEZ cefazolin
CF calcaneal fibular [ligament]; calcium leucovorin; calf blood flow; calibration factor; cancer-free; carbol-fuchsin; carbon filtered; carboxyfluorescein; cardiac failure; carotid foramen; carrier-free; cascade filtration; case file; Caucasian female; centrifugal force; characteristic frequency; chemotactic factor; chest and left leg [lead in electrocardiography]; Chiari-Frommel [syndrome]; chick fibroblast; Christmas factor; citrovorum factor; clotting factor; colicin factor; collected fluid; colonization factor; colony forming; complementary feeding; complement fixation; computed fluoroscopy; constant frequency; contractile force; coronary flow; correction factor; cough frequency; count fingers; counting finger; coupling factor; cycling fibroblast; cystic fibrosis
Cf californium
cf centrifugal force; bring together, compare [Lat. *confer*]; confidence factor
CFA cerebello-facio-articular [syndrome]; colonization factor antigen; colony-forming assay; common femoral artery; complement-fixing antibody; complete Freund's adjuvant; configuration frequency analysis; cryptogenic fibrosing alveolitis
CFAG cystic fibrosis antigen
CFB central fibrous body
CFC capillary filtration coefficient; cardiofaciocutaneous [syndrome]; colony-forming capacity; cardiofaciocutaneous [syndrome]; chlorofluorocarbon; colony-forming cell; continuous flow centrifugation
CFD cephalofacial deformity; computational fluid dynamics; craniofacial dysostosis

CF-DA carboxyfluorescein diacetate
CFDS craniofacial dyssynostosis
CFDU color-flow Doppler ultrasonography; color flow Doppler ultrasound
CFF critical flicker fusion [test]; critical fusion frequency; cystic fibrosis factor; Cystic Fibrosis Foundation
cff critical flicker fusion; critical fusion frequency
CFFA cystic fibrosis factor activity
CFH complement factor H; Council on Family Health
CFHL complement factor H-like [protein]
CFHP Council on Federal Health Programs
CFI chemotactic-factor inactivator; closed-clenched fist injury; color flow imaging; complement fixation inhibition
CFM chlorofluoromethane; close-fitting mask; craniofacial microsomia
CFMA Council for Medical Affairs
CFMDB Cystic Fibrosis Mutation Database
CFMG Commission on Foreign Medical Graduates
CFND craniofrontonasal dysostosis; craniofrontonasal dysplasia
CFNS chills, fever, night sweats; craniofrontonasal syndrome
CFO chief financial officer
CFP chronic false positive; Clinical Fellowship Program; culture filtrate protein; cyclophosphamide, fluorouracil, prednisone; cystic fibrosis of pancreas; cystic fibrosis protein
CFPC College of Family Physicians of Canada
CFPP craniofacial pattern profile
CFPR Canadian Familial Polyposis Registry
CFR case-fatality ratio; citrovorum-factor rescue; Code of Federal Regulations; complement-fixation reaction; coronary flow reserve; correct fast reaction; cycloc flow reduction
CFS cancer family syndrome; Chiari-Frommel syndrome; chronic fatigue syndrome; craniofacial stenosis; crush fracture syndrome; culture fluid supernatant; Cystic Fibrosis Society
CFSE crystal field stabilization energy
CFSTI Clearinghouse for Federal Scientific and Technical Information

CFT cardiolipin flocculation test; clinical full time; complement-fixation test

CFTR cystic fibrosis transmembrane conductance regulator

CFU colony-forming unit; coupling factor unit

cfu colony-forming unit

CFU-C CFU$_C$ colony-forming unit, culture

CFU-E, CFU$_E$ colony-forming unit, erythrocyte

CFU-EOS, CFU$_{EOS}$ colony-forming unit, eosinophil

CFU-F, CFU$_F$ colony-forming unit-fibroblastoid

CFU-G, CFU$_G$ colony-forming unit, granulocyte

CFU-GEMM, CFU$_{GEMM}$ colony forming unit, granulocyte, erythrocyte, macrophage, megakaryocyte

CFU-GM, CFU$_{GM}$ colony-forming unit, granulocyte macrophage

CFU-L, CFU$_L$ colony-forming unit, lymphocyte

CFU$_M$ colony-forming unit-megakaryocyte

CFU-MEG, CFU$_{MEG}$ colony-forming unit, megakaryocyte

CFUN cell function [UMLS]

CFU-NM, CFU$_{NM}$ colony-forming unit, neutrophil-monocyte

CFU-S, CFU$_S$ colony-forming unit, spleen; colony-forming unit, stem cells

CFV continuous flow ventilation

CFVS cerebrospinal fluid flow void sign

CFW Carworth farm [mouse], Webster strain

CFWM cancer-free white mouse

CFX cefoxitin; circumflex coronary artery

CFX-MARG marginal branch of the circumflex [coronary] artery

CFZ capillary free zone

CFz clofazimine

CFZC continuous-flow zonal centrifugation

CG cardiography; cardiogreen; central gray matter; choking gas; choriogenic gynecomastia; chorionic gonadotropin; chromogranin; chronic glomerulonephritis; cingulate gyrus; colloidal gold; control group; cryoglobulin; cystine guanine; cytosine-guanine-guanine; phosgene [choking gas]

cg center of gravity; centigram; chemoglobulin

CGA catabolite gene activator; color graphics adapter

CGAB congenital abnormality [UMLS]

CGAS Children's Global Assessment Scale

CGAT Canadian Genome and Technology [program]; chromatin granule amine transformer

CGB chronic gonadotropin, beta-unit

CGD Cattle Genome Database; chronic granulomatous disease

CGDE contact glow discharge electrolysis

CGE capillary gel electrophoresis

CGF cell generating factor

CGFH congenital fibrous histiocytoma

CGFNS Commission on Graduates of Foreign Nursing Schools

CGGE constant gradient gel electrophoresis

CGH chorionic gonadotropic hormone; comparative genome hybridization; congenital generalized hypertrichosis

CGI chronic granulomatous inflammation; Clinical Global Impression [scale]; common gateway interface [of the NCSA]; computer-generated imagery

CGKD complex glycerol kinase deficiency

CGL chronic granulocytic leukemia

c gl correction with glasses

CGM Center for Genetics in Medicine; central gray matter

cgm centigram

CGMC Center for Graphic Medical Communication

CGMMV cucumber green mottle mosaic virus

CGMP current good manufacturing practices

cGMP cyclic guanosine monophosphate

CGN chronic glomerulonephritis

CGNB composite ganglioneuroblastoma

CG/OQ cerebral glucose-oxygen quotient

CGP N-carbobenzoxy-glycyl-L-phenylalanine; chorionic growth hormone-prolactin; choline glycerophosphatide; circulating granulocyte pool; circulatory gene pool

CGRP calcitonin gene-related peptide

cGRP calcitonin gene-related peptide

CGRPR calcitonin gene related peptide receptor

CGS cardiogenic shock; catgut suture; causal genesis syndrome

CGS, cgs centimeter-gram-second [system]

CGT chorionic gonadotropin; cyclodextrin glucanotransferase

CGTT cortisone glucose tolerance test

CGVHD chronic graft-versus-host disease

CGW caregiver workstation

cGy centigray (1 rad)

CH case history; Chediak-Higashi [syndrome]; chiasma; Chinese hamster; chloral hydrate; cholesterol; Christchurch chromosome; chronic hepatitis; chronic hypertension; common hepatic [duct]; communicating hydrocele; community health; community hospital; completely healed; Conradi-Hünermann [syndrome]; continuous heparin [infusion]; cortical hamartoma; crown-heel [length]; cycloheximide; cystic hygroma; wheelchair

CH$_{50}$ 50% hemolyzing dose of complement

C$_H$ constant domain of H chain

C&H cocaine and heroin; coarse and harsh [breathing]

Ch chest; Chido [antibody]; chief; child; choline; Christchurch [syndrome]; chromosome

cH$^+$ hydrogen ion concentration

ch chest; child; chronic

CHA Canadian Hospital Association; Catholic Health Association; Chinese hamster; chronic hemolytic anemia; common hepatic artery; congenital hypoplasia of adrenal glands; congenital hypoplastic anemia; continuously heated acrosol; cyclohexyladenosine; cyclohexylamine

ChA choline acetylase

ChAC choline acetyltransferase

CHAD Cholesterol, Hypertension and Diabetes [study]; cold hemagglutinin disease; cyclophosphamide, hexamethylmelamine, Adriamycin (doxorubicin), and cisplatin

CHAF central hyperalimentation nutrition

CHAID chi-squared automatic interaction detector

CHAMP Cardiac Hospitalization Atherosclerosis Management Program; Children with HIV and Acquired AIDS Model Program; Children's Hospital Automated Medical Program; Combination Hemotherapy and Mortality Prevention [study]

CHAMPUS Civilian Health and Medical Program of Uniformed Services

CHAMPVA Civilian Health and Medical Program of Veterans Administration

CHANDS curly hair–ankylobleph—aron–nail dysplasia syndrome

Chang C Chang conjunctiva cells

CHANGE Chronic Heart Failure and Graded Exercise [study]

Chang L Chang liver cells

CHAOS Cambridge Heart Antioxidant Study; Cardiovascular Disease, Hypertension and Hyperlipidemia, Adult-onset Diabetes, Obesity, and Stroke [study]

CHAP Certified Hospital Admission Program; child health assessment program; Community Health Accreditation Program

CHAPS Carvedilol Heart Attack Pilot Study; 3[3-cholaminopropyl diethylammonio]-1-propane sulfonate

CHARGE coloboma, heart disease, atresia choanae, retarded growth and retarded development and/or CNS anomalies, genital hypoplasia, and ear anomalies and/or deafness [syndrome]

CHARM Candesartan in Heart Failure Assessment in Reduction of Mortality

CHART Continuous Hormones as Replacement Therapy [study]; Continuous Hyperfractionated Accelerated Radiotherapy Trial

CHAS Center for Health Administration Studies; Community Health Assessment Study

CHAT conversational hypertext access technology

ChAT choline acetyltransferase

CHB chronic hepatitis B; complete heart block; congenital heart block

ChB Bachelor of Surgery [Lat. *Chirurgiae Baccalaureus*]

CHBA congenital Heinz body hemolytic anemia

CHBHA congenital Heinz body hemolytic anemia

CHC chromosome condensation; community health center; community health computing; community health council

CH$_3$CCNU semustine

CHCL congenital healed cleft lip

CHCP correctional health care program

CHCS composite health care system

CHCT caffeine/halothane contracture test

CHD Chediak-Higashi disease; childhood disease; chronic hemodialysis; congenital or congestive heart disease; congenital hip dislocation; constitutional hepatic dysfunction; coronary heart disease; cyanotic heart disease

ChD Doctor of Surgery [Lat. *Chirurgiae Doctor*]

CHDM comprehensive hospital drug monitoring

ChE cholinesterase

che a gene involved in chemotaxis

CHEAPER Confirmation that Heparin is an Alternative to Promote Early Reperfusion in Acute Myocardial Infarction [study]

CHEC clearinghouse for emergency aid to the community; community hypertension evaluation clinic

CHED congenital hereditary endothelial dystrophy

CHEER Chest Pain Evaluation in Emergency Room [trial]

CHEF Chinese hamster embryo fibroblast; contour-clamped homologous electric field

CHEM chemical [UMLS]

chem chemistry, chemical; chemotherapy

ChemID Chemical Identification; Chemical Identification File

CHEMLINE Chemical Dictionary On-Line

Chemo chemotherapy

CHEMTREC Chemical Transportation Emergency Center

CHEP cricohyoidoepiglottoplexy

CHEPER Chest Pain Evaluation Registry [study]

CHERSS continuous high-amplitude EEG rhythmical synchronous slowing

CHESS chemical shift selective; Comprehensive or Computerized Health-Enhancement Support System

CHF chick embryo fibroblast; chronic heart failure; congenital hepatic fibrosis; congestive heart failure; Crimean hemorrhagic fever

CHFD controlled high flux dialysis

CHFDT congestive heart failure data tool

CHF-IES Congestive Heart Failure—Italian Epidemiological Study

CHF-STAT Congestive Heart Failure—Survival Trial of Antiarrhythmic Therapy

CHFV combined high-frequency ventilation

chg change, changed

CHGA chromogranin A

CHGB chromogranin B

CHH cartilage-hair hypoplasia

CHHS congenital hypothalamic hamartoma syndrome

CHI closed head injury; consumer health information; creatinine height index

chi chimera

χ Greek letter *chi*

χ^2 chi-squared statistic; chi-squared [test, measure goodness of fit]

χ_m magnetic susceptibility

χ_s electric susceptibility

Chi-A chimpanzee leukocyte antigen

CHIC Cardiovascular Health In Children [study]

CHID Combined Health Information [NIH] Database

CHILD congenital hemidysplasia with ichthyosiform erythroderma and limb defects [syndrome]

CHIM Center for Healthcare Information Management

CHIME College of Healthcare Information Management Executives; coloboma, heart anomaly, ichthyosis, mental retardation, ear abnormality

CHIMS community-based health information system

CHIN community health information network

CHINA chronic infectious neurotropic agent

CHIP child health improvement program; comprehensive health insurance plan; Coronary Health Improvement Project

CHIPASAT Children's Paced Auditory Serial Addition Task

CHIPPA community health planning agency

CHIPS catastrophic health insurance plans

Chir Doct Doctor of Surgery [Lat. *Chirurgiae Doctor*]

chirug surgical [Lat. *chirurgicalis*]

CHIS community health information system

CHL Chinese hamster lung; chlorambucil; chloramphenicol

Chl chloroform; chlorophyll

CHLA cyclohexyl linoleic acid

Chlb chlorobutanol

CHLD chronic hypoxic lung disease

chlor chloride

ChlVPP chlorambucil, vinblastine, procarbazine, prednisone

ChM Master of Surgery [Lat. *Chirurgiae Magister*]

CHMD clinical hyaline membrane disease

CHMIS community health management information system

CHN carbon, hydrogen, and nitrogen; child health nurse; child neurology; Chinese [hamster]; community health nurse

CHNS China Health and Nutrition Survey

CHO carbohydrate; Chinese hamster ovary; chorea; comprehensive health organization

Cho choline

C_{H_2O} water clearance

choc chocolate

CHOICE Caring for Hypertension on Initiation: Cost and Effectiveness [study]; Congestive Heart Failure Mortality: Investigation on Carvedilol's Efficacy

CHOICES Cancer, Heart Disease, Osteoporosis Interventions, and Community Evaluation Studies

CHOIR Center for Health Outcomes Improvement Research

CHOL, chol cholesterol

c hold withhold

CHOP cyclophosphamide, hydroxydaunomycin, Oncovin, and prednisone

CHP capillary hydrostatic pressure; charcoal hemoperfusion; Chemical Hygiene Plan; child psychiatry; Children's Health Project; community health plan; comprehensive health planning; coordinating hospital physician; cutaneous hepatic porphyria

ChP chest physician

CHPA community health planning agency; community health purchasing alliance

chpx chickenpox

CHQ chloroquinol

CHQCP Cleveland Health Quality Choice Project

CHR cerebrohepatorenal [syndrome]

Chr *Chromobacterium*

chr chromosome; chronic

c hr candle hour

c-hr curie-hour

ChRBC chicken red blood cell

CHREF Connecticut Healthcare Research and Education Foundation

CHRIS Cancer Hazards Ranking and Information System

CHRISTMAS Carvedilol Hibernation Reversible Ischemia Trial: Marker of Success

chron chronic

CHRONIC chronic disease, rheumatoid arthritis, neoplasms, infections, cryoglobulinemia [conditions in which rheumatoid factor is produced]

CHRPE congenital hypertrophy of the retinal pigment epithelium

CHRS cerebrohepatorenal syndrome; Christian syndrome

CHS Canada Health Survey; cardiovascular health study; central hypoventilation syndrome; Charleston Heart Study; Chediak-Higashi syndrome; Chinese Health Study; cholinesterase; chondroitin sulfate; community health study; compression hip screw; Congenital Heart Surgeons Society [study]; congenital hypoventilation syndrome; contact hypersensitivity; Copenhagen City Heart Study; coronary heart study

CHSD Children's Health Services Division

CHSO total hemolytic serum C activity

CHSP Clinton Health Security Plan

CHSS cooperative health statistics system

CHT chemotherapy; combined hormone therapy; contralateral head turning

ChTg chymotrypsinogen

ChTK chicken thymidine kinase

CHU closed head unit

CHUSPAN [treatment of] Churg-Strauss Syndrome and Polyarteritis Nodosa [study]

CHV canine herpes virus; centigrade heat unit

CHVF chemically viewed functionally [UMLS]

CHVS chemically viewed structurally [UMLS]

CI cardiac index; cardiac insufficiency; cation-independent; cell immunity; cell inhibition; cephalic index; cerebral infarction; chemical ionization; chemotactic index; chemotherapeutic index; chromatid interchange; chronic infection; clinical investigator; clomipramine; clonus index; cochlear implant; coefficient of intelligence; colloidal iron; color index; confidence interval; contamination index; contextual inquiry; continued insomnia; continuous improvement; continuous infusion; contraindication or contraindicated; convergence insufficiency; coronary insufficiency; corrected count increment; crystalline insulin; cumulative incidence; cytotoxic index

Ci curie

CIA chemiluminescent immunoassay; chymotrypsin inhibitor activity; colony-inhibiting activity; congenital intestinal aganglionosis

CIAIT Chinese Infarction Angiotensin Converting Enzyme Inhibitor Trial

CIBD chronic inflammatory bowel disease

CIBHA congenital inclusion-body hemolytic anemia

CIBIS Cardiac Insufficiency Bisoprolol Study

CIBP chronic intractable benign pain

CIBPS chronic intractable benign pain syndrome

CIC cardioinhibitor center; care improvement council; certification in infection control; circulating immune complex; clean intermittent catheterization; completely in the canal [hearing aid]; computing, information, and communication; constant initial concentration; crisis intervention center

Cic cicletanine

CICA cervical internal carotid artery

CICU cardiac intensive care unit; cardiovascular inpatient care unit; coronary intensive care unit

CID cellular immunodeficiency; center for infectious diseases; charge injection device; chick infective dose; combined immuno-deficiency disease; Cosmetic Ingredient Dictionary; cytomegalic inclusion disease

CID_{50} median chimpanzee infective dose

CIDEMS Center for Information and Documentation

CIDEP chemically induced dynamic electron polarization

CIDI composite international diagnostic interview

CIDNP chemically induced dynamic nuclear polarization

CIDP chronic idiopathic polyradiculopathy; chronic inflammatory demyelinating polyradiculoneuropathy; Clinical Initiatives Development Program

CIDS Canadian Implantable Defibrillator Study; Canadian Internal Defibrillator Study; cellular immunity deficiency syndrome; circular intensity differential scattering; continuous insulin delivery system

CIE Canberra interview for the elderly; cellulose ion exchange; congenital ichthyosiform erythroderma; counter-current immunoelectrophoresis; counterimmuno-electrophoresis; crossed immunoelectrophoresis

CIEP counterimmunoelectrophoresis

CIF cloning inhibitory factor

CIFC Council for the Investigation of Fertility Control

CIG cold-insoluble globulin

CIg intracytoplasmic immunoglobulin

cIgM cytoplasmic immunoglobulin M

CIH carbohydrate-induced hyperglyceridemia; Certificate in Industrial Health; children in hospital

CIHI Canadian Institute for Health Information

CIHR Canadian Institutes of Health Research

ci-hr curie-hour

CIHS central infantile hypotonic syndrome

CII Carnegie Interest Inventory; continuous intravenous infusion

CIIA common internal iliac artery

CIIP chronic idiopathic intestinal pseudo-obstruction

CIIPX [X-linked] chronic idiopathic intestinal pseudo-obstruction

CIM cimetidine; cortically induced movement; Cumulated Index Medicus

Ci/ml curies per milliliter

CI-MPR cation-independent mannose-6-phosphate receptor

CIMS chemical ionization mass spectrometry

CIN central inhibition; cervical intra-epithelial neoplasia; chronic interstitial nephritis; community information network

CIN1, CIN I cervical intraepithelial neoplasia, grade 1 (mild dysplasia)

CIN 2, CIN II cervical intraepithelial neoplasia, grade 2 (moderate-severe)

CIN 3, CIN III cervical intraepithelial neoplasia, grade 3 (severe dysplasia and carcinoma in situ)

C_{in} insulin clearance

CINAHL Cumulative Index to Nursing and Allied Health Literature

CINCA chronic infantile neurological cutaneous and auricular [syndrome]

CINDI Countrywide Integrated Noncommunicable Disease Intervention [study]

CINE chemotherapy-induced nausea and emesis

CINI Computers in Nursing Interactive

CIO chief information officer; corticoid-induced osteoporosis

CIOMS Council for International Organizations of Medical Sciences

CIP care information provision; chronic idiopathic polyradiculoneuropathy; chronic intestinal pseudo-obstruction; Collection de l'Institut Pasteur

CIPC Center for Injury Prevention and Control

CIPD continuous intermittent peritoneal dialysis

CIPF classic interstitial pneumonitis-fibrosis; clinical illness promoting factor

CIPN chronic inflammatory polyneuropathy

CIPSO chronic intestinal pseudo-obstruction

circ circuit; circular; circumcision; circumference

CIREN Crash Injury Research and Engineering Network

CIRF contrast-induced renal failure

CIRSE Cardiovascular and Interventional Radiological Society of Europe

circ & sens circulation and sensation

CIS capacity information system; carcinoma in situ; catheter-induced spasm; central inhibitory state; Chemical Information Service; clinical information system; computer-integrated surgery; continuous interleaved sampler; Coronary Intervention Study; cumulative impairment score

CI-S calculus index, simplified

CiS cingulate sulcus

CISC complex-instructional-set computing

CISCA$_{II}$B$_{IV}$ Cytoxan, Adriamycin, platinum, vinblastine, bleomycin

cis-DPP cisplatin

CISE Computer and Information Science and Engineering [National Science Foundation Directorate]

CISET Committee on International Science, Engineering, and Technology

CISH competitive in situ hybridization

CISP chronic intractable shoulder pain

CIS PT cisplatin

13-cis-RA 13-cis-retinoic acid

CISS chromosome in situ suppression; Common Internet Scheme Syntax

CIT citrate; combined intermittent therapy; conjugated-immunoglobulin technique; crossed intrinsic transfer

cit citrate

CITS Carey infant temperament scale

CITTS Central Illinois Thrombolytic Therapy Study

CIV continuous intravenous infusion

CIVII continuous intravenous insulin infusion

CIXA constant infusion excretory urogram

CJ conjunctivitis

CJA Creutzfeldt-Jakob agent

CJD Creutzfeldt-Jakob disease

CJS Creutzfeldt-Jakob syndrome

CjvO$_2$ jugular venous oxygen content

CK calf kidney; casein kinase; chemokine; chicken kidney; cholecystokinin; choline kinase; contralateral knee; creatine kinase; cyanogen chloride; cytokinin

ck check, checked

CKB creatine kinase, brain type

CKC cold-knife conization

CKD cone-kernal distribution

CKG cardiokymography

CKI cyclin-dependent kinase inhibitor

CKM creatine kinase, muscle type

CKMB creatine kinase, myocardial bound

CKMM creatine kinase, muscle type

CK-PZ cholecystokinin-pancreozymin

CKR chemokine receptor

CKRM clinical knowledge repository manager

CKS classic form of Kaposi sarcoma

CL capillary lumen; cardiolipin; cell line; centralis lateralis; central [venous] line; chemiluminescence; chest and left arm [lead in electrocardiography]; childhood leukemia; cholelithiasis; cholesterol-lecithin; chronic leukemia; cirrhosis of liver; clavicle; clear liquid; clearance; cleft lip; clinical laboratory; clomipramine; complete linkage; complex loading; confidence limit or level; contact lens; corpus luteum; corrected [echo long axis] length; cricoid lamina; criterion level; critical list; cycle length; cytotoxic lymphocyte

C-L consultation-liaison [setting]

C_L constant domain of L chain; lung compliance

Cl chloride; chlorine; clavicle; clear; clinic; *Clostridium*; closure; colistin

cl centiliter; clarified; clean; clear; cleft; clinic; clinical; clonus; clotting; cloudy

CLA cerebellar ataxia; Certified Laboratory Assistant; cervicolinguoaxial; closed loop algorithm [for infusion of catecholamine in heart stress test]; contralateral local anesthesia; cutaneous lichen amyloidosis; cutaneous lymphocyte antigen; cyclic lysine anhydride

Cl-a alternative chloride channel

ClAc chloroacetyl

CLAH congenital lipoid adrenal hyperplasia

CLam cervical laminectomy

CLAS Cholesterol-Lowering Atherosclerosis Study; classification [UMLS]; computerized laboratory alerting system; congenital localized absence of skin

CLASP Collaborative Low-Dose Aspirin Study in Pregnancy; Pre-eclampsia Prevention with Low-Dose Aspirin [study]

CLASS Clomethiazole Acute Stroke Study

class, classif classification

CLASSICS Clopidrogrel Aspirin Stent Interventional Cooperative Study

clav clavicle

CLB chlorambucil; clobazam; curvilinear body

CLBBB complete left bundle branch block

CLBP chronic low back pain

CLC Charcot-Leyden crystal; Clerc-Levy-Critesco [syndrome]

CLCA compact low-chromatin area

CLCD cleidocranial dysostosis

CLCN chloride channel

CL/CP cleft lip/cleft palate

Cl_{cr} creatinine clearance

CLCS colchicine sensitivity

CLD central low density; chloride diarrhea; chronic liver disease; chronic lung disease; congenital limb deficiency; crystal ligand field

CLE congenital lobar emphysema

CLEOPAD Clopidogrel in Peripheral Arterial Disease [study]

CLDH choline dehydrogenase

cldy cloudy

CLE centrilobular emphysema; continuous lumbar epidural [anesthesia]

CLED cystine-lactose-electrolyte-deficient [agar]

CLF cardiolipin fluorescent [antibody]; ceroid lipofuscinosis; cholesterol-lecithin flocculation

CLH chronic lobular hepatitis; cleft limb-heart [syndrome]; corpus luteum hormone; cutaneous lymphoid hyperplasia

CLI complement lysis inhibitor; corpus luteum insufficiency

CLIA Clinical Laboratories Improvement Act

CLIF cloning inhibitory factor; *Crithidia luciliae* immunofluorescence

CLIMS clinical laboratory information management system

clin clinic, clinical

CLINPROT Clinical Cancer Protocols

ClinQuery clinical query

CLINT clinical informatics network

CLIP capitolunate instability pattern; Cholesterol-Lowering Intervention Program; corticotropin-like intermediate lobe peptide

CLIPS C language integrated production system

CLL cholesterol-lowering lipid; chronic lymphatic leukemia; chronic lymphocytic leukemia; cow lung lavage

CLMA Clinical Laboratory Management Association

CLMF cytotoxic lymphocyte maturation factor

CLML Current List of Medical Literature

CLMV cauliflower mosaic virus

CLN ceroid lipofuscinosis

CLO cod liver oil

clo "clothing"—a unit of thermal insulation

CLOF clofibrate

CLON clonidine

Clon *Clonorchis*
CLOS common list processing language object system
Clostr *Clostridium*
CLOT Clinical Perspectives on Lysis of Thrombi [study]
CLOUT Clinical Outcomes with Ultrasound Trial; Core Laboratory Ultrasound Analysis Study
CLP cardiac laboratory panel; cecal ligation and puncture; chymotrypsin-like protein; cleft lip with cleft palate; constraining logic programming; paced cycle length
CL/P cleft lip with or without cleft palate
CL(P) cleft lip without cleft palate
ClP clinical pathology
CLS café-au-lait spot; classical least square; Clinical Laboratory Scientist; Coffin-Lowry syndrome; Cornelia de Lange syndrome
CLSC Centres Locaux de Services Communitaires [Quebec]
CLSE calf lung surfactant extract
CLSH corpus luteum stimulating hormone
CLSL chronic lymphosarcoma (cell) leukemia
CLT Certified Laboratory Technician; chronic lymphocytic thyroiditis; Clinical Laboratory Technician; clot lysis time; clotting time; lung-thorax compliance
CL$_{TB}$ total body clearance
CLT(NCA) Laboratory Technician Certified by the National Certification Agency for Medical Laboratory Personnel
CLU clusterin
CLV cassava latent virus; constant linear velocity
CL VOID clean voided specimen [urine]
CLZ clozapine
CM California mastitis [test]; calmodulin; capreomycin; carboxymethyl; cardiac monitoring; cardiac murmur; cardiac muscle; cardiomyopathy; carpometacarpal; castrated male; Caucasian male; cause of death [Lat. *causa mortis*]; cavernous malformation; cell membrane; center of mass; cerebral malaria; cerebral mantle; cervical mucosa or mucus; Chick-Martin [coefficient]; chloroquinemepacrine; chondromalacia; chopped meat [medium]; chronic meningitis; chylomicron; circular muscle; circulating monocyte; circumferential

measurement; classification-maximization; clindamycin; clinical medicine; clinical modification; coccidioidal meningitis; cochlear microphonic; combined modality; common migraine; complete medium; complications; condition median; conditioned medium; congenital malformation; congestive myocardiopathy; continuous murmur; contrast material; contrast medium; copulatory mechanism; costal margin; cow's milk; cytometry; cytoplasmic membrane; Master of Surgery [Lat. *Chirurgiae Magister*]; narrow-diameter endosseous screw implant [Fr. *crête manche*]
C-M cardiomyopathy
C/M counts per minute
C&M cocaine and morphine
Cm curium; minimal concentration
C$_m$ maximum clearance; membrane capacitance
cM *centi-morgan*
cm centimeter
cm^2 square centimeter
cm^3 cubic centimeter
CMA Canadian Medical Association; Certified Medical Assistant; chronic metabolic acidosis; cow's milk allergy; cultured macrophages
CMAC cerebellar model articulation controller
CMAP compound muscle (or motor) action potential
CMAR cell matrix adhesion regulator
Cmax, C$_{max}$ maximum concentration
CMB carbolic methylene blue; Central Midwives' Board; chloromercuribenzoate
CMBES Canadian Medical and Biological Engineering Society
CMC carboxymethylcellulose; care management continuity; carpometacarpal; cell-mediated cytolysis or cytotoxicity; chemical mismatch cleavage; chloramphenicol; chronic mucocutaneous candidiasis; critical micellar concentration
CMCC chronic mucocutaneous candidiasis
CMCJ carpometacarpal joint
CMCS computer-mediated communication system
CMCt care management continuity across settings
CMD campomelic dysplasia; camptomelic dwarfism; cartilage matrix deficiency; chief

medical director; childhood muscular dystrophy; common mental disorder; comparative mean dose; congenital muscular dystrophy; count median diameter; craniomandibular disorder

cmDNA cytoplasmic membrane-associated deoxyribonucleic acid

CME cervical mediastinal exploration; continuing medical education; Council on Medical Education; crude marijuana extract; cystoid macular edema

CMED central medical emergency dispatch center

CMF calcium-magnesium free; catabolite modular factor; chloromethylfluorescein; chondromyxoid fibroma; Christian Medical Fellowship; cold mitten fraction; cortical magnification factor; craniomandibulofacial; cyclophosphamide, methotrexate, and fluorouracil

CMFDA chloromethylfluorescein diacetate

CMFT cardiolipin microflocculation test

CMFV cyclophosphamide, methotrexate, fluorouracil, and vincristine

CMFVP cyclophosphamide, methotrexate, fluorouracil, vincristine, prednisone

CMG canine or congenital myasthenia gravis; chopped meat glucose [medium]; cystometrography, cystometrogram

CMGN chronic membranous glomerulonephritis

CMGS chopped meat-glucose-starch [medium]; Clinical Molecular Genetics Society

CMGT chromosome-mediated gene transfer

CMH cardiomyopathy, hypertrophic; community mental health [services or program]; congenital malformation of the heart

CMHC community mental health center

C/MHC community/migrant health center

CMHIS Community Mental Health Information System [Canada]

cmH₂O centimeters of water

CMHS Continuous Medicare History Sample

CMI carbohydrate metabolism index; care management integration; case mix index; cell-mediated immunity; cell multiplication inhibition; chronic mesenteric ischemia; circulating microemboli index; colonic motility index; combat medical informatics;

Commonwealth Mycological Institute; computed maxillofacial imaging; Cornell Medical Index

CMID cytomegalic inclusion disease

c/min cycles per minute

CMINET Chinese Medical Information Network

CMIO chief medical information officer

CMIR cell-mediated immune response

CMIS common management information services

CMISP common management information standards/protocol

CMIT Current Medical Information and Terminology

CMJ carpometacarpal joint

CMK chloromethyl ketone; congenital multicystic kidney

CML carboxymethyl lysine; cell-mediated lymphocytotoxicity; cell-mediated lympholysis; central motor latency; chronic myelocytic leukemia; chronic myelogenous leukemia; clinical medical librarian; clinical medical library

c/mL copies per milliliter

CMM cell-mediated mutagenesis; color Doppler M-mode; cutaneous malignant melanoma

cmm cubic millimeter

CMMC cervical myelomeningocele

CMME chloromethyl methyl ether

CMML chronic myelomonocytic leukemia

CMMoL chronic myelomonocytic leukemia

CMMS Columbia Mental Maturity Scale

CMN caudal mediastinal node; certification of medical necessity; cystic medial necrosis

CMNA complement-mediated neutrophil activation

CMN-AA cystic medial necrosis of ascending aorta

CMO cardiac minute output; Chief Medical Officer; comfort measures only; competitive medical organization; corticosterone methyloxidase

cMO centimorgan

CMOL chronic monocytic leukemia

CMOS compatible monolithic conductivity sensor; complementary metal-oxide semiconductor

CMP cardiomyopathy; cartilage matrix protein; chondromalacia patellae; collagen binding protein; competitive medical plan; comprehensive medical plan; cytidine monophosphate

CMPD chronic myeloproliferative disorder

cmpd compound, compounded

CMPGN chronic membranoproliferative glomerulonephritis

cmps centimeters per second

CMR cardiomodulorespirography; cerebral metabolic rate; chief medical resident; common medical record; chylomicron remnant; common mode rejection; cross-reacting material; crude mortality ratio

CMRG cerebral metabolic rate of glucose

CMRGlc combined metabolic rate of glucose

CMR$_{Glu}$ cerebral metabolic rate of glucose

CMRglu cerebral metabolic rate of glucose

CMRL cerebral metabolic rate of lactate

CMRNG chromosomal control of mechanisms of resistance of *Neisseria gonorrhoeae*

CMRO, CMRO$_2$ cerebral metabolic rate of oxygen consumption

CMRR common mode rejection ratio

CMS children's medical services; Christian Medical Society; chronic myelodysplastic syndrome; chromosome modification site; circulation, motion, sensation; clofibrate-induced muscular syndrome; Clyde Mood Scale; complement-mediated solubility; Copenhagen Male Study; cortical magnetic stimulation

cm/s centimeters per second

CMSD congenital myocardial sympathetic dysinnervation

cm/sec centimeters per second

CMSS circulation, motor ability, sensation, and swelling; Council of Medical Specialty Societies

CMT California mastitis test; cancer multistep therapy; catechol methyltransferase; certified medical transcriptionist; cervical motion tenderness; Charcot-Marie-Tooth [syndrome]; chemotherapy; circus movement tachycardia; complex motor unit; continuous memory test; controlled medical terminology; Council on Medical Television; Current Medical Terminology

CMT1 Charcot-Marie-Tooth [disease or neuropathy] type 1

CMTC cutis marmorata telangiectatica congenita

CMTD Charcot-Marie-Tooth disease

CMTIA Charcot-Marie-Tooth [disease or neuropathy] type IA

CMTIB Charcot-Marie-Tooth [disease or neuropathy] type IB

CMTL computer-mediated tutorial laboratory

CMTS Charcot-Marie-Tooth syndrome

CMTX Charcot-Marie-Tooth [syndrome], X-linked

CMU chlorophenyldimethylurea

CMUA continuous motor unit activity

CMV continuous mandatory ventilation; controlled mechanical ventilation; controlled medical vocabulary; conventional mechanical ventilation; cool mist vaporizer; cowpea mosaic virus; cucumber mosaic virus; cytomegalovirus

CMV-E cytomegalovirus encephalitis

CMV-MN cytomegalovirus mononucleosis

CMV-VE cytomegalovirus ventriculoencephalitis

CMX cefmenoxime

CN caudate nucleus; cellulose nitrate; charge nurse; child nutrition; chloroacetophenone; clinical nursing; cochlear nucleus; congenital nystagmus; cranial nerve; Crigler-Najjar [syndrome]; cyanogen; cyanosis neonatorum

C:N calorie:nitrogen [ratio]

C/N carbon/nitrogen [ratio]; carrier/noise [ratio]

CN⁻ cyanide anion

CN I first cranial nerve [olfactory]

CN II second cranial nerve [optic]

CN III third cranial nerve [oculomotor]

CN IV fourth cranial nerve [trochlear]

CN V fifth cranial nerve [trigeminal]

CN VI sixth cranial nerve [abducent]

CN VII seventh cranial nerve [facial]

CN VIII eighth cranial nerve [vestibulocochlear]

CN IX ninth cranial nerve [glossopharyngeal]

CN X tenth cranial nerve [vagus]

CN XI eleventh cranial nerve [accessory]

CN XII twelfth cranial nerve [hypoglossal]

CNA calcium nutrient agar; Canadian Nurses Association; certified nursing assistant

CNAF chronic nonvalvular atrial fibrillation

CNAG chronic narrow angle glaucoma

CNAP career nurse assistants' programs; compound nerve action potential

CNB cutting needle biopsy

CNBP cellular nucleic acid binding protein

CNC community nursing center

CNCbl cyanocobalamin

CNCC certified nurse in critical care

CND care need determination

CNDC chronic nonspecific diarrhea of childhood; chronic nonsuppurative destructive cholangitis

CNDI congenital nephrogenic diabetes insipidus

CNE chief nurse executive; chronic nervous exhaustion; concentric needle electrode

CNES chronic nervous exhaustion syndrome

C_{NET} net compliance

CNF chronic nodular fibrositis; congenital nephrotic syndrome of the Finnish [type]

CNFS craniofrontonasal syndrome

CNGC cyclic nucleotide gated channel

CNH central neurogenic hyperpnea; community nursing home

CNHD congenital nonspherocytic hemolytic disease

CNI center of nuclear image; chronic nerve irritation; community nutrition institute

CNIDR Clearinghouse for Networked Information Discovery and Retrieval

CNIS complex nonlinear least square; computerized nursing information system

CNK cortical necrosis of kidneys

CNL cardiolipin natural lecithin; chronic neutrophilic leukemia

CNM centronuclear myopathy; Certified Nurse-Midwife; combinatorial neural model; computerized nuclear morphometry

CNMDSA community nursing minimum data set, Australia

CNMT Certified Nuclear Medicine Technologist

CNO community nursing organization

cNOS constitutive nitric oxide synthase

CNP community nurse practitioner; continuous negative pressure; cranial nerve palsy; C-type natriuretic peptide; 2',3'-cyclic nucleotide 3'-phosphodiesterase

CNPase 2',3'-cyclic nucleotide 3'-phosphohydrolase

CNPV continuous negative pressure ventilation

CNQX 6-cyano-7-nitroquinoxaline-2,3-dione

CNR cannabinoid receptor; Center for Nursing Research; contrast-to-noise ratio; Council of Nurse Researchers

CNRC Children's Nutrition Research Center

CNRT corrected sinus node recovery time

CNS central nervous system; clinical nurse specialist; coagulase-negative staphylococci; congenital nephrotic syndrome; cutaneous nerve stimulator; sulfocyanate

CNSHA congenital nonspherocytic hemolytic anemia

CNS-L central nervous system leukemia

CNSLD chronic nonspecific lung disease

CNST coagulase-negative staphylococci

CNTF ciliary neutrophilic factor

CNTFR ciliary neutrophilic factor receptor

CNTHM conotruncal heart malformation

CNV choroidal neovascularization; contingent negative variation; cutaneous necrotizing vasculitis

CO carbon monoxide; cardiac output; castor oil; casualty officer; centric occlusion; cervical orthosis; cervicoaxial; choline oxidase; coccygeal; coenzyme; compound; control; corneal opacity; cross over; cyclophosphamide and vincristine

C/O check out; complains of; in care of

c/o complains of

CO_2 carbon dioxide

Co cobalt

Co I coenzyme I

Co II coenzyme II

COA Canadian Ophthalmological Association; Canadian Orthopaedic Association; certificate of authority; cervico-oculo-acusticus [syndrome]; condition on admission

CoA coenzyme A

COACH Canadian Organization for the Advancement of Computers in Health; cerebellar vermis hypoplasia/aplasia-oligophrenia-congenital ataxia-ocular colobomata-hepatic fibrosis [syndrome]

COAD chronic obstructive airway disease; clinician-oriented access to data

COAG chronic open angle glaucoma

coag coagulation, coagulated

COAL chronic obstructive airflow limitation

COAP cyclophosphamide, cytosine arabinose, vincristine, prednisone

coarct coarctation

CoASH uncombined coenzyme A

CoA-SPC coenzyme A-synthetizing protein complex

COAT Children's Orientation and Amnesia Test; Cooperative Osaka Adenosine Trial

COB chronic obstructive bronchitis; coordination of benefits

COBALT Continuous Infusion vs Bolus Alteplase Trial; Continuous Infusion vs Double-Bolus Administration of Alteplase

coban cohesive bandage

COBOL common business oriented language

COBRA common object request broker architecture; Comparison of Balloon vs Rotational Angioplasty; computer-operated birth defect recognition aid; Consolidated Omnibus Reconciliation Act

COBS cesarean-obtained barrier-sustained; chronic organic brain syndrome

COBT chronic obstruction of the biliary tract

COC cathodal opening contraction; coccygeal; combination oral contraceptive; commission on cancer

COCI Consortium on Chemical Information

COCl cathodal opening clonus

COCM congestive cardiomyopathy

COCP combined oral contraceptive pill

COCS Cornell-Oxford China Study

COD cause of death; cerebro-ocular dysplasia; chemical oxygen demand; codeine; collaborative organization design; condition on discharge

cod codeine

COD-MD cerebro-ocular dysplasia-muscular dystrophy [syndrome]

CODAS cerebro-oculo-dento-auriculo-skeletal [syndrome]

CODATA Committee on Data for Science and Technology

CODEC compression and decompression

CODS Charnes organizational diagnosis survey

coeff coefficient

COEPS cortical originating extra-pyramidal system

COER controlled onset, extended release

COF cutoff frequency

CoF cobra factor; cofactor

C of A coarctation of the aorta

COFS cerebro-oculo-facial-skeletal [syndrome]

COG center of gravity; cognitive function tests

CoGME Council on Graduate Medical Education

COGTT cortisone oral glucose tolerance test

COH carbohydrate; controlled ovarian hyperstimulation

CoHb carboxyhemoglobin

CoHgb carboxyhemoglobin

COHN Certified Occupational Health Nurse

COHR computer-based oral health record

COHSE Confederation of Health Service Employees

COI Central Obesity Index; certificate of insurance; conflict of interest; cost of illness

COIF congenital onychodysplasia of the index finger

COL central object library; colposcopy

col collection; colicin; collagen; colony; colored; column; strain [Lat. *cola*]

COLD chronic obstructive lung disease; computer output on laser disk

COLD A cold agglutinin titer

coll collateral; collection, collective; college; colloidal

collat collateral

COLTS Coronary Observational Long-Term Study

COM chronic otitis media; College of Osteopathic Medicine; component object model; computer-output microfilm

CoM center of noise

com comminuted; commitment

COMA Committee on Medical Aspects [food and nutrition]

COMAC/HRS/QA Community Concerted Action Programme on Quality Assurance in Health Care [European]

comb combination, combine

COMC carboxymethylcellulose

COME chronic otitis media with effusion

COMET Carvedilol or Metoprolol European Trial; Carvedilol or Metoprolol Evaluation Trial

comf comfortable

CoMFA comparative molecular shape analysis

comm, commun communicable

COMMIT Community Intervention Trial [for Smoking Cessation]; Comprehensive Multidisciplinary Interventional Trial [for Regression of Coronary Heart Disease]

COMP cartilage oligomeric matrix protein; complication; cyclophosphamide, vincristine, methotrexate, prednisone

comp comparative; compensation, compensated; complaint; complete; composition; compound, compounded; comprehension; compress; computer

COMPASS Comparative Trial of Saruplase vs Streptokinase; Computerized Online Medicaid Pharmaceutical Analysis and Surveillance System

compd compound, compounded

compl complaint; complete, completed, completion; complication, complicated

complic complication, complicated

compn composition

compr compression

COMS cerebrooculomuscular syndrome

comp stud comparative study

COMT catecholamine O-methyl transferase; certified ophthalmic medical technologist

COMTRAC computer-based case tracing

COMUL complement fixation murine leukosis [test]

CON certificate of need

Con concanavalin

con against [Lat. *contra*]; continuation, continue

Con A concanavalin A

Con A-HRP concanavalin A-horseradish peroxidase

CONC conceptual entity [UMLS]

c-onc cellular oncogene

conc, concentr concentrate, concentrated, concentration

COND cerebro-osteo-nephrodysplasia

cond condensation, condensed; condition, conditioned; conductivity; conductor

conf conference; confined; confinement; confusion

cong congested, congestion; gallon [Lat. *congius*]

congen congenital

CongHD congenital heart disease

coniz conization

conj conjunctiva, conjunctival

conjug conjugated, conjugation

CONPA-DRI I vincristine, doxorubicin, and melphalan

CONPA-DRI III conpa-dri I plus intensified doxorubicin

CONQUEST Computerized Needs-Oriented Quality Measurement Evaluation System

CONS coagulase-negative *Staphylococcus;* consultation; consultant

cons conservation; conservative; consultation

CONSENSUS Cooperative North Scandinavian Enalapril Survival Study

CONSORT Consolidated Standards of Reporting Trials

const constant

constit constituent

consult consultant, consultation

CONSUME Compliance of National Supplements Using Multiform Energy Sources [study]

cont against [Lat. *contra*]; bruised [Lat. *contusus*]; contains, contents; continue, continuation

contag contagion, contagious

contr contracted, contraction

contra contraindicated

contralat contralateral

contrib contributory

conv convalescence, convalescent, convalescing; convergence, convergent; convulsions, convulsive

converg convergence, convergent

CONVINCE Controlled Onset Verapamil Investigation for Cardiovascular Endpoints [study]; Controlled Onset Verapamil Investigation of Clinical Endpoints [study]

COO chief operating officer; cost of ownership [analysis]

COOD chronic obstruction outflow disease

COOH carboxy group; carboxy terminus

COOHTA Canadian Coordinating Office for Health Technology Assessment

COOP charts for primary care practices; cooperative

coord coordination, coordinated

COP capillary osmotic pressure; change of plaster; coefficient of performance; colloid oncotic pressure; colloid osmotic pressure; cryptogenic organizing pneumonitis; cyclophosphamide, Oncovin, and prednisone

COPA Council on Postsecondary Accreditation

COPAD cyclophosphamide, vincristine, Adriamycin, prednisone, cytarabine, asparagine, intrathecal methotrexate

COPC community oriented primary care

COPD chronic obstructive pulmonary disease

COPE chronic obstructive pulmonary emphysema

COPEM Committee on Pediatric Emergency Medicine

COPERNICUS Carvedilol Prospective Randomized Cumulative Survival [trial]

COP$_i$ colloid osmotic pressure in interstitial fluid

COPP cyclophosphamide, vincristine, procarbazine, prednisone; cyclophosphamide, Oncovin, procarbazine, prednisone

COP$_p$ colloid osmotic pressure in plasma

COPRO coproporphyrin; coproporphyrinogen

COPT circumoval precipitin reaction test; computerized oxygen therapy protocol

COPV canine oral papillomavirus

CoQ coenzyme Q

COR cardiac output recorder; comprehensive outpatient rehabilitation; conditional origin of replication; conditioned orientation reflex; consensual ophthalmotonic reaction; corrosion, corrosive; cortisone; cortex; crude odds ratio; custodian of records

CoR Congo red

cor body [Lat. *corpus*]; coronary; correction, corrected

CORA conditioned orientation reflex audiometry

CORALI coronarography and alimentation

CORAMI Cohort of Rescue Angioplasty in Myocardial Infarction

CORBA Common Object Request Broker Architecture

CORD Commissioned Officer Residency Deferment; Council of [Emergency Medicine] Residency Directors

CORDIS Cardiovascular Occupational Risk Factor Determination in Israel [study]

CORE Center for Organ Recovery and Education; Collaborative Organization for RheothRx Evaluation; comprehensive assessment and referral evaluation; concept reference

CORGENE Coronary Disease and Angiotensin Converting Enzyme I/D Genotype [study]

CORIS Coronary Risk Factor Study

CorPP coronary perfusion pressure

corr correspondence, corresponding

CORRECT Complete vs Restrictive Revascularization by Coronary Angioplasty Trial

CORSICA Chronic Occlusion Revascularization with Stent Implantation vs Coronary Angioplasty [study]

CORT corticosterone

cort bark [Lat. *cortex*]; cortex

CORTES Clivarin Assessment of Regression of Thrombus: Efficacy and Safety [study]; coordinate reduction time encoding system [ECG]

COS cheiro-oral syndrome; chief of staff; Clinical Orthopaedic Society; clinically observed seizures

CoS class of service

COSATI Committee on Scientific and Technical Information

COSHH Control of Substances Hazardous to Health Regulations [UK]

COSMIS Computer System for Medical Information Systems

COSSMHO [National] Coalition of Hispanic Health and Human Services Organizations

COST Cardiac Output Study Technology

COSTAR Computer-Stored Ambulatory Record

COSTART Common Standard Thesaurus of Adverse Reaction Terms

COSTEP Commissioned Officer Student Training and Extern Program

COSY correlated spectroscopy

COT colony overlay test; committee on trauma; content of thought; contralateral optic tectum; critical off-time

COTA Certified Occupational Therapy Assistant

COTAIM Continuation of Trial Antihypertensive Interventions and Management

COTD cardiac output by thermodilution

COTe cathodal opening tetanus

COTH Council of Teaching Hospitals and Health Systems

COTRANS Coordinated Transfer Application System

COTS commercial off-the-shelf [software or hardware]

COU cardiac observation unit

coul coulomb

COURAGE Clinical Outcomes Using Revascularization vs Aggressive Strategies; Clinical Outcomes Utilization Revascularization and Aggressive Drug Evaluation

COURT Contrast Media Utilization in High-Risk Percutaneous Transluminal Coronary Angioplasty [trial]

COV covariance; cross-over value

COVER Cover of Vaccination Evaluated Rapidly [UK]

COVESDEM costovertebral segmentation defect with mesomelia [syndrome]

CoVF cobra venom factor

COWS cold to opposite and warm to same side

COX cytochrome c oxidase; cyclooxygenase

CP candle power; capillary pressure; cardiac pacing; cardiac performance; cardiopulmonary; caudate putamen; cell passage; central pit; cephalic presentation; cerebellopontine; cerebral palsy; ceruloplasmin; chemically pure; chest pain; child psychiatry; child psychology; *Chlamydia pneumoniae*; chloropurine; chloroquine-primaquine; chondrodysplasia punctata; choroid plexus; chronic pain; chronic pancreatitis; chronic polyarthritis; chronic pyelonephritis; cicatricial pemphigoid; cleft palate; clinical pathology; clock pulse; closing pressure; cochlear potential; code of practice; cold pressor; color perception; combining power; compound; compressed; congenital porphyria; constant pressure; constrictive pericarditis; coproporphyrin; cor pulmonale; coracoid process; C peptide; creatine phosphate; creatine phosphokinase; cross-linked protein; crude protein; current practice; cyclophosphamide; cyclophosphamide and prednisone; cytosol protein; [viral] coat protein

C&P compensation and pension; complete and pain free [joint movement]; cystoscopy and pyelography

C/P cholesterol-phospholipid [ratio]

C+P cryotherapy with pressure

Cp ceruloplasmin; chickenpox; *Corynebacterium parvum;* peak concentration

C$_p$ constant pressure; phosphate clearance

cP centipoise

cp candle power; chemically pure; centipoise; compare

c$_p$ constant pressure

CPA Canadian Physiotherapy Association; Canadian Psychiatric Association; carboxypeptidase A; cardiopulmonary arrest; carotid phonoangiography; cerebellopontine angle; chlorophenylalanine; circulating platelet aggregate; complement proactivator; control, preoccupation, and addiction; costophrenic angle; cyclophosphamide; cyproterone acetate

C3PA complement-3 proactivator

CPAF chlorpropamide-alcohol flushing

C$_{pah}$ para-aminohippurate clearance

CP-ANN counterpropagation artificial neural network;

CPAP continuous positive airway pressure

CPAS Canadian Prinivil Atenolol Study

CPB carboxypeptidase B; cardiopulmonary bypass; cetylpyridinium bromide; competitive protein binding

CPBA competitive protein-binding analysis

CPBV cardiopulmonary blood volume

CPC central posterior curve; cerebellar Purkinje cell; cerebral palsy clinic; cerebral performance category; cetylpyridinium chloride; chest pain center; child protection center; chronic passive congestion; circumferential pneumatic compression; clinicopathological conference

CPCL congenital pulmonary cystic lymphangiectasia

CPCP chronic progressive coccidioidal pneumonitis

CPCR cardiopulmonary cerebral resuscitation

CPCS circumferential pneumatic compression suit; computer-based patient case simulation system

CPD calcium pyrophosphate deposition; cephalopelvic disproportion; cerebelloparenchymal disorder; childhood or congenital polycystic disease; chorioretinopathy and pituitary dysfunction; chronic peritoneal dialysis; chronic protein deprivation; citrate-phosphate-dextrose; contact potential difference; contagious pustular dermatitis; critical point drying; cyclobutane pyrimidine dimer; cyclopentadiene

cpd cigarettes per day; compound; cycles per degree

CPDA citrate-phosphate-dextrose-adenine

CPDD calcium pyrophosphate deposition disease; cis-platinum-diamine dichloride

cpd E compound E

cpd F compound F

CPDL cumulative population doubling level

CPDX cefpodoxime

CPDX-PR cefpodoxime proxetil

CPE cardiac pulmonary edema; chronic pulmonary emphysema; clinical progress exercise; compensation, pension, and education; complete physical examination; complicated pleural effusion; corona-penetrating enzyme; cytopathogenic effect

CPEO chronic progressive external ophthalmoplegia

CPEP Chicago Coronary Prevention Evaluation Program; clinical practice enhancement project

CPF clot-promoting factor; complication probability factor; contraction peak force; current patient file

CPG capillary blood gases; cardiopneumographic recording; carotid phonoangiogram; central pattern generator; clinical practice guidelines; computerized pattern generator

CPGN chronic proliferative glomerulonephritis

CPGs clinical practice guidelines

CPH Certificate in Public Health; chronic paroxysmal hemicrania; chronic persistent hepatitis; chronic primary headache; corticotropin-releasing hormone

CPHA Canadian Public Health Association; Commission on Professional and Hospital Activities

CPHA-PAS Commission on Professional and Hospital Activities—Professional Activity Study

CPHL Central Public Health Laboratory [UK]

CPHQ certified professional in healthcare quality

CPHRP Coronary Prevention and Hypertension Research Project

CPHS Centre for Public Health Sciences

CPI California Personality Inventory; Cancer Potential Index; common patient index; congenital palatopharyngeal incompetence; constitutional psychopathic inferiority; coronary prognosis index; cysteine proteinase inhibitor

CPIB chlorophenoxyisobutyrate

CPIP chronic pulmonary insufficiency of prematurity

CPIJH compass proximal interphalangeal joint hinge

CPIR cephalic-phase insulin release

CPK cell population kinetic [model]; creatine phosphokinase

CPK-BB creatine phosphokinase, brain-type

CPKD childhood polycystic kidney disease

CPL caprine placental lactogen; conditioned pitch level; congenital pulmonary lymphangiectasia

C/PL cholesterol/phospholipid [ratio]

cpl complete, completed

CPLM cysteine-peptone-liver infusion medium

CPLS cleft palate-lateral synechia syndrome

CPM calorie-protein malnutrition; central pontine myelinosis; chlorpheniramine maleate; confidence profile method; confined placental mosaicism; continuous passive motion; critical path method; cyclophosphamide

CP/M control program for microcomputers

C_{PM} circumference of papillary muscle

cpm counts per minute; cycles per minute

CPMG Carr-Purcell-Meiboom-Gill [sequence]

CPMP Committee for Proprietary Medicinal Products [EEC]; complete patient management problems

CPMS chronic progressive multiple sclerosis

CPMV cowpea mosaic virus

CPN causal probabilistic network; central parenteral nutrition; chronic polyneuropathy; chronic pyelonephritis

CPNE clinical performance nursing examination

CPNM corrected perinatal mortality

CPO contract provider organization; coproporphyrinogen oxidase

C-PORT Cardiovascular Patient Outcomes Research Team [trial]

CPOS chest pain order sheet

CPOTHA chest pain onset to hospital arrival

CPOU chest pain observation unit

CPP cancer proneness phenotype; canine pancreatic polypeptide; cerebral perfusion pressure; chest pain policy; dl-2[3-(2'-chlorophenoxy)phenyl] propionic [acid]; chronic pigmented purpura; coronary perfusion pressure; cyclopentenophenanthrene

CPPB continuous positive pressure breathing

CPPD calcium pyrophosphate dihydrate deposition [syndrome]; cisplatin; cost per patient day

CPPT Coronary Primary Prevention Trial

CPPV continuous positive pressure ventilation

CPQA certified professional in quality assurance

CPR cardiopulmonary reserve; cardiopulmonary resuscitation; centripetal rub; cerebral cortex perfusion rate; chlorophenyl red; computerized patient record; cortisol production rate; cumulative patency rate; customary, prevailing and reasonable [rate]

c-PR cyclopropyl

cpr computerized patient record

CPRAM controlled partial rebreathing anesthesia method

CPRCA constitutional pure red cell aplasia

CPRD Committee on Prosthetics Research and Development

CPRG Coronary Prevention Research Group

CPRI Computerized Patient Record Institute

CPRO coproporphyrinogen oxidase

CPRS Children's Psychiatric Rating Scale; Comprehensive Psychopathological Rating Scale; computerized patient record system

CPS Caerphilly Prospective Study; Cancer Prevention Study; carbamoylphosphate synthetase; cardioplegic perfusion solution; cardiopulmonary support; center for preventive services; centipoise; cervical pain syndrome; characters per second; chest pain syndrome; Child Personality Scale; Child Protective Services; chloroquine, pyrimethamine, and sulfisoxazole; chronic prostatitis syndrome; clinical performance score; Clinical Pharmacy Services; coagulase-positive *Staphylococcus*; complex partial seizures; concurrent planning system; constitutional psychopathic state; contagious pustular stomatitis; coronary perfusate solution; C-polysaccharide; cumulative probability of success; current population survey

cps counts per second; cycles per second

CPSA charged particle surface area

CPSC congenital paucity of secondary synaptic clefts [syndrome]; Consumer Products Safety Commission

CPSM Council for Professions Supplementary to Medicine

CPSO College of Physicians and Surgeons of Ontario

CPSP central poststroke pain

CPSTS Chinese Poststroke Treatment Study

CPT campothecin; carnitine palmityl transferase; carotid pulse tracing; chest physiotherapy; child protection team; ciliary particle transport; cold pressor test; combining power test; complex physical therapy; continuous performance task; continuous performance test; Current Procedural Terminology

CPTH chronic post-traumatic headache

CPTN culture-positive toxin-negative

CPTP culture-positive toxin-positive

CPTX chronic parathyroidectomy

CPU caudate putamen; central processing unit

CPUE chest pain of unknown etiology

CPV canine parvovirus; cytoplasmic polyhedrosis virus

CPVC common pulmonary venous channel

CPVD congenital polyvalvular disease

CPX cleft palate, X-linked; clinical practice examination; complete physical examination

CPXD chondrodysplasia punctata, X-linked dominant

CPXR chondrodysplasia punctata, X-linked recessive

CPZ cefoperazone; chlorpromazine; Compazine

CQ chloroquine; chloroquine-quinine; circadian quotient; conceptual quotient

CQI continuous quality improvement

CQIN clinical quality improvement network

CQI/TQM continuous quality improvement/total quality management

CQM chloroquine mustard

CQMS cost quality management system

CR calculation rate; calculus removed; calorie-restricted; cardiac rehabilitation; cardiac resuscitation; cardiac rhythm; cardiorespiratory; cardiorrhexis; caries-resistant; cathode ray; cellular receptor; centric relation; chemoradiation; chest and right arm [lead in electrocardiography]; chest roentgenogram, chest roentgenography; chief resident; child-resistant [bottle top]; choice reaction; chromium; chronic rejection; clinical record; clinical remission; clinical research; clot retraction; coefficient of fat retention; colon resection; colonization rate; colonization resistance; colony reared [animal]; colorectal; complement receptor; complete remission; complete response; compression ratio; computed radiography; computerized record; conditioned reflex, conditioned response; congenital rubella; Congo red; controlled release; controlled respiration; conversion rate; cooling rate; cortico-resistant; creatinine; cremaster reflex; cresyl red; critical ratio; crown-rump [measurement]

CR1 complement receptor type 1

C&R convalescence and rehabilitation

Cr chromium; cranium, cranial; creatinine; crown

CRA central retinal artery; Chinese restaurant asthma; chronic rheumatoid arthritis; constant relative alkalinity

CRABP cellular retinoic acid-binding protein

CRAC compliance-related acute complication

CRAD central retinal artery occlusion

CRADA Cooperative Research and Development Agreement [Army and NIH]

CRAFT Catheterization Rescue Angioplasty Following Thrombolysis [trial]; Controlled Randomized Atrial Fibrillation Trial

CRAG *Cryptococcus* antigen

CRAHCA Center for Research in Ambulatory Health Care Administration

CRAMS circulation, respiration, abdomen, motor, speech

cran cranium, cranial

CRAO central retinal artery occlusion

CRASH corpus callosum hypoplasia–retardation–adducted thumbs–spastic paraplegia–hydrocephalus [syndrome]

CRAW computed tomography acquisition workstation

CRB chemical, radiological, and biological; congenital retinal blindness; Cramer-Rao bound

CRBBB complete right bundle branch block

CRBC chicken red blood cell

CRBP cellular retinol-binding protein

CRC calcium release channel; cancer research campaign; cardiovascular reflex clinical research center; colorectal cancer; colorectal carcinoma; concentrated red blood cells; conditioning; contrast recovery coefficient; cross-reacting cannabinoids; cyclic redundancy check

CrCl creatinine clearance

CRCS cardiovascular reflex conditioning system

CRD carbohydrate-recognition domain; chronic renal disease; chronic respiratory disease; child restraint device; childhood rheumatic disease; chorioretinal degeneration; chronic renal disease; chronic respiratory disease; complete reaction of degeneration; complex repetitive discharge; cone-rod retinal dystrophy; congenital rubella deafness; crown-rump distance

CRDC Central Research and Development Committee

CR-DIP chronic relapsing demyelinating inflammatory polyneuropathy

CRDS Charles River Data System; client response documentation system

CRE cumulative radiation effect; creatinine; cyclic adenosine monophosphate-response element

creat creatinine

CREATE Cholesterol Research Education and Treatment Evaluation

CREB cyclic adenosine monophosphate responsive element-binding [protein]

CREDO Clopidogrel Reduction of Events During Extended Observation [study]

CREM center for rural emergency medicine; cyclic adenosine monophosphate-response element modulator

crem cremaster

CREOG Council on Resident Education in Obstetrics and Gynecology

crep crepitation; crepitus

CREST calcinosis, Raynaud phenomenon, esophageal involvement, sclerodactyly, and telangiectasia [syndrome]; Carotid Revascularization and Endarterectomy vs Stent Trial

CREW Coronary Regression with Estrogen in Women [study]

CRF case report form; chronic renal failure; chronic respiratory failure; coagulase-reacting factor; continuous reinforcement; corticotropin-releasing factor; cytokine receptor family

CRFK Crandell feline kidney cells

CRFR corticotropin-releasing factor receptor

CRG cardiorespirogram; central respiratory generator; collaborative review group

CRH corticotropin-releasing hormone

CRHBP corticosterone-releasing hormone binding protein

CRHL Collaborative Radiological Health Laboratory

CRHV cottontail rabbit herpes virus

CRI Cardiac Risk Index; catheter-related infection; chronic renal insufficiency; chronic respiratory insufficiency; Composite Risk Index; congenital rubella infection; corneal relaxing incision; cross-reaction idiotype

C-RI corecessive inheritance

CRIB clinical risk index for babies

CRIE crossed radioimmunoelectrophoresis

CRIP cysteine-rich intestinal protein

CRIS Calcium Antagonist Reinfarction Italian Study; clinically related information system

CRISP Cholesterol Reduction in Seniors Program [pilot study]; Computer Retrieval of Information on Scientific Projects [NIH database]; Consortium Research in Systems Performance; Consortium Research on Indicators of System Performance

Crit, crit critical; hematocrit

CRIYFS Cardiovascular Risk in Young Finns Study

CRL cell repository line; Certified Record Librarian; complement receptor location; complement receptor lymphocyte; crown-rump length

CRM Certified Reference Materials; counting rate meter; cross-reacting material; crown-rump measurement

CRM⁺ cross-reacting material-positive

CRMO chronic recurrent multifocal osteomyelitis

CRN complement requiring neutralization

CRNA Certified Registered Nurse Anesthetist

CRNF chronic rheumatoid nodular fibrositis

Cr Nn, cr nn cranial nerves

CRO cathode ray oscilloscope; centric relation occlusion; contract research organization

CROM cervical range of motion

CROME congenital cataracts-epileptic fits-mental retardation [syndrome]

CROP compliance, rate, oxygenation, and pressure

CROS contralateral routing of signals [hearing aid]

CRP chronic relapsing pancreatitis; corneal-retinal potential; coronary rehabilitation program; C-reactive protein; cross-reacting protein; cyclic adenosine monophosphate receptor protein; cysteine-rich protein

CrP creatine phosphate

CRPA C-reactive protein antiserum

CRPD chronic restrictive pulmonary disease

CRPF chloroquine-resistant *Plasmodium falciparum;* closed reduction and percutaneous fixation; contralateral renal plasma flow

CRPG central respiratory pattern generator

CRPS complex regional pain syndrome [type I and II]

CRPV cottontail rabbit papilloma virus

CRRN certified rehabilitation registered nurse

CRRT continuous renal replacement therapy

CrRT cranial radiotherapy

CRS Carroll rating scale for depression; catheter-related sepsis; caudal regression syndrome; cervical spine radiography;

Chinese restaurant syndrome; cis-acting repressive sequence; colon and rectum surgery; compliance of the respiratory system; congenital rubella syndrome; craniosynostosis; cryptidin-related sequence

CRSM cherry red spot myoclonus

CRSP comprehensive renal scintillation procedure

CRST calcinosis, Raynaud phenomenon, sclerodactyly, telangiectasia [syndrome]; corrected sinus recovery time

CRT cardiac resuscitation team; cathode-ray tube; certified; Certified Record Techniques; choice reaction time; chromium release test; complex reaction time; conformal radiation therapy; copper reduction test; corrected; corrected retention time; cortisone resistant thymocyte; cranial radiation therapy

crt hematocrit

CRTM cartilage matrix protein

CRTP Consciousness Research and Training Project

CRTT Certified Respiratory Therapy Technician

CRU cardiac rehabilitation unit; clinical research unit

CRUISE Can Routine Ultrasound Influence Stent Expansion? [study]

CRUSADE Coronary Reserve Utilization for Stent and Angiography: Doppler Endpoint [study]; Coronary Revascularization Ultrasound Angioplasty Device [trial]

CRV central retinal vein

CRVF congestive right ventricular failure

CRVO central retinal vein occlusion

CRYG gamma crystallin gene

CRYM crystallin

cryo cryogenic; cryoglobulin; cryoprecipitate; cryosurgery; cryotherapy

Cryoppt cryoprecipitate

CRYP cryptospiridiosis

crys, cryst crystal, crystaline

CS calf serum; campomelic syndrome; canalicular system; Capgras syndrome; carcinoid syndrome; cardiogenic shock; caries-susceptible; carotid sheath; carotid sinus; cat scratch; celiac sprue; central service; central supply; cerebral scintigraphy; cerebrospinal; cervical spine; cervical stimulation; cesarean section; chest strap; chief of staff; cholesterol stone; cholesterol

sulfate; chondroitin sulfate; chorionic somatomammotropin; chronic schizophrenia; cigarette smoker; citrate synthase; climacteric syndrome; clinical laboratory scientist; clinical stage; clinical status; clinic scheduling; Cockayne syndrome; complete stroke; compression syndrome; concentrated strength; conditioned stimulus; congenital syphilis; conjunctival secretion; conscious, consciousness; conscious sedation; conservative surgery; constant spring; contact sensitivity; continue same; contrast sensitivity; control serum; control subjects; convalescence, convalescent; coronary sclerosis; coronary sinus; corpus striatum; corticoid-sensitive; corticosteroid; countershock; crush syndrome; current smoker; current strength; Cushing syndrome; cyclic somatostatin; cycloserine; cyclosporine

C/S cesarean section; cycles per second

C&S calvarium and scalp; conjunctiva and sclera; culture and sensitivity

CS IV clinical stage 4

C4S chondroitin-4-sulfate

Cs case; cell surface; cyclosporine; static compliance

C$_s$ standard clearance; static compliance; static respiratory compliance

cS centistoke

cs catalytic subunit; chromosome; consciousness

CSA Canadian Standards Association; canavaninosuccinic acid; carbonyl salicylamide; cell surface antigen; chemical shift anisotropy; chondroitin sulfate A; chorionic somatomammotropin A; client server architecture; colony-stimulating activity; colony survival assay; compressed spectral assay; computerized spectral analysis; Controlled Substances Act; cross section area; cyclosporine A

CsA cyclosporine A

CSAA Child Study Association of America

CSAD corporate services administration department

CSAT center for substance abuse treatment

CSAVP cerebral subarachnoid venous pressure

CSB contaminated small bowel; craniosynostosis, Boston type

csb chromosome break
CSBF coronary sinus blood flow
CSBS contaminated small bowel syndrome
CSC blow on blow (administration of small amounts of drugs at short intervals) [Fr. *coup sur coup*]; collagen sponge contraceptive; corticostriatocerebellar; cryogenic storage container
CSCC cutaneous squamous cell carcinoma
CSCD Center for Sickle Cell Disease
CSCHDS Caerphilly and Speedwell Collaborative Heart Disease Studies
CSCI corticosterone side-chain isomerase
CSCR Central Society for Clinical Research
CSCV critical serum chemistry value
CSCW computer-supported collaborative work
CSD carotid sinus denervation; cat scratch disease; combined system disease; conditionally streptomycin dependent; conduction system disease; cortical spreading depression; craniospinal defect; critical stimulus duration
CSDB cat scratch disease bacillus
CSDMS Canadian Society of Diagnostic Medical Sonographers
CSE clinical-symptom/self-evaluation [questionnaire]; cone-shaped epiphysis; conventional spin-echo; cross-sectional echocardiography
C sect, C-section cesarean section
CSEP clinical sepsis; cortical somatosensory evoked potential
CSER cortical somatosensory evoked response
CSF cancer family syndrome; cerebrospinal fluid; cold stability factor; colony-stimulating factor; coronary sinus flow; critical success factor
CS-F colony-stimulating factor
CSFH cerebrospinal fluid hypotension
CSF-IR colony-stimulating factor I receptor
CSFP cerebrospinal fluid pressure
CSFR colony-stimulating factor receptor
CSFV cerebrospinal fluid volume
CSF-WR cerebrospinal fluid-Wassermann reaction
CSG cell surface glycoprotein; central sympathetic generator; cholecystography, cholecystogram; collaborative study group
csg chromosome gap

CSGBI Cardiac Society of Great Britain and Ireland
CSGBM collagenase soluble glomerular basement membrane
CSGE conformational sensitive gel electrophoresis
CSGTEI Collaborative Study Group Trial on the Effect of Irbesartan
CSH carotid sinus hypersensitivity; chronic subdural hematoma; combat support [army] hospital; cortical stromal hyperplasia
CSHA Canadian Study of Health and Aging
CSHCN children with special health care needs
CSHE California Society for Hospital Engineering
CSHH congenital self-healing histiocytosis
CSHN children with special health needs
CSHS Canadian Smoking Health Survey
CSI calculus surface index; cancer serum index; cavernous sinus infiltration; cervical spine injury; chemical shift imaging; cholesterol saturation index; computerized severity of illness [index]; coronary sinus intervention
CSICU cardiac surgical intensive care unit
CSIF cytokine synthesis inhibitory factor
CSII continuous subcutaneous insulin infusion
CSIIP continuous subcutaneous insulin infusion pump
CSIN Chemical Substances Information Network
CSIS clinical supplies and inventory system
CSL cardiolipin synthetic lecithin; corticosteroid liposome
CSLM confocal scanning microscopy
CSLU chronic stasis leg ulcer
CSM cardiosynchronous myostimulator; carotid sinus massage; cerebrospinal meningitis; circulation, sensation, motion; Committee on Safety of Medicines; confined space medicine, Consolidated Standards Manual; corn-soy milk
CSMA chronic spinal muscular atrophy
CSMAP celiac-superior mesenteric artery portography
C-SMART Cardiomyoplasty–Skeletal Muscle Assist Randomized Trial
CSMA/CD carrier sense multiple access and collision detection

CSMB Center for the Study of Multiple Births

CSMMG Chartered Society of Massage and Medical Gymnastics

CSMP chloramphenicol-sensitive microsomal protein

CSMSS Collaborative Social and Medical Services System

CSMT chorionic somatomammotropin

CSN cardiac sympathetic nerve; carotid sinus nerve

CSNA congenital sensory neuropathy with anhidrosis [syndrome]

CSNB congenital stationary night blindness

CS(NCA) Clinical Laboratory Scientist Certified by the National Certification Agency for Medical Laboratory Personnel

CSNK casein kinase

CSNRT, cSNRT corrected sinus node recovery time

CSNS carotid sinus nerve stimulation

CSNU cystinuria

CSO claims services only; common source outbreak; craniostenosis; craniosynostosis; ostium of coronary sinus

CSOM chronic suppurative otitis media

CSOP coronary sinus occlusion pressure

CSP carotid sinus pressure; cavum septi pellucidi; cell surface protein; cerebrospinal protein; Chartered Society of Physiotherapy; chemistry screening panel; chondroitin sulfate protein; circumsporozoite protein; Cooperative Statistical Program; criminal sexual psychopath; cyclosporin

CSPG chondroitin sulfate proteoglycan

Csp, C-spine cervical spine

CSPI Center for Science in the Public Interest

CSPINE corticosteroid use, seropositive RA, peripheral joint destruction, involvement of cervical nerves, nodules (rheumatoid), established disease [cervical spine disease risk factors]

CSPS continual skin peeling syndrome

CSpT corticospinal tract

CSQ Coping Strategies Questionnaire

CSR central supply room; chart-stimulated recall [test]; Cheyne-Stokes respiration; continued stay review; corrected sedimentation rate; corrected survival rate; cortisol secretion rate; cumulative survival rate

CSRP cysteine-rich protein

CSRS cardiac surgery reporting system

CSS Cancer Surveillance System; carotid sinus stimulation; carotid sinus syndrome; cavernous sinus syndrome; central sterile section; central sterile supply; chewing, sucking, swallowing; chronic subclinical scurvy; Churg-Strauss syndrome; client satisfaction scale; clinical support system; Copenhagen Stroke Study; cranial sector scan; critical care system

CSSA Carotid Stent-Supported Angioplasty [trial]

CSSAE Communication Skills Self-Assessment Exam

CSSCD Cooperative Study of Sickle Cell Disease

CSSD central sterile supply department

CSSRD Cooperative Systematic Study of Rheumatic Diseases

CSSU central sterile supply unit

CST cardiac stress test; cardiovascular self-assessment tool; cavernous sinus thrombosis; certified surgical technologist; chemostatin; Christ-Siemens Touraine [syndrome]; compliance, static; computer scatter tomography; contraction stress test; conversational speech task; convulsive shock therapy; corticospinal tract; cosyntropin stimulation test; cystatin

C$_{st}$ static compliance

cSt centistoke

C$_{stat}$ static compliance

CSTB Computer Science and Telecommunications Board [National Academy of Sciences]

CSTE Council of State and Territorial Epidemiologists

CSTI Clearinghouse for Scientific and Technical Information

CSTM cervical prevertebral soft tissue measurement

CSTP Committee for Scientific and Technological Policy

Cst,rs static compliance of respiratory system

CSTT cold-stimulation time test

CSU casualty staging unit; catheter specimen of urine; central statistical unit; clinical specialty unit

CSUF continuous slow ultrafiltration

CSV chick syncytial virus

CSW Certified Social Worker; current sleep walker

CSWG Clinical Systems Working Group

CT calcitonin; calf testis; cardiac tamponade; cardiothoracic [ratio]; carotid tracing; carpal tunnel; cell therapy; cerebral thrombosis; cerebral tumor; cervical traction; cervicothoracic; chemotherapy; chest tube; chicken tumor; *Chlamydia trachomatis*; chlorothiazide; cholera toxin; cholesterol, total; chordae tendineae; chronic thyroiditis; chymotrypsin; circulation time; classic technique; closed thoracotomy; clotting time; coagulation time; coated tablet; cobra toxin; cognitive therapy; coil test; collecting tubule; colon, transverse; combined tumor; compressed tablet; computed tomography; connective tissue; continue treatment; continuous-flow tub; contraceptive technique; contraction time; controlled temperature; Coombs test; corneal transplant; coronary thrombosis; corrected transposition; corrective therapy; cortical thickness; cough threshold; crest time; cystine-tellurite; cytotechnologist; cytotoxic therapy; unit of attenuation [number]

C/T compression/traction [ratio]

C&T color and temperature

Ct carboxyl terminal

ct carat; chromatid; count

C$_{T-1824}$ T-1824 (Evans blue) clearance

CTA Canadian Tuberculosis Association; center for total access; chemotactic activity; chromotropic acid; Committee on Thrombolytic Agents; computed tomography of the abdomen; computed tomographic angiography; congenital trigeminal anesthesia; cyanotrimethyl-androsterone; cystine trypticase agar; cytoplasmic tubular aggregate; cytotoxic assay

CTAB cetyltrimethyl-ammonium bromide

CTAC Cancer Treatment Advisory Committee

CTAF Canadian Trial of Atrial Fibrillation; conotruncal anomaly face [syndrome]

CTAFS conotruncal anomaly face syndrome

cTAL cortical thick ascending limb

CTAP computed tomography in arterial portography; connective tissue activating peptide

CTAT computerized transaxial tomography

CTB ceased to breathe; cholera toxin B

ctb chromated break

CTC chlortetracycline; Clinical Trial Certificate; computed tomographic colography; computer-aided tomographic cisternography; consent to continue; cultured T cells

CTCL cutaneous T-cell lymphoma

ctCO$_2$ carbon dioxide concentration

CTD carpal tunnel decompression; chest tube drainage; congenital thymic dysplasia; connective tissue disease; cumulative trauma disorder

CT&DB cough, turn, and deep breathe

ctDNA chloroplast deoxyribonucleic acid

CTE calf thymus extract; cultured thymic epithelium

CTEM conventional transmission electron microscopy

CTF cancer therapy facility; certificate; Colorado tick fever; cytotoxic factor

ctf certificate

CTFE chlorotrifluoroethylene

CTFS complete testicular feminization syndrome

CTG cardiotocography; cervicothoracic ganglion; chymotrypsinogen

C/TG cholesterol-triglyceride [ratio]

ctg chromated gap

CTGA complete transposition of great arteries

CTH ceramide trihexoside; chronic tension headache; cystathionase

CTh carrier-specific T-helper [cell]

CTHD chlorthalidone

CTI cardiac troponin I; coffee table injury; computers in teaching initiatives

CTL cervico-thoraco-lumbar; control; cytolytic C lymphocyte; cytotoxic T-lymphocyte

CTLL cytotoxic lymphoid line

CTLSO cervicothoracolumbosacral orthosis

CTM cardiotachometer; Chlortrimeton; cricothyroid muscle; computed tomographic myelography

CTMC connective tissue mast cell

CTMM computed tomographic metrizamide myelography

CTMM-SF California Test of Mental Maturity–Short Form

CTMR clinical treatment and medical research

CTN calcitonin; clinical trials notification; computer tomography number; continuous noise

cTn-I cardiac troponin I

cTNM TNM (*q.v.*) staging of tumors as determined by clinical noninvasive examination

CTO cervicothoracic orthosis

CTOPP Canadian Trial of Physiological Pacing

CTP California Test of Personality; citrate transport protein; clinical terms project; comprehensive treatment plan; cytidine triphosphate; cytosine triphosphate

C-TPN cyclic total parenteral nutrition

CTPP cerebral tissue perfusion pressure

CTPVO chronic thrombotic pulmonary vascular obstruction

CTR cardiothoracic ratio; carpal tunnel release; central tumor registry; Connecticut Tumor Registry

ctr central; center; centric

CTRB chymotrypsinogen B

CTRD Cardiac Transplant Research Database

CTRL chymotrypsin-like [protease]

CTRS certified therapeutic recreation specialist

CTRX ceftriaxone

CTS carpal tunnel syndrome; clinical trials support [program]; Collaborative Transplant Study; composite treatment score; computed tomographic scan; contralateral threshold shift; corticosteroid

CTSB cathepsin B

CTSD cathepsin D

CTSE cathepsin E

CTSG cathepsin G

CTSH cathepsin H

CTSL cathepsin L

CTSNFR corrected time of sinoatrial node function recovery

CTSP Cooperative Triglyceride Standardization Program

CTSS cathepsin S; closed tracheal suction system

CTT cefotetan; central tegmental tract; central transmission time; compressed tablet triturate; computed transaxial tomography; critical tracking time

CTTAC clinical trials and treatment advisory committee

CTU cardiac-thoracic unit; centigrade thermal unit; constitutive transcription unit

CTV cervical and thoracic vertebrae; clinical target volume

CTVDR conformal treatment verification, delivery and recording [system]

CTW central terminal of Wilson; combined testicular weight

CTX cefotaxime; ceftriaxone; cerebrotendinous xanthomatosis; chemotaxis; clinical trials exemption scheme; costotendinous xanthomatosis; cytoxan

CTx cardiac transplantation; conotoxin

CTZ chemoreceptor trigger zone; chlorothiazide

CU cardiac unit; casein unit; cause unknown or undetermined; chymotrypsin unit; clinical unit; color unit; contact urticaria; convalescent unit

C$_u$ urea clearance

cu cubic

CUA cost-utility analysis [ratio]

CUAVD congenital unilateral absence of vas deferens

CuB copper band

CUBA Cutting Balloon vs Conventional Balloon Angioplasty [study]

CUC chronic ulcerative colitis

cu cm cubic centimeter

CUD cause undetermined; congenital urinary deformity

CuD copper deficiency

CUE confidential unit exclusion; cumulative urinary excretion

CUG Computer-Stored Ambulatory Record User's Group; cystidine, uridine, and guanidine; cystourethrogram, cystourethrography

CUI concept unique identifier [UMLS]; Cox-Uphoff International [tissue expander]

cu in cubic inch

cult culture

cum cumulative

cu m cubic meter

CUMITECH Cumulative Techniques and Procedures in Clinical Microbiology

cu mm cubic millimeter

CUMULVS collaborative user migration, user library for visualization and steering

CUP carcinoma unknown primary

CUR cystourethrorectal

cur cure, curative; current

CURE Clopidogrel in Unstable Angina to Prevent Recurrent Ischemic Events [trial]; Columbia University Restenosis Elimination [trial]

CURL compartment of uncoupling of receptors and ligands

CURN Conduct and Utilization of Research in Nursing

CurrMIT Curriculum Management and Information Tool

CUS carotid ultrasound examination; catheterized urine specimen; contact urticaria syndrome

CuS copper supplement

CUSA Cavitron ultrasonic aspirator

CUSSN computer use in social service network

CuTS cubital tunnel syndrome

CV cardiac volume; cardiovascular; care vigilance; carotenoid vesicle; cell volume; central venous; cephalic vein; cerebrovascular; cervical vertebra; Chikungunya virus; chorionic villi; closing volume; coefficient of variation; color vision; concentrated volume; conducting vein; conduction velocity; conjugata vera; contrast ventriculography; conventional ventilation; corpuscular volume; costovertebral; cresyl violet; crystal violet; cutaneous vasculitis; cyclic voltometry or voltamogram

C/V coulomb per volt

Cv specific heat at constant volume

C$_v$ coefficient of variation; constant volume

cv cultivar

CVA cardiovascular accident; cerebrovascular accident; chronic villous arthritis; common variable agammaglobulinemia; costovertebral angle; cyclophosphamide, vincristine, and Adriamycin

CVAH congenital virilizing adrenal hyperplasia

CVAP cerebrovascular amyloid peptide

CVAT costovertebral angle tenderness

CVB chorionic villi biopsy

CVC central venous catheter

CV cath central venous catheter

CVCT cardiovascular computed tomography

CVD cardiovascular disease; Center for Vaccine Development; collagen vascular disease; color-vision-deviant

CVELTP Comox Valley Electronic Lab Transfer Project [Canada]

CVF cardiovascular failure; central visual field; cervicovaginal fluid; cobra venom factor

CVFn cardiovascular function

CVG contrast ventriculography; coronary venous graft; cutis verticis gyrata

CVG/MR cutis verticis gyrata/mental retardation [syndrome]

CVH cerebroventricular hemorrhage; cervicovaginal hood; combined ventricular hypertrophy; common variable hypogammaglobulinemia

CVHD chronic valvular heart disease

CVI cardiovascular incident; cardiovascular insufficiency; cerebrovascular incident; cerebrovascular insufficiency; chronic venous insufficiency; common variable immunodeficiency; content validity index

CVICU cardiovascular intensive care unit

CVID common variable immunodeficiency

CVIS cardiovascular imaging system

CVK computerized videokeratography

CVL central venous line

CVLM caudal ventrolateral medulla; caudoventrolateral medulla

CVLT California Verbal Learning Test; clinical vascular laboratory

CVM cardiovascular monitor; cerebral venous malformation; cyclophosphamide, vincristine, and methotrexate

CVMP Committee on Veterans Medical Problems

CVO central vein occlusion; central venous oxygen; Chief Veterinary Officer; circumventricular organ; credentialing verification organization

CVO$_2$ central venous oxygen content or saturation

CVOD cerebrovascular obstructive disease

CVP cardioventricular pacing; cell volume profile; central venous pressure; cyclophosphamide, vincristine, and prednisone

cvPO$_2$, cvP$_{O_2}$ cerebral venous partial pressure of oxygen

CVR cardiovascular-renal; cardiovascular-respiratory; cephalic vasomotor response; cerebrovascular resistance

CVRD cardiovascular-renal disease

CVRMED computer vision, virtual reality, and robotics in medicine

CVRR cardiovascular recovery room

CVRS cardiovascular and respiratory elements of trauma score

CVS cardiovascular surgery; cardiovascular system; challenge virus strain; chorionic villi sampling; clean voided specimen; coronavirus susceptibility; current vital signs

CVSMC cultured vascular smooth muscle cells

CVST cerebral venous sinus thrombosis

CVST-T Cerebral Venous Sinus Thrombosis Trial

CVT cardiovascular technologist; central venous temperature; cerebral venous thrombosis; congenital vertical talus

CVTR charcoal viral transport medium

CVVH continuous veno-venous hemofiltration

CVVHD continuous veno-venous hemodialysis

CVVHDF continuous venovenous hemodiafiltration

CW cardiac work; case work; cell wall; chemical warfare; chemical weapon; chest wall; children's ward; clockwise; continuous wave; crutch walking

Cw crutch walking

C/W compare with; consistent with

CWBTS capillary whole blood true sugar

CWC chest wall compliance

CWD cell wall defect; continuous-wave Doppler

CWDF cell wall-deficient form [bacteria]

CWEQ conditions of work effectiveness scale

CWF Cornell Word Form

CWH cardiomyopathy and wooly haircoat [syndrome]

CWHB citrated whole human blood

CWI cardiac work index

CWL cutaneous water loss

CWM cardiological workspace manager

CWMS color, warmth, movement sensation

CWOP childbirth without pain

CWP childbirth without pain; coal worker's pneumoconiosis

CWPEA Childbirth Without Pain Education Association

CWS cell wall skeleton; chest wall stimulation; child welfare service; children's clinical workstation; clinician's workstation; cold water-soluble; cotton wool spots

CWT circuit weight training; cold water treatment; continuous wavelet transform

Cwt, cwt hundredweight

CWW clinic without walls

CWXSP Coal Workers' X-ray Surveillance Program

CX cervix; chest x-ray; connexin; critical experiment

Cx cervix; circumflex; clearance; complaint; complex; convex

cx cervix; complex; connexin; culture; cylinder axis

CXB3S Coxsackie B3 virus susceptibility

CxCor circumflex coronary [artery]

CXMD canine X-linked muscular dystrophy

CXR, CxR chest x-ray

CY casein-yeast autolysate [medium]; cyclophosphamide

Cy cyanogen; cyclophosphamide; cyst; cytarabine

cy, cyan cyanosis

CyA cyclosporine A

CYC cyclophosphamide; cytochrome C

cyc cyclazocine; cycle; cyclotron

CYCAZAREM Cyclophosphamide vs Azathioprine during Remission of Systemic Vasculitis [trial]

CYCLO, Cyclo cyclophosphamide; cyclopropane

Cyclo C cyclocytidine hydrochloride

CYCLOPS cyclically ordered phase sequence; Cyclophosphamide in Systemic Vasculitis

Cyd cytidine

CYE charcoal yeast extract [agar]

CYH chymase

CYL casein yeast lactate

cyl cylinder; cylindrical lens

CYM chymase, mast cell

CYMP chymosin, pseudogene

CYN cyanide

CYP cyclophilin; cyproheptadine; cytochrome P

CYPA cyclophilin A

CYPC cyclophilin C

CYPH cyclophilin

CYS cystoscopy
Cys cyclosporine; cysteine
Cys-Cys cystine
CysLT1 cysteinyl leukotriene 1
CYSTO cystogram
cysto cystoscopy
CYT cytochrome
Cyt cytoplasm; cytosine
cyt cytochrome; cytology, cytological; cytoplasm, cytoplasm

Cyto cytotechnologist
cytol cytology, cytological
CY-VA-DIC cyclophosphamide, vincristine, Adriamycin, and dacarbazine
CZ cefazolin
Cz central midline placement of electrodes in electroencephalography
CZI crystalline zine insulin
C$_{zn}$ zinc clearance
CZP clonazepam

D absorbed dose aspartic acid; cholecalciferol; coefficient of diffusion; dacryon; dalton; date; daughter; day; dead; dead air space; debye; deceased; deciduous; decimal reduction time; degree; density; dental; dermatology, dermatologist, dermatologic; deuterium; deuteron; development; deviation; dextro; dextrose; diabetic; diagnosis; diagonal; diameter; diaphorase; diarrhea; diastole; diathermy; died; difference; diffusion, diffusing; dihydrouridine; dilution [rate]; diopter; diplomate; dipyridamole; disease; dispense; displacement [loop]; distal; distance [focus-object]; diuresis; diurnal; divergence; diversity; diverticulum; divorced; doctor; dog; donor; dorsal; drive; drug; dual; duct; duodenum, duodenal; duration; dwarf; electric displacement; mean dose; right [Lat. *dexter*]; unit of vitamin D potency

D̄ mean dose

D₁ diagonal one; first dorsal vertebra

1-D one-dimensional

D₂ diagonal two; second dorsal vertebra

2-D two-dimensional

2,4-D 2,4-dichlorophenoxyacetic acid

D/3 distal third

3-D three-dimensional

D₃₋₁₂ third to twelfth dorsal vertebrae

D4 fourth digit

4-D four-dimensional

D₁₀ decimal reduction time

d atomic orbital with angular momentum quantum number 2; day [Lat. *dies*]; dead; deceased; deci-; decrease, decreased; degree; density; deoxy; deoxyribose; dextro-; dextrorotatory; diameter; diastasis; died; diopter; distal; distance [between radiographic grids or between subject and film or casette]; diurnal; dorsal; dose; doubtful; duration; dyne; right [Lat. *dexter*]

Δ see *delta*

δ see *delta*

1/d once a day

2/d twice a day

DA dark adaptation; dark agouti [rat]; daunomycin; degenerative arthritis; delayed action; Dental Assistant; deoxyadenosine; descending aneurysm; descending aorta; developmental age; dextroamphetamine; diabetic acidosis; differential amplifier; differential analyzer; differentiation antigen; digital angiography; digital to analogue [converter]; diphenylchlorarsine; Diploma in Anesthetics; direct agglutination; disability assistance; disaggregated; discriminant analysis; distal arthrogryposis; dopamine; drug addict, drug addiction; drug administration; ductus arteriosus

DA1 distal arthrogryposis type 1

DA2 distal arthrogryposis type 2

D/A date of accident; date of admission; digital-to-analog [converter]; discharge and advise

D-A donor-acceptor

D&A dilatation and aspiration; drugs and allergy

Da dalton

da daughter; day; deca-

d(A) primary donor

DAA decompensated autonomous adenoma; dementia associated with alcoholism; dialysis-associated amyloidosis; diaminoanisole

DAAF deoxyribonucleic acid amplification fingerprinting; Digoxin in Acute Atrial Fibrillation [study]

DAAO diaminoacid oxidase

D(A-a)O₂ alveolar arterial oxygen gradient

DAB days after birth; 3,3'-diaminobenzidine; dysrhythmic aggressive behavior

DABA 2,4-diaminobutyric acid

DABP D site albumin promoter binding protein

DAC derived air concentration; digital-to-analog converter; disaster assistance center; Division of Ambulatory Care

dac dacryon

DACCM department of anesthesiology and critical care medicine

DACL Depression Adjective Check List

DACM N-(7-diamethylamino-4-methyl-3-coumarinyl) maleimide

DACMD deputy associate chief medical director

DACS data acquisition and control system

DACT dactinomycin; daily activity [UMLS]

DAD delayed afterdepolarization; diffuse alveolar damage; dispense as directed

DADA dichloroacetic acid diisopropylammonium salt

DADDS diacetyldiaminodiphenylsulfone

DADS Director Army Dental Service

DAE diphenylanthracene endoperoxide; diving air embolism; dysbaric air embolism

DA/ES data analysis expert system

DAF decay-accelerating factor; delayed auditory feedback; drug-adulterated food

DAG diacylglycerol; dianhydrogalactitol; directed acyclic graph; dystrophin-associated glycoprotein

DAGK diacylglycerol kinase

DAGT direct antiglobulin test

DAH disordered action of the heart

DAHEA Department of Allied Health Education and Accreditation

DAHM Division of Allied Health Manpower

DAI diffuse axonal injury

DAIDS Division of Acquired Immunodeficiency Syndrome (AIDS) [NIH]

DAIS Diabetes Atherosclerosis Intervention Study

DAISY Diabetes Autoimmunity Study in the Young

DAIT Division of Allergy, Immunology and Transplantation [NIH]

Dal, dal dalton

DALA delta-aminolevulinic acid

DALE Drug Abuse Law Enforcement

DALY(s) disability-adjusted life year(s)

DAM database access module; data-associated message; degraded amyloid; diacetyl monoxime; diacetylmorphine

dam decameter

DAMA discharged against medical advice

DAMAD Diabetic Microangiopathy Modification with Aspirin vs Dipyridamole

DAMET Diet and Moderate Exercise Trial

DAMOS drug application methodology with optical storage

dAMP deoxyadenosine monophosphate; deoxyadenylate adenosine monophosphate

D and C dilatation and curettage

DAN data acquisition in neurophysiology; diabetic autonomic neuropathy

DANAMI Danish Multicenter Study of Acute Myocardial Infarction

DANS 1-dimethylaminonaphthalene-5-sulfonyl chloride

DANTE delays altered with nutation for tailored excitation

DAO diamine oxidase

DAo descending aorta

DAOM depressor anguli oris muscle

DAP data acquisition processor; data architecture project; depolarizing afterpotential; diabetes-associated peptide; diaminopimelic acid; diaminopyridine; diastolic aortic pressure; dihydroxyacetone phosphate; dipeptidylaminopeptidase; direct latex agglutination pregnancy [test]; dose area product; Draw-a-Person [test]; Drug Action Programme [WHO]

D-AP5 D-2-amino-5-phosphonovaleric acid

D-AP7 D-2-amino-7-phosphonoheptanoic acid

DAP&E Diploma of Applied Parasitology and Entomology

DAPI 4,6-diamino-2-phenylindole

DAPPAF Dual-Site Atrial Pacing for Prevention of Atrial Fibrillation [trial]

DAPRE daily adjustable progressive resistive exercise

DAPRU Drug Abuse Prevention Resource Unit

DAPT diaminophenylthiazole; direct agglutination pregnancy test

DAQ Diagnostic Assessment Questionnaire

DAR death after resuscitation; diacereine; differential absorption ratio

DARE Database of Abstracts of Reviews of Effectiveness

DARP drug abuse rehabilitation program

DARPA Defense Advanced Research Project Agency [Department of Defense]

DART Developmental and Reproductive Toxicology [NLM database]; Diet and Reinfarction Trial; Dilation vs Ablation Revascularization Trial

D/ART Depression, Awareness, Recognition, and Treatment [NIMH hotline]

DARTS Diabetes Audit and Research in Tayside Scotland; Drug and Alcohol Rehabilitation Testing System

DAS dead air space; Death Anxiety Scale; delayed anovulatory syndrome; dextroamphetamine sulfate; Dietary Alternatives Study; digital angiography segmentation; double addition of serum; Dyadic adjustment scale

DASD direct access storage device

DASH Delay in Accessing Stroke Healthcare [trial]; Dietary Approaches to Stop Hypertension [trial]; Distress Alarm for the Severely Handicapped

DASI Duke activity status index

DASS Dilazep Aspirin Stroke Study

DAST diethylaminosulfur trifluoride; drug abuse screening test; drug and alcohol screening test

DAT delayed-action tablet; dementia Alzheimer's type; dental aptitude test; diacetylthiamine; diet as tolerated; differential agglutination titer; Differential Aptitude Test; diphtheria antitoxin; direct agglutination test; direct antiglobulin test; Disaster Action Team; dopamine transporter

DATA Diltiazem as Adjunctive Therapy to Activase [study]

DATE dental auxiliary teacher education

DATOS Diet and Antismoking Trial of Oslo Study

DATP deoxyadenosine triphosphate

dATP deoxyadenosine monophosphate

DATTA diagnostic and therapeutic technology assessment

DAU 3-deazauridine; Dental Auxiliary Utilization

dau daughter

DAUs drug abuse testing and urines

DAV data valid; Disabled American Veterans; duck adenovirus

DAVF dural arteriovenous fistula

DAVIT Danish Verapamil Infarction Trial

DAVM dural arteriovenous malformation

DAvMED Diploma in Aviation Medicine

DAVP deamino-arginine vasopressin

DAWN Drug Abuse Warning Network

DAZ deleted in azospermia

DB database; date of birth; deep breath; dense body; dextran blue; diabetes, diabetic; diagonal band; diet beverage; direct bilirubin; disability; distobuccal; double-blind [study]; double buffer [board]; Dutch belted [rabbit]; duodenal bulb

Db diabetes, diabetic

D$_b$ database; body density

dB, db decibel

db database; date of birth; diabetes, diabetic

DBA database administrator; Diamond-Blackfan anemia; dibenzanthracene; *Dolichos biflorus* agglutinin

DBAE dihydroxyborylaminoethyl

DBB diagonal band of Broca

DBC dibencozide; distal balloon catheter; dye-binding capacity

DB&C deep breathing and coughing

DBCL dilute blood clot lysis [method]

DBCP dibromochloropropane

DBD definite brain damage; deoxyribonucleic acid-binding domain; dibromodulcitol

DBDG distobuccal developmental groove

DB/DS database of data sets

dB/dt change of magnetic flux with time

DBE deep breathing exercise; dibromoethane

DBED penicillin G benzathine

dbEST Database of Expressed Sequence Taga [NLM]

dbGSS Database on Genome Survey Sequences [NLM]

DBH dopamine beta-hydroxylase

DbH diagnosis by hybridization

DBI development at birth index; phenformin hydrochloride

DBil direct bilirubin

DBIOC database input/output control

DBIR Directory of Biotechnology Information Resources

dBk decibels above 1 kilowatt

DBLE Double Bolus Lytic Efficacy [trial]

DBM database management; dibromomannitol; dobutamine

dBm decibels above 1 milliwatt

dBMAN database manager

DBMS database management system

DBO distobucco-occlusal

db/ob diabetic obese [mouse]

DBP diastolic blood pressure; dibutylphthalate; distobuccopulpal; Döhle body panmyelopathy; vitamin D-binding protein

DBPOFC double-blind placebo-controlled oral food challenge

DBR distorted breathing rate

DBRI dysfunctional behavior rating instrument

DBRPC double-blind randomized placebo-controlled

DBS deep brain stimulation; Denis Browne splint; despeciated bovine serum; Diamond-Blackfan syndrome; dibromosalicil; diminished breath sounds; direct bonding system; Division of Biological Standards; double blind study; double-burst stimulus; dysgenesis of corpus callosum

DBSP dibromosulphthalein

dbSTS database of Sequence Tagged Sites [NLM]

DBSV deconvolution based on shape variation

DBT dry bulb temperature

DBW desirable body weight

dBW decibels above 1 watt

DC daily census; data communication; data conversion; decrease; deep compartment; defining characteristic; dendritic cell; Dental Corps; deoxycholate; descending colon; dextran charcoal; diagonal conjugate; diagnostic center; diagnostic cluster; diagnostic code; differentiated cell; diffusion capacity; digit copying; digital computer; dilatation and curettage; dilation catheter; diphenylcyanoarsine; direct Coombs' [test]; direct current; discharge, discharged; discontinue, discontinued; distal colon; distocervical; Doctor of Chiropractic; donor cells; dopachrome; dorsal column; dressing change; duodenal cap; Dupuytren contracture; duty cycle; dyskeratosis congenita; electric defibrillator using DC discharge

Dc critical dilution rate

D/C discontinue

D/c discontinue; discharge

DC65 Darvon compound 65

D&C dilatation and curettage; drugs and cosmetics

dC deoxycytidine

dc decrease; direct current; discharge; discontinue

DCA deoxycholate-citrate agar; deoxycholic acid; desoxycorticosterone acetate; dichloroacetate; directional coronary atherectomy

DCABG double coronary artery bypass graft

DCAF dilated cardiomyopathy and atrial fibrillation

DCB dichlorobenzidine

DCBE double contrast barium enema

DCBF dyamic cardiac blood flow

DCbN deep cerebellar nucleus

DCC day care center; deleted in colorectal cancer; device communication controller; dextran-coated charcoal; diameter of cylindrical collimator; N,N'-dicyclohexylcarbodiimide; digital compact casette; disaster control center; dorsal cell column; double concave; dysgenesis of corpus callosum

DCCMP daunomycin, cyclocytidine, 6-mercaptopurine, and prednisolone

DC$_{CO2}$ diffusing capacity for carbon dioxide

DCCT Diabetes Control and Complications Trial

DCCV direct current cardioversion

DCD Diploma in Chest Diseases; dynamic cooling device

D/c'd, dc'd discontinued

D/CDK D-type cyclin-dependent kinase

DCE desmosterol-to-cholesterol enzyme; distributed computing environment

DCET dicarboxyethoxythiamine

DCF 2'-deoxycoformycin; dichlorofluorescein; direct centrifugal flotation; dopachrome conversion factor

DCFDA 2',7'-dichlorofluorescein diacetate

DCFH dichlorofluorescein

DCFH-DA dichlorofluorescein diacetate

DCG dacryocystography; deoxycorticosterone glucoside; diagnosis cost-related group; disodium cromoglycate; dynamic electrocardiography

DCGE denaturation gradient gel electrophoresis

DCH delayed cutaneous hypersensitivity; Diploma in Child Health

DCh Doctor of Surgery [Lat. *Doctor Chirurgiae*]

DCHA docosahexaenoic acid

DCHEB dichlorohexafluorobutane

DCHN dicyclohexylamine nitrite

DChO Doctor of Ophthalmic Surgery

DCI dichloroisoprenaline; dichloroisoproterenol; digital cardiac imaging; Doppler color imaging; duplicate coverage inquiry

DCIP dichlorophenolindophenol

DCIS ductal carcinoma in situ

DCK, dCK deoxycytidine kinase

DCL dicloxacillin; diffuse or disseminated cutaneous leishmaniasis; digital case library

DCLHb diaspirin cross-linked hemoglobin

DCLS deoxycholate citrate lactose saccharose

DCM dichloromethane; dichloromethotrexate; dilated cardiomyopathy; Doctor of Comparative Medicine; dyssynergia cerebellaris myoclonica

DCMADS [Washington] DC Metropolitan Area Drug Study

DCML dorsal column medial lemniscus

DCMP daunomycin, cytosine arabinoside, 6-mercaptopurine, and prednisolone

dCMP deoxycytidine monophosphate

DCMT Doctor of Clinical Medicine of the Tropics

DCMX 2,4-dichloro-m-xylenol

DCN data collection network; deep cerebral nucleus; delayed conditioned necrosis; depressed, cognitively normal; dorsal cochlear nucleus; dorsal column nucleus; dorsal cutaneous nerve

DCNU chlorozotocin

DCO Diploma of the College of Optics

D$_{CO}$ diffusing capacity for carbon monoxide

DCOG Diploma of the College of Obstetricians and Gynaecologists

DCOP distal coronary occlusion pressure

DCOR dopachrome oxidoreductase

DCP dicalcium phosphate; Diploma in Clinical Pathology; Diploma in Clinical Psychology; District Community Physician; dual chamber pacemaker; dynamic compression plate

DCR dacryocystorhinostomy; data conversion receiver; direct cortical response

DCRT Division of Computer Research and Technology [NIH]

3-DCRT three-dimensional conformal radiation therapy

DCS decompression sickness; dense canalicular system; diffuse cortical sclerosis; dorsal column stimulation, dorsal column stimulator; dynamic condylar screw; dynamic contrast-enhanced subtraction; dynamic contrast-enhanced tomography; dyskinetic cilia syndrome

dcSSc diffuse cutaneous systemic sclerosis

DCT detached ciliary tuft; direct Coombs' test; discrete cosine transform; distal convoluted tubule; diurnal cortisol test; dynamic computed tomography

3DCT, 3D-CT 3-dimensional computed tomography

DCTMA desoxycorticosterone trimethylacetate

dCTP deoxycytidine triphosphate

DCTPA desoxycorticosterone triphenylacetate

DCTS dynamic carpal tunnel syndrome

DCV diagnostic content validity; distribution of conduction velocities

D$_{2CV}$ Doppler 2-chamber view

D$_{4CV}$ Doppler 4-chamber view

DCX double charge exchange

DCx double convex

DD dangerous drug; Darier disease; data definition; data dictionary; day of delivery; D-dimer; death domain; degenerated disc; degenerative disease; delusional disorder; depth dose [x-ray]; detrusor dyssynergia; developmental disability; diastrophic dysplasia; died of the disease; differential diagnosis; differential display; digestive disorder; Di Guglielmo disease; disc diameter; discharge diagnosis; discharged dead; dog dander; double diffusion; drug dependence; dry dressing; Duchenne dystrophy; Dupuytren disease

D&D design and development

D6D delta-6-desaturase

dd dideoxy

DDA Dangerous Drugs Act; dideoxyadenosine; digital differential analysis

ddA 2',3'-dideoxyadenosine

DDase deoxyuridine diphosphatase

ddATP dideoxyadenosine triphosphate

DDAVP, dDAVP 1-deamino-8-D-arginine vasopressin; 1-desamino-8-D arginine vasopressin

DDC dangerous drug cabinet; dideoxycytidine; 3,5-diethoxycarbonyl-1,4-dihydrocollidine; dihydroxyphenylalanine decarboxylase; diethyl-dithiocarbamate; direct display console; diverticular disease of the colon

DDc double concave

ddC dideoxycytidine

DDD AV universal [pacemaker]; defined daily dose; degenerative disc disease; dehydroxydinaphthyl disulfide; dense deposit disease; Denver dialysis disease; dichlorodiphenyl-dichloroethane; dihydroxydinaphthyl disulfide; dorsal dural deficiency; Dowling-Degos disease

DDD CT double-dose-delay computed tomography

DDDD-CAT Drug Delivery Device Dispatch in Coronary Angioplasty Trial

DDE dichlorodiphenyldichloroethylene; dynamic data exchange

DDEB dominantly inherited dystrophic epidermolysis bullosa

DDF demographic data form

ddF dideoxy fingerprinting

DDG deoxy-D-glucose

ddGTP dideoxyguanidine triphosphate

DDH developmental dysplasia of the hip; Diploma in Dental Health; dissociated double hypertropia

DDI dynamic data icon

DDI, ddI dideoxyinosine

DDIB Disease Detection Information Bureau

DDKase deoxynucleoside diphosphate kinase

DDL data definition language

DDM Diploma in Dermatological Medicine; Doctor in Dental Medicine; Dyke-Davidoff-Masson [syndrome]

DDMR Dam-directed DNA mismatch repair

dDNA denatured deoxyribonucleic acid

DDNTP, ddNTP dideoxynucleotide triphosphate

DDO Diploma in Dental Orthopaedics

DDP cisplatin; density-dependent phosphoprotein; difficult denture patient; digital data processing; distributed data processing

DDPA Delta Dental Plans Association

DD-PCR, DDPCR differential display polymerase chain reaction

DDQ database directed query

DDR diastolic descent rate; Diploma in Diagnostic Radiology; DNA damage response

DDRB Doctors' and Dentists' Review Body

DDRP DNA damage responsive protein

DDRT diseases, disorders and related topics

DDS damaged disc syndrome; dendrodendritic synaptosome; dental distress syndrome; depressed DNA synthesis; dialysis disequilibrium syndrome; diaminodiphenylsulfone; directional Doppler sonography; Director of Dental Services; disability determination service; Disease-Disability Scale; Doctor of Dental Surgery; dodecyl sulfate; double decidual sac; dystrophy-dystocia syndrome

DDSc Doctor of Dental Science

DDSI digital damage severity index

DDSO diaminodiphenylsulfoxide

DDSS Defense Dental Standard System; Diagnostic Decision Support System [software]

DDST Denver Developmental Screening Test

DDST-R Denver Developmental Screening Test-Revised

DDT dichlorodiphenyltrichloroethane; dithiothreitol; ductus deferens tumor; dynamic data table

Ddt deceleration time

DDTC diethyldithiocarbamate

DDTN dideoxy-didehydrothymidine

ddTTP dideoxythymidine triphosphate

DDU dermo-distortive urticaria; duplex Doppler ultrasound

dDVH differential dose-volume histogram

D/DW dextrose in distilled water

D 5% DW 5% dextrose in distilled water

DDx differential diagnosis

DE deprived eye; design effect; diagnostic error; dialysis encephalopathy; digestive energy; dose equivalent; dream elements; drug evaluation; duration of ejection

D&E diet and elimination; dilation or dilatation and evacuation

2DE two-dimensional echocardiography

D=E dates equal to examination

DEA dehydroepiandrosterone; diethanolamine; Drug Enforcement Administration

DEAD Dying Experience at Dartmouth

DEAE diethylaminoethyl [cellulose]

DEAE-D diethylaminoethyl dextran

DEAFF detection of early antigen fluorescent foci

DEALE declining exponential approximation of life expectancy [method]

DEATH Dying Experience at the Hitchcock

DEB diepoxybutane; diethylbutanediol; Division of Environmental Biology; dystrophic epidermolysis bullosa

deb debridement

DEBA diethylbarbituric acid

DEBATE Doppler Endpoints Balloon Angioplasty Trial, Europe

debil debilitation

DEBRA Dystrophic Epidermolysis Bulosa Research Association

DEBS dominant epidermolysis bullosa simplex

DEC decrease; deoxycholate citrate; diagnostic episode cluster; diethylcarbamazine; dynamic environmental conditioning

Dec, dec decant

dec deceased; deciduous; decimal; decompose, decomposition; decrease, decreased

DECA Demographic and Echonomic Characteristics of the Aged [database]

decd deceased

DECG differentiated ECG

decoct decoction

DECODE Diabetes Epidemiology, Collaborative Analysis of Diagnostic Criteria in Europe

decomp decompensation; decomposition, decompose

decr decrease, decreased

D-ECST Dutch-European Cerebral Sinus Thrombosis [trial]

DECU decubitus [ulcer]

decub lying down [Lat. *decubitus*]

DED date of expected delivery; death effector domain [cell]; defined exposure dose; delayed erythema dose

DEEDS Data Elements for Emergency Department Systems

DEEG depth electroencephalogram, depth electroencephalography

DEER Diet and Exercise in Elevated Risk [trial]

DEF decayed primary teeth requiring filling, decayed primary teeth requiring extraction, and primary teeth successfully filled; dose-effect factor

def defecation; deficiency, deficient; deferred

DEFIANT Doppler Flow and Echocardiography in Functional Cardiac Insufficiency Assessment of Nisoldipine Therapy [trial]

defib defibrillation

DEFIBRILAT Defibrillator as Bridge to Later Transplantation [study]

defic deficiency, deficient

DEFN Danubian endemic familial nephropathy

DEF$_{NT}$ dose-effect factor for normal tissue

deform deformed, deformity

DEFT direct epifluorescent filter technique

DEF$_T$ dose-effect factor for tumor

DEG diethylene glycol

Deg, deg degeneration, degenerative; degree

degen degeneration, degenerative

DEH dysplasia epiphysealis hemimelica

DEHP di(2-ethylhexyl)phthalate

DEHR distributed electronic health record

DEHS Division of Emergency Health Services

DEHT developmental hand function test

dehyd dehydration, dehydrated

DEJ, dej dentino-enamel junction; dermoepidermal junction

del deletion; delivery; delusion

DELFIA dissociated enhanced lantanide fluoroimmunoassay

deliq deliquescence, deliquescent

DELIRIUM drugs–electrolytes–low temperature and lunacy–intoxication and intracranial processes–retention of urine or feces–infection–unfamiliar surroundings–myocardial infarction [causes of delirium]

Delt deltoid

DELTA dietary effects on lipoproteins and thrombogenic activity

Δ Greek capital letter *delta*

δ Greek lower case letter *delta*; immunoglobulin D

DEM demerol; diethylmaleate

Dem Demerol

DEMO dynamic essential modeling

DEN denervation; dengue; dermatitis exfoliativa neonatorum; Device Experience Network [of the CDRH]; diethylnitrosamine

denat denatured

DENT Dental Exposure Normalization Technique

Dent, dent dentistry, dentist, dental, dentition

DENTALPROJ Dental Research Projects

DEP depression emulation program [computer simulation]; dielectrophoresis; diethylpropanediol; dilution end point

dep dependent; deposit

DEPA diethylene phosphoramide

DEPC diethyl pyrocarbonate

depr depression, depressed

DEPS distal effective potassium secretion

DEP ST SEG depressed ST segment

DEPT distortionless enhancement by polarization transfer

dept department

DEQ Depression Experiences Questionnaire

DER disulfiram-ethanol reaction; dual energy radiography

DeR degeneration reaction

der derivative [chromosome]

DERI Diabetes Epidemiology Research International [study]

deriv derivative, derived

Derm, derm dermatitis, dermatology, dermatologist, dermatological; dermatome

DERS dependent error regression smoothing

DES Danish Enoxaparin Study; dementia rating scale; dermal-epidermal separation; desmin; dialysis encephalopathy syndrome; diethylstilbestrol; diffuse esophageal spasm; disequilibrium syndrome; doctor's emergency service

desat desaturated

desc descendant; descending

Desc Ao descending aorta

desq desquamation

DESIRE Debulking and Stenting in Restenosis Elimination [trial]

DESS double-echo steady state

DEST Denver Eye Screening Test; dichotic environmental sounds test; differentially expressed sequence tag

DESTINI Doppler Endpoint Stent International Investigation; Duke University Clinical Cardiology Study Elective Stent Trial: A Cost Containment Initiative

DeSyGNER Decision Systems Group Nucleus of Extensible Resources

DET diethyltryptamine; dipyridamole echocardiography test

DETC diethyldithiocarbamate

Det-6 detroid-6 [human sternal marrow cells]

determ determination, determined

detn detention

detox detoxification

DEUV direct electronic urethrocystometry

DEV deviant, deviation; duck embryo vaccine or virus

dev development; deviation

devel development

DevPd developmental pediatrics

DEW diagnostic encyclopedia workstation

DEX dexamethasone

Dex dextrose

dex dexterity; dextrorotatory; right [Lat. *dexter*]

DEXA dual-energy x-ray absorptiometry

DF decapacitation factor; decontamination factor; deferoxamine; defibrillation; deficiency factor; defined flora [animal]; degree of freedom; diabetic father; dietary fibers; digital fluoroscopy; discriminant function; disseminated foci; distribution factor, dorsiflexion; dysgonic fermenter

Df *Dermatophagoides farinae*; discrimination factor

df degrees of freedom

DF-2 dysgonic fermenter 2

DFA direct fluorescent antibody; discriminant function analysis; dorsiflexion assistance

DFB dinitrofluorobenzene; dysfunctional bleeding

DFC developmental field complex; dry-filled capsule

DFD defined formula diets; developmental field defect; diisopropyl phosphorofluoridate

DFDT difluoro-diphenyl-trichloroethane

DFE diffuse fasciitis with eosinophilia; distal femoral epiphysis

DFECT dense fibroelastic connective tissue

3DFEM three-dimensional finite element method

2D-FFT 2-dimensional fast Fourier transform

DFG direct forward gaze

DFHom Diploma of the Faculty of Homeopathy

DFI disease-free interval

DFIB defibrillation

DFL digital film library

DFM decreased fetal movement

DFMC daily fetal movement count

DFMO difluoromethylornithine

DFMR daily fetal movement record

DFO, DFOM deferoxamine

DFP diastolic filling period; diisopropyl-fluorophosphate

DF^{32}P radiolabeled diisopropylfluorophosphate

DFPP double filtration plasmapheresis

DFR diabetic floor routine; digital fluororadiography

DFS disease-free survival; distributed file system

DFSP dermatofibrosarcoma protuberans

DFT defibrillation threshold; dementia of frontal type; diagnostic function test; discrete Fourier transform

DFT$_3$ dialyzable fraction of triiodothyronine

DFT$_4$ dialyzable fraction of thryoxine

2DFT two-dimensional Fourier transform

3DFT three-dimensional Fourier transform

DFU dead fetus in utero; dideoxyfluorouridine

DFV diarrhea with fever and vomiting

DG dentate gyrus; deoxyglucose; desmoglein; diacylglycerol; diagnosis; diastolic gallop; DiGeorge [anomaly or syndrome] diglyceride; distogingival

2DG 2-deoxy-*D*-glucose

Dg dentate gyrus

dg decigram; diagnosis

DGA DiGeorge anomaly

DGAVP desglycinamide-9-[Arg-8]-vasopressin

DGBG dimethylglyoxal bisguanyl-hydrazone

DGCR DiGeorge chromosome region; DiGeorge critical region

DGE delayed gastric emptying

dge drainage

DGF duct growth factor

DGGE denaturing gradient gel electrophoresis

DGI dentinogenesis imperfecta; disseminated gonococcal infection

dGI dorsal giant interneuron

DGIM Division of General Internal Medicine

DGLA dihomogamma-linolenic acid

dGMP deoxyguanosine monophosphate

DGMS Division of General Medical Sciences

DGN diffuse glomerulonephritis

DGNA delayed gamma neutron activation

DGO Diploma in Gynaecology and Obstetrics

DGP 2,3-diglycerophosphate; Dutch General Practices Study

DGPG diffuse proliferative glomerulonephritis

DGS decompression sickness; developmental Gerstmann syndrome; diabetic glomerulosclerosis; DiGeorge sequence; DiGeorge syndrome; disease guidance systems; dysplasia-gigantism syndrome

DGSCR DiGeorge syndrome critical region

DGSX X-linked dysplasia gigantism syndrome

dGTP deoxyguanosine triphosphate

DGU uracil deoxyribonucleic acid glycosylase

DGV dextrose-gelatin-Veronal [buffer]

DG/VCF DiGeorge/velocardiofacial [syndrome]

DH daily habits; day hospital; dehydrocholate; dehydrogenase; delayed hypersensitivity; department of health; dermatitis herpetiformis; developmental history; diaphragmatic hernia; disseminated histoplasmosis; dominant hand; dorsal horn; drug history; ductal hyperplasia; Dunkin-Hartley [guinea pig]

D/H deuterium/hydrogen [ratio]

DHA dehydroacetic acid; dehydroascorbic acid; dehydroepiandrosterone; dihydroacetic acid; dihydroxyacetone; district health authority

DHAD mitoxantrone hydrochloride

DHAOS Dutch Hypertension and Offspring Study

DHAP dihydroxyacetone phosphate

DHAP-AT dihydroxyacetone phosphate acyltransferase

DHAS dehydroandrostenedione

DHB duck hepatitis B

DHBE dihydroxybutyl ether

DHBG dihydroxybutyl guanine

DHBS dihydrobiopterin synthetase

DHBV duck hepatitis B virus

DHC dehydrocholesterol; dehydrocholate; delivery of health care

DHCA deep hypothermia and circulatory arrest; dihydroxycholestanoic acid

DHCC dehydrocholecalciferol

DHCCP Department of Health and Social Security Hypertension Care Computing Project

DHCP decentralized hospital computer program

DHCS Department of Health and Community Services [Australia]

DHD district health department

DHE dihematoporphyrin ether; dihydroergocryptine; dihydroergotamine; distributed healthcare environment

DHEA dehydroepiandrosterone

DHEAS dehydroepiandrosterone sulfate

DHEC dihydroergocryptine

DHES Division of Health Examination Statistics

DHESN dihydroergosine

DHEW Department of Health, Education, and Welfare

DHF dengue hemorrhagic fever; dihydrofolate; dorsihyperflexion

DHF/DSS dengue hemorrhagic fever/dengue shock syndrome

DHFR dihydrofolate reductase

DHFRase dihydrofolate reductase

DHFRP dihydrofolate reductase pseudogene

DHFS Diet–Heart Feasibility Study

DHg Doctor of Hygiene

DHGG deaggregated human gammaglobulin

DHHS Department of Health and Human Services

DHI Dental Health International; dihydroxyindole

DHIA dehydroisoandrosterol

DHIAP Defense Healthcare Information Assurance Program

DHIC dihydroisocodeine

DHICA 5,6-dihydroxyindole-2-carboxylic acid

DHIS district health information system; Duke Hospital Information System

DHL diffuse histiocytic lymphoma

DHLD dihydrolipoamide dehydrogenase

DHM dihydromorphine

DHMA 3,4-dihydroxymandelic acid

DHMO dental health maintenance organization

DHO dihydro-orotate

DHODH dihydro-orotate dehydrogenase

DHP dehydrogenated polymer; dihydroprogesterone; 1,4-dihydropyridine; dual heuristic programming

DHPA dihydroxypropyl adenine

DHPCCB dihydropyrimidine calcium channel blocker

DHPDH dihydropyrimidine dehydrogenase

DHPG dihydroxyphenylglycol; dihydroxypropoxymethylguanine

DHPR dihydropteridine reductase

DHR delayed hypersensitivity reaction; Department of Human Resources; disclarge homologous region

DHS delayed hypersensitivity; diabetic hyperosmolar state; document handling system; duration of hospital stay; dynamic hip screw

D-5-HS 5% dextrose in Harman's solution

DHSM dihydrostreptomycin

DHSS Department of Health and Social Security; dihydrostreptomycin sulfate

DHT dehydrotestosterone; dihydroergotoxine; dihydrotachysterol; dihydrotestosterone; dihydrothymine; dihydroxytryptamine; discrete Hartley transform

5,7-DHT 5,7-dihydroxytryptamine

DHTP dihydrotestosterone propionate

DHTR dihydrotestosterone receptor

DHU dihydroxyuracil

DHUA Division of Health and Utilization Analysis

DHy, DHyg Doctor of Hygiene

DHZ dihydralazine

DI date of injury; date interviewed; defective interfering [particle]; dental informatics; dentinogenesis imperfecta; deoxyribonucleic acid index; deterioration index; detrusor instability; diabetes insipidus; diagnostic imaging; dialyzed iron; disability insurance; disto-incisal; document index; dorsoiliac; double indemnity; drug information; drug injection; drug interactions; duct injection; dyskaryosis index

5'DI 5'-deiodinase

DIA depolarization-induced automaticity; diabetes; diaphorase; diazepam; Drug Information Association

DiA Diego antigen

dia diakinesis; diathermy

diab diabetes, diabetic

DIACOMP Diabetes Complications [study]

DiaComp diabetes computer-aided [management]

DIAG diagnostic procedure [UMLS]

Diag diagnosis

diag diagonal; diagnosis; diagram

diam diameter

DIAMOND Danish Investigation of Arrhythmia and Mortality on Dofetilide

DIAMOND-CHF Danish Investigation of Arrhythmia and Mortality on Dofetilide in Congestive Heart Failure

DIAMOND-MI Danish Investigation of Arrhythmia and Mortality on Dofetilide in Myocardial Infarction

diaph diaphragm

dias diastole, diastolic

diath diathermy

DIB diagnostic interview for borderlines; difficulty in breathing; disability insurance benefits; dot immunobinding; duodeno-ileal bypass

DIBAL diisobytylaluminum

diBr-HQ 5,7-dibromo-8-hydroxy-quinidine

DIC dicarbazine; differential interference contrast microscopy; diffuse intravascular coagulation; direct isotope cystography; disseminated intravascular coagulation; drug information center

dic dicentric [chromosome]

DICA diagnostic interview of children and adolescents

DICD dispersion-induced circular dichroism

DICO diffusing capacity of carbon monoxide

DICOM digital imaging and communication in medicine

DICPM distributed information, computation, and process management

DID dead of intercurrent disease; dissociative identity disorder; double immunodiffusion

DIDD dense intramembranous deposit disease

DiDi Diltiazem in Dilated Cardiomyopathy [trial]

DIDMOA diabetes insipidus-diabetes mellitus-optic atrophy [syndrome]

DIDMOAD diabetis insipidus, diabetes mellitus, otpic atrophy, deafness [syndrome]

DIDS 4,4'diisothiocyanostilbene-2,2-disulfonate

DIE died in emergency department

diEMG diaphragmatic electromyography

DIET Dietary Intervention: Evaluation of Technology [study]

DIF diffuse interstitial fibrosis; direct immunofluorescence; dose increase factor

DIFF, diff difference, differential; diffusion

diff diagn differential diagnosis

DIFP diffuse interstitial fibrosing pneumonitis; diisopropyl fluorophosphonate

dif-PIPE diffuse persistent interstitial pulmonary emphysema

DIG digitalis; Digitalis Investigation Group; digoxin; drug-induced galactorrhea

dig digitalis; digoxigenin; digoxin

DIGAF Digoxin in Atrial Fibrillation [study]

DIGAMI Diabetes Mellitus, Insulin Glucose Infusion in Acute Myocardial Infarction

DIH digoxin-induced hyperkalemia; Diploma in Industrial Health

DIHE drug-induced hepatic encephalopathy

diHETE dihydroxyeicosatetraenoic acid

DIHPPA di-iodohydroxyphenylpyruvic acid

D_{ii} input delay

D_{ij} transfer delay

DIL, Dil Dilantin; drug-induced lupus [erythematosus]

Dil dilatation, dilated

dil dilute, dilution, diluted

dilat dilatation

DILCACOMP Diltiazem Captopril Comparative Study

DILD diffuse infiltrative lung disease; diffuse interstitial lung disease

DILDURANG Diltiazem Duration in Angina [study]

DILE drug-induced lupus erythematosus

DILPLACOMP Diltiazem Placebo Comparative Trial

DILS diffuse infiltrative lymphocytosis syndrome

DIM divalent ion metabolism; domain information model; medium infective dose [Lat. *dosis infectionis media*]

dim dimension; diminished

DiMe [childhood] Diabetes Mellitus [in Finland]

DIMIT 3,5-dimethyl-3'-isopropyl-L-thyronine

DIMOAD diabetes insipidus, diabetes mellitus, optic atrophy, deafness

DIMS disorders of initiating and maintaining sleep

DIMSE DICOM message service element

DIMT Dutch Ibopamine Multicenter Trial

DIN, din damage inducible [gene]

DIP desquamative interstitial pneumonitis; diffuse interstitial pneumonitis; diisopropyl phosphate; diisopropylamine; diphtheria; distal interphalangeal; drip infusion pyelogram; dual-in-line package; dynamic integral proctography

Dip diplomate

dip diploid; diplotene

DIPA diisopropylamine

DIPAL Dipyridamole in Peripheral Arteriopathy [study]

DipBact Diploma in Bacteriology

DIPC diffuse interstitial pulmonary calcification

DipChem Diploma in Chemistry

DipClinPath Diploma in Clinical Pathology

DIPF diisopropylphosphofluoridate

diph diphtheria

diph-tet diphtheria-tetanus [toxoid]

diph-tox AP alum precipitated diphtheria toxoid

DIPI defective interfering particle induction

DIPJ distal interphalangeal joint

DIPPER distributed Internet protocol performance [test system]

Dipy dipyridamole

DIR double isomorphous replacement

Dir, dir director; direction, directions

DIRD drug-induced renal disease

DIRECT Diabetes Intervention: Reaching and Educating Communities Together; Direct Myocardial Revascularization in Regeneration of Endomyocardial Channels Trial

DIRLINE Directory of Information Resources Online [NLM database]

DIRS Dutch Invasive Reperfusion Study

DIS departmental information system; Diagnostic Interview Schedule; Diagnostic Interview Survey; draft international standard

DI-S debris index, simplified

dis disability, disabled; disease; dislocation; distal; distance

DISC Diagnostic Interview Schedule for Children; Dietary Intervention Study in Children; digital interchange standards for cardiology

disc discontinue

disch discharge, discharged

DISC-HSV disabled infectious single-cycle herpes simplex virus

dis eval disability evaluation

DISH Dietary Intervention Study of Hypertension; diffuse idiopathic skeletal hyperostosis; disseminated idiopathic skeletal hyperostosis

DISI dorsal intercalated segment instability

disinfect disinfection

disl, disloc dislocation, dislocated

disod disodium

disp dispensary, dispense

DISS disease or syndrome [UMLS]; distributed image spreadsheet

diss dissolve, dissolved

dissem disseminated, dissemination

DIST Dutch Iliac Stent Trial

dist distal; distill, distillation, distilled; distance; distribution; disturbance, disturbed

DISTRESS Dispatch Stent Restenosis Study

DIT deferoxamine infusion test; defining issues test; diet-induced thermogenesis; diiodotyrosine; drug-induced thrombocytopenia

dit dictyate

dITP deoxyinosine triphosphate

div divergence, divergent; divide, divided, division

DIVBC disseminated intravascular blood coagulation

DIVC disseminated intravascular coagulation

DJD degenerative joint disease

DJOA dominant juvenile optic atrophy

DJS Dubin-Johnson syndrome

DK dark; decay; diabetic ketoacidosis; diet kitchen; diseased kidney; dog kidney [cells]

dk deka

DKA diabetic ketoacidosis

DKB deep knee bends

DKC dyskeratosis congenita

dkg dekagram

DKI dextrose potassium insulin

dkl decaliter

dkm dekameter

DKP dikalium phosphate

DKTC dog kidney tissue culture

DKV deer kidney virus

DL danger list; data language; De Lee [catheter]; deep lobe; description logic; developmental level; diagnostic laparoscopy; difference limen; diffusion lung [capacity]; digital library; dipole layer; direct laryngoscopy; disabled list; distolingual; equimolecular mixture of the dextrorotatory and levorotatory enantiomorphs; lethal dose [Lar. *dosis lethalis*]

DL, D-L Donath-Landsteiner [antibody]

D_L diffusing capacity of the lungs

dl deciliter

DLa distolabial

DLaI distolabioincisal

DLaP distolabiopulpal

DL&B direct larygoscopy and bronchoscopy

DLBD diffuse Lewy body disease

DLC Dental Laboratory Conference; differential leukocyte count; dual-lumen catheter

DLCL diffuse large cell lymphoma

DLCO carbon monoxide diffusion in the lung; single-breath diffusing capacity

DL_{CO2} carbon dioxide diffusion in the lungs

DL_{CO}^{SB} single-breath carbon monoxide diffusing capacity of the lungs

DL_{CO}^{SS} steady-state carbon monoxide diffusing capacity of the lungs

DLD dihydrolipoamide dehydrogenase

dld d-lactate dehydrogenase [gene]

D-LDH D-lactate dehydrogenase

DLE delayed light emission; dialyzable leukocyte extract; discoid lupus erythematosus; disseminated lupus erythematosus

D_1LE diagonal 1 lower extremity

D_2LE diagonal 2 lower extremity

DLF Disabled Living Foundation; dorsolateral funiculus

DLG distolingual groove

Dlg, dlg disc large

Dlg-R disc large related

DLI Digital Libraries Initiative; distolinguoincisal; double label index

DLIS digoxin-like immunoreactive substance

DLK diffuse lamellar keratitis

DLL dihomo-gammalinoleic acid

DLLI dulcitol lysine lactose iron

DLMD Duchenne-like muscular dystrophy

DLMP date of last menstrual period

DLNMP date of last normal menstrual period

DLO Diploma in Laryngology and Otology; distolinguo-occlusal

D_{LO2} diffusing capacity of the lungs for oxygen

DLP delipidized serum protein; direct linear plotting; dislocation of patella; distolinguopulpal; dysharmonic luteal phase

DLPFC dorsolateral prefrontal cortex

DLR digital luminescence radiography

D/LR dextrose in lactated Ringer solution

D_5LR dextrose in 5% lactated Ringer solution

DLST dihydrolipoamide S-succinyltransferase

DLT digital library technology; dihydroepiandrosterone loading test; direct linear transformation; dose-limiting toxicity; double lung transplantation; double-lumen endotracheal tube

DLTS digoxin-like immunoreactive substance

DLV defective leukemia virus; delavirdine

DLW dry lung weight

DM defined medium; dermatomyositis; Descemet's membrane; dextromaltose; dextromethorphan; diabetes mellitus; diabetic mother; diastolic murmur; distal metastases; dopamine; dorsomedial; double minute [chromosome]; duodenal mucosa; dry matter; dystrophia myotonica

D_M membrane component of diffusion

dm decimeter; diabetes mellitus; dorsomedial

dm^2 square decimeter

dm^3 cubic decimeter

DMA department of medical assistance; dimethylamine; dimethylaniline; dimethylarginine; direct memory access; director of medical affairs

DMAB dimethylaminobenzaldehyde

DMAC N,N-dimethylacetamide; disseminated *Mycobacterium avium* complex

DMAD dimethylaminodiphosphate

DMAE dimethylaminoethanol

DMAEM N,N'-dimethylaminoethyl methacrylate

DMAPN dimethylaminopropionitrile

DMARD disease-modifying anti-rheumatic drug

D_{max} maximum denaturation; maximum diameter

DMB diffusional microburet

DMBA 7,12-dimethylbenz[a]anthracene

DMC demeclocycline; di(p-chlorophenyl) methylcarbinol; direct microscopic count; duration of muscle contraction; Dyggve-Melchior-Clausen [syndrome]

DMCC direct microscopic clump count

DMCL dimethylclomipramine

DMCO Disease Management and Clinical Outcomes

DMCS Diagnostic Marker Cooperative Study

DMCT, DMCTC dimethylchlortetracycline

DMD disease-modifying drug; Doctor of Dental Medicine; Duchenne muscular dystrophy; dystonia musculorum deformans

DMD/BMD Duchenne/Becker muscular dystrophy

DMDC dimethyldithiocarbamate; 2'-deoxy-2'-methylidencytidine

DMDT dimethoxydiphenyl trichloroethane

DMDZ desmethyldiazepam

DME degenerative myoclonus epilepsy; dimethyl diester; dimethyl ether; diphasic meningoencephalitis; direct medical education; director of medical education; Division of Medical Education [AAMC]; dropping mercury electrode; drug-metabolizing enzyme; Dulbecco modified Eagle [medium]; durable medical equipment

DMEM Dulbecco modified Eagle medium

DMF decayed, missing, and filled [teeth]; N,N-dimethylformamide; diphasic milk fever

DMFT decayed, missing, and filled teeth

DMG dimethylglycine

DMGBL dimethyl-gammabutyrolactone

DMGT deoxyribonucleic acid-mediated gene transfer

DMH diffuse mesangial hypercellularity; 1,2-dimethylhydrazine; dorsal medial hypothalamic [nucleus]

DMHD dimenhydrinate

DMI Defense Mechanism Inventory; Diagnostic Medical Instruments; diaphragmatic myocardial infarction; direct migration inhibition

DMID Division of Microbiology and Infectious Diseases [NIH]

DMIM Defense Medical Information Management

D_{min} minimum diameter

dmin double minute

DMIS Defense Medical Information System

DMJ Diploma in Medical Jurisprudence

DMKA diabetes mellitus ketoacidosis

DMKase deoxynucleoside monophosphate kinase

DML data manipulation language; distal motor latency

DMLP Dutch Medical Language Processor

DMM dimethylmyleran; disproportionate micromelia

DMN dimethylnitrosamine; dorsal motor nucleus; Duchenne muscular dystrophy; dysplastic melanocytic nevus

DMNA dimethylnitrosamine

DMNL dorsomedial hypothalamic nucleus lesion

DMNX dorsal motor nucleus of the vagus nerve

DMO 5,5-dimethyl-2,4-oxazolidinedione (dimethadione)

D_{mo2} membrane diffusing capacity for oxygen

DMOA diabetes mellitus–optic atrophy [syndrome]

DMOD disease model

DMOOC diabetes mellitus out of control

DMP diffuse mesangial proliferation; dimercaprol; dimethylphthalate

DMPA depot medroxyprogesterone acetate

DMPC dimyristyl phosphatidyl choline

DMPE, DMPEA 3,4-dimethoxyphenylethylamine

DMPP dimethylphenylpiperazinium

DMPS dysmyelopoietic syndrome

DMR depolarizing muscle relaxant; differentially methylated region; Diploma in Medical Radiology; direct myocardial revascularization; distributed medical record

DM-R decayed plus missing teeth, minus replaced teeth

DMRD Diploma in Medical RadioDiagnosis

DMRE Diploma in Medical Radiology and Electrology

DMRF dorsal medullary reticular formation

DMRT Diploma in Medical Radio Therapy

DMS delayed match-to-sample; delayed microembolism syndrome; demarcation membrane system; department of medicine and surgery; dermatomyositis; diagnostic medical sonographer; diffuse mesangial sclerosis; dimethylsulfate; dimethylsulfoxide; District Management Team; Doctor of Medical Science; drug misuse statistics; dysmyelopoietic syndrome

DMSA dimercaptosuccinic acid; disodium monomethanearsonate

DMSO dimethyl sulfoxide

DMSS data mining surveillance system

DMT dermatophytosis; N,N-dimethyltryptamine; Doctor of Medical Technology; dynamometer muscle testing

DMTU dimethylthiourea

DMU dimethanolurea

DMV diurnal mood variations; Doctor of Veterinary Medicine; dorsal motor nucleus of the vagus nerve

DMWP distal mean wave pressure

DN Deiter's nucleus; dextrose-nitrogen; diabetic neuropathy; dibucaine number; dicrotic notch; DiFrancesco-Noble [equation]; dinitrocresol; Diploma in Nursing; Diploma in Nutrition; District Nurse; Doctor of Nursing; do not [resuscitate]; duodenum

D/N dextrose/nitrogen [ratio]

D&N distance and near [vision]

Dn dekanem

dn decinem

DNA deoxyribonucleic acid; did not answer

DNA DSB DNA double-strand break

DNAP DNA phosphorus

DNA-PK DNA–protein kinase

DNAR do not attempt resuscitation

DNASE, DNAse, DNase deoxyribonuclease

DNB dinitrobenzene; Diplomate of the National Board [of Medical Examiners]; dorsal nonadrenergic bundle

DNBP dinitrobutylphenol

DNC did not come; dinitrocarbanilide; dinitrocresol; Disaster Nursing Chairman

DNCB dinitrochlorobenzene

DNCM cytoplasmic membrane-associated deoxyribonucleic acid

DND died a natural death

DNE Director of Nursing Education; Doctor of Nursing Education

DNET dysembryoplastic neuroepithelial tumor

DNFB dinitrofluorobenzene

DNH do-not-hospitalize [order]

DNIC diffuse noxious inhibitory control

DNK did not keep [appointment]

DNKA did not keep appointment

DNLL dorsal nucleus of lateral lemniscus

DNMS delayed nonmatch-to-sample; Director of Naval Medical Services

DNMT deoxyribonucleic acid methyltransferase

Dnmt DNA methyltransferase gene

DNO District Nursing Officer

DNOC dinitroorthocresol

DNP deoxyribonucleoprotein; dinitrophenol

DNPH dinitrophenylhydrazine

DNPM dinitrophenol-morphine

DNQX 6,7-dinitroquinoxaline-2,3-dione

DNR daunorubicin; do not resuscitate; dorsal nerve root

DNS deviated nasal septum; diaphragmatic nerve stimulation; did not show [for appointment]; Dietitians in Nutrition Support; Doctor of Nursing Services; domain name system [electronic mail addressing system]; dysplastic nevus syndrome

D/NS dextrose in normal saline [solution]

D5NS 5% dextrose in normal saline [solution]

D₅NSS 5% dextrose in normal saline solution

DNT did not test; dysembryoplastic neuroepithelial tumor

DNTM disseminated nontuberculous mycobacterial [infection]

dNTP deoxyribonucleoside triphosphate

DNTT terminal deoxynucleotidyltransferase

DNV dorsal nucleus of vagus nerve; double-normalized value

DO diamine oxidase; digoxin; Diploma in Ophthalmology; Diploma in Osteopathy; dissolved oxygen; disto-occlusal; Doctor of Ophthalmology; Doctor of Optometry; Doctor of Osteopathy; doctor's orders; drugs only

D$_O$ oxygen diffusion

D$_{O2}$ oxygen delivery

DOA date of admission; dead on arrival; Department of Agriculture; depth of anesthesia; differential optical absorption; dominant optic atrophy

DOAC Dubois oleic albumin complex

DOB date of birth; doctor's order book

Dob dobutamine

DObstRCOG Diploma of the Royal College of Obstetricians and Gynaecologists

DOC date of conception; deoxycholate; deoxycorticosterone; died of other causes; disorders of cornification; dissolved organic carbon; distributed object computing; Doctros Ought to Care [project]

doc doctor; document, documentation

DOCA deoxycorticosterone acetate

DOCG deoxycorticosterone glucoside

DOCLINE Documents On-Line

DOCS deoxycorticosteroids

DOcSc Doctor of Ocular Science

DOCUSER Document Delivery User [NLM database]

DOD date of death; dementia syndrome of depression; depth of discharge; died of disease; dissolved oxygen deficit

DoDCPR Department of Defense computerized patient record

DOE date of examination; Department of Defense; desoxyephedrine; direct observation evaluation; dyspnea on exertion

DOES disorders of excessive sleepiness

DOF, dof degree of freedom

DOFCOSY double-quantum filtered correlated spectroscopy

DOFISK Dose Finding of Streptokinase [trial]

DOFOS disturbance of function occlusion syndrome

DOG deoxyglucose; difference of gaussians; distraction osteogenesis

DoG difference of gaussians

DOH department of health

DOHyg Diploma in Occupational Hygiene

DOI date of injury; died of injuries; digital object identifier

DO$_2$I oxygen delivery index

DOIA Dermatological Online Atlas

Dol dolichol

dol pain [Lat. *dolor*]

DOLLS [Lee] double-loop locking suture

DOLV double outlet left ventricle

DOM deaminated O-methyl metabolite; department of medicine; dimethoxymethylamphetamine; dissolved organic matter; dominance, dominant

dom dominant

DOMA dihydromandelic acid

DOMF 2'7'-dibromo-4'-(hydroxymercuri) fluorescein

DOMIOS Determinants of Myocardial Infarction Onset [study]

DOMS Diploma in Ophthalmic Medicine and Surgery

DON Director of Nursing; diazooxonorleucine

DONALD dissection of neck arteries: long-term follow-up determination

DOOR deafness, onycho-osteodystrophy, mental retardation [syndrome]

DOP dioctyl phthalate; Directory of Physicians

DOPA, dopa dihydroxyphenylalanine

DOPAC dihydrophenylacetic acid

DOPAMINE dihydroxyphenylethylamine

dopase dihydroxyphenylalanine oxidase

DOPC determined osteogenic precursor cell; dioleoyl-phosphatidyl choline

DOPE dioleoyl-phosphatidyl ethanolamine

DOph Doctor of Ophthalmology

DOPP dihydroxyphenylpyruvate

DOPS diffuse obstructive pulmonary syndrome; dihydroxyphenylserine; dioleoyl-phosphatidyl serine

dor dorsal

DORNA desoxyribonucleic acid

Dors dorsal

DOrth Diploma in Orthodontics; Diploma in Orthoptics

DORV double outlet right ventricle

DOS day of surgery; deoxystreptamine; disk operating system; Doctor of Ocular Science; Doctor of Optical Science; dysosteosclerosis

dos dosage, dose

DOSC Dubois oleic serum complex

DOSPO documentation system for pediatric oncology

DOSS distal over-shoulder strap; dioctyl sodium sulfosuccinate; docusate sodium

DOT date of transfer; Dictionary of Occupational Titles; directly observed therapy

DOTC Dameshek's oval target cell

DOTES dosage record and treatment emergent symptoms

DOTMA di-oleoyloxopropyl-trimethyl-ammonium chloride

DOTS directly observed therapies; directly observed treatment, short course

DOUBLE Double Bolus Lytic Efficacy [trial]

DOUBTFUL double quantum transition for finding unresolved lines

DOUBTLESS Doppler and Ultrasound-Guided Balloon Therapeutics for Coronary Lesions [study]

DOX doxorubicin

Dox doxorubicin

DOX-SL stealth ribosomal doxorubicin

DP data processing; deep pulse; definitive procedure; degradation product; degree of polymerization; dementia praecox; dementia pugillistica; dental prosthodontics, dental prosthesis; desmoplakin; dexamethasone pretreatment; diastolic pressure; diazepam; diffuse precipitation; diffusion pressure; diffusion pressure deficit; digestible protein; diphosgene; diphosphate; dipropionate; directional preponderance; disability pension; discrimination power; distal pancreatectomy; distal phalanx; distal pit; distopulpal; docking protein; Doctor of Pharmacy; Doctor of Podiatry; donor's plasma; dorsalis pedis

D/P dialysate-to-plasma [ratio]

Dp duplication; dyspnea

D_p pattern difference

DPA D-penicillamine; Department of Public Assistance; diphenylalanine; dipicolinic acid; dipropylacetic acid; direct provider agreement; dual photon absorptiometry; dynamic physical activity

DPAHC durable power of attorney for health care

DPB days post-burn; diffuse panbronchiolitis

DPBP diphenylbutylpiperidine

DPC delayed primary closure; deoxyribonucleic acid [DNA] probe chromatography; deoxyribonucleic acid [DNA] protein cross-links; desaturated phosphatidylcholine; diethylpyrocarbonate; direct patient care; discharge planning coordinator; distal palmar crease

dpc days post coitum

DPCRT double-blind placebo-controlled randomized clinical trial

DPD Department of Public Dispensary; depression pure disease; desoxypyridoxine; diffuse pulmonary disease; diphenamid; Diploma in Public Dentistry

DPDL diffuse poorly differentiated lymphocytic lymphoma

dP/dt first derivative of pressure measured over time

dpdt double-pole double-throw [switch]

dP/dV pressure per unit change in volume

DPE dipiperidinoethane

DPEP dipeptidase

DPF Dental Practitioners' Formulary; dilsopropyl fluorophosphate

DPFC distal flexion palmar crease

DPFR diastolic pressure-flow relationship

DPG 2,3-diphosphoglycerate; displacement placentogram

2,3-DPG 2,3-diphosphoglycerate

2,3-DPGM 2,3-diphosphoglycerate mutase

DPGN diffuse proliferative glomerulonephritis

DPGP diphosphoglycerate phosphatase

DPH Department of Public Health; diphenhydramine; diphenylhexatriene; diphenylhydantoin; Diploma in Public Health; Doctor of Public Health; Doctor of Public Hygiene; dopamine beta-hydrolase

DPhC Doctor of Pharmaceutical Chemistry

DPhc Doctor of Pharmacology

DPHN Doctor of Public Health Nursing

DPhys Diploma in Physiotherapy

DPhysMed Diploma in Physical Medicine

DPI daily permissible intake; days post inoculation; dietary protein intake; diphtheria-pertussis immunization; disposable personal income; drug prescription index; Dynamic Personality Inventory

DPJ dementia paralytica juvenilis

DPKC diagnostic problem-knowledge coupler

DPL diagnostic peritoneal lavage; dipalmitoyl lecithin; distopulpolingual

DPLa distopulpolabial

DPLN diffuse proliferative lupus nephritis

DPLS differentially polarized light scattering

DPM Diploma in Psychological Medicine; discontinue previous medication; Doctor of Physical Medicine; Doctor of Podiatric Medicine; Doctor of Preventive Medicine; Doctor of Psychiatric Medicine; dopamine

dpm disintegrations per minute

DPN dermatosis papulosa nigra; diabetic polyneuropathy; diphosphopyridine nucleotide; disabling pansclerotic morphea; dorsal parabrachial nucleus

DPNB dorsal penile nerve block

DPNH reduced diphosphopyridine nucleotide

DPO dimethoxyphenyl penicillin

DPP Diabetes Prevention Program; differential pulse polarography; digital pulse plethysmography; dimethylphenylpenicillin; dipeptidylpeptidase; distal photoplethysmography

dpp decapentaplegic

DPPC dipalmitoylphosphatidylcholine; double-blind placebo-controlled trial

DPPD diphenylphenylenediamine

DpPHR duodenum-preserving pancreatic head resection

DPR dietary prevention of recurrent myocardial infarction; drug price review; dynamic perception resolution

DPS delayed primary suture; descending perineum syndrome; dimethylpolysiloxane; Division of Provider Studies [database]; dysesthetic pain syndrome

dps disintegrations per second

dpst double-pole single-throw [switch]

DPSWF discrete prolate spheroidal wave function

DPT Demerol, Phenergan, and Thorazine; dermatopontin; Diabetes Prevention Trial; dichotic pitch discrimination test; diphtheria-pertussis-tetanus [vaccine]; diphtheritic pseudotabes; dipropyltryptamine; dumping provocation test

Dpt house dust mite

DPTA diethylenetriamine penta-acetic acid

DPTI diastolic pressure time index

DPTPM diphtheria-pertussis-tetanus-poliomyelitis-measles [vaccine]

Dptr diopter

DPUF Doppler ultrasound flowmeter

DPV disabling positional vertigo

DPVS Denver peritoneovenous shunt

DPW Department of Public Welfare; distal phalangeal width

DQ deterioration quotient; developmental quotient

3DQCT three-dimensional computed tomography

DQE detective quantum efficiency

DR death receptor [cell], degeneration reaction; delivery room; deoxyribose; diabetic retinopathy; diagnostic radiology; digital radiography; direct repeat; distal recurrence; distribution ratio; doctor; dopamine receptor; dorsal raphe; dorsal root; dose ratio; drug receptor

Dr doctor

dR dextroribose, deoxyriboside

dr dorsal root; drain; dram; dressing

DRA dextran-reactive antibody

DRACOG Diploma of Royal Australian College of Obstetricians and Gynaecologists

DRACR Diploma of Royal Australasian College of Radiologists

DRAM dynamic random access memory

dr ap dram, apothecary

DRASTIC Dutch Renal Artery Stenosis Intervention Cooperative Study

DRAT differential rheumatoid agglutination test

DRB daunorubicin

DRBC denaturated red blood cell; dog red blood cell; donkey red blood cell

DRC damage risk criterion; dendritic reticulum cell; diagnostic reporting console; digitorenocerebral [syndrome]; dorsal root, cervical; dynamic range compression

DRCOG Diploma of Royal College of Obstetricians and Gynaecologists

DRCPath Diploma of Royal College of Pathologists

DRD dihydroxyphenylalanine-responsive dystonia; dorsal root dilator; dystrophia retinae pigmentosa–dysostosis [syndrome]

DRD$_2$ dopamine D$_2$ receptor

DRD$_3$ dopamine D$_3$ receptor

DRD$_4$ dopamine D$_4$ receptor

DRE damage response element [DNA]; digital rectal examination

DREF dose rate effectiveness factor

DREN Department of Defense Research and Engineering Network

DRES dynamic random element stimuli

DRESS depth-resolved surface-coil spectroscopy

DREZ dorsal root entry zone

DRF Daily Rating Form; daily replacement factor; Deafness Research Foundation; dose reduction factor

DRFS Dundee Rank Factor Score [risk factors in coronary heart disease]

DRG diagnosis-related group; Division of Research Grants [NIH]; dorsal respiratory group; dorsal root ganglion; duodenal-gastric reflux gastropathy

drg drainage

DrHyg Doctor of Hygiene

DRI defibrillation response interval; discharge readiness inventory

dRib deoxyribose

DRID double radial immunodiffusion; double radioisotope derivative

DRIN direct reconstructor interface

DRIP delirium and drugs-restricted mobility and retention-infection, inflammation and impaction-polyuria [causes of urinary incontinence]

DRL dorsal root, lumbar; drug-related lupus

D5RL 5% dextrose in Ringer lactate [solution]

DRME Division of Research in Medical Education

Dr Med Doctor of Medicine

DRMF directional recursive median filtering

DRMS drug reaction monitoring system

DrMT Doctor of Mechanotherapy

DRN dorsal raphe nucleus

DRNDP diribonucleoside-3',3'-diphosphate

DRnt diagnostic roentgenology

DRO differential reinforcement of other behavior; Disablement Resettlement Officer

DRP digoxin reduction product; dorsal root potential; drug-related problems; dystrophia retinae pigmentosa–dysostosis [syndrome]; dystrophin-related protein

dRp deoxyribose-phosphate

dRPase, dRpase deoxyribophosphodiesterase

DrPH Doctor of Public Health; Doctor of Public Hygiene

DRPLA dentorubral-pallidoluysian atrophy

DRQ discomfort relief quotient

DRR digitally reconstructed radiograph; dorsal root reflex; dysjunction regulator region

DRS descending rectal septum; diagnostic review station; diffuse reflectance spectroscopy; disability rating scale; Diltiazem Reinfarction Study; drowsiness; Duane retraction syndrome; dynamic renal scintigraphy; Dyskinesia Rating Scale

drsg dressing

DRSP drug-resistant *Streptococcus pneumoniae*

DRST Delayed Recognition Span Test

DRT dorsal root, thoracic

3-DRTP three dimensional radiation treatment planning

DRUGS Doctor, Recreational User, Gynaecological Sensitivities [study]

DRUJ distal radioulnar joint

dRVVT dilute Russell viper venom time

DRY donryu [rat]

DS Dahl strain [rat]; dead air space; dead space; deep sedative; deep sleep; defined substrate; dehydroepiandrosterone sulfate; delayed sensitivity; dendritic spine; density standard; dental surgery; dermatan sulfate; dermatology and syphilology; desynchronized sleep; Devic syndrome; dextran sulfate; dextrose-saline; diameter stenosis; diaphragm stimulation; diastolic murmur; differential stimulus; diffuse scleroderma; dilute strength; dioptric strength; disaster services; discrimination score; disoriented; disseminated sclerosis; dissolved solids; Doctor of Science; donor's serum; Doppler sonography; double-stranded; double strength; double stringency; Down syndrome; drug store; dry swallow; dumping syndrome; duplex scan; duration of systole

D/S dextrose/saline

D&S dermatology and syphilology

D-5-S 5% dextrose in saline solution

ds double stranded [DNA]

%DS percent diameter stenosis

D1S first year dental student

D2S second year dental student

D3S third year dental student

D4S fourth year dental student

DSA density spectral array; destructive spondyloarthropathy; digital subtraction angiography; dynamic scalable architecture

DSACT, D-SACT direct sinoatrial conduction time

DSAF Decision Support Access Facility [Bureau of Data Management and Strategy Facilities, BDMS]

DSAP disseminated superficial actinic porokeratosis

DSAS discrete subaortic stenosis

DSB, dsb double-strand break [DNA]

Dsb single-breath diffusion capacity

DSBL disabled

DSBR double-strand break repair

DSBT donor-specific blood transfusion

DSC de Sanctis-Cacchione [syndrome]; desmocollin; digital scan converter; disodium chromoglycate; Doctor of Surgical Chiropody; Down syndrome child

DSc Doctor of Science

DSCF Doppler-shifted constant frequency

DSCG disodium chromoglycate

DSCR developmental self-care requisites

DSCT dorsal spinocerebellar tract

DSD Déjerine-Sottas disease; depression spectrum disease; discharge summary dictated; dry sterile dressing

DS-DAT Discomfort Scale for Dementia of the Alzheimer Type

DSDDT double sampling dye dilution technique

dsDNA double-stranded deoxyribonucleic acid

DSE dobutamine stress echocardiography; Doctor of Sanitary Engineering

DSG decision system group; desmoglein; dry sterile gauze

Dsg desmoglein

DSH deliberate self harm; dexamethasone suppressible hyperaldosteronism; disproportionate share hospital

DSHR delayed skin hypersensitivity reaction

DSI deep shock insulin; Depression Status Inventory; desmocollin-specific insertion; disulfide isomerase; Down Syndrome International

DSIM Doctor of Science in Industrial Medicine

DSIP delta sleep-inducing peptide

DSL distal sensory latency

DSL MU distal sensory latency–median-ulnar

dslv dissolve

DSM dextrose solution mixture; Diagnostic and Statistical Manual [of Mental Disorders]; Diploma in Social Medicine; drink skim milk

DSM, dsm disease-specific mortality

DSM-III-R Diagnostic and Statistical Manual [of Mental Disorders], Third Edition, Revised

DSM-IV Diagnostic and Statistical Manual [of Mental Disorders], Fourth Edition

DSMA diet and stress management in angina

DSMB Data Safety Monitoring Board [FDA]

DSMC data and safety monitoring committee

DSNI deep space neck infection

DSO digital storage oscilloscope; distal subungual onychomycosis

DSP decreased sensory perception; delayed sleep phase; desmoplakin; dibasic sodium phosphate; digital subtraction phlebography; display

DSPC disaturated phosphatidylcholine

DSPCR, DS-PCR double stringency polymerase chain reaction

DSPN distal sensory polyneuropathy; distal symmetrical polyneuropathy

DSR distal spleno-renal; double simultaneous recording; dynamic spatial reconstructor

dsRNA double-stranded ribonucleic acid

DSRS distal splenorenal shunt

DSS [computer-based] decision support system; Déjerine-Sottas syndrome; dengue shock syndrome; digital storage system; dioctyl sodium sulfosuccinate; Disability Status Scale; discrete subaortic stenosis; docusate sodium; dosage-sensitive sex [reversal]; double simultaneous stimulation

DSSc Diploma in Sanitary Science

DSSEP dermatomal somatosensory evoked potential

DSSI Duke social support index

DSST Digit Symbol Substitution Task

DST desensitization test; dexamethasone suppression test; dihydrostreptomycin; disproportionate septal thickening; donor-specific transfusion

DS-TRIEL Decision Support [cancer clinical] Trial Eligibility

DSUH directed suggestion under hypnosis

DSur Doctor of Surgery

DSVP downstream venous pressure

DSWI deep surgical wound infection
DT database tomography; deceleration time; defibillation threshold; definitive type; differential technique; delirium tremens; dental technician; depression of transmission; dietetic [services]; dietetic technician; digitoxin; diphtheria-tetanus [toxoid]; discharge tomorrow; dispensing tablet; distance test; dorsalis tibialis; double tachycardia; duration of tetany; dye test
D/T date of treatment; total ratio of deaths
d/t due to
dT deoxythymidine
dt due to; dystonic
DTA decision to abort; differential thermal analysis; diphtheria toxin A
DTaP diphtheria-tetanus-pertussis [vaccine]
DTB dedicated time block
DTBC d-tubocurarine
DTBN di-t-butyl nitroxide
DTC day treatment center; differential thyroid carcinoma
dTc d tubocurarine
DTCD Diploma in Tuberculosis and Chest Diseases
DTCH Diploma in Tropical Child Health
DTD diastrophic dysplasia; document type definition
DTDase deoxyuridine triphosphate diphosphohydrolase
DTDES dynamic template driven data entry system
dTDP deoxythymidine diphosphate
DTE desiccated thyroid extract
DTF detector transfer function
D-TGA dextraposed transposition of great arteries
DTH delayed-type hypersensitivity; Diploma in Tropical Hygiene
DTI diffusion tensor imaging; dipyridamole-thallium imaging; Doppler tissue imaging
DTIA Doppler tissue imaging acceleration
DTIC dacarbazine; dimethyltriazenyl imidazole carboxamide
DTICH delayed traumatic intracerebral hemorrhage
DTIE Doppler tissue imaging energy
D time dream time
DTIV Doppler tissue imaging velocity
DTLA Detroit Test of Learning Aptitudes

DTM dermatophyte test medium; Diploma in Tropical Medicine
DTM&H Diplomate of Tropical Medicine and Hygiene
DTMP deoxythymidine monophosphate
DTMS Drug Therapy Monitoring System
DTN diphtheria toxin, normal
DTNB 5,5'-dithiobis-(2-nitrobenzoic) acid
DTO data terminal operator; deodorized tincture of opium
DTP diphtheria-tetanus-pertussis [vaccine]; distal tingling on percussion; Tinel's sign
DTPA diethylenetriaminepentaacetic acid
DTPa diphtheria-tetanus-acellular pertussis [vaccine]
DTPBw diphtheria-tetanus whole cell pertussis [vaccine]
DTPH Diploma in Tropical Public Health
dTPM deoxythymidine monophosphate
DTR deep tendon reflex; dietetic technician registered
DTRTT digital temperature recovery time test
DTS dense tubular system; diphtheria toxin sensitivity; distributed time service; donor transfusion, specific
DT's delirium tremens
DTT diagnostic and therapeutic team; diphtheria tetanus toxoid; direct transverse traction; dithiothreitol
dTTP deoxythymidine triphosphate
DTUS diathermy, traction, and ultrasound
DT-VAC diphtheria-tetanus vaccine
DTVM Diploma in Tropical Veterinary Medicine
DTVMI developmental test of visual motor integration
DTVP developmental test of visual perception
DTX detoxification
DTZ diatrizoate
DU decubitus ulcer; density unknown; deoxyuridine; dermal ulcer; diagnosis undetermined; diazouracil; dog unit; duodenal ulcer; duroxide uptake; Dutch [rabbit]
dU deoxyuridine
du dial unit; duplication [chromosome]
DUA dorsal uterine artery
DUB dysfunctional uterine bleeding
DUCCS Duke University Clinical Cardiology Study

DUDP Drug Use and Drug Prevention [study]

dUDP deoxyuridine dephosphate

DUE drug use evaluation

D₁UE diagonal 1 upper extremity

D₂UE diagonal 2 upper extremity

DUET Dispatch Urokinase Efficacy Trial

DUF Doppler ultrasonic flowmeter; drug use forecast

DUFSS Duke-University of North Carolina Functional Social Support [questionnaire]

DUHP Duke-University Health Profile

DUI driving under the influence

DUL diffuse undifferentiated lymphoma

dulc sweet [Lat. *dulcis*]

dUMP deoxyuridine monophosphate

duod duodenum, duodenal

dup duplication

DUQUES Duke University quantitative/qualitative evaluation system

DUR drug use review; drug utilization review

Dur during, duration

dur during

DURAC duration of anticoagulation

DUS diagnostic ultrasonography; Doppler flow ultrasound

DUSN diffuse unilateral subacute neuroretinitis

DUSOCS Duke social support and stress scale

DUSOI Duke University severity of illness [index]

dut deoxyuridine triphosphatase [gene]

DUTCH-TIA Dutch Transient Ischemic Attack Study

dUTP deoxyuridine triphosphate

dUTPase deoxyuridine triphosphatase

DUV damaging ultraviolet [radiation]

DV dependent variable; diagnostic variable; difference in volume; digital vibration; dilute volume; distemper virus; domestic violence; domiciliary visit; dorsoventral; double vibration; double vision; ductus venosus

3-DV three dimensional visualization

D&V diarrhea and vomiting

dv double vibrations

DVA developmental venous anomaly; distance visual acuity; duration of voluntary apnea; vindesine

DVB divinylbenzene

DVC divanillylcyclohexane; dorsal vagal complex

DVCC Disease Vector Control Center

DVD dissociated vertical deviation

DV&D Diploma in Venereology and Dermatology

dVDAVP 1-deamine-4-valine-D-arginine vasopressin

DVE duck virus enteritis

DVH Diploma in Veterinary Hygiene; Division for the Visually Handicapped; dose volume histogram

DVI deep venous insufficiency; diastolic velocity integral; digital vascular imaging; Doppler velocity index; AV sequential [pacemaker]

DVIS digital vascular imaging system

DVIU direct-vision internal urethrotomy

DVL deep vastus lateralis

DVM digital voltmeter; Doctor of Veterinary Medicine

DVMS Doctor of Veterinary Medicine and Surgery

DVN dorsal vagal nucleus

DVP deep venous pressure; Doppler velocity profile

DVR digital vascular reactivity; Doctor of Veterinary Radiology; double valve replacement; double ventricular response

DVS Doctor of Veterinary Science; Doctor of Veterinary Surgery

DVSc Doctor of Veterinary Science

DVT Danish Verapamil Trial; deep venous thrombosis

DVT/PE deep venous thrombosis/pulmonary embolism

DW daily weight; deionized water; dextrose in water; distilled water; doing well; dry weight

D/W dextrose in water

D5W 5% dextrose in water

D₅W 5% dextrose in water

D10W 10% aqueous dextrose solution

dw dwarf [mouse]

DWA died from wounds by the action of the enemy

DWCE density-weighted contrast enhancement

DWD died with disease

DWDL diffuse well-differentiated lymphocytic lymphoma

DWDM dense wave division multiplexing

DWECNP Dr. Welford's Electronic Chart Notes Program

DWI driving while impaired; driving while intoxicated

DWM Dandy-Walker malformation

DWML deep white matter lesion

DWS Dandy-Walker syndrome; disaster warning system

DWT dichotic word test; discrete wave transform

dwt pennyweight

DWV Dandy-Walker variant

DX DNA region X chromosome; dextran; dicloxacillin

Dx, dx diagnosis

D&X dilation and extraction

DXA dual [energy] x-ray absorptiometry

dx cath diagnostic catheterization

DXD discontinued

DxDx differential diagnosis

DXM dexamethasone

DXP digital x-ray prototype

DxPLAIN Massachusetts General Hospital's expert diagnostic system

DXPNET Digital X-Ray Prototype Network

DXR deep x-ray

DXRT deep x-ray therapy

DXT deep x-ray therapy; dextrose

dXTP deoxyxanthine triphosphate

D_{xx} input delay

D_{xy} transfer delay

DY dense parenchyma

Dy dysprosium

dy dystrophia muscularis [mouse]

dyn dynamic; dynamometer; dyne

DYNAMO dynamic decision modeling [system]

DYS dysautonomia

dysp dyspnea

DZ diazepam; dizygotic; dizziness

dZ impedance change

dz disease; dozen

dZ/dt time-dependent impedance change

DZM dorsal zone of membranelle

DZP diazepam

E air dose; cortisone [compound E]; each; eating; edema; elastance; electric charge; electric field vector; electrode potential; electromotive force; electron; embryo; emmetropia; encephalitis; endangered [animal]; endogenous; endoplasm; enema; energy; *Entamoeba*; enterococcus; enzyme; eosinophil; epicondyle; epinephrine; error; erythrocyte; erythroid; erythromycin; *Escherichia;* esophagus; ester; estradiol; ethanol; ethyl; examination; exhalation; expectancy [wave]; expected frequency in a cell of a contingency table; experiment, experimenter; expiration; expired air; exposure; extract, extracted, extraction; extraction fraction; extralymphatic; eye; glutamic acid; internal energy; kinetic energy; mathematical expectation; redox potential; stereodescriptor to indicate the configuration at a double bond [Ger. *entgegen* opposite]; unit [Ger. *Einheit*]

E* lesion on the erythrocyte cell membrane at the site of complement fixation

Ē average beta energy

E_0 electric affinity

E_1 estrone

E_2 17β-estradiol

E_3 estriol

E_4 estetrol

4E four-plus edema

$E°$ standard electrode potential

e base of natural logarithms, approximately 2.7182818285; egg transfer; ejection; electric charge; electron; elementary charge; exchange

e^- negative electron

e^+ positron

ε see *epsilon*

η see *eta*

EA early antigen; educational age; egg albumin; electric affinity; electrical activity; electroacupuncture; electroanesthesia; electrophysiological abnormality; embryonic antibody; endocardiographic amplifier; Endometriosis Association; enteral alimentation; enteroanastomosis; enzymatically active; epiandrosterone; episodic ataxia; erythrocyte antibody; erythrocyte antiserum; esophageal atresia; estivo-autumnal; ethacrynic acid

E/A early to late diastolic filling ratio; emergency admission

E&A evaluate and advise

E_a energy of aggregation

ea each

Eα kinetic energy of alpha particles

EAA electroacupuncture analgesia; Epilepsy Association of America; essential amino acid; excitatory amino acid; extrinsic allergic alveolitis

EAAC excitatory amino acid carrier

EAB elective abortion; Ethics Advisory Board

EABV effective arterial blood volume

EAC Ehrlich ascites carcinoma; electroacupuncture; epithelioma adenoides cysticum; erythema annulare centrifugum; erythrocyte, antibody, complement; external auditory canal

EACA epsilon-aminocaproic acid

EACD eczematous allergic contact dermatitis

EACH essential access community hospital

EACSS European and Australian Cooperative Stroke Study

EACT educational activity [UMLS]

EAD early afterdepolarization; Enterprise Access Directory; extracranial arterial disease

EA-D early antigen, diffuse

E-ADD epileptic attentional deficit disorder

EADS early amnion deficit spectrum or syndrome

EAE experimental allergic encephalomyelitis; experimental autoimmune encephalitis

EAEC enteroadherent *Escherichia coli*

EAFT European Atrial Fibrillation Trial

EAG electroarteriography

EAGAR Estrogen and Graft Atherosclerosis Research Trial

EAggEC enteroaggregative *Escherichia coli*

EAHF eczema, asthma, and hay fever

EAHLG equine antihuman lymphoblast globulin

EAHLS equine antihuman lymphoblast serum

EAI Emphysema Anonymous, Inc.; erythrocyte antibody inhibition

EAK ethyl amyl ketone

EAM episodic ataxia with myokymia; external acoustic meatus

EAMG experimental autoimmune myasthenia gravis

EAMI exercise training in anterior myocardial infarction

EAN experimental allergic neuritis

EAO experimental allergic orchiitis

EAP electric acupuncture; employee assistance program; epiallopregnanolone; Epstein-Barr associated protein; erythrocyte acid phosphatase; evoked action potential

EAQ eudismic affinity quotient

EAR European Association of Radiology

EA-R early antigen, restricted

Ea R reaction of degeneration [Ger. *Entartungs-Reaktion*]

EARIIA East Anglian Regional Health Authority

EARS European Atherosclerosis Research Study

EARR extended aortic root replacement

EAS Edinburgh Artery Study; endarterectomized aortic segment

EASI European Antiplatelet Stent Investigation; European applications in surgical interventions

EAST Eastern Association for the Surgery of Trauma; elevated-arm stress test; Emory angioplasty vs. surgery trial; external rotation, abduction stress test

EAT Eating Attitudes Test; Ehrlich ascites tumor; electro-aerosol therapy; epidermolysis acuta toxica; experimental autoimmune thymitis; experimental autoimmune thyroiditis

EATC Ehrlich ascites tumor cell

EAV entity-attribute-value [data organization]; equine abortion virus; equine arteritis virus

EAVC enhanced atrioventricular conduction

EAVM extramedullary arteriovenous malformation

EAVN enhanced atrioventricular nodal [conduction]

EB elective abortion; electron beam; elementary body; emotional behavior; endometrial biopsy; epidermolysis bullosa; Epstein-Barr [virus]; esophageal body; estradiol benzoate; Evans blue

EBA epidermolysis bullosa acquisita; epidermolysis bullosa atrophicans; orthoethoxybenzoic acid

EBC esophageal balloon catheter

EBCDIC Extended Binary Coded Decimal Interchange Code

EBCT electron-beam computed tomography

EBD epidermolysis bullosa dystrophica

EBDCT Cockayne-Touraine type of epidermolysis bullosa dystrophica

EBDD epidermolysis bullosa dystrophica dominant

EBDR epidermolysis bullosa dystrophica recessiva

EBF erythroblastosis fetalis; exclusive breast feeding

E-BFU erythroid blood forming unit

EBG electroblepharogram, electroblepharography

EBH epidermolysis bullosa hereditaria

EBHC evidence-based healthcare

EBI emetine bismuth iodide; erythroblastic island; estradiol binding index

EB-IORT intraoperative electron beam boost

EBK embryonic bovine kidney

EBL erythroblastic leukemia; estimated blood loss

eBL endemic Burkitt lymphoma

EBL/S estimated blood loss during surgery

EBM electrophysiologic behavior modification; epidermal basement membrane; epidermolysis bullosa, macular type; evidence-based medicine; expressed breast milk

EBMS Engineering and Biology in Medicine Society

EBMWG evidence-based medicine working group

EBNA Epstein-Barr virus-associated nuclear antigen

EBO Ebola [disease or virus]

E/BOD electrolyte biochemical oxygen demand

EBO-R Ebola Reston virus

EBP error-back propagation; estradiol-binding protein

EBRI Employee Benefits Research Institute

EBRT electron beam radiotherapy; external beam radiation therapy

EBS elastic back strap; electric brain stimulation; Emergency Bed Service; epidermolysis bullosa simplex

EBSS Earle's balanced salt solution

EBT electron beam tomography; external beam therapy

EBV effective blood volume; Epstein-Barr virus; estimated blood volume

EBv Epstein-Barr virus

EBVS Epstein-Barr virus susceptibility

EBZ epidermal basement zone

EC effective concentration; ejection click; electrochemical; electron capture; embryonal carcinoma; emergency center; endemic cretinism; endocrine cells; endothelial cell; energy charge; enteric coating; entering complaint; enterochromaffin; entorhinal cortex; Enzyme Commission; epidermal cell; epirubicin/cyclophosphamide; epithelial cell; equalization-cancellation; error correction; *Escherichia coli*; esophageal carcinoma; ethyl chloride; excitation-contraction; experimental control; expiratory center; extended care; exterior coat; external carotid [artery]; external conjugate; extracellular; extracellular concentration; extracorporeal; extracranial; eye care; eyes closed

E-C ether-chloroform [mixture]

E/C endocystoscopy; enteric-coated; estrogen/creatinine ratio

Ec ectoconchion; entorhinal cortex

EC$_{50}$ median effective concentration

ECA electrical control activity; electrocardioanalyzer; endothelial cytotoxic activity; enterobacterial common antigen; epidemiological catchment area; esophageal carcinoma; ethacrynic acid; ethylcarboxylate adenosine; external carotid artery

E$_{Ca}$ calcium reversal potential

ECAA European Concerted Action on Anticoagulation [study]

E-CABG endarterectomy and coronary artery bypass graft

E-CAD E-cadherin

ECAO enteric cytopathogenic avian orphan [virus]

ECAP European Concerted Action Project

ECAQ elderly cognitive assessment questionnaire

ECASS European Cooperative Acute Stroke Study

ECAT European Concerted Action on Thrombosis [study]

ECAT AP European Concerted Action on Thrombosis: Angina Pectoris [study]

ECBD exploration of common bile duct

ECBO enteric cytopathogenic bovine orphan [virus]

ECBS Expert Committee on Biological Standardization [WHO]

ECBV effective circulating blood volume

ECC electrocorticogram, electrocorticography; electronic claim capture; embryonal cell carcinoma; emergency cardiac care; emergency care center; encoding combinatorial chemistry; endocervical cone; endocervical curettage; estimated creatinine clearance; external cardiac compression; extracorporeal circulation

ECCE Effects of Captopril on Cardiopulmonary Exercise [study]; extracapsular cataract extraction

ECCL encephalocraniocutaneous lipomatosis

ECCLS European Committee for Clinical Laboratory Standards

ECCO enteric cytopathogenic cat orphan [virus]; European Culture Collection Organisation

ECCO$_2$ extracorporeal carbon dioxide

ECCO$_2$R extracorporeal carbon dioxide removal

ECCOMAC European Concerted Community Action Programmes

ECD ectrodactyly; electrochemical detector; electron capture detector; endocardial cushion defect; enzymatic cell dispersion; equivalent current dipole; ethylcysteinate dimer

E/CDK cyclin E dependent kinase

ECDO enteric cytopathic dog orphan [virus]

ECE equine conjugated estrogen

ECEO enteric cytopathogenic equine orphan [virus]

ECETOC European Centre for Ecotoxicity and Toxicology of Chemicals

ECF effective capillary flow; eosinophilic chemotactic factor; erythroid colony formation; extended care facility; extracellular fluid

ECFA, ECF-A eosinophilic chemotactic factor of anaphylaxis

ECFC eosinophilic chemotactic factor complement

ECFMG Educational Commission on Foreign Medical Graduates; Educational Council for Foreign Medical Graduates

ECFMS Educational Council for Foreign Medical Students

E-CFU erythroid colony-forming unit

ECFV extracellular fluid volume

ECFVD extracellular fluid volume depletion

ECG electrocardiogram, electrocardiography

ECGF endothelial cell growth factor

ECGS endothelial cell growth supplement

ECH educator contact hour

ECHO echocardiography; enteric cytopathic human orphan [virus]; Etoposide, cyclophosphamide, Adriamycin, and vincristine

EchoCG echocardiography

Echo-Eg echoencephalography

Echo-VM echoventriculometry

ECHSCP Exeter Community Health Services Computer Project

ECI electrocerebral inactivity; eosinophil chemotaxis index; eosinophilic cytoplasmic inclusions; extracorporeal irradiation

ECIB extracorporeal irradiation of blood

EC/IC extracranial/intracranial

ECICD European Consortium for Intensive Care Data

ECIL extracorporeal irradiation of lymph

ECIS equipment control information system

ECK extracellular potassium

ECL electrochemoluminescent; emitter-coupled logic; enterochromaffin-like [type]; euglobin clot lysis

ECLAP European Collaboration on Low-Dose Aspirin in Polycythemia Vera

ECLS extracorporeal life support

ECM electronic claims management; embryonic chick muscle; erythema chronicum migrans; experimental cerebral malaria; external cardiac massage; extracellular material; extracellular matrix

ECML extracellular membrane layer

ECMO enteric cytopathic monkey orphan [virus]; extracorporeal membrane oxygenation

ECN equipment control number

E co *Escherichia coli*

ECochG electrocochleography

ECOG Eastern Cooperative Oncology Group

ECoG electrocorticogram, electrocorticography

E COLI eight nerve action potential, cochlear nucleus, olivary complex (superior), lateral lemniscus, inferior colliculus [hearing test]

E coli Escherichia coli

ECP ectrodactyly-cleft palate [syndrome]; effector cell precursor; endocardial potential; eosinophil cationic protein; erythrocyte coproporphyrin; erythroid committed precursor; *Escherichia coli* polypeptide; estradiol cyclopentane propionate; external cardiac pressure; external counterpulsation; free cytoporphyrin of erythrocytes

ECPA Electronic Communication Privacy Act

ECPO enteric cytopathic porcine orphan [virus]

ECPOG electrochemical potential gradient

ECPR external cardiopulmonary resuscitation

ECR effectiveness-cost ratio; electrocardiographic response; emergency care research; emergency chemical restraint; European Congress of Radiology

ECRB extensor carpi radialis brevis

ECRHS European Community Respiratory Health Survey

ECRI Emergency Care Research Institute

ECRL extensor carpi radialis longus

ECRO enteric cytopathogenic rodent orphan [virus]

ECR-SCSI European Committee for Recommendation-Standard on Computer Aspects of Diagnostic Imaging

ECS elective cosmetic surgery; electrocerebral silence; electroconvulsive shock, electroshock; endocervical swab; endothelial cells; extracellular solids; extracellular space

ECSG European Cooperative Study Group

ECSO enteric cytopathic swine orphan [virus]

ECSP epidermal cell surface protein

ECSS European Coronary Surgery Study

ECST European carotid surgery trial

ECSURF economic evaluation of surfactant

ECSYSVAS European Community Systemic Vasculitis [trials]

ECT electroconvulsive therapy; emission computed tomography; enteric coated tablet; euglobulin clot test; European compression technique

ect ectopic, ectopy

ECTA esophageal gastric tube airway; Everyman's Contingency Table Analysis

ECU environmental control unit; extended care unit; extensor carpi ulnaris

ECV epithelial cell vacuolization; extracellular volume; extracorporeal volume

ECVAM European Centre for the Validation of Alternative Methods

ECVD extracellular volume of distribution

ECW extracellular water

ED early-decision [applicant]; early differentiation; ectodermal dysplasia; ectopic depolarization; effective dose; Ehlers-Danlos [syndrome]; elbow disarticulation; electrodialysis; electron diffraction; embryonic death; emergency department; emotional disorder, emotionally disturbed; end-diastole; enteric drainage; entering diagnosis; Entner-Doudoroff [pathway]; enzyme deficiency; epidural; epileptiform discharge; equine dermis [cells]; erectile dysfunction; erythema dose; ethyl dichlorarsine; ethynodiol; event definition; evidence of disease; exertional dyspnea; exponential distribution; extensive disease; extensor digitorum; external diameter; extra-low dispersion

E-D ego-defense; Ehlers-Danlos [syndrome]

ED$_{50}$ median effective dose

E$_d$ depth dose

ed edema

EDA ectodermal dysplasia, anhidrotic; electrodermal activity; electrodermal audiometry; electrolyte-deficient agar; electron donor acceptor; electronic design automation; end-diastolic area; exploratory data analysis

EDAM electron-dense amorphous material

EDAP emergency department approved for pediatrics

EDAX energy dispersive x-ray analysis

EDB early dry breakfast; electron-dense body; Enrollment Database [Medicare]; extended definition beta; extensor digitorum brevis

EDBP erect diastolic blood pressure

EDC emergency decontamination center; end-diastolic count; estimated date of conception; expected date of confinement; expected delivery, cesarean; extensor digitorum communis

ED&C electrodesiccation and curettage

EDCF endothelium-derived contracting factor

EDCI energetic dynamic cardiac insufficiency

EDCP eccentric dynamic compression plate [osteosynthesis]

EDCS end-diastolic chamber stiffness; end-diastolic circumferential stress

EDD effective drug duration; electron dense deposit; end-diastolic dimension; esophageal detection device; estimated due date; expected date of delivery

EDDA expanded duty dental auxiliary

EDDS electronic development delivery system

EDE effective dose equivalent

EDECS emergency department expert charting system

edent edentia, edentulous

EDF eosinophil differentiation factor; erythroid differentiation factor; extradural fluid

EDG electrodermography

EDGE Evaluation of Dispatch Catheter for Vein Graft Revascularization

EDH epidural hematoma

EDHEP European Donor Hospital Education Program

EDHF endothelium-derived hyperpolarizing factor

EDI eating disorder inventory; electronic data interchange

EDIC Echocardiography Dobutamine International Cooperative Study; Epidemiology of Diabetes Intervention and Complications

EDIM epizootic diarrhea of infant mice

E-diol estradiol

EDIT Early Defibrillator Implantation Trial; Early Diabetes Intervention Trial

EDL end-diastolic length; end-diastolic load; Essential Drug List [WHO]; estimated date of labor; extensor digitorum longus

ED/LD emotionally disturbed and learning disabled

ED LOS emergency department length of stay

EDM early diastolic murmur; esophageal Doppler monitoring; Essential Drugs and Medicines [WHO]; extramucosal duodenal myotomy

EDMA ethylene glycol dimethacrylate

EDMD emergency physician; Emery-Dreifuss muscular dystrophy

EDN electrodesiccation; eosinophil-derived neurotoxin

EDNA Emergency Department Nurses Association

EDNF endogenous digitalis-like natriuretic factor

EDOC estimated date of confinement

EDOU emergency department observation unit

EDP electron dense particle; electronic data processing; end-diastolic pressure

EDQ extensor digiti quinti

EDR early diastolic relaxation; effective direct radiation; electrodermal response; endothelium-dependent relaxation

EDRES Effects of Debulking on Restenosis [trial]

EDRF endothelium-derived relaxing factor

EDS edema disease of swine; egg drop syndrome; Ehlers-Danlos syndrome; Emery-Dreifus syndrome; energy-dispersive spectrometry; epigastric distress syndrome; essential data set; excessive daytime sleepiness; extradimensional shift

EDSR electronic document storage and retrieval

EDSS expanded disability status scale

EDT end-diastolic thickness; erythrocyte density test

EDTA ethylenediamine tetraacetic acid

EDTR emergency department-based trauma response

EDTU emergency diagnostic and treatment unit

Educ education

EDV end-diastolic volume; epidermodysplasia verruciformis

EDVI end-diastolic volume index

EDVX X-linked epidermodysplasia verruciformis

EDWTH end-diastolic wall thickness

EDX, EDx electrodiagnosis

EDXA energy-dispersive x-ray analysis

EE embryo extract; end-to-end; end expiration; energy expenditure; *Enterobacteriaceae* enrichment [broth]; equine encephalitis; ethinyl estradiol; expressed emotion; external ear; eye and ear

E&E eye and ear

E-E erythema-edema [reaction]

EEA electroencephalic audiometry; end-to-end anastomosis

EEC ectrodactyly–ectodermal dysplasia–clefting [syndrome]; enteropathogenic *Escherichia coli*

EECD endothelial-epithelial corneal dystrophy

EECG electroencephalography

EED experimental emergency department

EEE eastern equine encephalitis; eastern equine encephalomyelitis; experimental enterococcal endocarditis; external eye examination

EEEP end-expiratory esophageal pressure

EEEV eastern equine encephalomyelitis virus

EEG electroencephalogram, electroencephalography

EEGA electroencephalographic audiometry

EEG-CSA electroencephalography with computerized spectral analysis

EEGL low-voltage electroencephalography

EEGV1 electroencephalographic variant pattern 1

EELS electron energy loss spectroscopy

EELV end-expiratory lung volume

EEM ectodermal dysplasia, ectrodactyly, macular dystrophy [syndrome]; erythema exudativum multiforme

EEMCO European Group for Efficacy Measurements on Cosmetics and Other Tropical Products

EEME, EE3ME ethinylestradiol-3-methyl ether

EEMG evoked electromyogram

EENT eye, ear, nose, and throat

EEP end-expiratory pressure; equivalent effective photon

EEPI extraretinal eye position information

EER electroencephalographic response; extended entity-relationship

EES erythromycin ethylsuccinate; ethyl ethanesulfate

EESG evoked electrospinogram

EET epoxyeicosatrienoic [acid]

EEV endocardial ventriculotomy

EF ectopic focus; edema factor; ejection fraction; elastic fibril; electric field; elongation factor; embryo-fetal; embryo fibroblasts; emergency facility; encephalitogenic factor; endothoracic fascia; endurance factor; eosinophilic fasciitis; epithelial focus; equivalent focus; erythroblastosis fetalis; erythrocyte fragmentation; exposure factor; extrafine; extended field [radiotherapy]; extrinsic factor

EFA Epilepsy Foundation of America; essential fatty acid; extrafamily adoptee

EFAD essential fatty acid deficiency

EFAS embryofetal alcohol syndrome

EFC elastin fragment concentration; endogenous fecal calcium; ephemeral fever of cattle

EFCC European Federation of Coding Centres

EFD estimated fluid deficit

EFDA expanded function dental assistant

EFE endocardial fibroelastosis

EFERF Enalapril Felodipine Extended Release Factorial Study

EFF electromagnetic field focusing

eff effect; efferent; efficiency; effusion

effect effective

effer efferent

EFFU epithelial focus-forming unit

EFH explosive follicular hyperplasia

EFICAT Ejection Fraction in Carvedilol-treated Transplant Candidates [study]

EFL effective focal length

EFM elderly fibromyalgia; electronic fetal monitoring; external fetal monitor

EFMI European Federation of Medical Informatics

EFP early follicular phase; effective filtration pressure; endoneural fluid pressure

EFR effective filtration rate

EFS electric field stimulation; European Fraxiparin Study; event-free survival

EFT Embedded Figures Test

EFV extracellular fluid volume

EFVC expiratory flow-volume curve

EFW estimated fetal weight

EFZ efavirenz

EG enteroglucagon; eosinophilic granuloma; esophagogastrectomy; ethylene glycol; external genitalia

eg for example [Lat. *exempli gratia*]

EGA enhanced graphics adaptation; estimated gestational age

EGAD Expressed Gene Anatomy Database

EGBUS external genitalia, Bartholin, urethral, Skene glands

EGC early gastric cancer; epithelioid-globoid cell

EGD esophagogastroduodenoscopy

EGDF embryonic growth and development factor

EGDT early goal-directed therapy

EGF early graft failure; endothelial growth factor; epidermal growth factor

EGFR, EGF-R epidermal growth factor receptor

EGF-URO epidermal growth factor, urogastrone

EGG electrogastrogram

EGH equine growth hormone

EGHIN Ellen Gartenfeld Health Information Network

EGIR European Group for the Study of Insulin Resistance

EGL eosinophilic granuloma of the lung

EGLT euglobin lysis time

EGM electrogram; extracellular granular material

EGME ethylene glycol monomethyl ether

EGN experimental glomerulonephritis

EGOT erythrocytic glutamic oxaloacetic transaminase

EGR early growth response; erythema gyratum repens

E-GR erythrocyte glutathione reductase

EGR-2 early growth response [protein]

EGRA equilibrium-gated radionuclide angiography

EGRAC erythrocyte glutathione reductase activity coefficient

EGS electrogalvanic stimulation; electron gamma-shower; external guide sequence

EGT ethanol gelation test

EGTA esophageal gastric tube airway; ethyleneglycol-bis-(β-aminoethylether)-N,N,N',N'-tetraacetic acid

EH enlarged heart; epidural hematoma; epidermolytic hyperkeratosis; epoxide hydratase; esophageal hiatus; essential hypertension; external hyperalimentation

E/H environment and heredity

E&H environment and heredity

E$_h$ redox potential

eh enlarged heart

EHA Emotional Health Anonymous; Environmental Health Agency

EHAA epidemic hepatitis-associated antigen

EHB elevate head of bed

EHBA extrahepatic biliary atresia

EHBD extrahepatic bile duct

EHBF estimated hepatic blood flow; exercise hyperemia blood flow; extrahepatic blood flow

EHC enterohepatic circulation; enterohepatic clearance; essential hypercholesterolemia; ethylhydrocupreine hydrochloride; extended health care; extrahepatic cholestasis

EHCW emergency health care worker

EHD electrohemodynamics; epizootic hemorrhagic disease

EHDP ethane-1-hydroxy-1,1-diphosphate

EHDV epizootic hemorrhagic disease virus

EHEC enterohemorrhagic *Escherichia coli*

EHF epidemic hemorrhagic fever; exophthalmos-hyperthyroid factor; extreme high frequency

EHG electrohysterogram, electrohysterography

EHH esophageal hiatal hernia

EHI employer's health insurance; environmental health indicator

EHIBCC European Health Industry Business Communications Council

EHIV exposure to human immunodeficiency virus

EHK epidermolytic hyperkeratosis

EHL effective half-life; electrohydraulic lipotripsy; endogenous hyperlipidemia; Environmental Health Laboratory; essential hyperlipemia; extensor hallucis longus

EHME employee health maintenance examination

EHMS electrohemodynamic ionization mass spectometry

EHNA 9-erythro-2-(hydroxy-3-nonyl) adenine

EHO environmental health officer; extrahepatic obstruction

EHP di-(20-ethylhexyl) hydrogen phosphate; Environmental Health Perspectives; excessive heat production; extrahigh potency

EHPAC Emergency Health Preparedness Advisory Committee

EHPH extrahepatic portal hypertension

EHPT Eddy hot plate test

EHQ Eating Habits Questionnaire

EHR electronic healthcare record

EHS environmental health and safety

EHSDS experimental health services delivery system

EHT electrohydrothermoelectrode; essential hypertension

EHV electric heart vector; equine herpes virus

EHVT Edinburgh Heart Valve Trial

EI earliness index; Edmonton injector; electrical injury; electrolyte imbalance; electron impact; electron ionization; emotionally impaired; energy index; energy intake; enzyme inhibitor; eosinophilic index; Evans index; excretory index

E/I expiration/inspiration [ratio]

E$_I$ ionic reversal potential

e-I early inspiratory

EIA electroimmunoassay; enzyme immunoassay; enzyme-linked immunosorbent assay; equine infectious anemia; erythroimmunoassay; excessive inappropriate aggression; exercise induced asthma; external iliac artery; an interface between a computer and a system for transmitting digital information

EIAB extracranial-intracranial arterial bypass

EIAV equine infectious anemia virus

EIB electrophoretic immunoblotting; eosinophilic intracytoplasmic inclusion body; exercise-induced bronchospasm

EIC elastase inhibition capacity; enzyme inhibition complex; extensive intraductal component

EICESS European Intergroup Cooperative Ewing's Sarcoma Study

EID egg infectious dose; electroimmunodiffusion; emergency infusion device

EIEC enteroinvasive *Escherichia coli*
EIEE early infantile epileptic encephalopathy
EIES Electronic Information Exchange System
EIF erythrocyte initiation factor; eukaryotic initiation factor
eIF erythrocyte initiation factor; eukaryotic initiation factor
eIF4E eukaryotic initiation factor 4E
EIHDW Evaluation of Ischemic Heart Disease in Women [study]
EII electrical impedance imaging
EIM equity implementation model; excitability-inducing material
EIMS electron ionization mass spectrometry
EINECS European Inventory of Existing Commercial Chemical Substances
EIP end-expiratory pause; extensor indicis proprius
EIPS endogenous inhibitor of prostaglandin synthase
eIPV enhanced inactivated poliomyelitis vaccine
EIRnv extra incidence rate of non-vaccinated groups
EIRP effective isotropic radiated power
EIRv extra incidence in vaccinated groups
EIS Environmental Impact Statement; Epidemic Intelligence Service; European Infarction Study
EIT electrical impedance tomography; erythroid iron turnover
EIU enzyme immunoassay unit
EIV external iliac vein
EIVA equine infectious anemia virus
EIW electronic information warehouse
EJ elbow jerk; external jugular
EJB ectopic junctional beat
EJM epilepsy juvenile myoclonic
EJP excitation junction potential
EJV external jugular vein
EK enterokinase; erythrokinase
E$_K$ potassium reversal potential
EKC epidemic keratoconjunctivitis
EKG electrocardiogram, electrocardiography
EKLF erythroid Krüppel-like factor
EKS epidemic Kaposi sarcoma
EKV erythrokeratodermia variabilis
EKY electrokymogram, electrokymography

EL early latent; elbow; electroluminescence; erythroleukemia; exercise limit; external lamina
El elastase
el elixir
ELA elastase; elastomer-lubricating agent; endotoxin-like activity
ELAM endothelial leukocyte adhesion molecule
ELAS extended lymphadenopathy syndrome
ELAT Embolism in Left Atrial Thrombi [study]
ELAV embryonic lethal, abnormal vision
ELB early light breakfast; elbow
elb elbow
ELBW extremely low birth weight
ELCA Excimer Laser Coronary Angioplasty [registry]
ELD egg lethal dose
elec electricity, electric
elect elective; electuary
ELECTZ electrosurgical loop excision of the cervical transformation zone
ELEM equine leukoencephalomalacia
elem elementary
elev elevation, elevated, elevator
ELF elective low forceps; extremely low frequency
ELG eligibility [database]
ELH egg-laying hormone
ELHE Evaluation of Losartan in Hemodialysis [study]
ELI exercise lability index
ELIA enzyme-linked immunoassay
ELICT enzyme-linked immunocytochemical technique
ELIEDA enzyme-linked immunoelectron diffusion assay
ELIRA enzyme-linked immunoreceptor assay
ELISA enzyme-linked immunosorbent assay
ELISK excimer laser intrastromal keratomileusis
ELITE Evaluation of Losartan in the Elderly [study]
elix elixir
ELL elongation factor homologous to mixed lineage leukemia
ELM external limiting membrane; extravascular lung mass

ELN elastin; electronic noise
ELND elective lymph node dissection
ELOD expected average lod [score]
ELOP estimated length of program
ELOS estimated length of stay
ELP elastase-like protein; endogenous limbic potential
ELS Eaton-Lambert syndrome; electron loss spectroscopy; enzymatic labile site; extended least square; extralobar sequestration
ELSA European Lacidipine Study on Atherosclerosis; European Longitudinal Study on Aging
ELSI ethical, legal, and social issues
ELSS emergency life support system
ELT endless loop tachycardia; euglobulin lysis time
ELV erythroid leukemia virus
ELVD Exercise in Left Ventricular Dysfunction [trial]
ELVD-CHF Exercise in Left Ventricular Dysfunction and Chronic Heart Failure [trial]
elx elixir
EM early memory; ejection murmur; electromagnetic; electron micrograph; electron microscopy, electron microscope; electrophoretic mobility; Embden-Meyerhof [pathway]; emergency medicine; emmetropia; emotional disorder, emotionally disturbed; ergonovine maleate; erythema migrans; erythema multiforme; erythrocyte mass; erythromycin; esophageal manometry; esophageal motility; estramusine; expectation-maximization [algorithm]; extensive metabolizer; extracellular matrix
E/M electron microscope, electron microscopy; evaluation and management
E&M endocrine and metabolic
Em emmetropia
E$_m$ mid-point redox potential
EMA electronic microanalyzer; emergency medical assistance, emergency medical assistant; emergency medical attendant; endothelial monocyte antigen; epithelial membrane antigen
EMAB endothelial monocyte antigen B
E-mail electronic mail
EMAP evoked muscle action potential
E$_{max}$ maximum effect, maximum energy
EMB embryology; endomyocardial biopsy; engineering in medicine and biology; eosin-methylene blue; ethambutol; explosive mental behavior
emb embolism; embryo; embryology
EMBASE Excerpta Medica Database
EMBL European Molecular Biology Laboratory
EMBO European Molecular Biology Organization
embryol embryology
EMC electromagnetic compatibility; electron microscopy; emergency medical care; emergency medical condition; emergency medical coordinator; encephalomyocarditis; essential mixed cryoglobulinemia
EMCR electronic medical care record
EMC&R emergency medical care and rescue
EMCRO Experimental Medical Care Review Organization
EMD emergency medical dispacher; emergency medical doctor; Emery-Dreifuss muscular dystrophy; esophageal mobility disorder
EMDIS European Marrow Donor Information System
EMDR eye movement desensitization and reprocessing
EMEDI European Medical Electronic Data Interchange [group]
EMEM Eagle minimal essential medium
EMER electromagnetic molecular electron resonance
emer emergency
EMF electromagnetic flowmeter; electromotive force; Emergency Medicine Foundation; endomyocardial fibrosis; equivalent molecules of immunofluorescence; erythrocyte maturation factor; evaporated milk formula
emf electromotive force
EMG electromyogram, electromyography; eye movement gauge; exomphalos-macroglossia-gigantism [syndrome]
EMG(int) integrated electromyographic [value]
EMGN extramembranous glomerulonephritis
EMG/NCV electromyography/nerve conduction velocity [test]
EMI electromagnetic immunity; electromagnetic interference; emergency medical information

EMIAT European Myocardial Infarction Amiodarone Trial; European Myocardial Infarction Arrhythmia Trial

EMIC emergency maternal and infant care; Environmental Mutagen Information Center [NLM]

EMICBACK Environmental Mutagen Information Center Backfile [NLM database]

EMIP European Myocardial Infarction Project

EMIP-FR European Myocardial Infarction Project—Free Radicals

EMIT enzyme multiplied immunoassay technique; European Mivazerol Trial

EMJH Ellinghausen-McCullough-Johnson-Harris [medium]

EML erythema nodosum leprosum

EMLA eutectic mixture of local anesthetics

EMM erythema multiforme major

EMMA eye movement measuring apparatus

EMO Epstein-Macintosh-Oxford [inhaler]; exophthalmos, myxedema circumscriptum praetibiale, and osteoarthropathia hypertrophicans [syndrome]

emot emotion, emotional

EMP electric membrane property; electromagnetic pulse; Embden-Meyerhof pathway; European Myocardial Infarction Project; external membrane potential or protein; extramedullary plasmacytoma; malignant proliferation of eosinophils

EMPAR Enoxaparin Maxepa Prevention of Angioplasty Restenosis [study]

EMPhMA European Pharmaceutical Marketing Association

EMPIRE Economics of Myocardial Perfusion Imaging in Europe [study]

EMPS exertional muscle pain syndrome

EMR educable mentally retarded; electromagnetic radiation; electronic medical record; emergency mechanical restraint; emergency medicine resident; essential metabolism ratio; eye movement record

EMRA Emergency Medicine Residents Association

EMRC European Medical Research Council

EMRD emergency medicine residency director

EMRS electronic medical record system

EMS early morning specimen; early morning stiffness; electrical muscle stimulation; Electronic Medical Service; emergency medical services; endometriosis; eosinophilia myalagia syndrome; ethyl methane-sulfonate; European Multicenter Study

EMSA electrophoretic mobility shift assay; Emergency Medical Services Agency

EMSC emergency medical services for children

EMSS emergency medical services system

EMT emergency medical tag; emergency medical team; emergency medical technician; emergency medical treatment; endocardial mapping technique

EMTA endomethylene tetrahydrophthalic acid

EMT-A emergency medical technician-ambulance; emergency medical technician providing basic life support or cardiopulmonary resuscitation

EMTALA Emergency Medical Treatment and Active Labor Act

EMT-B basic emergency medical technician

EMT-D emergency medical technician providing basic life support or defibrillation

EMT-I emergency medical technician-intermediate

EMT-M or **EMT-MAST** emergency medical technician–military antishock trousers

EMT-P emergency medical technician-paramedic

EMTS electromagnetic tracking system

EMT-W emergency medical technician-wilderness

EMU early morning urine; energy-mode ultrasound

emu electromagnetic unit

emul emulsion

EMV eye, motor, voice [Glasgow coma scale]; equine morbillivirus

EMVC early mitral valve closure

EMY emergency medicine resident year

EN endoscopy; enrolled nurse; enteral nutrition; epidemic nephritis; erythema nodosum

En, en enema

ENA Emergency Nurses' Association; epithelial neutrophil-activating [protein]; extractable nuclear antigen

E$_{Na}$ sodium reversal potential
ENaC epithelial sodium channel
ENASA Enoxaparin and/or Aspirin in Unstable Angina [trial]
ENC encounter; endotoxin neutralizing capacity; environmental control
ENCORE Evaluation of Nifedipine and Cerivastatin on Recovery of Endothelial Function [trial]
END early neonatal death; endocrinology; endorphin; endothelin; endurance
end endoreduplication
ENDIT European Nicotinamide Diabetes Intervention Trial
Endo endocardial, endocardium; endocrine, endocrinology; endodontics; endonuclease; endotracheal
endo endoscopy
ENDOR electron nuclear double resonance
Endo X endonuclease X
ENDPT end-point of flow velocity after angioplasty; evaluation of Doppler parameters during percutaneous transluminal coronary angioplasty
ENDR endothelin receptor
ENDRB endothelin receptor B
ENDT electroneurodiagnostic technologist
ENE ethylnorepinephrine
ENeG electroneurography
enem enema
ENG electroneurography, electroneurograph; electronystagmogram, electronystagmography
Eng English
ENI elective neck irradiation
ENK enkephalin
ENL erythema nodosum leproticum
ENO, Eno enolase
ENOG, ENoG electroneuronography
eNOS endothelial nitric oxide synthase
ENOXART enoxaparin in arterial surgery
ENP electromagnetic pulse; ethyl-p-nitrophenylthiobenzene phosphate; excellence for nursing practice; extractable nucleoprotein
ENR eosinophilic nonallergic rhinitis; extrathyroid neck radioactivity
ENRICAD Enhancing Recovery in Coronary Heart Disease [trial]
ENRICHD Enchancing Recovery in Coronary Heart Disease Patients [trial]

ENS enteral nutritional support; epidermal nevus syndrome; ethylnorsuprarenin
ENT ear, nose, and throat; enzootic nasal tumor; extranodular tissue
ent enterotoxin
ent A enterotoxin A
ENTICES Enoxaparin and Ticlopidine after Elective Stenting [study]
Entom entomology
ENTY entity [UMLS]
ENU N-ethyl–nitrosourea
Env envelope [protein]
env, environ environment, environmental
ENVR environmental effect [UMLS]
ENX endonexin
enz enzyme, enzymatic
EO early-onset; eosinophil; ethylene oxide; eyes open
E$_o$ skin dose
EOA effective orifice area; erosive osteoarthritis; esophageal obturator airway; examination, opinion, and advice
EOAD early-onset Alzheimer disease
EOB emergency observation bed; explanation of benefits
EOC emergency observation center
EOCA early onset cerebellar ataxia
EOD entry on duty; every other day
EOF end of file
E of M error of measurement
EOG electro-oculogram, electro-oculography; electro-olfactogram, electro-olfactography
EOGBS early onset group B streptococcal [infection]
EOJ extrahepatic obstructive jaundice
EOL end-of-life
EOM electro-optic modulator; end of message; equal ocular movement; external otitis media; extraocular movement; extraocular muscle
EoM equation of motion
EOMA emergency oxygen mask assembly
EOMB explanation of Medicare benefits
EOMI extraocular muscles intact
EOM NL extraocular eye movements normal
EOP efficiency of plating; emergency outpatient
EOR European Organization for Research; exclusive operating room

EORTC European Organization for Research and Treatment of Cancer
EOS end of study; eosinophil; European Orthodontic Society
eos, eosin eosinophil
Eosm effective osmolarity
EOT effective oxygen transport
EOU epidemic observation unit
EOx eye oximeter
EP echo planar; ectopic pregnancy; edible portion; electrophoresis; electrophysiologic; electroprecipitin; emergency physician; emergency procedure; endogenous pyrogen; endoperoxide; endorphin; end point; enteropeptidase; environmental protection; enzyme product; eosinophilic pneumonia; epicardial electrogram; epirubicin; epithelium, epithelial; epoxide; erythrocyte protoporphyrin; erythrophagocytosis; erythropoietic porphyria; erythropoietin; esophageal pressure; European Pharmacopoeia; evoked potential; expert panel; extramustine phosphate; extreme pressure
E$_p$ proton energy
EPA eicosapentaenoic acid; empiric phrase association; Environmental Protection Agency; erect posterior-anterior; erythroid potentiating activity; extrinsic plasminogen activator
EPAP expiratory positive airway pressure
EPAQ Extended Personal Attitudes Questionnaire
EPA/RCRA Environmental Protection Agency Resource Conservation and Recovery Act
EPB extensor pollicis brevis
EPC end-plate current; epilepsia partialis continua; external pneumatic compression
EPCA external pressure circulatory assistance
EPCG endoscopic pancreatocholangiography
EPCOT European Prospective Cohort on Thrombophilia
EPCRLS European Pancreatic Cancer Reference Library System
EPCS emergency portocaval shunt
EPD energy-protein deficit
EPDML epidemiology, epidemiologic
EPE erythropoietin-producing enzyme
EPEC enteropathogenic *Escherichia coli*
EPEG etoposide

EPESE epidemiologic studies of the elderly; established populations for epidemiologic studies of the elderly
EPF early pregnancy factor; endocarditis parietalis fibroplastica; endothelial proliferating factor; established program financing; estrogenic positive feedback; exophthalmos-producing factor
EPG eggs per gram [count]; electropalatography; electropneumography, electropneumogram; ethanolamine phosphoglyceride
EPH edema-proteinuria-hypertension; episodic paroxysmal hemicrania; extensor proprius hallucis
EPI echo planar imaging; electronic portal imaging; Emotion Profile Index; epilepsy; epinephrine; epithelium, epithelial; Estes Park Institute; evoked potential index; Expanded Programme of Immunization [WHO]; extrapyramidal involvement; extrinsic pathway inhibitor
EPIC Echocardiography Persantine International Cooperative Study; Echo Persantine Italian Cooperative Study; European Prevalence of Infection in Intensive Care Study; European Prospective Investigation into Cancer and Nutrition Study; European Prototype for Integrated Care; Evaluation of 7E3 for the Prevention of Ischemic Complications
EPICORE Epidemiology Coordinating Research Centre
EPICS Early Postmenopausal Intervention Cohort Study
EPID electronic portal imaging device
EPIDS Early Post-Myocardial Infarction Intravenous Dipyridamole Study
epid epidemic
epil epilepsy, epileptic
EPILOG Evaluation of Percutaneous Transluminal Coronary Angioplasty to Improve Long-Term Outcome with Abciximab Glycoprotein IIb/IIIa Blockade [trial]
epineph epinephrine
epis episiotomy
EPISODE Evaluation Peripheral Intramuscular Sonography on Dotter Effect
EPI/STAR echo planar imaging with signal targeting and alternating radiofrequency
EPISTENT EPILOG STENT Trial; Evaluation of IIb/IIIa Platelet Inhibitor for Stenting

epith epithelium

EPIV enhanced potency inactivated polio vaccine

EPIX Emergency Preparedness Information Exchange [Canada]

EPL effective patient's life; equivalent path length; essential phospholipid; extensor pollicis longus; extracorporeal piezoelectric lithotriptor

EPM electron probe microanalysis; electrophoretic mobility; energy-protein malnutrition

EPMR progressive epilepsy with mental retardation

EPO eosinophil peroxidase; erythropoiesis; erythropoietin; evening primrose-oil; exclusive provider organization; expiratory port occlusion

Epo erythropoietin

EPOB employee per occupied bed

EPOCH Erythropoietin in Chinese Hamster Ovary [study]

EPOR erythropoietin receptor

EPP end-plate potential; equal pressure point; erythropoietic protoporphyria

epp end-plate potential

EPPB end positive-pressure breathing

EPPS Edwards Personal Preference Schedule

EPQ Eysenck Personality Questionnaire

EPR early progressive resistance; effective poor radius; electron paramagnetic resonance; electronic patient record; electrophrenic respiration; emergency physical restraint; estradiol production rate; extraparenchymal resistance

EPRCSS European Prospective Randomized Coronary Surgery Study

EPROM erasable programmable read-only memory

EPROU Electronic Patient Record System at Osaka University Hospital

EPRS electronic patient record system; European Prospective Randomized Study

EPS ear-patella-short stature [syndrome]; elastosis perforans serpiginosa; electrophysiologic study; enzyme pancreatic secretion; exophthalmos-producing substance; extracellular polysaccharide; extrapyramidal side effects; extrapyramidal symptom, extrapyramidal syndrome

ep's epithelial cells

EPSC excitatory postsynaptic current

EPSDT early and periodic screening diagnosis and treatment program

EPSE extrapyramidal side effects

EPSEM equal probability of selection method

EPSI echo planar spectroscopic imaging

ε Greek letter *epsilon*; heavy chain of IgE; permittivity; specific absorptivity

EPSP excitatory postsynaptic potential

EPSS E-point septal separation

EPT early pregnancy test

EPTE existed prior to enlistment

EPTFE, ePTFE expanded polytetrafluoroethylene

EPTS existed prior to service

EPV encephaloclastic proliferative vasculopathy; entomopoxvirus

EPXMA electron probe x-ray microanalyzer

EQ educational quotient; encephalization quotient; energy quotient; equal to

Eq, eq equation; equivalent

EQA external quality assessment

EQAM Ervin quality assessment measure

EQOL economics and quality of life

EQS electroquasistatic

equip equipment

EQUIPP Evaluation of Quinapril in Primary Practice [trial]

equiv equivalency, equivalent

ER efficiency ratio; epigastric region; ejection rate; electroresection; emergency room; endoplasmic reticulum; enhanced reactivation; enhancement ratio; environmental resistance; equine rhinopneumonia; equivalent roentgen [unit]; erythrocyte receptor; estradiol receptor; estrogen receptor; etretinate; evoked response; expiratory reserve; extended release; extended resistance; external resistance; external rotation

ER⁻ decreased estrogen receptor

ER⁺ increased estrogen receptor

E/R entity/relationship

Er erbium; erythrocyte

E_r repulsive energy

er endoplasmic reticulum

ERA echo record access study; electrical response activity; electroencephalic response audiometry; Electroshock Research Association; Enoxaparin Restenosis after Angioplasty [study]; entity relationship attribute; estrogen receptor assay; Estrogen Replacement in Atherosclerosis [study]; estradiol receptor assay; evoked response audiometry; extended relational algebra

ERA-ICA estradiol receptor assay immunocytochemical analysis

ERAS electronic residency application service

ERASME Efficacy of Renal Artery Stent Multicentre Evaluation

ERBAC Excimer Laser, Rotablator and Balloon Angioplasty Comparison [study]

ERBF effective renal blood flow

ERC endoscopic retrograde cholangiography; enteric cytopathic human orphan-rhinocoryza [virus]; erythropoietin-responsive cell; ethical review committee; European Resuscitation Council

Erc erythrocyte

ERCC excision repair cross-complementing

ERCP endoscopic retrograde cholangiopancreatography

ERD evoked response detector

ERDA Energy Research and Development Administration

ERE external rotation in extension

EREP event related evoked potential

eRF eukaryotic release factor

ERF Education and Research Foundation; external rotation in flexion; Eye Research Foundation

E-RFC E-rosette forming cell

ERFS electrophysiological ring finger splinting

ERG electron radiography; electroretinography, electroretinogram

ERHD exposure-related hypothermic death

ERI E-rosette inhibitor

ERIA electroradioimmunoassay

ERIC Educational Resource Information Center; Educational Resource Information Clearinghouse

ERICA European Risk and Incidence: A Coordinated Analysis

ERISA Employee Retirement Income Security Act

ERK extracellular signal-regulated kinase

ERM electrochemical relaxation method; extended radical mastectomy; ezrin, radixin, and moesin

ERMSa embryonal rhabdomyosarcoma

ERNA early return to normal activities [after acute myocardial infarction]; efferent renal nerve activity; equilibrium radionuclide angiocardiography

ERNST European Resuscitation Nimodipine Study

ERO$_2$ oxygen extraction ratio

ERP early receptor potential; effective refractory period; elodoisin-related peptide; endoscopic retrograde pancreatography; enzyme-releasing peptide; equine rhinopneumonitis; estrogen receptor protein; event-related potential

Er-PBMC E-rosette-negative peripheral blood mononuclear cell

ERPC evacuation of retained products of conception

ERPF effective renal plasma flow

ERPLV effective refractory period of left ventricle

ERS enamel-renal syndrome; endoscopic retrograde sphincterectomy

ERSP event-related slow potential

ERSPC European Randomized Study of Screening for Prostatic Cancer

ERT emergency room thoracotomy, emergent resuscitative thoracotomy; esophageal radionuclide transit; estrogen replacement therapy; examination room terminal; external radiation therapy

ERTAS extended reticulo-thalamic activating system

ERTOCS, ERTOS European Randomised Trial of Ovarian Cancer Screening

ERU endorectal ultrasound

ERV equine rhinopneumonitis virus; expiratory reserve volume

ERY erysipelas

Ery *Erysipelothrix*

ES ejection sound; elastic stocking; electrical stimulus, electrical stimulation; electroshock; embryonic stem; emergency service; emission spectrometry; endometritis-salpingitis; endoscopic sphincterotomy; end-systole; end-to-side; English-speaking; enzyme substrate; epileptic seizures; epileptic syndrome; erythromycin stearate; esophageal, esophagus; esophageal scintigraphy; esterase; evoking strength; Ewing sarcoma; exfoliation syndrome; expert system; Expectation Score; experimental study; exterior surface; extrasystole

Es einsteinium; estrid

E$_s$ shear energy

ESA Electrolysis Society of America; electronic signature authentication; endocardial surface area; epidermal surface antigen; esterase; esterase A

ESADDI estimated safe and adequate daily dietary intake

ESAT esterase activator

ESB electrical stimulation of the brain; enhanced skill building [program]; esterase B

ESBY Electrical Stimulation vs Coronary Artery Bypass [study]

ESC electromechanical slope computer; endosystolic count; epidural spinal cord; erythropoietin-sensitive stem cell; esterase C

ESCA electron spectroscopy for chemical analysis

ESCALAT Efegatran and Streptokinase to Canalize Arteries Like Accelerated Tissue Plasminogen Activator [study]

ESCALATE Efegatran and Streptokinase to Canalize Arteries Like Accelerated Tissue Plasminogen Activator [study]

ESCC epidural spinal cord compression

Esch *Escherichia*

ESCN electrolyte and steroid cardiopathy with necrosis

ESCOBAR Emergency Stenting Compared to Conventional Balloon Angioplasty Randomized Trial

ESD electronic submission document; electronic summation device; electrostatic discharge; emission spectrometric device; end-systolic dimension; esterase-D; exoskeletal device

ESDI enhanced small device interface

ESE electrostatic unit [Ger. *electrostatische Einheit*]; exercise stress echocardiography

ESETCID European Study of Epidemiology and Treatment of Cardiac Inflammatory Diseases

ESF edge spread function; electron scatter function; electrosurgical filter; erythropoietic stimulating factor

ESFL end-systolic force-length relationship

ESG electrospinogram; estrogen; exfoliation syndrome glaucoma

ESGE European Society for Gastrointestinal Endoscopy

ESHEL Association for Planning and Development of Services for the Aged in Israel

ESHG European Society of Human Genetics

ESHR elder spontaneously hypertensive rat

ESI elastase-specific inhibitor; emergency severity index; enzyme substrate inhibitor; epidural steroid injection

ESIMV expiratory synchronized intermittent mandatory ventilation

ESL end-systolic length; extracorporeal shockwave lithotripsy

ESLD end-stage liver disease

ESLF end-stage liver failure

ESM ejection systolic murmur; endolymphatic stromal myosis; endoscopic specular microscope; ethosuximide

ESMIR Echocardiographic Selection of Patients for Mitral Regurgitation [study]

ESMIS Emergency Medical Services Management Information System

ESN educationally subnormal; estrogen-stimulated neurophysin

ESnet Energy Sciences Network [Department of Energy]

ESN(M) educationally subnormal-moderate

ESN(S) educationally subnormal-severe

ESO electrospinal orthosis

eso esophagoscopy; esophagus

ESOCAP European Study of Community Acquired Pneumonia

ESP early systolic paradox; echo spacing; effective sensory projection; effective systolic pressure; endometritis-salpingitis-peritonitis; end-systolic pressure; eosinophil stimulation promoter; epidermal soluble protein; especially; evoked synaptic potential; extrasensory perception

ESPA electrical stimulation–produced analgesia; extended sib pair analysis

ESPC enhanced spectral pathology component

ESPRIM European Study Prevention Research of Infarct with Molsidomine

ESPRIT Efficacy Safety Prospective Randomized Ibopamine Trial; European and Australian Stroke Prevention in Reversible

Ischemia Trial; European Study of the Prevention of Reocclusion after Initial Thrombolysis; European Study Programme for the Relevance of Immunology in Liver Transplantation

ESPS European Secondary Prevention Study; European Stroke Prevention Study

ESPVR end-systolic pressure-volume relationship

ESQ early signs questionnaire

ESR Einstein stoke radius; electric skin resistance; electron spin resonance; equipment service report; erythrocyte sedimentation rate; estrogen receptor

ESRD end-stage renal disease

ESRF end-stage renal failure

ESS earth and space sciences; elementary sulcal surface; empty sella syndrome; endostreptosin; erythrocyte-sensitizing substance; euthyroid sick syndrome; evolutionary stable energy; excited skin syndrome; squamous self-healing epithelioma

ess essential

ESSENCE Efficacy Safety Subcutaneous Enoxaparin in Non-Q-Wave Coronary Events [study]

ESSEX European Scimed Stent Experience

EST Early Stroke Trial; electric shock threshold; electroshock therapy; endodermal sinus tumor; endometrial sinus tumor; endoscopic sphincterectomy; esterase; exercise stress test; expressed sequence tag

est ester; estimation, estimated

esth esthetics, esthetic

ESU electrosurgical unit; electrostatic unit

E-sub excitor substance

ESUE emergency screening ultrasound examination

ESV end-systolic volume; esophageal valve

ESVEM Electrophysiologic Study vs Electrocardiographic Monitoring

ESVH endoscopic saphenous vein harvesting

ESVI end-systolic volume index

ESVS endoscopic vascular surgery; epiurethral suprapubic vaginal suspension

ESWL extracorporeal shock wave lithotripsy

ESWS end-systolic wall stress

E_{syn} reversal potential

ET educational therapy; effective temperature; ejection time; embryo transfer; endothelin; endotoxin; endotracheal; endotracheal tube; end-tidal; endurance time; enterotoxin; epidermolytic toxin; epithelial tumor; esophageal temperature; esotropia; essential thrombocythemia; essential tremor; ethanol; etiocholanolone test; etiology; eustachian tube; examination terminal; exchange transfusion; exercise test; exercise treadmill; exfoliative toxin; expiration time; exploratory thoracoscopy

ET_3 erythrocyte triiodothyronine

ET_4 effective thyroxine [test]

Et ethyl; etiology

et and [Lat. *et*], end-tidal

E/T effect to target [ratio]

E:T effect to target [ratio]

ET-1 endothelin-1

ETA electron transfer agent; endotracheal airways; endotracheal aspiration; ethionamide

ET-A endothelin A

ET_A endothelin A

η Greek letter *eta*; absolute viscosity

ETAB extrathoracic assisted breathing

ETAF epidermal thrombocyte activating factor

et al and others [Lat. *et alii*]

ETAR equivalent tissue air ratio

ET-B endothelin B

ET_B endothelin B

ETC electron transport chain; emergency trauma care; esophageal tracheal combitude; estimated time of conception

ET_c corrected ejection time

ETCC emergency team coordination course

$ETCO_2$ end-tidal carbon dioxide [concentration]

ETD eustachian tube dysfunction

ETDRS Early Treatment Diabetic Retinopathy Study

ETEC enterotoxin of *Escherichia coli*, enterotoxic *Escherichia coli*

ETF electron-transferring flavoprotein; eustachian tube function

ETFB electron transfer flavoprotein, beta polypeptide

ETH elixir terpin hydrate; ethanol; ethmoid

eth ether

ETHC elixir terpin hydrate with codeine

ETHR education, training, and human resources

ETI endotracheal intubation

ETIC Environmental Teratology Information Center

ETICBACK Environmental Toxicology Information Center Backfile

ETIO etiocholanolone

etiol etiology

ETK erythrocyte transketolase

ETKTM every test known to man

ETL echo train length; expiratory threshold load

ETM erythromycin

ETNet Educational Technology Network

EtNU ethyl nitrosourea

ETO estimated time of ovulation

Eto ethylene oxide

ETOH, EtOH ethyl alcohol

ETOX ethylene oxide

ETP electron transport particle; entire treatment period; ephedrine, theophylline, phenobarbital; eustachian tube pressure

ETPCO$_2$ end-tidal partial carbon dioxide [concentration]

ETR effective thyroxine ratio; electronic textbook of radiology; endothelin receptor

ETS educational testing service; electrical transcranial stimulation; environmental tobacco smoke; event timing system; expiration time signal

ETT endotracheal tube; epinephrine tolerance test; exercise tolerance test; exercise treadmill test; extrathyroidal thyroxine

ETU emergency and trauma unit; emergency treatment unit

ETV extravascular thermal volume

ETX etiology

EU Ehrlich unit; elementary unit; emergency unit; endotoxin unit; entropy unit; enzyme unit; esterase unit; etiology unknown; expected utility

Eu europium; euryon

EUA examination under anesthesia

EUCLID European Diabetes Controlled Trial of Lisinopril in Insulin-Dependent Diabetes Mellitus

EUCROMIC European Collaborative Research on Mosaicism in Chorionic Virus Sample

EUHID encrypted universal health care identifier

EUL expected upper limit

EUM external urethral meatus

EUP extrauterine pregnancy

EURAGE European Community Concerted Action on Aging

EURALIM European Alimentation Study

EURAMIC European Community Multicenter Study on Antioxidants, Myocardial Infarction and Breast Cancer

EURID European Registry for Implantable Cardioverter Defibrillators

EURO-ART European Angiojet Rapid Thrombectomy [study]

EUROASPIRE European Action on Secondary Prevention by Intervention to Reduce Events

EUROCARE European Carvedilol Restenosis Trial

EUROCARDI European Concerted Action for the Rapid Diagnosis of Myocardial Infarction

EURO-CAT European Cancer After Transplant [project]; European Register of Congenital Anomalies and Twins

EURODIAB ACE European Diabetes: Aetiology of Childhood Diabetes on an Epidemiological Basis

EURODIAB IDDM European Diabetes Centers Study of Complications in Patients with Insulin-dependent Diabetes Mellitus

EURODIAB TIGER European Diabetes: Type I Genetic Epidemiology Resources

EURO-DIRECT European Direct Myocardial Revascularization in Regeneration of Endomyocardial Channels Trial

EUROHAZCON Congenital Anomalies Near Hazardous Waste Landfill Sites in Europe [study]

EURONET European On-Line Network

EUROPA European Trial of Reduction of Cardiac Events with Perindopril in Stable Coronary Artery Disease

EuroQol European quality of life [scale]

EUROSCOP European Registry Society Study of Chronic Obstructive Pulmonary Diseases

EUROSTROKE European Collaborative Study of Incidence and Risk Factors for Ischemic and Hemorrhagic Stroke

EUROTOX European Committee on Chronic Toxicity Hazards

EUROWINTER European Study on Cold Exposure and Winter Mortality from Ischemic Heart Disease

EUS endoscopic ultrasound; external urethral sphincter

Eust eustachian

EUV extreme ultraviolet laser

EV ejected volume; electric vehicle; emergency vehicle; enterovirus; epidermodysplasia verruciformis; estradiol valerate; eustachian valve; evoked potential [response]; excessive ventilation; expected utility; expected value; extravascular

Ev, ev eversion

eV, ev electron volt

EVA Epidemiological Study on Vascular and Cognitive Aging; ethyl violet azide; ethylene vinyl acetate; European Vascular Agency [study]

evac evacuate, evacuated, evacuation

EVADE Experience with Left Ventricular Assist Device with Exercise [trial]

eval evaluate, evaluated, evaluation

eval stud evaluation study

evap evaporation, evaporated

EVB electronic view box; esophageal variceal bleeding

EVC, EvC Ellis-van Creveld [syndrome]

EVCI expected value of clinical information

EVD extravascular [lung] density

ever eversion, everted

EVF ethanol volume fraction

EVFMG exchange visitor foreign medical graduate

EVG electroventriculography

EVGLI European Working Group on *Legionella* Surveillance Centre

EVIL exposure to selected viruses in research laboratories

EVL electronic visualization laboratory

EVLW extravascular lung water

EVM electronic voltmeter; extravascular mass

EVNT event [UMLS]

EVOC emergency vehicle operator course

EVP episcleral venous pressure; evoked visual potential

EVR evoked visual response; exudative vitreoretinopathy

EVRS early ventricular repolarization syndrome

EVS eligibility verification system; endovaginal sonography

EVTV extravascular thermal volume

EVXX exudative vitreoretinopathy, X-linked

EW emergency ward; estrogen withdrawal

E-W Edinger-Westphal [nucleus]

EWA estrogen replacement for women with coronary artery disease; exponentially-weighted average

EWAs erythrocytes without antigens

EWB estrogen withdrawal bleeding

EWGCP European Working Group on Cardiac Pacing

EWHO elbow-wrist-hand orthosis

EWL egg-white lysozyme; evaporation water loss

EWPHE European Working Party on Hypertension in the Elderly

EWKY elder Wistar-Kyoto rat

EWR European Wallstent Registry

EWS Ewing sarcoma

EWSR Ewing sarcoma breakpoint region

EX exfoliation; exsmoker

E(X) expected value of the random variable X

ex exacerbation; examination, examined, examiner; example; excision; exercise; exophthalmos; exposure; extraction

EXA electronic X-ray archives

exac exacerbation

EXACT Extended Release Adalat Canadian Trial

EXACTO Excimer Laser Angioplasty in Coronary Total Occlusion

EXAFS extended x-ray absorption fine structure

exam examination, examine, examined

EXBF exercise hyperemia blood flow

exc excision

EXCEL Expanded Clinical Evaluation of Lovastatin [trial]

exch exchange

EXCITE Evaluation of Oral Xemilofiban in Controlling Thrombotic Events

excr excretion

ExEF ejection fraction during exercise

EXELFS extended electron-loss line fine structure

exer exercise

EXERT Exercise Rehabilitation Trial

exg exogenous

EXO exonuclease; exophoria
exog exogenous
exoph exophthalmia
exos exostosis
exp expansion; expectorant; experiment, experimental; expiration, expired; exponential function; exposure
EXPAPS Exeter Primary Angioplasty Pilot Study
exp lap exploratory laparotomy
expect expectorant
exper experiment, experimental
ExPGN extracapillary proliferative glomerulonephritis
expir expiration, expiratory, expired
expl exploratory
Expl Lap exploratory laparotomy
exptl experimental

EXREM external radiation-emission man [dose]
EXS external support
EXT exercise testing
Ext extraction, extract
ext extension; extensive; extensor; exterior; external; extract; extreme, extremity
extr extract
EXTRA Evaluation of XT Stent for Restenosis of Native Arteries
extrav extravasation
ext rot external rotation
extub extubation
EXU excretory urogram
exud exudate, exudation
EY egg yolk; epidemiological year
EYA egg yolk agar
Ez eczema

F bioavailability; a cell that donates F factor in bacterial conjugation; a conjugative plasmid in F+ bacterial cells; degree of fineness of abrasive particles; facies; factor; Fahrenheit; failure; false; family; farad; Faraday constant; fascia; fasting; fat; father; feces; fellow; female; fermentation; fertility; fetal; fiat; fibroblast; fibrous; field of vision; filament; *Filaria*; fine; finger; flexion; flow; fluorine; flux; focal [spot]; focus; foil; fontanel; foramen; force; form, forma; formula; fornix; fossa; fraction, fractional; fracture; fragment; free; French [catheter]; frequency; frontal; frontal electrode placement in electroencephalography; function; fundus; *Fusiformis*; *Fusobacterium*; gilbert; Helmholz free energy; hydrocortisone [compound F]; inbreeding coefficient; left foot electrode in vectorcardiography; phenylalanine; variance ratio

F_0, F_1 coupling factor

F_1, F_2 **etc.** first, second, etc., filial generation; years of fellowship study

FI, FII, etc. factors I, II, etc.

F344 Fischer 344 [rat]

°F degree on the Fahrenheit scale

F' a hybrid F plasmid

F$^-$ a bacterial cell lacking an F plasmid

F$^+$ a bacterial cell having an F plasmid

f atomic orbital with angular momentum quantum number 3; farad; father; female; femto; fiber, fibrous; fingerbreadth; fission; flexion; fluid; focal; foot; form, forma; formula; fostered [experimental animal]; fraction; fracture; fragment; frequency; frontal; function; fundus; numerical expression of the relative aperture of a camera lens

FA factor analysis; false aneurysm; Families Anonymous; Fanconi anemia; far advanced; fatty acid; febrile antigen; femoral artery; fetal age; fibrinolytic activity; fibroadenoma; fibrosing alveolitis; field ambulance; field assessment; filterable

agent; filtered air; first aid; flip angle; fluorescent antibody; fluorescent assay; fluoroalanine; folic acid; follicular area; food allergy; forearm; fortified aqueous [solution]; free acid; Freund adjuvant; Friedreich ataxia; functional activity; functional administration

F/A fetus active

fa fatty [rat]

FAA folic acid antagonist; formaldehyde, acetic acid, alcohol

FA-A Fanconi anemia A [gene]

FAAN Fellow of the American Academy of Nursing

FAB fast atom bombardment; formalin ammonium bromide; fragment, antigen-binding [of immunoglobulins]; French-American-British [carcinoma staging]; functional arm brace

FA-B Fanconi anemia B [gene]

Fab fragment, antigen-binding [of immunoglobulins]

F(ab')$_2$ fragment, antigen-binding [of immunoglobulins]

Fabc fragment, antigen and complement binding [of immunoglobulins]

FABER flexion in abduction and external rotation

FABF femoral artery blood flow

FAB-MS fast atom bombardment-mass spectrometry

FABP fatty acid-binding protein; folate-binding protein

FAC familial adenomatosis coli; femoral arterial cannulation; ferric ammonium citrate; fetal abdominal circumference; 5-fluorouracil, Adriamycin, and cyclophosphamide; foamy alveolar cast; fractional area changes; free available chlorine; functional aerobic capacity

FA-C Fanconi anemia C [gene]

Fac factor

fac facility; to make [Lat. *facere*]

FACA Fanconi anemia complementation group A; Fellow of the American College of Anesthetists; Fellow of the American College of Angiology; Fellow of the American College of Apothecaries

FACAI Fellow of the American College of Allergy and Immunology

FACAS Fellow of the American College of Abdominal Surgeons

FACB Fanconi anemia complementation group B

Facb fragment, antigen, and complement binding

FACC Fanconi anemia complementation group C; Fellow of the American College of Cardiologists

FACCT Foundation for Accountability

FACD Fanconi anemia complementation group D; Fellow of the American College of Dentists

FACEP Fellow of the American College of Emergency Physicians

FACES unique facies, anorexia, cachexia, and eye and skin lesions [syndrome]

FACET Flosequinan Angiotensin Converting Enzyme-Inhibitor [ACEI] Trial; Fosinopril Amlodipine Cardiovascular Events Trial

FACFP Fellow of the American College of Family Physicians

FACFS Fellow of the American College of Foot Surgeons

FACG Fellow of the American College of Gastroenterology

FACH forceps to after-coming head

FACHA Fellow of the American College of Health Administrators; Fellow of the American College of Hospital Administrators

FACHE Fellow of the American College of Healthcare Executives

FACIT fibril-associated collagen with interrupted triple helices

FACL fatty acid coenzyme ligase

FACLM Fellow of the American College of Legal Medicine

FACMTA Federal Advisory Council on Medical Training Aids

FACN Fellow of the American College of Nutrition

FACNHA Foundation of American College of Nursing Home Administrators

FACO Fellow of the American College of Otolaryngology

FACOG Fellow of the American College of Obstetricians and Gynecologists

FACOS Fellow of the American College of Orthopaedic Surgeons

FACOSH Federal Advisory Committee on Occupational Safety and Health

FACP Fellow of the American College of Physicians

FACPE Fellow of the American College of Physician Executives

FACPM Fellow of the American College of Preventive Medicine

FACR Fellow of the American College of Radiology

FACS Fellow of the American College of Surgeons; fluorescence-activated cell sorter

FACSM Fellow of the American College of Sports Medicine

FACT Flannagan Aptitude Classification Test; functional assessment of cancer therapy

FACT-B functional assessment of cancer therapy–breast

FACTS Functional Angiometric Correlation with Thallium Scintigraphy [trial]

FACWA familial amyotrophic chorea with acanthocytosis

FAD familial Alzheimer dementia; familial autonomic dysfunction; fetal activity-acceleration determination; flavin adenine dinucleotide

FA-D Fanconi anemia D [gene]

FADF fluorescent antibody dark field

FADH$_2$ reduced form of flavin adenine dinucleotide

FADIR flexion in adduction and internal rotation

FADN flavin adenine dinucleotide

FADS fetal akinesia deformation sequence

FAE fetal alcohol effect

FA-E Fanconi anemia E [gene]

FAEES fatty acid ethyl ester synthase

FAES Foundation for Advanced Education in the Sciences

FAF fatty acid free; fibroblast-activating factor

FAH Federation of American Hospitals

Fahr Fahrenheit

FAI first aid instruction; free androgen index; functional aerobic impairment; functional assessment inventory

FAJ fused apophyseal joint

FAK focal adhesion kinase

FALG fowl antimouse lymphocyte globulin

FALP fluoro-assisted lumbar puncture

FALS familial amyotrophic lateral sclerosis

FAM 5-fluorouracil, Adriamycin, and mitomycin C; fuzzy associative memory

Fam, fam family, familial

FAMA Fellow of the American Medical Association; fluorescent antibody to membrane antigen

FAM-A functional area model–activity

FAM-D functional area model of data

FAME fatty acid methyl ester

FAMG family group [UMLS]

fam hist family history

FAMIS Fosinopril in Acute Myocardial Infarction Study

FAMMM familial atypical multiple mole–melanoma [syndrome]

FAMOUS Fragmin Advanced Malignancy Outcome Study

FAN fuchsin, amido black, and naphthol yellow

FANA fluorescent antinuclear antibody

F and R force and rhythm [of pulse]

FANEL Federation for Accessible Nursing Education and Licensure

FANPT Freeman Anxiety Neurosis and Psychosomatic Test

FANTASTIC Full Anticoagulation vs Aspirin Ticlopidine After Stent Implantation [study]; Full Anticoagulation vs Ticlopidine Plus Aspirin After Stent Implantation [study]

FAOF family assessment of occupational functioning

FAP familial adenomatous polyposis; familial amyloid polyneuropathy; fatty acid polyunsaturated; fatty acid poor; femoral artery pressure; fibrillating action potential; Fibrinolytics vs Primary Angioplasty [trial]; fixed action potential; French-American-British [staging of neoplastic diseases]; frozen animal procedure; functional ambulation profile

FAPA Fellow of the American Psychiatric Association; Fellow of the American Psychoanalytical Association

FAPHA Fellow of the American Public Health Association

FAPIS Flecainide and Propafenone Italian Study

FAPS Felodipine Atherosclerosis Prevention Study; French Aortic Plaque Study

FAPY formamidopyrimidine

FAQ frequently asked question; functional asessment questionnaire

FAR fatal accident rate; Federal acquisitions regulation; fractional albumin rate; fresh bone marrow

far faradic

FARE Federation of Alcoholic Rehabilitation Establishments

FARS Fatality Analysis Reporting System

FAS fatty acid synthetase; Federation of American Scientists; fetal akinesia sequence; fetal alcohol syndrome

FASA Federated Ambulatory Surgery Association

FASB Financial Accounting Standards Board

FASC free-standing ambulatory surgical center

fasc fasciculus, fascicular

FASEB Federation of American Societies for Experimental Biology

FASHP Federation of Associations of Schools of the Health Professions

FAST Fitness, Arthritis and Seniors Trial; flow-assisted, short-term [balloon catheter]; fluorescent antibody staining technique; fluoro-allergosorbent test; focused abdominal sonography for trauma; Fourier acquired steady state; Frenchay Aphasia Screening Test; functional assessment stages

FASTEST Femoral Artery Stent Study

FAST-MI Field Ambulance Study of Thrombolysis in Myocardial Infarction

FAT family attitudes test; fluorescent antibody technique; fluorescent antibody test

FAT$_{DPA}$ fat dual photon absorptiometry

FATIMA Fraxiparin Anticoagulant Therapy in Myocardial Infarction Study in Amsterdam

Fat$_{IVNA}$ fat in vitro neutron activation analysis

FATS face and thigh squeeze [position for bag mask ventilation]; Familial Atherosclerosis Treatment Study

FAT$_{UWW}$ fat underwater weighing

FAV facio-auriculovertebral [sequence]; feline ataxia virus; floppy aortic valve; fowl adenovirus

FAVS facio-auriculo-vertebral spectrum

FAX, fax facsimile

FAZ Fanconi-Albertini-Zellweger [syndrome]; foveal avascular zone; fragmented atrial activity zone

FB feedback; fiberoptic bronchoscopy; fingerbreadth; foreign body; *Fusobacterium*
FBA fecal bile acid
FBAO foreign-body airway obstruction
FBC full blood count
FBCOD foreign body of the cornea, oculus dexter (right eye)
FBCOS foreign body of the cornea, oculus sinister (left eye)
FBCP familial benign chronic pemphigus
FBD functional bowel disorder
FbDP fibrin degradation products
FBE full blood examination
FBEC fetal bovine endothelial cell
FBF forearm blood flow; full breast feeding
FBG fasting blood glucose; fibrinogen; foreign body granulomatosis
fbg fibrinogen
FBH familial benign hypercalcemia
FBHH familial benign hypocalciuric hypercalcemia
FBI flossing, brushing, and irrigation
FBL follicular basal lamina
FBLN fibulin
FBM felbamate; fetal breathing movements; fractional or fractal brownian motion
FBN Federal Bureau of Narcotics; fibrillin
FBP femoral blood pressure; fibrin breakdown product; filtered back projection [algorithm]; folate-binding protein; fructose-1, 6-biphosphatase
FBPsS Fellow of the British Psychological Society
FBPM forward-backward Prony method [spectral analysis of heart sounds]
FBR fetal breathing rate
FBS fasting blood sugar; feedback system; fetal bovine serum
FBSC Frederick Biomedical Supercomputing Center [NIH]
FBSS failed back surgery syndrome
FC family coping; fasciculus cuneatus; fast component [of a neuron]; febrile convulsions; feline conjunctivitis; ferric chloride; ferric citrate; fibrocyte; finger clubbing; finger counting; flow compensation; fluorocarbon; fluorocytosine; Foley catheter; foster care; fowl cholera; free cholesterol; frontal cortex; functional castration
5-FC 5-fluorocytosine

Fc centroid frequency; fraction/centrifuge; fragment, crystallizable [of immunoglobulin]
Fc' a fragment of an immunoglobulin molecule produced by papain digestion
fc foot candles
F + C flare ;pl cells
FCA ferritin-conjugated antibodies; Freund's complete adjuvant; functional capacity assessment
FCAH familial cytomegaly adrenocortical hypoplasia [syndrome]
FCAP Fellow of the College of American Pathologists
FCAT Federative Committee on Anatomical Terminology
F cath Foley catheter
FCC follicular center cells
fcc face-centered-cubic
f/cc fibers per cubic centimeter of air
FCCA familial congenital cardiac abnormality
FCCH family child care home
FCCL follicular center cell lymphoma
FCCSET Federal Coordinating Committee for Science, Engineering and Technology
FCD feces collection device; fibrocystic disease; fibrocystic dysplasia; focal cytoplasmic degradation
FCE fibrocartilaginous embolism
FCF fetal cardiac frequency; fibroblast chemotactic factor
FCFC fibroblast colony-forming cell
FCH faculty contact hour; family care home; fetal cystic hygroma
FCHL familial combined hyperlipidemia
FChS Fellow of the Society of Chiropodists
FCHSP flight crew health stabilization program [NASA]
FCI fixed-cell immunofluorescence; folded cell index; food chemical intolerance
FCIM Federated Council for Internal Medicine
fCJD familial Creutzfeldt-Jakob disease
FCL fibroblast cell line
fcly face lying
FCM flow cytometry; fuzzy C-means [clustering algorithm]
FCMC familial chronic mucocutaneous candidiasis; family centered maternity care
FCMD Fukuyama congenital muscular dystrophy

FCMS Fellow of the College of Medicine and Surgery; Foix-Chavany-Marie syndrome

FCMW Foundation for Child Mental Welfare

FCO Fellow of the College of Osteopathy

FCP F-cell production; final common pathway; Functional Communication Profile

FCPN fuzzy coloured Petri net

FCPS Fellow of the College of Physicians and Surgeons

FCR flexor carpi radialis; fractional catabolic rate

FcR Fc receptor

FCRA fecal collection receptacle assembly; Fellow of the College of Radiologists of Australasia

FCRC Frederick Cancer Research Center

FCS faciocutaneoskeletal syndrome; fecal containment system; feedback control system; fetal calf serum; foot compartment syndrome

FCSP Fellow of the Chartered Society of Physiotherapy

FCST Fellow of the College of Speech Therapists

FCSW female commercial sex worker

FCT food composition table; fucosyl transferase

FCU flexor carpi ulnaris

FCx frontal cortex

FCXM flow cytometric cross-matching

FD familial dysautonomia; family doctor; fan douche; fatal dose; fetal danger; fibrin derivative; fibrous dysplasia; focal distance; Folin-Denis [assay]; follicular diameter; foot drop; forceps delivery; fractal dimension; freeze drying; mixed disk

Fd the amino-terminal portion of the heavy chain of an immunoglobulin molecule; ferredoxin

fd fundus

FD$_{50}$ median fatal dose

FDA fluorescein diacetate; Food and Drug Administration; right frontanterior [position of the fetus]

FDAM fuzzy logic based decision analysis module

FDAW film digitizer acquisition workstation

FDB familial defective apolipoprotein B

FDBL fecal daily blood loss

FDC factor-dependent cell [line]; fluorodeoxyglucose; follicular dendritic cell

FD&C Food, Drug and Cosmetic Act; food, drugs, and cosmetics

FDCPA Food, Drug, and Consumer Product Agency

FDD fluorescent differential display; Food and Drugs Directorate

FDDC ferric dimethyldithiocarbonate

FDDI fiber distributed data interface; film distribution data interface

FDDS Family Drawing Depression Scale

FDE female day-equivalent; final drug evaluation

FDF fast death factor; fractional dimension filtering

FDFQ Food/Drink Frequency Questionnaire

FDFT farnesyldiphosphate farnesyltransferase

FDG F-deoxyglucose; [clinical] features of differential diagnosis; fluorine 18-labeled deoxyglucose; fluorodeoxyglucose [scan]

fdg feeding

FDGF fibroblast-derived growth factor

FGD-PET fluorodeoxyglucose positron emission tomography

FDH familial dysalbuminemic hyperthyroxinemia; focal dermal hypoplasia; formaldehyde dehydrogenase

FDI first dorsal interosseous [muscle]; International Dental Federation [Fédération Dentaire Internationale]

FDIU fetal death in utero

FDL flexor digitorum longus

FDLMP first day of last menstrual period

FDLO fluorescent dye-labeled oligonucleotide

FDLV fer de lance virus

FDM fetus of diabetic mother; fibrous dysplasia of the mandible; finite differentiation method; fluoro-deoxyglucose

FDMP fluid depth at Morison's pouch

FDNB fluorodinitrobenzene

FDO Fleet Dental Officer

FDP fibrin degradation product; fibrinogen degradation product; flexor digitorum profundus; frontodextra posterior [position of fetus]; fructose-1,6-diphosphate

FDPase fructose-1,6-diphosphatase

FDPS farnesyl diphosphate synthetase

FDPSL farnesyl diphosphate synthetase-like

FDQB flexor digiti quinti brevis

FDR first-degree relative; fractional disappearance rate

FDS Fellow in Dental Surgery; fiber duodenoscope; flexor digitorum superficialis

FDSRCSEng Fellow in Dental Surgery of the Royal College of Surgeons of England

FDT frontodextra transversa [position of fetus]

FDTD finite difference time domain [method]

FdUrd fluorodeoxyuridine

(F)dUTP fluorescent deoxyuridine triphosphate

FDV Friend disease virus

FDZ fetal danger zone

FE fatty ester; fecal emesis; fetal erythroblastosis; fetal erythrocyte; fluid extract; fluorescent erythrocyte; finite element [algorithm]; forced expiration; formaldehyde-ethanol; frequency-encoded; frozen embryo

Fe female; ferret

fe female

feb fever [Lat. *febris*]

FEBP fetal estrogen-binding protein

FEBS Federation of European Biochemical Societies

FEB SZ febrile seizures

FEC fixed excitation codebook; forced expiratory capacity; free erythrocyte coproporphyrin; freestanding emergency center; Friend erythroleukemia cell

FECH ferrochelatase

FECG fetal electrocardiogram

F$_{ECO2}$ fractional concentration of carbon dioxide in expired gas

FECP free erythrocyte coproporphyrin

FECSR flexion–extension cervical spine radiography

FECT fibroelastic connective tissue

FECU factor [VIII] correctional unit

FECV feline enteric coronavirus

FECVC functional extracellular fluid volume

FED fish eye disease

FeD iron deficiency

Fed federal

FedNets Federal agency networks

FEDRIP Federal Research in Progress [database]

FedStats Federal statistics

FEE forced equilibrating expiration

FEEG fetal electroencephalography

FEER field echo with even echo rephasing

FEF forced expiratory flow

FEF$_{25-75}$ forced expiratory flow at 25–75% of forced vital capacity

FEF$_{50}$ forced expiratory flow at 50% of forced vital capacity

FEF$_{50}$/FIF$_{50}$ ratio of expiratory flow to inspiratory flow at 50% of forced vital capacity

FEFV forced expiratory flow volume

FEGO International Federation of Gynecology and Obstetrics

FEH focal epithelial hyperplasia

FEHBARS Federal Employee Health Benefit Acquisition Regulations

FEHBP Federal Employee Health Benefits Program

FEHBP-MSA Federal Employees Health Benefits Program–Medical Savings Account

Fe+^{2}Hgb ferromethemoglobin

Fe+^{3}Hgb ferrimethemoglobin

FEIBA factor eight bypassing activity

FEKG fetal electrocardiogram

FEL familial erythrophagocytic lymphohistiocytosis

FELASA Federation of European Laboratory Animal Science Association

FELC Friend erythroleukemia

FeLV feline leukemia virus

FEM female; femur, femoral; finite element method [algorithm]

fem female; femur, femoral

FEMA Federal Emergency Management Agency

FEMINA Felodipine ER and Metoprolol in the Treatment of Angina Pectoris

fem intern at inner side of the thighs [Lat. *femoribus internus*]

FEN flap endonuclease [protein]

Fen fenfluramine

FENa, FE$_{Na}$ fractional excretion of sodium

FEO familial expansile osteolysis

FE$_{O2}$, F$_{EO2}$ fractional concentration of oxygen in expired gas

FEOBV fluoroethoxybenzylvesamicol

FEP fluorinated ethylene-propylene; free erythrocyte protoporphyrin; front-end processing; front-end processor

FEPB functional electronic peroneal brace

FEPP free erythrocyte protoporphyrin

FER flexion, extension, rotation; fractional esterification rate; functional entity-relationship

fert fertility, fertilized

FES family environment scale; fat embolism syndrome; flame emission spectroscopy; forced expiratory spirogram; functional electrical stimulation

Fe/S iron/sulfur [protein]

FESO₄ ferrous sulfate

FESS functional endoscopic sinus surgery

FEST Fosinopril Efficacy/Safety Trial; Fosinopril on Exercise Tolerance [study]; Framework for European Services in Telemedicine

FeSV feline sarcoma virus

FET field-effect transistor; forced expiratory time

FETE Far Eastern tick-borne encephalitis

FETs forced expiratory time in seconds

FEUO for external use only

FEV familial exudative vitreoretinopathy; forced expiratory volume

fev fever

FEV1, FEV₁ forced expiratory volume in one second

FEV₁% ratio of FEV₁ to FVC

FEVB frequency ectopic ventricular beat

FEVR familial exudative vitreoretinopathy

FF degree of fineness of abrasive particles; fat-free; father factor; fecal frequency; fertility factor; field of Forel; filtration fraction; fine fiber; fine focus; finger flexion; finger-to-finger; fixation fluid; flat feet; flip-flop; fluorescent focus; follicular fluid; force fluids; forearm flow; forward flexion; foster father; free fraction; fresh frozen; fundus firm

F2F face-to-face

ff⁺ fertility inhibition positive

ff⁻ fertility inhibition negative

FFA Fellow of the Faculty of Anaesthetists; free fatty acid

FFAP free fatty acid phase

FFARCS Fellow of the Faculty of Anaesthetists of the Royal College of Surgeons

FFB fat-free body; flexible fiberoptic bronchoscopy

FFC fixed flexion contracture; fluorescence flow cytometry; free from chlorine

FFCM Fellow of the Faculty of Community Medicine

FFD Fellow in the Faculty of Dentistry; finger-to-floor distance; focus-film distance; free-form deformations

FFDCA Federal Food, Drug, and Cosmetic Act

FFDD focal facial dermal dysplasia

FFDSRCS Fellow of the Faculty of Dental Surgery of the Royal College of Surgeons

FFDW fat-free dry weight

FFE fast field echo; fecal fat excretion

FFF degree of fineness of abrasive particles; field-flow fractionation; flicker fusion frequency

FFG free fat graft

FFHC federally funded health center

FFHom Fellow of the Faculty of Homeopathy

FFI family function index; fatal familial insomnia; free from infection; fundamental frequency indicator

FFIT fluorescent focus inhibition test

FFL flexible fiberoptic laryngoscopy

FFM fat-free mass; fundus flavimaculatus

FFMDXA fat-free mass dual energy x-ray absorptiometry

FFMHYD fat-free mass hydrodensitometry

FFOM Fellow of the Faculty of Occupational Medicine

FFP freedom from progression; fresh frozen plasma

FFR Fellow of the Faculty of Radiologists

FFROM full and free range of motion

FFS fat-free solids; fee-for-service, femorofacial syndrome

FFT fast Fourier transform; flicker fusion test or threshold

FFU femur-fibula-ulna [syndrome]; focal forming unit

FFW fat-free weight

FFWC fractional free water clearance

FFWW fat-free wet weight

FG fasciculus gracilis; fast-glycolytic [fiber]; Feeley-Gorman [agar]; fibrinogen; Flemish giant [rabbit]

fg femtogram

FGA fibrinogen alpha

FGB fibrinogen beta

FGC fibrinogen gel chromatography

FGD fatal granulomatous disease

FgDP fibrinogen degradation products

FGDS fibrogastroduodenoscopy

FGDY faciogenital dysplasia

FGF father's grandfather; fibroblast growth factor; fresh gas flow

FGF1 fibroblast growth factor 1 [acidic]

FGF2 fibroblast growth factor 2 [basic]

FGFA fibroblast growth factor, acidic

FGFB fibroblast growth factor, basic

FGFR fibroblast growth factor receptor

FGG fibrinogen gamma; focal global glomerulosclerosis; fowl gamma-globulin

FGGM finite generalized gaussian mixture

FGH formylglutathione hydrolase

FGL fasting gastrin level

FGM father's grandmother; female genital mutilation

FGN fibrinogen; focal glomerulonephritis; fractional gaussian noise

FGP fundic gland polyp

FGR familial glucocorticoid resistance

FGS fibrogastroscopy; focal glomerular sclerosis; formal genesis syndrome

FGT fluorescent gonorrhea test

FH facial hemihyperplasia; familial hypercholesterolemia; familial hypertension; family history; fasting hyperbilirubinemia; favorable histology; femoral hernia; femoral hypoplasia; fetal head; fetal heart; fibromuscular hyperplasia; follicular hyperplasia; Frankfort horizontal [plane]; fumarate hydratase

FH+ family history positive

FH− family history negative

FH₄ tetrahydrofolic acid

fh fostered by hand [experimental animal]

FHA familial hypoplastic anemia; Fellow of the Institute of Hospital Administrators; filamentous hemagglutinin

FHADES Farm Hazard and Demographic Enumeration Survey

FH/BC frontal horn/bicaudate [ratio]

FHC familial hypercholesterolemia; familial hypertrophic cardiomyopathy; family health center; Ficoll-Hypaque centrifugation; Fuchs heterochromic cyclitis

FHD familial histiocytic dermatoarthritis; family history of diabetes

FHF fetal heart frequency; fulminant hepatic failure

fHg free hemoglobin

FHH familial hypocalciuric hypercalcemia; fawn-hooded hypertensive [rat]; fetal heart heard

FHI Fuchs' heterochromic iridocyclitis

FHIP family health insurance plan

FHIS Farm Health Interview Survey

FHIT fragile histidine triad [gene]

FHL flexor hallucis longus; functional health literacy; functional hearing loss

FHM familial hemiplegic migraine; fathead minnow [cells]

FHN family history negative

FHNH fetal heart not heard

FHP family history positive; functional health pattern

FHPMHP family history of physical and mental health problems

FHPSAT functional health pattern screening assessment screening tool

FHR familial hypophosphatemic rickets; fetal heart rate

FHRDC family history research diagnostic criteria

FHRNST fetal heart rate nonstress test

FHRS Familial Hypercholesterolemia Regression Study

FHS Family Heart Study; fetal heart sound; fetal hydantoin syndrome; Floating Harbor syndrome; Framingham Heart Study

FHSA Family Health Service Authority [UK]

FHT fast Hartley transform; fetal heart; fetal heart tone

FHTG familial hypertriglyceridemia

FH-UFS femoral hypoplasia-unusual facies syndrome

FHV falcon herpesvirus

FHVP free hepatic vein pressure

FHx family history

FI fasciculus intrafascicularis; fever caused by infection; fibrinogen; fixed interval; flame ionization; follicular involution; food intolerance; forced inspiration; frontoiliac

FIA fistula in ano; fluorescent immunoassay; focal immunoassay; Freund incomplete adjuvant

FIAC 2'-fluoro-5-iodo-aracytosine

FIB Fellow of the Institute of Biology; fibrin; fibrinogen; fibrositis; fibula

fib fiber; fibrillation; fibrin; fibrinogen; fibula

FIC finite-sample information criterion; Fogarty International Center; fractional inhibitory concentration

FICA Federal Insurance Contributions Act

FICD Fellow of the Institute of Canadian Dentists; Fellow of the International College of Dentists

FiCO$_2$, FI$_{CO2}$ fractional concentration of carbon dioxide in inspired gas

FICS Fellow of the International College of Surgeons

FICSIT Frailty and Injuries: Cooperative Studies of Intervention Techniques

FICU fetal intensive care unit

FID flame ionization detector; free induction decay; fungal immunodiffusion

FIDD fetal iodine deficiency disorder

FIF feedback inhibition factor; fibroblast interferon; forced inspiratory flow; formaldehyde-induced fluorescence

FIF$_{50}$ forced inspiratory flow at 50% of forced vital capacity

FIFO first in, first out

FIFR fasting intestinal flow rate

FIG Flosequinan Investigator Group

FIGD familial idiopathic gonadotropin deficiency

FIGE field inversion gel electrophoresis

FIGLEAF Fine Grained Lexical Analysis Facility

FIGLU, FIGlu formiminoglutamate, formiminoglutamic acid

FIGLU-uria formiminoglutaminaciduria

FIGO International Federation of Gynecology and Obstetrics

FIH familial isolated hypoparathyroidism; fat-induced hyperglycemia

fil filament; filial

filt filter, filtration

FIM field ion microscopy; fimbria; functional independence measure

FIMG familial infantile myasthenia gravis

FIMLT Fellow of the Institute of Medical Laboratory Technology

FIN fine intestinal needle

FINCC familial idiopathic nonarteriosclerotic cerebral calcification

FIND finding [UMLS]

FINESS First International New Intravascular Rigid-Flex Endovascular Stent Study

FINMONICA Finnish Monitoring Trends and Determinants in Cardiovascular Diseases

FINRISK Finland Cardiovascular Risk Study

FI$_{O2}$ forced inspiratory oxygen; fractional concentration of oxygen in inspired gas

FiO$_2$ fractional concentration of oxygen in inspired gas

FIP feline infectious peritonitis

FIPA familial intestinal polyatresia [syndrome]

FIPS Federal information processing standards; Frankfurt Isoptin Progression Study

FIPV feline infectious peritonitis virus

FIQ full-scale intelligence quotient

FIR far infrared; finite impulse response; fold increase in resistance; fractional intramural retention

FIRDA frontal, intermittent delta activity

FIRST Flolan International Randomized Survival Trial

FIS fatigue interview schedule; forced inspiratory spirogram; free induction signal

fis fission

FISAC Federal Information Services and Application Council

FISH Finnish Isradipine Study in Hypertension; fluorescence in situ hybridization

FISP fast imaging with steady state precession

FISS Fraxiparine in Stroke Study

fist fistula

FIT fluorescein isothiocyanate; Fracture Intervention Trial; fusion inferred threshold

FITC fluorescein isothiocyanate

FIUO for internal use only

FIV feline immunodeficiency virus; forced inspiratory volume

FIV$_1$ forced inspiratory volume in one second

FIVC forced inspiratory vital capacity

FIVE familial isolated vitamin E [deficiency]

FIXAg factor IX antigen

FJN familial juvenile nephrophthisis

FJRM full joint range of movement

FJS finger joint size

FK feline kidney

FK506 tacrolimus [drug]

FKBP FK 506 [macrolide] binding protein

FKT Fukunaga-Koontz transform

FL false lumen; fatty liver; feline leukemia; femur length; fibers of Luschka; fibroblast-like; filtration leukapheresis; focal length; follicular lymphoma; Friend leukemia;

frontal lobe; full liquid [diet]; functional length

FL-2 feline lung [cells]

Fl fluid; fluorescence

fl femtoliter; filtered load; flexion, flexible; fluorescent; flow; fluid; flutter; foot lambert

FLA fluorescent-labeled antibody; left frontoanterior [position of the fetus] [Lat. *fronto-laeva anterior*]

flac flaccidity, flaccid

FLAIR fluid attenuated inversion recovery

FLAP 5-lipoxygenase activating protein

FLARE Fluvastatin Angioplasty Restenosis [trial]

FLASH fast low angle shot; fluorescence in situ hybridization

FLC family life cycle; fatty liver cell; fetal liver cell; Friend leukemia cell

FLD fibrotic lung disease

fld fluid

fl dr fluid dram

FLE fiducial localization error

FLEX Federation Licensing Examination

flex flexor, flexion

FLG filaggrin

FLEQUIN Flecainide Compared to Oral Quinidine [study]

FLEXOR Focused Lesion Expansion Optimizes Result [trial]

FLIC functional living index-cancer

FLICC Federal Library and Information Center Committee

FLK funny looking kid

FLKS fatty liver and kidney syndrome

FLM fasciculus longitudinalis medialis; fraction of labeled mitosis

FLO Fourier linear combiner

floc flocculation

Flops floating point operations per second

fl oz fluid ounce

FLP left frontoposterior [position of the fetus] [Lat. *fronto-laeva posterior*]; functional limitations profile

FLR funny looking rash

FLS fatty liver syndrome; Fellow of the Linnean Society; fibrous long-spacing [collagen]; flow-limiting segment

FLSP fluorescein-labeled serum protein

FLT left frontotransverse [position of the fetus] [Lat. *fronto-laeva transversa*]

FLU 5-fluorouracil; flunitrazepam; fluphenazine; flutamide

flu influenza

FLUENT Fluvastatin Long-Term Extension Trial

fluor fluorescence; fluorescent; fluorometry; fluoroscopy

fluoro fluoroscope, fluoroscopy

FLV feline leukemia virus; Friend leukemia virus; fuzzy linguistic value

FM face mask; facilities management; family medicine; fat mass; feedback mechanism; fetal movement; fibrin monomer; fibromuscular; filtered mass; flavin mononucleotide; flowmeter; foramen magnum; forensic medicine; foster mother; frequency modulation; functional movement

Fm fermium

fM full mutation

f-M free metanephrine

fm femtometer

FMA Frankfort mandibular plane angle

FMAT fetal movement acceleration test

f_{max} maximum frequency

FMC family medicine center; flight medicine clinic; focal macular choroidopathy; foundation for medical care

FMCG fetal magnetocardiography

FMD facility medical director; family medical doctor; fibromuscular dysplasia; foot and mouth disease; frontometaphyseal dysplasia

FMDI frequency modulation detection interference

FMDV foot and mouth disease virus

FME full mouth extraction

Fmed median frequency

FMEG fetal magnetoencephalography

FMEL Friend murine erythroleukemia

FMEN familial multiple endocrine neoplasia

F-met, fMet formyl methionine

FMF familial Mediterranean fever; fetal movement felt; flow microfluorometry; forced midexpiratory flow

FMFD V familial multiple coagulation factor deficiency V

FMFM full mutation/full methylation

FMG five-mesh gauze; foreign medical graduate

FMGEMS Foreign Medical Graduate Examination in Medical Sciences

FMH family medical history; fat-mobilizing hormone; feto-maternal hemorrhage; fibromuscular hyperplasia

FMI fat mass index; Foods and Moods Inventory

FMIBMA fiber movement induced biological movement artifacts

FML flail mitral leaflet; fluorometholone

FMLA Family and Medical Leave Act

FMLP N-formyl-methionyl-leucyl-phenylalanine; formylpeptide

f-MLP N-formyl-methionyl-leucyl-phenylalanine

FMN first malignant neoplasm; flavin mononucleotide; frontomaxillonasal [suture]

FMNH, FMNH$_2$ reduced form of flavin mononucleotide

FMO flavin monooxygenase; Fleet Medical Officer; Flight Medical Officer

fmol femtomole

FMP faculty mentorship program; first menstrual period; fructose monophosphate

FMPM full mutation/partial methylation

FMPP familial male precocious puberty

FMR fragile site mental retardation [syndrome]; Friend-Moloney-Rauscher [antigen]

F MRI fluorine magnetic resonance imaging

fMRI functional magnetic resonance imaging

FMRP fragile site mental retardation [syndrome] protein

FMS fat-mobilizing substance; Fellow of the Medical Society; fibromyalgia syndrome; Finnish Multicenter Study; Fragmin Multicenter Study; full mouth series

FMT Fragmin Multicenter Trial; frequency modulation detection threshold

FMTC familial medullary thyroid cancer

FMU first morning urine

F-MuLV Friend murine leukemia virus

FMX full mouth x-ray

FN false negative; fecal nitrogen; fibronectin; FitzHugh–Nagumo [model]; fluoride number

F-N finger to nose

fn function

FNA fine-needle aspiration

FNAB fine-needle aspiration biopsy

FNAC fine-needle aspiration cytology

FNB fine needle biopsy; food and nutrition board

FNC fatty nutritional cirrhosis

FNCJ fine needle catheter jejunostomy

FND febrile neutrophilic dermatosis; frontonasal dysplasia

f-NE free norepinephrine

Fneg false negative

FNF false-negative fraction; femoral neck fracture

FNFMG foreign national foreign medical school graduate

FNH focal nodular hyperplasia

FNIC Food and Nutrition Information Center [National Agricultural Library]

FNL fibronectin-like

f-NM free normetanephrine

FNP family nurse practitioner

FNR false-negative rate; fibronectin receptor

FNRA fibronectin receptor alpha

FNRB fibronectin receptor beta

FNRBL fibronectin receptor beta-like

FNS frontier nursing service; functional neuromuscular stimulation

FNT false neurochemical transmitter; farnesyltransferase

FNTA farnesyltransferase alpha

FNTB farnesyltransferase beta

FNZ flunarizine

FO fiberoptic; fish oil; foot arthrosis; foramen ovale; forced oscillation; fronto-occipital

Fo fomentation, fomenting

FOA Federation of Orthodontic Associations

FOAR facio-oculo-acoustico-renal [syndrome]

FOAVF failure of all vital forces

FOB fecal occult blood; feet out of bed; fiberoptic bronchoscopy; foot of bed; functional observational battery

FOBT fecal occult blood test

FOC fronto-occipital circumference

FOCAL formula calculation

FOD focus-to-object distance; free of disease

F-ODN fluorescein-labeled oligodeoxyribonucleotide

FOG fast oxidative glycolytic [fiber]

FOL folate

FOLR folate receptor

FOM figure-of-merit

FOMi 5-fluorouracil, vincristine, and mitomycin C

F-OMP fluorescein-labeled oligonucleoside methylphosphonate

FOOB fell out of bed

FOOD Feed or Ordinary Diet [trial]

FOOSH fell onto [his or her] outstretched hand

FOP fibrodysplasia ossificans progressiva; forensic pathology

FOPR full outpatient rate

F-OPT fluorescein-labeled oligonucleoside phosphorothioate

For foramen; forensic

for foreign; formula

FORECAST Fractional Flow Reserve or Relative Fractional Velocity Reserve Evaluation of Coronary Artery Stenosis vs Thallium

FORIMG foreign national international medical school graduate

form formula

FORT Fish Oil Restenosis Trial

FORTRAN formula translation

FOS fiberoptic sigmoidoscopy; fractional osteoid surface; Framingham Offspring Study

FOSIT Fosamax International Trial

Fos-R foscarnet-resistant

Fos-R HIV foscarnet-resistant human immunodeficiency virus [HIV]

FOSS Framingham Offspring–Spouse Study

FOV field of view

FOX ferrous xylenol orange

FP false positive; family physician; family planning; family practice; family practitioner; Fanconi pancytopenia; femoropopliteal; fetoprotein; fibrinopeptide; field pronouncement; filling pressure; filter paper; fixation protein; flank pain; flash point; flavin phosphate; flavoprotein; flexor profundus; flow probe; fluid percussion; fluid pressure; fluorescence polarization; fluticazone propionate; food poisoning; forearm pronated; freezing point; frontoparietal; frozen plasma; full period; fusion peptide; fusion point

F1P, F-1-P fructose-1-phosphate

F6P, F-6-P fructose-6-phosphate

Fp fibrinopeptide; frontal polar electrode placement in electroencephalography

fp flexor pollicis; foot-pound; forearm pronated; freezing point

FPA Family Planning Association; Federal Privacy Act; fibrinopeptide A or alpha; filter paper activity; fluorophenylalanine

FpA fibrinopeptide A or alpha

FPB femoral popliteal bypass; fibrinopeptide B or beta; flexor pollicis brevis

FpB fibrinopeptide B or beta

FPBC false-positive blood culture

FPC familial polyposis coli; family planning clinic; fish protein concentrate

FPCA family practice comfort assessment

FpCA 1-fluoromethyl-2-p-chlorophenylethylamine

FPD feto-pelvic disproportion; flame photometric detector

FPDM fibrocalculous pancreatic diabetes mellitus

FPE fatal pulmonary embolism; field placement error; final prediction error

FPF false positive fraction; fibroblast pneumocyte factor

FPG fasting plasma glucose; fluorescence plus Giemsa; focal proliferative glomerulonephritis

FPGA field programmable gate array

FPGS folylpolyglutamate synthetase

FPH$_2$ reduced form of flavin phosphate

FPHE formaldehyde-treated pyruvaldehyde-stabilized human erythrocytes

FPHT fosphenytoin

FPI femoral pulsatility index; fluid percussion injury; formula protein intolerance; Freiburg Personality Identification Questionnaire

FPIA fluorescence polarization immunoassay

FPK fructose phosphokinase

FPL fasting plasma lipids; flexor pollicis longus

FPLC fast protein liquid chromatography

FPM filter paper microscopic [test]; full passive movements

fpm feet per minute

FPN ferric chloride, perchloric acid, and nitric acid [solution]; fuzzy Petri net

FPO faciopalatoosseous [syndrome]; Federation of Prosthodontic Organizations; freezing point osmometer

FPP faculty practice plan; free portal pressure

FPPH familial primary pulmonary hypertension

FPR false-positive rate; finger peripheral resistance; fluorescence photobleaching recovery; N-formylpeptide receptor; fractional proximal resorption
FPRA first pass radionuclide angiogram
FPRH N-formylpeptide homolog
FPS farnesylpyrophosphate synthetase; Fellow of the Pathological Society; Fellow of the Pharmaceutical Society; fetal PCB (polychlorinated biphenyl) syndrome; footpad swelling
fps feet per second; frames per second
FPSL farnesylpyrophosphate synthetase-like
FPSTS false-positive serologic test for syphilis
FPV feline pseudoleukopenia virus; fowl plague virus
FPVB femoral popliteal vein bypass
FQHC federally qualified health center
FR faculty rater; failure rate; film-screen radiograph; fasciculus retroflexus; febrile reaction; feedback regulation; Fischer-Race [notation]; fixed ratio; flocculation reaction; flow rate; fluid restriction; fluid resuscitation; fluid retention; free radical; frequency of respiration; frequent relapses
F2R [blood coagulation] factor II receptor
F&R force and rhythm [pulse]
Fr fracture; francium; franklin [unit charge]; French; frequency or frequent
Fr1 first fraction
f$_R$ respiratory frequency
F( )R:Ag factor ( ) related antigen
F( )R:C factor ( ) related cofactor activity
FRA fibrinogen-related antigen; fluorescent rabies antibody
fra fragile [site]
FRAC Food Research and Action Center
frac fracture
fract fracture
FRAME Fund for the Replacement of Animals in Medical Experiments
FRAMI Fragmin in Acute Myocardial Infarction [study]
FRAP fluorescence recovery after photobleaching
FRAT free·radical assay technique
FRAX fragile [chromosome] X
fra(X) chromosome X fragility; fragile X chromosome, fragile X syndrome
FRAXA fragile X syndrome A

FRAXE fragile X syndrome E
FRAXIDIS Fraxiparine in Post-Hospital Discharge [study]
FRAXIS Fraxiparine in Ischemic Syndromes [study]
FRAX-MR fragile X-mental retardation [syndrome]
FRAXODI Fraxiparine Once Daily Injection [study]
Fr BB fracture of both bones
FRC Federal Radiation Council; frozen red cells; functional reserve capacity; functional residual capacity
FRCD Fellow of the Royal College of Dentists; fixed ratio combination drug
FRCGP Fellow of the Royal College of General Practitioners
FRCOG Fellow of the Royal College of Obstetricians and Gynaecologists
FRCP Fellow of the Royal College of Physicians
FRCPA Fellow of the Royal College of Pathologists of Australia
FRCPath Fellow of the Royal College of Pathologists
FRCP(C) Fellow of the Royal College of Physicians of Canada
FRCPE Fellow of the Royal College of Physicians of Edinburgh
FRCPI Fellow of the Royal College of Physicians of Ireland
FRCPsych Fellow of the Royal College of Psychiatrists
FRCS Fellow of the Royal College of Surgeons
FRCS(C) Fellow of the Royal College of Surgeons of Canada
FRCSEd Fellow of the Royal College of Surgeons of Edinburgh
FRCSEng Fellow of the Royal College of Surgeons of England
FRCSI Fellow of the Royal College of Surgeons of Ireland
FRCVS Fellow of the Royal College of Veterinary Surgeons
FRD fumarate dehydrogenase
frd fumarate dehydrogenase [gene]
FRDA Friedreich ataxia
FRDA-Acad Acadian Friedreich ataxia
FRD A fumarate dehydrogenase A
FRD B fumarate dehydrogenase B
FRD C fumarate dehydrogenase C

FRD D fumarate dehydrogenase D

FRE Fischer rat embryo; flow-related enhancement

FREIR Federal Research on Biological and Health Effects of Ionizing Radiation

frem fremitus

freq frequency

FRES Fellow of the Royal Entomological Society

FRESCO Florence Randomized Elective Stenting in Acute Coronary Occlusion [study]

FRESH food re-education for elementary school health [program]

FRET fluorescence resonance energy transfer

FRF Fertility Research Foundation; follicle-stimulating hormone-releasing factor

FRFC functional renal failure of cirrhosis

FRH follicle-stimulating hormone-releasing hormone

FRh fetal rhesus monkey [kidney cell]

FRhK fetal rhesus monkey kidney [cell]

FRHS fast-repeating high sequence

FRIC Fragmin in Unstable Coronary Artery Disease [trial]

frict friction

FRIPHH Fellow of the Royal Institute of Public Health and Hygiene

FRISC Fragmin During Instability in Coronary Artery Disease [trial]

FRISC II Fragmin and/or Revascularization during Instability in Coronary Artery Disease [trial]

FRJM full range joint movement

FRMedSoc Fellow of the Royal Medical Society

FRMS Fellow of the Royal Microscopical Society

FRNS Fryns syndrome

FRO floor reaction orthosis

FROC free receiver operating characteristic

FROG French Rotablator Group [study]

FROM full range of movements

FROST French Optimal Stenting Trial

FRP follicle-stimulating hormone releasing protein; functional refractory period

FRS Fellow of the Royal Society; ferredoxin-reducing substance; first rank symptom; furosemide

FRSH Fellow of the Royal Society of Health

FRT Family Relations Test; full recovery time

Fru fructose

FRV full-length retroviral [sequence]; functional residual volume

Frx fracture

FS factor of safety; Fanconi syndrome; Felty syndrome; fibromyalgia syndrome; field stimulation; Fisher syndrome; food service; forearm supination; fractional shortening; fracture site; fragile site; Friesinger score; frozen section; full scale [IQ]; full soft [diet]; full strength; full sensitivity; function study; human foreskin [cells]; simple fracture

F/S female, spayed [animal]; frozen section

FSA flexible spending account

FSB fetal scalp blood

FSBA fluorosulfonylbenzoyladenosine

FSBP finger systolic blood pressure

FSBT Fowler single breath test

FSC finite sample criterion; Food Standards Committee; forward scatter

FSD focus-skin distance

FSE fast spin echo; feline spongiform encephalopathy; filtered smoke exposure

FSE-IR fast spin echo–inversion recovery [imaging]

FSF fibrin stabilizing factor; front surface fluorescence

FSG fasting serum glucose; focal segmental sclerosis

FSGHS focal segmental glomerular hyalinosis and sclerosis

FSGN focal sclerosing glomerulonephritis

FSGS focal segmental glomerulosclerosis

FSH fascioscapulohumeral; focal and segmental hyalinosis; follicle-stimulating hormone

FSHB follicle-stimulating hormone, beta chain

FSHD facioscapulohumeral muscular dystrophy

FSH/LR-RH follicle-stimulating hormone and luteinizing hormone releasing hormone

FSHR follicle-stimulating hormone receptor

FSH-RF follicle-stimulating hormone-releasing factor

FSH-RH follicle-stimulating hormone-releasing hormone

FSHSMA facioscapulohumeral spinal muscular atrophy

FSI foam stability index; Food Sanitation Institute; functional status index

FSIQ full-scale intelligence quotient

FSL fasting serum level

FSM finite state machine

FSMB Federation of State Medical Boards

FSN functional stimulation, neuromuscular

FSOP free-standing surgical outpatient facility

FSP familial spastic paraplegia; fibrin split products; fibrinogen split products; fine suspended particles

F-SP special form [Lat. *forma specialis*]

FSQ Functional Status Questionnaire

FSR Fellow of the Society of Radiographers; film screen radiography; force sensing resistor; force sensing retractor; fragmented sarcoplasmic reticulum; fusiform skin revision

FSRS functional status rating system

FSS focal segmental sclerosis; Freeman-Sheldon syndrome; French steel sound

FST foam stability test

FSU family service unit; functional spine unit

FSV feline fibrosarcoma virus; forward stroke volume; functional subunit

FSW field service worker

FT Fallot tetralogy; false transmitter; family therapy; fast twitch; fatigue trial; fibrous tissue; fingertip; follow through; Fourier transform; free testosterone; free thyroxine; full term; function test

FT₃ free triiodothyronine

FT_3 free triiodothyronine

FT₄ free thyroxine

FT_4 free thyroxine

Ft ferritin

fT free testosterone

ft foot, feet

FTA fluorescent titer antibody; fluorescent treponemal antibody

FTA-ABS, FTA-Abs fluorescent treponemal antibody, absorbed [test]

FTAG, F-TAG fast-binding target-attaching globulin

FTAS familial testicular agenesis syndrome

FTAT fluorescent treponemal antibody test

FTBD fit to be detained; full-term born dead

FTBE focal tick-borne encephalitis

FTBI fractionated total body irradiation

FTBS Family Therapist Behavioral Scale

FTC Federal Trade Commission; Fibrinolysis Trialists Collaboration; follicular thyroid carcinoma; frequency threshold curve; frequency tuning curve

ftc foot candle

FTD femoral total density; frontotemporal dementia

FTDS familial testicular dysgenesis syndrome

FTE full-time equivalent

FTEE full-time employe equivalent

FTF finger to finger

FTFT fast time frequency transform

FTG full-thickness graft

FTH ferritin heavy chain; fracture threshold

FTI free thyroxine index

FT₃I free triiodothyronine index

FT_3I free triiodothyronine index

FT₄I free thyroxine index

FT_4I free thyroxine index

FTIR Fourier transform infrared; functional terminal innervation ratio

FTKA failed to keep appointment

FTL ferritin light chain

ftL foot lambert

FTLB full-term live birth

ft lb foot pound

FTLV feline T-lymphotropic lentivirus

FTM fluid thioglycolate medium; fractional test meal

FTMS Fourier transform mass spectrometry

FTN finger to nose

FTNB full-term newborn

FTND full-term normal delivery

FTO fructose-terminated oligosaccharide

FTP file transfer protocol [sending and receiving files from remote computers on the internet]

FTQ Fagerström Tolerance Questionnaire

FTR fractional tubular reabsorption

FTS family tracking system; feminizing testis syndrome; fetal tobacco syndrome; fissured tongue syndrome; flexortenosynovitis; thymulin [Fr. *facteur thymique sérique*]

FTSG full thickness skin graft

FTT failure to thrive; fat tolerance test; Fibrinolytic Therapy Trialist [collaboration]

FTU fluorescence thiourea

FTVD full term vaginal delivery

FU fecal urobilinogen; fetal urobilinogen; fluorouracil; follow-up; flux unit [ion]; fractional urinalysis; fundus

Fu Finsen unit

F/U follow-up, fundus of umbilicus

F&U flanks and upper quadrants

5-FU 5-fluorouracil

FUB functional uterine bleeding

FUC fucosidase

Fuc fucose

FUCA fucosidase alpha

FUCA1 alpha-L-fucosidase gene

FUDR, FUdR fluorodeoxyuridine

FUF functional unification formalism

FUFA free volatile fatty acid

FULL fully formed anatomical structure [UMLS]

FUM 5-fluorouracil and methotrexate; fumarate; fumigation

FUMIR 5-fluorouracil, mitomycin C, radiation

FUMP fluorouridine monophosphate

FUN follow-up note

FUNC functional concept [UMLS]

funct function, functional

FUO fever of unknown origin

FUOV follow-up office visit

FUR 5-fluorouracil and radiation; fluorouracil riboside; fluorouridine; follow-up report; furin membrane-associated receptor

FUS feline urologic syndrome; first-use syndrome; fusion

FUT fibrinogen uptake test; fucosyl transferase

FUTP fluoridine triphosphate

FV femoral vein; fluid volume; Friend virus

FVA Friend virus anemia

FVC false vocal cord; femoral vein cannulation; forced vital capacity

FVCC First Virtual Congress of Cardiology

FVE forced volume expiration

FVIC forced inspiratory vital capacity

FVL femoral vein ligation; flow volume loop; force, velocity, length

FVOP finger venous opening pressure

FVP Friend virus polycythemia

FVR feline viral rhinotracheitis; forearm vascular resistance

FVS fetal valproate syndrome

FVT follicular-variant-translocation

FW Felix-Weil [reaction]; Folin-Wu [reaction]; fragment wound

Fw F wave

fw fresh water

FWA Family Welfare Association

FWB full weight bearing

FWHM full width at half maximum [resolution or measurement]

FWPCA Federal Water Pollution Control Administration

FWR Felix-Weil reaction; Folin-Wu reaction

FWTM full width tenth maximum

FX factor X; fluoroscopy; fornix; fracture frozen section

Fx fracture

fx fracture; friction

Fx-dis fracture-dislocation

FXN function

FXS fragile X syndrome

fx/V$_T$ frequency/tidal volume [ratio]

FY fiscal year; full year

FYI for your information

FYMS fourth-year medical student

FZ focal zone; furazolidone

Fz frontal midline placement of electrodes in electroencephalography

FZS Fellow of the Zoological Society

G acceleration [force]; conductance; free energy; gallop; ganglion; gap; gas; gastrin; gauge; gauss; genome, genomic; geometric efficiency; giga; gingiva, gingival; glabella; globular; globulin; glucose; glycine; glycogen; goat; gold inlay; gonidial; good; goose; grade; Grafenberg spot; gram; gravida; gravitation constant; Greek; green; guanidine; guanine; guanosine; gynecology; unit of force of acceleration

G₀ quiescent phase of cells leaving the mitotic cycle

G₁ presynthetic gap [phase of cells prior to DNA synthesis]

G₂ postsynthetic gap [phase of cells following DNA synthesis]

GI primigravida

GII secundigravida

GIII tertigravida

G° standard free energy

g force [pull of gravity]; gap; gauge; gender; grain; gram; gravity; group; ratio of magnetic moment of a particle to the Bohr magneton; standard acceleration due to gravity, 9.80665 m/s^2

ᵍ relative centrifugal force

γ see *gamma*

GA Gamblers Anonymous; gastric analysis; gastric antrum; general anesthesia; general angiography; general appearance; genetic algorithm; gentisic acid; germ-cell antigen; gestational age; gibberellic acid; gingivoaxial; glucoamylase; glucose; glucose/acetone; glucuronic acid; Golgi apparatus; gramicidin A; granulocyte adherence; granuloma annulare; guessed average; gut-associated; gyrate atrophy

G/A globulin/albumin [ratio]

Ga gallium; granulocyte agglutination

ga gauge

GAA gossypol acetic acid

GAAS Goldberg Anorectic Attitude Scale

GABA, gaba gamma-aminobutyric acid

GABAₐ gamma-aminobutyric acid A

GABAв gamma-aminobutyric acid B

GABAT, GABA-T gamma-aminobutyric acid transaminase

GABHS group A beta-hemolytic streptococcus

GABI German Angioplasty Bypass Intervention [trial]; German Angioplasty Bypass Surgery Investigation

GABOA gamma-amino-beta-hydroxybutyric acid

GABRA gamma-aminobutyric acid alpha receptor

GACELISA immunoglobulin G [IgG] capture enzyme-linked immunosorbent assay [ELISA]

GACT government activity [UMLS]

GAD generalized anxiety disorder; glutamic acid decarboxylase

GADH gastric alcohol dehydrogenase

GADS gonococcal arthritis/dermatitis syndrome

GAEIB Group of Advisors on the Ethical Implications of Biotechnology [European Economic Community]

GAF global assessment of functioning [scale]

GAFG goal attainment follow-up guide

GAG glycosaminoglycan; group-specific antigen gene

GAH glyceraldehyde

GAHS galactorrhea-amenorrhea hyperprolactinemia syndrome

GAIN Glycine Antagonist GV150526 in Acute Stroke [trial]

GaIN Georgia Interactive Network for Medical Information

GAIPAS General Audit Inpatient Psychiatric Assessment Scale

GAIT-ER-AID Gait Explanation and Reasoning Aid [computer gait analysis system]

GAL galactose; galactosyl; glucuronic acid lactone

Gal galactose

gal galactose; gallon

GALBP galactose-binding protein

GALC, GalC galactocerebroside

GALE galactose epimerase

GALK galactokinase

GalN galactosamine

GalNAc *N*-acetylgalactosamine

GALNS galactosamine-4-sulfatase

Gal-1-P galactose-1-phosphate

GalR galanin receptor

GALT galactose-1-p-uridyltransferase; gut-associated lymphoid tissue

GALV gibbon ape leukemia virus

Galv, galv galvanic

γ Greek letter *gamma*; a carbon separated from the carboxyl group by two other carbon atoms; a constituent of the gamma protein plasma fraction; heavy chain of immunogammaglobulin; a monomer in fetal hemoglobin; photon

γG immunoglobulin G

GAM geographical analysis machine

GAME immunoglobulins G, A, M, and E

GAMIS German-Austrian Myocardial Infarction Study

GAMM generalized abstract medical model

GAMP German-Austrian Multicenter Project

GAMS German-Austrian Multicenter Study

GAN giant axon neuropathy

G and D growth and development

gang, gangl ganglion, ganglionic

GANS granulomatous angiitis of the nervous system

GAO general accounting office

GAP glottal area patency; D-glyceraldehyde-3-phosphate; growth associated protein; guanosine triphosphatase-activating protein

GAPD glyceraldehyde-3-phosphate dehydrogenase

GAPDH glyceraldehyde-3-phosphate dehydrogenase

GAPDP glyceraldehyde-3-phosphate dehydrogenase pseudogene

GAPO growth retardation, alopecia, pseudoanodontia, and optic atrophy [syndrome]

GAPST global average peri-stimulus time

GARS German-Austrian Reinfarction Study; glycine amide phosphoribosyl synthetase

GART genotype antiretroviral resistance test

GAS galactorrhea-amenorrhea syndrome; gastric acid secretion; gastrin; gastroenterology; general adaptation syndrome; generalized arteriosclerosis; global anxiety score; global assessment scale; goal attainment scale; group A *Streptococcus*; growth arrest-specific [gene]

GASA growth-adjusted sonographic age

GASCIS German-Austrian Space-occupying Cerebellar Infarction Study

GASP Group Against Smoking Pollution [study]

gastroc gastrocnemius [muscle]

GAT gelatin agglutination test; geriatric assessment team; Gerontological Apperception Test; group adjustment therapy

GATR group attribute [UMLS]

GAUS German Activator Urokinase Study

GAWTS genomic amplification with transcript sequencing

GAXS German and Austrian Xamoterol Study

GB gallbladder; gigabyte; glial bundle; goof balls; Guillain-Barré [syndrome]

Gb gilbert; gigabit

gB glycoprotein B

GBA ganglionic blocking agent; gingivobuccoaxial

GBAP glucocerebrosidase pseudogene

GBD gallbladder disease; gender behavior disorder; glass blower's disease; Global Burden of Disease [study]; granulomatous bowel disease

GBG glycine-rich beta-glycoprotein; gonadal steroid-binding globulin

GBH gamma-benzene hexachloride; graphite benzalkonium-heparin

GBHA glyoxal-bis-(2-hydroxyanil)

GBI globulin-binding insulin

GBIA Guthrie bacterial inhibition assay

GBL glomerular basal lamina

GBM glioblastoma multiforme; glomerular basement membrane

GBP gabapentin; galactose-binding protein; gastric bypass; gated blood pool

GBpd gigabits per day

Gbps gigabits per second

Gbq gigabequerel

GBS gallbladder series; gastric bypass surgery; group B *Streptococcus*; general biopsychosocial screening; Guillain-Barré syndrome; glycerine-buffered saline [solution]

GBSS Gey's balanced saline solution; Guillain-Barré-Strohl syndrome

GC ganglion cell; gas chromatography; general circulation; general closure; general condition; generalizability coefficient; genetic counseling; geriatric care; germinal center; giant cell; glucocerebrosidase; glucocorticoid; goblet cell; Golgi cell; gonococcus; gonorrhea; granular casts; granulomatous colitis; granulosa cell; group-specific component; guanine cytosine; guanylcyclase

Gc galactocerebroside; gigacycle; gonococcus; group-specific component

gC glycoprotein C

GCA gastric cancer area; giant cell arteritis

g-cal gram calorie

GCAP germ-cell alkaline phosphatase

GCB gonococcal base

GC-B guanylate cyclase B

gCBF global cerebral blood flow

GCBM glomerular capillary basement membrane

GCD graft coronary disease

GCF growth-rate-controlling factor

GCFT gonococcal/gonorrhea complement fixation test

GCG galactosyl ceramide beta-galactosidase; Genetics Computer Group; glucagon

GCGR glucagon receptor; glucocorticoid receptor

GCH granular clinical history

GCI glottal closure instant; General Cognitive Index

GCIIS glucose controlled insulin infusion system

GCK glomerulocystic kidney; glucokinase

GCL giant-cell lesion; globoid cell leukodystrophy

GCLO gastric *Campylobacter*-like organism

GCM Gorlin-Chaudhry-Moss [syndrome]

g-cm gram-centimeter

gCMRO$_2$ global cerebral oxygen uptake

GC-MS gas chromatography-mass spectrometry

GCN geometric constraint network; giant cerebral neuron

GCNA Genetic Confidentiality and Nondiscrimination Act

GCNF glial cell-derived neurotrophic factor

g-coef generalizability coefficient

GCOP glucocorticoid-induced osteoporosis

GCP geriatric cancer population; German Cardiovascular Prevention [study]; good clinical practices; granulocyte chemotactic protein

GCPS Greig cephalopolysyndactyly syndrome

GCR glucocorticoid receptor; Group Conformity Rating

GCRC General Clinical Research Center [of NIH]

GCRG giant-cell reparative granuloma

GCRS gynecological chylous reflux syndrome

GCS general clinical services; Gianotti-Crosti syndrome; Glasgow Coma Scale; glucocorticosteroid; glutamylcysteine synthetase; glycine cleavage system

GCSA Gross cell surface antigen

GCSE generalized convulsive status epilepticus

G-CSF granulocyte colony-stimulating factor

GCSFR granulocyte colony-stimulating factor receptor

GCSP glycine cleavage system protein

GCT general care and treatment; germ-cell tumor; giant cell thyroiditis; giant cell tumor

GC(T)A giant cell (temporal) arteritis

GCU gonococcal urethritis

GCV ganciclovir; great cardiac vein

GCVF great cardiac vein flow

GCV-TP ganciclovir triphosphate

GCW glomerular capillary wall

GCWM General Conference on Weights and Measures

GCY gastroscopy

GD gadolinium; gastroduodenal; Gaucher disease; general diagnostics; general dispensary; gestational day; Gianotti disease; gonadal dysgenesis; Graves disease; growth and development; growth delay

Gd gadolinium

gD glycoprotein D

gD2 glycoprotein D2

G&D growth and development

GDA gastroduodenal artery; germine diacetate; Graves disease autoantigen

GDB gas density balance; Genome Database; guide dogs for the blind

GDC giant dopamine-containing cell; General Dental Council; Guglielmi detachable coils [x-ray imaging]

Gd-CDTA gadolinium-cyclohexane-diamine-tetraacetic acid

GDCMS German Dilated Cardiomyopathy Study

Gd-DOTA gadolinium-tetra-azacyclo-dodecatetraacetic acid

Gd-DTPA gadolinium-diethylene-triamine-pentaacetic acid

Gd-EDTA gadolinium diethylene-triamine-pentaacetic acid

GDEP general dielectrophoretic [force]

GDF gel diffusion precipitin; growth and differentiation factor

GDH glucose dehydrogenase; glutamate dehydrogenase; glycerophosphate dehydrogenase; glycol dehydrogenase; gonadotropin hormone; growth and differentiation hormone

GDID genetically determined immunodeficiency disease

g/dl grams per deciliter

GDM gestational diabetes mellitus

GDMO General Duties Medical Officer

GDMS glow discharge mass spectrometry

gDNA genomic deoxyribonucleic acid

GDNF giant cell line-derived neutrophilic factor; glial-derived neurotrophic cell

GDP gel diffusion precipitin; gross domestic product; guanosine diphosphate

GDS General Dental Service [UK]; geriatric depression scale; Global Deterioration Scale; Gordon Diagnostic System [for attention disorders]; gradual dosage schedule; guanosine diphosphate dissociation stimulator

GDT geometrically deformable template

GDU gastroduodenal ulcer

GDW glass-distilled water

GDXY XY gonadal dysgenesis

GE gastric emptying; gastroemotional; gastroenteritis; gastroenterology; gastroenterostomy; gastroesophageal; gastrointestinal endoscopy; gel electrophoresis; generalized epilepsy; generator of excitation; gentamicin; glandular epithelium; gradient-echo [imaging]

Ge germanium

Ge⁻ Gerbich negative

G-E gradient-echo [imaging]

G/E granulocyte/erythroid [ratio]

gE glycoprotein E

GEA gastric electrical activity; gastroepiploid artery

GEART Gemfibrozil Atherosclerosis Regression Trial

GEB gum elastic bougie

GEC galactose elimination capacity; glomerular epithelial cell

GECC Government Employees' Clinic Centre

GEE generalized estimating equation

GEF gastroesophageal fundoplication; glossoepiglottic fold; gonadotropin enhancing factor

GEH glycerol ester hydrolase

GEJ gastroesophageal junction

gel gelatin

GELIA German Experience with Low-Intensity Anticoagulation

GEMISCH Generalized Medical Information System for Community Health

GEMS generic error-modeling system

GEMSS glaucoma-lens ecopia-microspherophakia-stiffness-shortness syndrome

GEMT German Eminase Multicenter Trial

GEN gender; generation

Gen genetics, genetic; genus

gen general; genital

GENESIS Genes in Stroke [study]

genet genetic, genetics

GENE-TOX Genetic Toxicology [database]

genit genitalia, genital

GENNET Genetic Network

GENOA Genetics of Atherosclerosis [study]

GENOVA generalized analysis of variance

GENPS genital neoplasm-papilloma syndrome

GENT gentamicin

GEP gastroenteropancreatic; gustatory evoked potential

GEPG gastroesophageal pressure gradient

GEPIC granulocyte elastase alpha-1 proteinase inhibitor complex

GER gastroesophageal reflux; geriatrics; granular endoplasmic reticulum

Ger geriatric(s); German

GERD gastroesophageal reflux disease

geriat geriatrics, geriatric
GeriROS geriatric review of systems
GERL Golgi-associated endoplasmic reticulum lysosome
Geront gerontology, gerontologist, gerontologic
GERRI geriatric evaluation by relative rating instrument
GES gastroesophageal sphincter; glucose-electrolyte solution
GEST, gest gestation; gestational
GET gastric emptying time; general endotracheal [anesthesia]; graded treadmill exercise test
GEU geriatric evaluation unit
Gev giga electron volt
GEWS Gianturco expandable wire stent
GEX gas exchange
G$_{exg}$ exogenous glucose
GF gastric fistula; gastric fluid; germ-free; glass factor; glomerular filtration; gluten-free; grandfather; growth factor; growth failure
gf gram-force
GFA glial fibrillary acidic [protein]
GF-AAS graphite furnace atomic absorption spectroscopy
GFAP glial fibrillary acidic protein
GFAT glutamine:fructose-6-phosphate amidotransferase
GFCI ground-fault circuit-interrupter
GFD gingival fibromatosis-progressive deafness [syndrome]; gluten-free diet
GFFS glycogen and fat-free solid
GFH glucose-free Hanks [solution]
GFI glucagon-free insulin; goodness-of-fit index; ground-fault interrupter
GFL giant follicular lymphoma
Gflops gigaflops [billions of floating point operations per second]
GFP gamma-fetoprotein; gel-filtered platelet; glomerular filtered phosphate; green fluorescent protein
GFR glomerular filtration rate
GFRP growth factor response protein
GFS global focal sclerosis; guafenesin
GG gamma globulin; genioglossus; glycylglycine
gG glycoprotein G
gg gynogenetic
GGA general gonadotropic activity
GGC gamma-glutamyl carboxylase

GGCS gamma-glutamyl cysteine synthetase
GGE generalized glandular enlargement; gradient gel electrophoresis
GGED Graphical Gene-Expression Database
GGFC gamma-globulin-free calf [serum]
GGG glycine-rich gamma-glycoprotein
GGH glycine-glycine-histidine
GGM glucose-galactose malabsorption
GGMRF generalized gaussian Markov random field
GG or S glands, goiter, or stiffness [of neck]
GGPNA gamma-glutamyl-p-nitroanilide
GGR global genomic repair
GGT gamma-glutamyl transferase; gamma-glutamyl transpeptidase; geranylgeranyltransferase
GGTB glycoprotein 4-beta-galactosyl transferase
GGTP gamma-glutamyl transpeptidase
GGV generalized gross validation
GGVB gelatin, glucose, and veronal buffer
GH general health; general hospital; genetic hemochromatosis; genetic hypertension; genetically hypertensive [rat]; geniohyoid; growth hormone
GHA Group Health Association
GHAA Group Health Association of America
GHAT German Hip Arthroplasty Trial
GHB gamma hydroxybutyrate
GHb glycated hemoglobin
GHBA gamma-hydroxybutyric acid
GHBP growth hormone binding protein
GHC group health cooperative
GHD growth hormone deficiency
GHDD ghosal hematodiaphyseal dysplasia
GHDNet Global Health Disaster Network
GHF growth hormone factor
GHL growth hormone-like
GHNet Global Health Network
GHP growth hormone promotor [locus]; group health plan
GHPM general health policy model
GHPQ General Health Perception Questionnaire
GHQ General Health Questionnaire
GHR granulomatous hypersensitivity reaction

GHRA geriatric health risk appraisal [survey]

GHRF growth hormone-releasing factor

GHRFR growth hormone-releasing releasing factor

GH-RH growth hormone-releasing hormone

GHRHR growth hormone-releasing hormone receptor

GHRI general health rating index

GH-RIF growth hormone-release inhibiting factor

GH-RIH growth hormone-release inhibiting hormone

GHT generalized Hough transform

GHV goose hepatitis virus; growth hormone variant

GHz gigahertz

GI gastrointestinal; gelatin infusion [medium]; giant interneuron; gingival index; globin insulin; glomerular index; glucose intolerance; granuloma inguinale; growth inhibition

G$_i$ inhibitory guanine nucleotide-binding protein

gi gill

GIA gastrointestinal anastomosis

GIB gastrointestinal bleeding

GIBF gastrointestinal bacterial flora

GIBS generalized interative Bayesian simulation

GICA gastrointestinal cancer

GID gender identity disorder

GIF gastric intrinsic factor; growth hormone-inhibiting factor

GIFB growth hormone inhibitory factor, brain

GIFIC graphical interface for intensive care

GIFT gamete intrafallopian transfer; granulocyte immunofluorescence test

GIGO garbage in, garbage out

GIH gastrointestinal hemorrhage; growth-inhibiting hormone

GIHINA Genetic Information Health Insurance Nondiscrimination Act

GII gastrointestinal infection

GIK Glucose-Insulin-Kalium [pilot trial]; glucose-insulin-potassium [solution]

GIM general internal medicine; gonadotropin-inhibiting material

GIMC general internal medicine clinic

GINA Global Initiative for Asthma

Ging, ging gingiva, gingival

g-ion gram-ion

GIP gastric inhibitory polypeptide; giant cell interstitial pneumonia; glucose-dependent insulinotropic peptide; gonorrheal invasive peritonitis

GIPR gastric inhibitory polypeptide receptor

GIPSI Gradual Inflation at Optimum Pressure vs Stent Implantation [study]

GIR global improvement rating

GIS gas in stomach; gastrointestinal series; geographic information system; guaranteed income supplement

GISSI Grupo Italiano per lo Studio della Streptochinasi nell'Infarto Miocardico

GIST gastrointestinal stromal tumor

GIT gastrointestinal tract

GITS gastrointestinal therapeutic system

GITSG gastrointestinal tumor study group

GITT gastrointestinal transit time; glucose insulin tolerance test

GJ gap junction; gastric juice; gastrojejunostomy

gJ glycoprotein J

GJA-S gastric juice aspiration syndrome

GK galactokinase; glomerulocystic kidney; glycerol kinase

GKD glycerol kinase deficiency

GKI glucose potassium insulin

GL gland; glomerular layer; glycolipid; glycosphingolipid; glycyrrhizin; graphics library; greatest length; gustatory lacrimation

Gl glabella

gL glycoprotein L

gl gill; gland, glandular

g/l grams per liter

4GL fourth generation [computer] language

GL-4 glycophospholipid

GLA galactosidase A; gamma-linolenic acid; gingivolinguoaxial

glac glacial

GLAD gold-labelled antigen detection

gland glandular

GLAT galactose + activator

GLB galactosidase beta

GLC gas-liquid chromatography

Glc glucose

glc glaucoma

GlcA gluconic acid

GLCB beta-glucuronidase

GLCLC glutamylcysteine synthase

GLC-MS gas-liquid chromatography-mass spectrometry

GlcN glucosamine

GlcNAc N-acetylglucosamine

GlcUA D-glucuronic acid

GLD globoid-cell leukodystrophy; glutamate dehydrogenase

GLDH glutamic dehydrogenase

GLH germinal layer hemorrhage; giant lymph node hyperplasia

GLI glicentin; glioblastoma; glucagon-like immunoreactivity

GLIF guideline interchange format

GLIM generalized linear interactive model

GLM general linear model

GLN glutamine

Gln glucagon; glutamine

GLNH giant lymph node hyperplasia

GLNN galanin

GlnRS glutaminyl transfer ribonucleic acid synthase

GLO glyoxylase

GLO1 glyoxylase 1

glob globular; globulin

GLOM glenoid labrum ovoid mass

GLP glucagon-like peptide; glucose-L-phosphate; glycolipoprotein; good laboratory practice; group living program

GLPR glucagon-like peptide receptor

GLR generalized likelihood ratio; graphic level recorder

GLRA glycine receptor alpha

GLRB glycine receptor beta

GLS generalized least square [estimator]; generalized lymphadenopathy syndrome

GLTN glomerulotubulonephritis

GLTT glucose-lactate tolerance test

GLU glucose; glucuronidase; glutamate; glutamic acid

Glu glucuronidase; glutamic acid; glutamine

glu glucose; glutamate

GLU-5 five-hour glucose tolerance test

GLUC glucosidase

gluc glucose

GLUD glutamate dehydrogenase

GLUDP glutamate dehydrogenase pseudogene

GLUL glutamate (ammonia) ligase

GluproRS glupropyl transfer ribonucleic acid synthase

GLUR glutamate receptor

GluR glutamate receptor

GLUT glucose transporter

GLV gibbon ape leukemia virus; Gross leukemia virus

GLVR gibbon ape leukemia virus receptor

Glx glucose; glutamic acid

GLY, gly glycine

glyc glyceride

GlyCAM glycosylation-dependent cell adhesion molecule

GM gastric mucosa; Geiger-Müller [counter]; general medicine; genetic manipulation; geometric mean; giant melanosome; gram; grand mal [epilepsy]; grandmother; grand multiparity; granulocyte-macrophage; graph-based model; Grateful Med [NLM database]; gray matter; growth medium

GM+ gram-positive

GM⁻ gram-negative

G-M Geiger-Müller [counter]

G/M granulocyte/macrophage

Gm an allotype marker on the heavy chains of immunoglobins

gM glycoprotein M

gm gram

g-m gram-meter

GMA glyceral methacrylate

GMB gastric mucosal barrier; granulomembranous body

GMBF gastric mucosa blood flow

GMC general medical clinic; general medical council; giant migratory contraction; grivet monkey cell

gm cal gram calorie

gm/cc grams per cubic centimeter

GMCD grand mal convulsive disorder

GM-CFU granulocyte-macrophage colony forming unit

GM-CSA granulocyte-macrophage colony-stimulating activity

GM-CSF, (GM)-CSF granulocyte-macrophage colony-stimulating factor

GMD geometric mean diameter; glycopeptide moiety modified derivative

GME graduate medical education

GMENAC Graduate Medical Education National Advisory Committee

GMF glial maturation factor

GMH germinal matrix hemorrhage

GMK green monkey kidney [cells]

GML gut mucosa lymphocyte

g/ml grams per milliliter
gm/l grams per liter
gm-m gram-meter
GMN gradient moment nulling
GMO genetically modified organism
g-mol gram-molecule
GMP genetically modified product; glucose monophosphate; good manufacturing practice; granule membrane protein; guanosine monophosphate
3':5'-GMP guanosine 3':5'-cyclic phosphate
GMPR guanine monophosphate reductase
GMPS guanosine 5'-monophosphorothioate
GMR gallops, murmurs, rubs; gradient motion rephasing
GMRH germinal matrix related hemorrhage
GMRI gated magnetic resonance imaging
GMS General Medical Service; geriatric mental state; Gilbert-Meulengracht syndrome; Gomori methenamine silver [stain]; goniodysgenesis-mental retardation short stature [syndrome]; glyceryl monostearate
GM&S general medicine and surgery
GMSC General Medical Services Committee
GMSP Galen Model for Surgical Procedures
GMT geometric mean titer; gingival margin trimmer; Göteborg Metoprolol Trial
GMV gram molecular volume
GMW gram molecular weight
GN gaze nystagmus; glomerulonephritis; glucose nitrogen [ratio]; gnotobiote; graduate nurse; gram-negative; guanine nucleotide
G/N glucose/nitrogen ratio
Gn gnathion; gonadotropin
GNA general nursing assistance
GNAT guanine nucleotide-binding protein, alpha-transducing
GNAZ guanosine nucleotide-binding alpha Z polypeptide
GNB ganglioneuroblastoma; gram-negative bacillus; guanine nucleotide-binding [protein]
GNBM gram-negative bacillary meningitis
GNBT guanine nucleotide-binding protein, beta transducing
GNC general nursing care; General Nursing Council; geriatric nurse clinician

GND Gram-negative diplococci
GNDF giant cell-derived neurotropic factor
GNDFR giant cell-derived neurotropic factor-responsive
GNID gram-negative intracellular diplococci
GNP geriatric nurse practitioner; gerontologic nurse practitioner
GNR gram-negative rods
GnRF gonadotropin-releasing factor
GnRH gonadotropin-releasing hormone
GnRHR gonadotropin-releasing hormone receptor
GNRP guanine-nucleotide releasing protein
GNS German Nutrition Study
G/NS glucose in normal saline [solution]
GNSWA Genetic Nurses and Social Worker's Association
GNTP Graduate Nurse Transition Program
GNUDI gerontological nursing U-diagnose instrument
GO gastro-[o]esophageal; geroderma osteodysplastica; glutamic oxylacetic [acid]; gonorrhea, glucose oxidase
G&O gas and oxygen
Go gonion
GOA generalized osteoarthritis
GOAT Galveston Orientation and Amnesia Test
GOBAB gamma-hydroxy-beta-amino-butyric acid
GOBI Growth and Development Charting the Road to Health, Oral Rehydration Therapy, Breast Feeding, Immunization [WHO program]
GOE gas, oxygen, and ether
GOG Gynecologic Oncology Group
GOH geroderma osteodysplastica hereditaria
GΩ gigaohm [one billion ohms]
GOMBO growth retardation–ocular abnormalities–microcephaly–brachycephaly–oligophrenia [syndrome]
GON gonococcal ophthalmia neonatorum
GOND glaucomatous optic nerve damage
GOQ glucose oxidation quotient
GOR gastroesophageal reflux; general operating room
GOS Glasgow outcome score; gum optical shield

GOSIP Government Open Systems Inter-communications Profile

GOT aspartate aminotransferase; glucose oxidase test; glutamate oxaloacetate transaminase; goal of treatment

GOTM glutamic-oxaloacetic transaminase, mitochondrial

GOTS geriatric outpatient telephone screening

GP gangliocytic paraganglioma; gastroplasty; general paralysis, general paresis; general practice, general practitioner; genetic prediabetes; geometric progression; globus pallidus; glucose phosphate; glutamic pyruvic [acid]; glutathione peroxidase; glycerophosphate; glycopeptide; glycophorin; glycoprotein; Goodpasture syndrome; gram-positive; guinea pig; gutta percha

G-P Grassbeger-Procaccia [algorithm]

G/P gravida/para

G-1-P glucose-1-phosphate

G3P, G-3-P glyceraldehyde-3-phosphate; glycerol-3-phosphate

G6P, G-6-P glucose-6-phosphate

Gp glycoprotein

G$_p$ guanine nucleotide-binding protein

gp gene product; glycoprotein; group

GPA Goodpasture antigen; grade point average; Group Practice Association; guinea pig albumin

GPAIS guinea pig anti-insulin serum

G6Pase, G-6-Pase glucose-6-phosphatase

GPB glossopharyngeal breathing; glycophorin B

GPC gastric parietal cell; gel permeation chromatography; giant papillary conjunctivitis; glycophorin C; granular progenitor cell; guinea pig complement

GPCI geographic practice cost index

GPD glucose-6-phosphate dehydrogenase; glycerol-phosphate dehydrogenase

G3PD glucose-3-phosphate dehydrogenase

G6PD, G-6-PD glucose-6-phosphate dehydrogenase

G-6-PDA glucose-6-phosphate dehydrogenase enzyme variant A

G6PDH, G-6-PDH glucose-6-phosphate dehydrogenase reduced

G6PDL glucose-6-phosphate dehydrogenase-like

GPE guinea pig embryo; granulocyte colony-stimulating factor promoter element

GPEBP granulocyte colony-stimulating factor promoter element binding protein

GPEP General Professional Education of the Physician

GP/ES gait pathology expert system [automatic data preprocessing]

GPET graphic plan evaluation tool

GPF glomerular plasma flow; granulocytosis-promoting factor

GPGG guinea pig gamma-globulin

GPh Graduate in Pharmacy

GPHN giant pigmented hairy nevus

GP-HPLC gel permeation high-performance liquid chromatography

GPHV guinea pig herpes virus

GPI general paralysis of the insane; glucose phosphate isomerase; glycoprotein I; glycosylphosphatidylinositol; guinea pig ileum

GpIbβ glycoprotein Ib beta

GPII General Practice Immunisation Incentives [Australia]

GPIMH guinea pig intestinal mucosal homogenate

GPIPID guinea pig intraperitoneal infectious dose

GPK guinea pig kidney [antigen]

GPKA guinea pig kidney absorption [test]

GPLV guinea pig leukemia virus

Gply gingivoplasty

GPM general preventive medicine; giant pigmented melanosome

GPm medial globus pallidus

GPMAL gravida, para, multiple births, abortions, and live births

GPN graduate practical nurse

GPNA Genetic Privacy Nondiscrimination Act

GPOA primary open angle glaucoma

GPP generalist physician program; gross primary production

GPPQ General Purpose Psychiatric Questionnaire

GPPT Göteborg Primary Prevention Trial

GPRBC guinea pig red blood cell

GPS Goodpasture syndrome; gray platelet syndrome; guinea pig serum; guinea pig spleen

GPT General Population Trial; glutamate-pyruvate transaminase; glutamic-pyruvic transaminase; guanosine triphosphate

GpTh group therapy

GPU guinea pig unit

GPUT galactose phosphate uridyl transferase

GPWW group practice without wall

GPX glutathione peroxidase

GPx glutathione peroxidase

GQAP general question-asking program

GR gamma-rays; gastric resection; general research; generalized rash; glucocorticoid receptor; glutathione reductase; gravity resistance

gr grade; graft; grain; gram; gravity; gray; gross

gr⁻ gram-negative

gr⁺ gram-positive

GR II Gianturco Roubin Second Generation Coronary Stent Trial

GRA gated radionuclide angiography; glucocorticoid-remedial aldosteronism; gonadotropin-releasing agent

GRABS group A beta-hemolytic streptococcal pharyngitis

GRACE Gianturco Roubin Stent in Acute Closure Evaluation

grad gradient; gradually; graduate

GRAE generally regarded as effective

GRAIL GALEN Representation and Integration Language; gene recognition and assembly link

GRAMI Gianturco Roubin Second Generation Coronary Stent in Acute Coronary Infarction

gran granule, granulated

GRAND Glaxo Receptor Antagonist Against Nottingham Deep Vein Thrombosis Study

GRANDDAD growth delay-aged facies-normal development-deficiency of subcutaneous fat [syndrome]

GRAPE Glycoprotein Receptor Antagonist Potency Evaluation [study]

GRAS generally recognized as safe

GRASP Glaxo Restenosis and Symptoms Project

GRASS gradient recalled acquisition in a steady state

GRASSIC Grampian Asthma Study of Integrated Care

grav gravid

grav I pregnancy one, primigravida

grav II pregnancy two, secundagravida

GRB growth factor receptor-binding protein

GRD gastroesophageal reflux disease; gender role definition

grd ground

GRE glucocorticoid response element; gradient-recalled echo; Graduate Record Examination

GREAT Genome Recognition and Exon Assembly Tool; Grampian Region Early Antistreplase Trial

GRECC Geriatric Research and Education Clinical Center

GRECO German Recanalization of Coronary Occlusion [trial]; German Recombinant Plasminogen Activator [study]

GRF gastrin-releasing factor; genetically related macrophage factor; Gibbs random field; gonadotropin-releasing factor; growth hormone-releasing factor

GRG glucocorticoid receptor gene; glycine-rich glycoprotein; guidelines review group

GRH growth hormone-releasing hormone

GRHR gonadotropic-releasing hormone receptor

GRIA glutamate receptor, ionotropic, ampa

GRID gay-related immunodeficiency [syndrome]

GRIF growth hormone release-inhibiting factor

GRIK glutamate receptor, ionotropic, kainate

GRINA glutamate receptor, ionotropic, N-methyl-D-aspartate A

GRINB glutamate receptor, ionotropic, N-methyl-D-aspartate B

GRIPS Göttingen Risk, Incidence and Prevalence Study

GRMP granulocyte membrane protein

GRN granules; granulin

GrN gram-negative

Grn green

gRNA guide ribonucleic acid

GRO growth-related [protein]

GROB growth-related protein beta

GROD granular osmophilic deposit

GROG growth-related protein gamma

GROU group [UMLS]

GRP gastrin-releasing peptide; glucose-regulated protein

GrP gram-positive

Gr₁P₀AB₁ one pregnancy, no births, one abortion

GRPR gastrin-releasing peptide receptor

GRPS glucose-Ringer-phosphate solution

GRS Golabi-Rosen syndrome

GRV ground reaction vector

GRW giant ragweed [test]

gr wt gross weight

GS gallstone; Gardner syndrome; gastric shield; general surgery; gestational score; Gilbert syndrome; glomerular sclerosis; glutamine synthetase; goat serum; Goldenhar syndrome; Goodpasture syndrome; graft survival; granulocytic sarcoma; grip strength; group section; group-specific

G6S glucosamine-6-sulfatase

gs group specific

G/S glucose and saline

g/s gallons per second

GSA general somatic afferent; Gerontological Society of America; group-specific antigen; Gross virus antigen; guanidinosuccinic acid

Gsα G protein stimulatory alpha subunit

GSBG gonadal steroid-binding globulin

G-SBS guanosine substrate-binding strand

GSC gas-solid chromatography; gravity settling culture

GSCN giant serotonin-containing neuron

GSD genetically significant dose; Gerstmann-Sträussler disease; glutathione synthetase deficiency; glycogen storage disease

GSD-0 glycogen storage disease-zero

GSE general somatic efferent; gluten-sensitive enteropathy

GSF galactosemic fibroblast; genital skin fibroblast

GSFR granulocyte colony-stimulating factor receptor

GSH glomerulus-stimulating hormone; golden Syrian hamster; reduced glutathione; L-alpha-glutamyl-L-cysteinyl-glycine

GSH-Px glutathione peroxidase

GSI global severity index

GSM group sequential method

GSN gelsolin; giant serotonin-containing neuron

GSoA Gerontological Society of America

GSP galvanic skin potential

GSR galvanic skin response; generalized Shwartzman reaction; glutathione reductase

GSS gamete-shedding substance; General Social Survey; Gerstmann-Sträussler-Scheinker [disease]; glutathione synthetase

GSSD Gerstmann-Sträussler-Scheinker disease

GSSG oxidized glutathione

GSSG-R glutathione reductase

GSSR generalized Sanarelli-Shwartzman reaction

GST glutathione-S-transferase; gold salt therapy; gold sodium thiomalate; graphic stress telethermometry; group striction

GSTA glutathione-S-transferase, alpha

GST1L glutathione-S-transferase-1-like

GSTM glutathione-S-transferase, mu

GSV gestational sac volume

GSVD general evoked potential value decomposition

GSVT greater saphenous vein thrombophlebitis

GSW gunshot wound

GSWA gunshot wound, abdominal

GT gait training; galactosyl transferase; gastrostomy; generation time; genetic therapy; gingiva treatment; Glanzmann thrombasthenia; glucose therapy; glucose tolerance; glucose transport; glucuronyl transferase; glutamyl transpeptidase; glycityrosine; granulation tissue; great toe; greater trochanter; group tensions; group therapy

GT1-GT10 glycogen storage disease, types 1 to 10

gt drop [Lat. *gutta*]

g/t granulation time; granulation tissue

G&T gowns and towels

GTA gene transfer agent; Glanzmann thrombasthenia; glycerol teichoic acid

GTB gastrointestinal tract bleeding

GTD gestational trophoblastic disease

GTDS Giesen Tumor Documentation System

GTEM gigahertz transverse electromagnetic [cell]

GTF general transcription factor; glucose tolerance factor; glucosyl-transferase

GTH gonadotropic hormone

GTHR generalized thyroid hormone resistance

GTI grid tiler

GTM generalized tendomyopathy

GTN gestational trophoblastic neoplasia; glomerulotubulonephritis; glyceryl trinitrate

GTO Golgi tendon organ

GTP glutamyl transpeptidase; guanosine triphosphate

GTPase guanosine triphosphatase

gt-PET ground-truth positron emission tomography

GTR galvanic tetanus ratio; granulocyte turnover rate

GTS Gilles de la Tourette syndrome; glucose transport system

GTT gelatin-tellurite-taurocholate [agar]; glucose tolerance test

GTV gross tumor volume

GU gastric ulcer; genitourinary; glucose uptake; glycogenic unit; gonococcal urethritis; gravitational ulcer; guanethidine

GUA group of units of analysis

Gua guanine

GUARANTEE Global Unstable Angina Registry and Treatment Evaluation

GUCA guanylate cyclase activator

GUD genitourinary dysplasia

GUI graphic user interface

GUIDE Guidance by Ultrasound Imaging for Decision Endpoints [trial]

GUIDE II Guidance by Ultrasound for Interventional Decision Endpoints II [trial]

GUK guanylate kinase

GULHEMP general physique, upper extremity, lower extremity, hearing, eyesight, mentality, and personality

GUM genitourinary medicine

GUNM Georgetown University Nursing Model

Guo guanosine

GUS genitourinary sphincter; genitourinary system

GUSTO Globus Ubiquitous Supercomputing Testbed Organization

GUSTO-I Global Utilization of Streptokinase and Tissue Plasminogen Activator for Occluded Coronary Arteries [trial]

GUSTO-IIa Global Use of Strategies to Open Occluded Arteries

GUSTO-IIb Global Use of Strategies to Open Occluded Arteries in Acute Coronary Syndromes [trial]

GUSTO-III Global Use of Strategies to Open Occluded Coronary Arteries [trial]

GUSTO-IV Global Use of Streptokinase and Tissue Plasminogen Activator for Occluded Arteries [trial]

GV gastric volume; gas ventilation; gentian violet; germinal vesicle; granulosis virus; griseoviridan; Gross virus

GVA general visceral afferent [nerve]

GVB gelatin-Veronal buffer

GVBD germinal vesicle breakdown

GVE general visceral efferent [nerve]

GVF good visual fields; gradient vector flow

GVG gamma-vinyl-gamma-aminobutyric acid

GVH, GvH graft-versus-host

GVHD, GvHD graft-versus-host disease

GVHR, GvHR graft-versus-host reaction

GVL graft versus leukemia

G vs HD graft versus host disease

GVTY gingivectomy

GW germ warfare; gigawatt; glycerin in water; gradual withdrawal; group work; guidewire

G/W glucose in water

GWAFD Genée-Wiedemann acrofacial dysostosis

GWB general well-being [schedule]

GWE glycerol and water enema

GWG generalized Wegener granulomatosis

GWN gaussian white noise

GWUHP George Washington University Health Plan

GX glycinexylidide

GXD Gene-Expression Database

GXT graded exercise test

Gy gray

GY-1 graduate year one

GYN, Gyn, gyn gynecologic, gynecologist, gynecology

GZ Guilford-Zimmerman [test]

H bacterial antigen in serologic classification of bacteria [Ger. *Hauch*, film]; deflection in the His bundle in electrogram [spike]; dose equivalent; draft [Lat. *haustus*]; electrically induced spinal reflex; enthalpy; fucosal transferase-producing gene; heart; heavy [strand]; height; hemagglutination; hemisphere; hemolysis; *Hemophilus;* henry; heparin; heroin; high; hippocampus; histidine; *Histoplasma;* histoplasmosis; Holzknecht unit; homosexual; horizontal; hormone; horse; hospital; Hounsfield unit; hour; human; hydrogen; hydrolysis; hygiene; hyoscine; hypermetropia; hyperopia; hypodermic; hypothalamus; magnetic field strength; magnetization; mustard gas; oersted; the region of a sarcomere containing only myosin filaments [Ger. *heller*, lighter] [band]

H⁺ hydrogen ion

[H⁺] hydrogen ion concentration

H₀ null hypothesis

H1, ¹H, H¹ protium

H₁ alternative hypothesis

H2, ²H, H² deuterium

H₂ blockers histamine blockers

H3, ³H, H³ tritium

h hand-rearing [of experimental animals]; heat transfer coefficient; hecto; height; henry; hour [Lat. *hora*]; human; hundred; hypodermic; negatively staining region of a chromosome; Planck constant; secondary constriction; specific enthalpy

H1/2 half-value layer

4H hypothalamic hamartoblastoma-hyperphalangeal hypoendocrine-hypoplastic anus [syndrome]

HA H antigen; Hakim-Adams [syndrome]; halothane anesthesia; Hartley [guinea pig]; headache; health affairs; health alliance; hearing aid; height age; hemadsorption; hemagglutinating antibody; hemagglutination; hemagglutinin; hemolytic anemia; hemophiliac with adenopathy; hepatic adenoma; hepatic artery; hepatitis A; hepatitis-associated; heterophil antibody; Heyden antibiotic; high anxiety; hippocampal asymmetry; hippuric acid; histamine; histocompatibility antigen; Horton arteritis; hospital administration; hospital admission; hospital apprentice; Hounsfield unit; human albumin; hyaluronic acid; hydroxyapatite; hyperalimentation; hyperandrogenism; hypersensitivity alveolitis; hypothalamic amenorrhea

H/A head to abdomen; headache

HA2 hemadsorption virus 2

Ha absolution hypermetropia; hafnium; hamster; Hartmann number

ha hectare

HAA hearing aid amplifier; hemolytic anemia antigen; hepatitis-associated antigen; hospital activity analysis

HA Ag hepatitis A antigen

HAART highly active antiviral therapy

HAAS Honolulu-Asia Aging Study

hAAT human α-1-antitrypsin

HAB histoacryl blue

HABA 2(4'-hydroxyazobenzene) benzoic acid

HABF hepatic artery blood flow

HACCP hazard analysis and critical control point system [food safety]

HACE high-altitude cerebral edema

HACEK *Haemophilus, Actinobacillus, Cardiobacterium, Eikinella, Kingella*

HACER hypothalamic area controlling emotional response

HAChT high affinity choline transport

HACR hereditary adenomatosis of the colon and rectum

hACSP human adenylate cyclase-stimulating protein

HACS hyperactive child syndrome

HACT health care activity [UMLS]

HAD health care alternatives development; hemadsorption; hospital administration, hospital administrator; hospital anxiety and depression [scale]; human immunodeficiency virus-associated dementia

HAd hemadsorption; hospital administrator

HADH hydroxyacyl CoA dehydrogenase

HAd-I hemadsorption-inhibition

HADS hospital anxiety and depression scale

HAE health appraisal examination; hearing aid evaluation; hepatic artery embolism; hereditary angioneurotic edema

HAF hyperalimentation fluid

HaF Hageman factor

HAFP human alpha-fetoprotein

HAG heat-aggregated globulin

HAGG hyperimmune antivariola gamma-globulin

HAGH hydroxyacyl-glutathione hydrolase

HAHS Harvard Alumni Health Study

HAHTG horse antihuman thymus globulin

HAI hemagglutination inhibition; hepatic arterial infusion; hospital-acquired infection

H&A Ins health and accident insurance

HAIR-AN hyperandrogenism, insulin resistance, and acanthosis nigricans [syndrome]

HaK hamster kidney

HAL Heart Attacks in London [study]; hepatic artery ligation; hypoplastic acute leukemia

hal halogen; halothane

HALC high affinity-low capacity

HALF Homocysteine, Atherosclerosis, Lipid and Familial Hypercholesterolemia [study]

HALFD hypertonic albumin-containing fluid demand

halluc hallucinations

HALO Halotestin

HALP hyperalphalipoproteinemia

HALT Hypertension and Lipid Trial

HALT MI Hu23F2G Anti-Adhesion to Limit Cytotoxic Injury Following Acute Myocardial Infarction [study]

HaLV hamster leukemia virus

HAM hearing aid microphone; helical axis in motion; human albumin microsphere; human alveolar macrophage; human T-cell lymphotropic virus associated myelopathy; hypoparathyroidism, Addison disease, and mucocutaneous candidiasis [syndrome]

HAm human amnion

HAMA Hamilton anxiety [scale]; human anti-murine antibody

HAMD Hamilton depression [scale]

HAMIT Heparin in Acute Myocardial Infarction Trial

Ha-MSV Harvey murine sarcoma virus

HAN heroin-associated nephropathy; hyperplastic alveolar nodule

HANA hemagglutinin neuraminidase

H and E hematoxylin and eosin [stain]

HANDI Hemophilia and AIDS/HIV Network for the Dissemination of Information

Handicp handicapped

HANE hereditary angioneurotic edema; Hydrochlorothiazide, Atenolol, Nitrendipine, Enalapril [study]

HANES Health and Nutrition Examination Survey

hANF human atrial natriuretic factor

h ANP human atrial natriuretic peptide

HAODM hypoplasia anguli oris depressor muscle

HAP Handicapped Aid Program; Hazardous Air Pollutants [List]; hazardous air pollution; health alliance plan; heredopathia atactica polyneuritiformis; high-altitude peristalsis; histamine acid phosphate; hospital-acquired pneumonia; hospital admissions program; humoral antibody production; hydrolyzed animal protein; hydroxyapatite

HAp hydroxyapatite

HAPA hemagglutinating anti-penicillin antibody

HAPC high-amplitude peristaltic contraction; hospital-acquired penetration contact

HAPE high-altitude pulmonary edema

HAPI Heparin as an Alternative to Promote Patency in Acute Myocardial Infarction [study]

HAPORT Heart Attack Patient Outcome Research Team [study]

HAPPHY Heart Attack Primary Prevention in Hypertension

HAPS hepatic arterial perfusion scintigraphy

HaPV hamster polyomavirus

HAPVC hemi-anomalous pulmonary venous connection

HAPVD hemi-anomalous pulmonary venous drainage

HAPVR hemi-anomalous pulmonary venous return

HAQ health assessment questionnaire

HAR high-altitude retinopathy

HARD hydrocephalus-agyria-retinal dysplasia [syndrome]

HARD +/– E hydrocephalus-agyria-retinal dysplasia plus or minus encephalocele [syndrome]

HAREM heparin assay rapid easy method

HARH high-altitude retinal hemorrhage

HARM harmonics from the injected signal; heparin assay rapid method

HAROLD Hypertension and Ambulatory Recording in the Old

HARP Harvard Atherosclerosis Reversibility Project; homeless and at-risk population; hospital admission risk profile

HARS histidyl-ribonucleic acid [RNA] synthetase

HART Heparin-Aspirin Reperfusion Trial; Hypertension Audit of Risk Factor Therapy [study]

HART II Heparin and Reperfusion Therapies [study]

HARTS Hoechst Adverse Reaction Terminology System

HAS Hamilton Anxiety Scale; health advisory service; Helsinki Ageing Study; Hemostatic System Activation Substudy; highest asymptomatic [dose]; Hirulog Angioplasty Study; hospital administrative service; hospital advisory service; human albumin solution; hydrocephalus due to stenosis of the aqueduct of Sylvius; hyperalimentation solution; hypertensive arteriosclerotic

HASCVD hypertensive arteriosclerotic cardiovascular disease

HASHD hypertensive arteriosclerotic heart disease

HASI Hirulog Angioplasty Study Investigators

HASP Hospital Admissions and Surveillance Program

HASS highest anxiety subscale score

HAT Halsted Aphasia Test; head, arm, trunk; heparin-associated thrombocytopenia; heterophil antibody titer; histone acetyltransferase; hospital arrival time; hypoxanthine, aminopterin, and thymidine; hypoxanthine, azaserine, and thymidine

3-HAT 3-hydroxyanthranilic acid

HATG horse antihuman thymocyte globulin

HATH Heterosexual Attitudes Toward Homosexuality [scale]

HATT heparin-associated thrombocytopenia and thrombosis

HATTS hemagglutination treponemal test for syphilis

HAU hemagglutinating unit

HAV hemadsorption virus; hepatitis A virus

HAVOC Hematoma and Vascular Outcome Complications [study]

HAWIC Hamburg-Wechsler Intelligence Test for Children

HAZMAT hazardous material

HAZR hazardous substance [UMLS]

HAZUS hazard loss estimation

HB health board; heart block; heel to buttock; held back; hemoglobin; hepatitis B; His bundle; hold breakfast; housebound; hybridoma bank; hyoid body

Hb hemoglobin

HBA heated blood agar [test]

HbA hemoglobin A, adult hemoglobin

HbA$_{1c}$ hemoglobin A$_{1c}$

HBA$_1$ glycosylated hemoglobin

HBAb hepatitis B antibody

HBABA hydroxybenzeneazobenzoic acid

HBAg hepatitis B antigen

HB$_s$AG hepatitis B surface virus

HBB hemoglobin beta-chain; hospital blood bank; hydroxybenzyl benzimidazole

HbBC hemoglobin binding capacity

HBBW hold breakfast blood work

HBC hereditary breast cancer

HB$_c$, HBC, HBc hepatitis B core [antigen]

HbC hemoglobin C

HBCAB hepatitis B core antibody

HB$_c$Ag, HBcAg, HBCAG hepatitis B core antigen

HBCG heat-aggregated Calmette-Guérin bacillus

HbCO carboxyhemoglobin

Hb CS hemoglobin Constant Spring

HbCV *Haemophilus influenzae* conjugate vaccine

HBD has been drinking; homozygous-by-descent; hydroxybutyric dehydrogenase; hypophosphatemic bone disease

HbD hemoglobin D

HBDH hydroxybutyrate dehydrogenase

hBDNF human brain derived neurotrophic factor

HBDT human basophil degranulation test

HBE His bundle electrogram

HbE hemoglobin E

HB$_e$ hepatitis B early antigen

HB$_e$Ag, HbeAg, HBEAG hepatitis B early antigen

HB-EGF heparin-binding epidermal growth factor

HBF hand blood flow; hemispheric blood flow; hemoglobinuric bilious fever; hepatic blood flow; hypothalamic blood flow

HbF fetal hemoglobin, hemoglobin F

Hbg hemoglobin

HBGF heparin-binding growth factor

HBGM home blood glucose monitoring

HBGR hemoglobin-gamma regulator

HbH hemoglobin H

HBHC hospital-based home care

HBHCT hospital-based home care team

Hb-Hp hemoglobin-haptoglobin [complex]

HBI high serum-bound iron

HBIG, HBIg hepatitis B immunoglobulin

HBL hepatoblastoma

HBLA human B-cell lymphocyte antigen

HBLV human B-cell lymphotropic virus

HBM health belief model; hypertonic buffered medium

HbM hemoglobin Milwaukee

HbMet methemoglobin

HBMP Human Brain Map Project

hBMP human brain natriuretic peptide

HBO hyperbaric oxygen, hyperbaric oxygenation

HbO oxyhemoglobin

HbO$_2$ oxyhemoglobin

HBOC hereditary breast-ovarian cancer

HBOT hyperbaric oxygen therapy

HBP heartbeat period; hepatic binding protein; high blood pressure; hospital-based practice

HbP primitive hemoglobin

HBr hydrobromic acid

HbR reduced hemoglobin

HBS hepatitis B surface [antigen]; hyperkinetic behavior syndrome

HB$_s$ hepatitis B surface [antigen]

HbS hemoglobin S, sickle-cell hemoglobin

HBSAg IgG antibody to HBsAg

HB$_s$Ag, HBsAg, HBSAG hepatitis B surface antigen

HBsAg/adr hepatitis B surface antigen manifesting group-specific determinant *a* and subtype-specific determinants *d* and *r*

HBSC hematopoietic blood stem cell

HBSS Hank's balanced salt solution

HbSS hemoglobin SS

HBT human brain thromboplastin; human breast tumor

Hb$_{tot}$ total hemoglobin

HBV hepatitis B vaccine; hepatitis B virus; high biological value

HBV-MN membranous nephropathy associated with hepatitis B virus

HBVS hepatitis B virus integration site

HBW Healthbeat Wales [study]; high birth weight

HbZ hemoglobin Z, hemoglobin Zürich

HC hair cell; hairy cell; handicapped; head circumference; head compression; health care; healthy control; heat conservation; heavy chain; hemoglobin concentration; hemorrhagic colitis; heparin cofactor; hepatic catalase; hepatitis C; hepatocellular; hereditary coproporphyria; hippocampus; histamine challenge; histochemistry; home care; Hospital Corps; house call; Huntington chorea; hyaline casts; hydraulic concussion; hydrocarbon; hydrocortisone; hydroxycorticoid; hyoid cornu; hypercholesterolemia; hypertrophic cardiomyopathy

H&C hot and cold

Hc hydrocolloid

4HC 4-hydroperoxy-cyclophosphamide

HCA heart cell aggregate; hepatocellular adenoma; home care aide; hierarchical clustering analysis; Hospital Corporation of America; hydrocortisone acetate; hypothermic circulatory arrest

HCa high calcium [diet]

HCAP handicapped

HCA/W home care aide or worker

HCB hexachlorobenzene

HCC healthcare related common component; hepatitis contagiosa canis; hepatocellular carcinoma; history of chief complaint; hospital computer center; hydroxycholecalciferol

25-HCC 25-hydroxycholecalciferol

HCCA healthcare commuting area

HCCAA hereditary cysteine C amyloid angiopathy

HCCS hereditary cancer consulting service

HCD health care delivery; heavy-chain disease; high-calorie diet; high-carbohydrate diet; homologous canine distemper

HCE healthcare establishment; healthcare expertise; hypoglossal carotid entrapment

HCF [fetal] head-to-cervix force; heparin cofactor; hereditary capillary fragility;

highest common factor; hypocaloric carbohydrate feeding

HCFA Health Care Financing Administration (pronounced Hickfa)

hCFSH human chorionic follicle-stimulating hormone

HCG, hCG human chorionic gonadotropin

HCH Health Care for the Homeless; hexachlorocyclohexane; hemochromatosis; hygroscopic condenser humidifier

HCHP Harvard Community Health Plan

HCHWA hereditary cerebral hemorrhage with amyloidosis

HCHWA-D hereditary cerebral hemorrhage with amyloidosis–Dutch type

HCI Health Commons Institute; human collagenase inhibitor; human-computer interface

HcImp hydrocolloid impression

HCIS Health Care Information System

HCK hematopoietic cell kinase

HCL hairy-cell leukemia; human cultured lymphoblasts

HCl hydrogen chloride

HCLF high carbohydrate, low fiber [diet]

HCM health care management; hypertrophic cardiomyopathy

HCMM hereditary cutaneous malignant melanoma

HCMV human cytomegalovirus

HCN health communication network; hereditary chronic nephritis

HCO health care organization

HCO₃⁻ bicarbonate

HCOP health center opportunity program

HCP handicapped; hematopoietic cell phosphatase; hepatocatalase peroxidase; hereditary coproporphyria; hexachlorophene; high cell passage

H&CP hospital and community psychiatry

HCPCS Health Care Financing Administration common procedural collecting system; Health Care Financing Administrators Common Procedure Coding System

HCPH hematopoietic cell phosphatase

HCPOTP health care professionals other than physicians

HCPP health care prepayment plan

HCQI health care quality improvement (pronounced Hicky)

HCQIA Health Care Quality Improvement Act

HCR heme-controlled repressor; host-cell reactivation; hysterical conversion reaction

HCRE Homeopathic Council for Research and Education

hCRH human corticotropin-releasing hormone

Hcrit hematocrit

HCS Hajdu-Cheney syndrome; Hazard Communication Standard; health care support; high confidence [information] system; hourglass contraction of the stomach; human chorionic somatotropin; human cord serum

17-HCS 17-hydroxycorticosteroid

hCS human chorionic somatomammotropin

HCSD Health Care Studies Division

hCSM human chorionic somatomammotropin

HCSS hypersensitive carotid sinus syndrome

HCT health check test; helical computed tomography; hematocrit; historic control trial; homocytotrophic; human calcitonin; hydrochlorothiazide; hydroxycortisone

Hct hematocrit

hCT human calcitonin; human chorionic thyrotropin

HCTA health care technology assessment

HCTC Health Care Technology Center

HCTD hepatic computed tomography density

HCTS high cholesterol and tocopherol supplement

HCTU home cervical traction unit

HCTZ hydrochlorothiazide

HCU healthcare unit; homocystinuria; hyperplasia cystica uteri

HCUP Hospital Cost and Utilization Project [database]

HCV hepatitis C virus; hog cholera virus

HCVD hypertensive cardiovascular disease

HCVS human coronavirus sensitivity

HCW health care worker

Hcy homocysteine

HD Haab-Dimmer [syndrome]; Hajna-Damon [broth]; Hansen disease; hard disk; hearing distance; heart disease; helix destabilizing [protein]; hemidesmosome; hemidiaphragm; hemodialysis; hemolytic disease;

hemolyzing dose; hemorrhagic dengue; herniated disc; high density; high dose; hip disarticulation; Hirschsprung disease; histopathologic damage; Hodgkin disease; homeodomain; hormone-dependent; house dust; human diploid [cells]; Huntington disease; hydatid disease; hydrodensitometry; hydroxydopamine

H&D Hunter and Driffield [curve]

HD$_{50}$ 50% hemolyzing dose of complement

HDA heteroduplex analysis; Huntington Disease Association; hydroxydopamine

HDAC histone deacetylase

HDAd helper-dependent adenovirus

HD-AF hemidesmosome-anchoring filament

HDAg hepatitis delta antigen

HDARAC high-dose cytarabine

HDBH hydroxybutyric dehydrogenase

HDC hand drive control; Health Care Financing Administration [HCFA] Data Center; histidine decarboxylase; human diploid cell; hypodermoclysis

HDCS human diploid cell strain

HDCT high-dose chemotherapy

HDCV human diploid cell rabies vaccine

HDD hard disk device; high-dosage depth; Higher Dental Diploma

HDDRISC Heart Disease and Diabetes Risk Indicators in a Screened Cohort [study]

HDES Heidelberg Diet and Exercise Study

HDF hemodiafiltration; host defense factor; human diploid fibroblast

HDFP Hypertension Detection and Follow-up Program

^{3}II-DFP tritiated diisopropyl-fluorophosphonate

HDG high-dose group

HDH heart disease history

Hdh huntingtin; Huntington disease homolog

3H-DHE tritiated dihydroergocriptine

HDI Hamilton depression inventory; hemorrhagic disease of infants; hexamethylene diisocyanate; hospital discharge index

HDIVIG high-dose intravenous immunoglobulin

HDL high-density lipoprotein

HDLBP high-density lipoprotein binding protein

HDL-C high-density lipoprotein-cholesterol complex

HDL-c high-density lipoprotein-cell surface

HDLP high-density lipoprotein

HDLS hereditary diffuse leukoencephalopathy with spheroids

HDLW distance from which a watch ticking is heard by left ear

HDM house dust mite

HDMP high-dose methylprednisolone

HDMTX high-dose methotrexate

HDMTX-CF high-dose methotrexate citrovorum factor

HDMTX-LV high-dose methotrexate leucovorin

HDN health data network; hemolytic disease of the newborn

hDNA heteroduplex deoxyribonucleic acid [DNA]; hybrid deoxyribonucleic acid

HDP hexose diphosphate; high-density polyethylene; hydrogen diphosphonate; hydroxydimethylpyrimidine

HDPAA heparin-dependent platelet-associated antibody

HDPE high-density polyethylene

HDR high-dose radiation; high dose rate

HDRBC head-damaged red blood cells

HDRF Heart Disease Research Foundation

HDRS Hamilton Depression Rating Scale

HDRV human diploid rabies vaccine

HDRW distance from which a watch ticking is heard by right ear

HDS Hamilton Depression Scale; Health Data Services; health delivery system; Healthcare Data Systems; herniated disc syndrome; Hospital Discharge Survey; Hypertension in Diabetes Study

HDSCR health deviation self-care requisites

HDU hemodialysis unit; high dependency unit

HDV hepatitis D virus; hepatitis delta virus

HDZ hydralazine

HE half-scan with extrapolation; hard exudate; hektoen enteric [agar]; hemagglutinating encephalomyelitis; hematoxylin-eosin [stain]; hemoglobin electrophoresis; hepatic encephalopathy; hereditary eliptocytosis; high exposure; hollow enzyme; human enteric; hydroxyethyl [cellulose];

hyperextension; hypertensive encephalopathy; hypogonadotropic eunuchoidism

H&E hematoxylin and eosin [stain]; hemorrhage and exudate; heredity and environment

He heart

HEA hexone-extracted acetone; human erythrocyte antigen

HEADDFIRST Hemicraniectomy and Durotomy from Massive Hemispheric Infarctions: A Proposed Multicenter, Prospective Randomized Study

HEADLAMP Health and Environment Analysis for Decision-Making: Linkage and Monitoring Project

HEAL health education assistance loan

HealSB Health Standards Board

HEALTH ABC Dynamics of Health, Aging and Body Composition [study]

HealthSTAR Health Services, Technology, Administration, and Research [NLM database]

HEAP heparin and early patency

HEART Healing and Early Afterload Reducing Therapy [study]; Health Education and Research Trial; Hyperlipidemia, Epidemiology, Atherosclerosis Risk-Factor Trial; Hypertension and Ambulatory Recording Venetia Study

HEAT human erythrocyte agglutination test

HEB hemato-encephalic barrier

HEC hamster embryo cell; Health Education Council; human endothelial cell; hydroxyergocalciferol; hydroxyethyl cellulose

HECC high-end computing and computation

HECCWG High End Computing and Computation Working Group

HED hereditary ectodermal dysplasia; hydrotropic electron-donor; hydroxyephedrine; hypohidrotic ectodermal dysplasia; unit skin dose [of x-rays] [Ger. *Haut-Einheits-Dosis*]

HEDH hypohidrotic ectodermal dysplasia-hypothyroidism [syndrome]

HEDIS health employer data and information set

HEENT head, ears, eyes, nose, and throat

HEEP health effects of environmental pollutants

HEF hamster embryo fibroblast; human embryo fibroblast

HeFT heart failure trial

HEG hemorrhagic erosive gastritis

HEHR highest equivalent heart rate

HEI Health Effects Institute; high-energy intermediate; homogenous enzyme immunoassay; human embryonic intestine [cells]

HEIR health effects of ionizing radiation; high-energy ionizing radiation

HEIS high-energy ion scattering

HEK human embryo kinase; human embryonic kidney

HEL hen egg white lysozyme; human embryonic lung; human erythroleukemia

HeLa Helen Lake [human cervical carcinoma cells]

Heliox helium and oxygen

HELF human embryo lung fibroblast

HELLIS Health, Literature, Library and Information Services

HELLP hemolysis, elevated liver enzymes, and low platelet count [syndrome]

HELP Hawaii early learning profile; Health Education Library Program; Health Emergency Loan Program; Health Evaluation and Learning Program; Health Evaluation Through Logical Processing; Heart European Leaders Panel [study]; heat escape lessening posture; heparin-induced extracorporeal low-density lipoprotein precipitation [treatment]; Heroin Emergency Life Project; Hospital Equipment Loan Project; Hospitalized Elderly Longitudinal Project

HELP NSAID *Helicobacter* Eradication for Lesion Prevention with Nonsteroidal Anti-inflammatory Drugs [study]

HELPS Hypertension, Exercise and Lifestyle Programs for Seniors [study]

HELVETICA Hirudin in European Restenosis Prevention Trial vs Heparin Treatment in Percutaneous Transluminal Coronary Angioplasty

HEM high-electrolyte meal; hematology, hematologist; hematuric; hemophilia; hemorrhage; hemorrhoids

HEMA Health Education Media Association; 2-hydroxyethyl methacrylate

hemat hematology, hematologist

HEMB hemophilia B

hemi hemiparesis, hemiparalysis; hemiplegia

HEMO, hemo hemodialysis

HEMOA Hemophilia A Mutation Database

HEMOSTAT Hemostasis with ProstarXL vs Angioseal After Coronary Intervention Trial

HEMPAS hereditary erythrocytic multinuclearity with positive acidified serum

HEMRI hereditary multifocal relapsing inflammation

HEMS hospital engineering management system

HEN home enteral nutrition

HeNe helium neon [laser]

HEP hemolysis end point; hepatoerythropoietic porphyria; high egg passage [virus]; high-energy phosphate; human epithelial cell; Hypertension in Elderly Persons [trial]

Hep hepatic; hepatitis

hEP human endorphin

HEp-1 human cervical carcinoma cells

HEp-2 human laryngeal tumor cells

HEPA high-efficiency particulate air [filter]

HEP A hepatitis A

HEP B hepatitis B

HEPBsAg hepatitis B surface antigen

HEP C hepatitis C

HEP D hepatitis D

HEPES N-2-hydroxyethylpiperazine-N-2-ethanesulfonic [acid]

HEPM human embryonic palatal mesenchymal [cell]

HEPOD hereditary expansile polyostotic dysplasia

HER hemorrhagic encephalopathy of rats; hernia

hered heredity, hereditary

HERN Human T-cell Leukemia Virus European Research Network

hern hernia, herniated

HERO Hirulog Early Reperfusion/Occlusion [study]

HEROICS How Effective are Revascularization Options in Cardiogenic Shock? [trial]

HERS Health Evaluation and Referral Service; Heart and Estrogen-Progestin Replacement Study; Human Immunodeficiency Virus [HIV] Research Study; hemorrhagic fever with renal syndrome; Hysterectomy Educational Resources and Services [Foundation]

HERT hospital emergency response team

HES health examination survey; hematoxylin-eosin stain; human embryonic skin; human embryonic spleen; hydroxyethyl starch; hypereosinophilic syndrome; hyperprostaglandin E syndrome

HeSCA Health Sciences Communications Association

HET Health Education Telecommunications; helium equilibration time

Het heterophil

het heterozygous

HETE hydroxy-eicosatetraenoic [acid]

HETP height equivalent to a theoretical plate; hexaethyltetraphosphate

HEV health and environment; hemagglutinating encephalomyelitis virus; hepatitis E virus; hepato-encephalomyelitis virus; high endothelial venule; high endothelial vessel; human enteric virus

HeV hepatitis virus

HEW [Department of] Health, Education, and Welfare

HEX hexaminidase; hexosaminidase

Hex hexamethylmelamine

HEXA Hexosaminidase A Locus Database

HEX A, hex A hexosaminidase A

HEX B, hex B hexosaminidase B

HEX C, hex C hexosaminidase C

HF Hageman factor; haplotype frequency; hard filled [capsule]; hay fever; head of fetus; head forward; heart failure; helper factor; hemofiltration; hemorrhagic factor; hemorrhagic fever; Hertz frequency; high fat [diet]; high flow; high frequency; human fibroblast; hydrogen fluoride; hyperflexion

Hf hafnium; hippocampal formation

hf half; high frequency

HFAK hollow-fiber artificial kidney

HFB human fetal brain

HFC hard filled capsule; high-frequency current; histamine-forming capacity

HFD hemorrhagic fever of deer; high-fiber diet; high-flux dialysis; high forceps delivery; hospital field director; human factors design

HFDA high film density area

HFDK human fetal diploid kidney

HFDL human fetal diploid lung

HFE, HFe hemochromatosis

HFEC human foreskin epithelial cell

HFF human foreskin fibroblast

HFG hand-foot-genital [syndrome]

HFGC human fetal glial cell

HFH hemifacial hyperplasia

HFHV high frequency, high volume

HFI hereditary fructose intolerance; human fibroblast interferon

HFIS high-frequency insertion system [electrosurgery]

HFIF human fibroblast interferon

HFJV high-frequency jet ventilation

HFL human fetal lung

HFM hand, foot and mouth [disease]; hemifacial microsomia

HFMA Healthcare Financial Management Association

HFO high-frequency oscillator; high-frequency oscillatory [ventilation]

HFO-A high-frequency oscillatory [ventilation]-active [expiratory phase]

HFOV high-frequency oscillatory ventilation

HFP hexafluoropropylene; high-frequency pulsation; hypofibrinogenic plasma

HFPPV high-frequency positive pressure ventilation

HFPV high-frequency percussive ventilation

HFR high-frequency recombination

Hfr heart frequency; high frequency

HFRND high frequency and responsibility nursing diagnosis

HFRS hemorrhagic fever with renal syndrome

HFS hemifacial spasm; Hospital Financial Support

hfs hyperfine structure

hFSH, HFSH human follicle-stimulating hormone

HFSP Hanukah factor serine protease

HFST hearing for speech test

HFT high-frequency transduction; high-frequency transfer

Hft high-frequency transfer

HFU hand-foot-uterus [syndrome]

HFV high-frequency ventilation

HG hand grip; herpes gestationis; Heschl's gyrus; high glucose; human gonadotropin; human growth; hypoglycemia

hg hectogram; hemoglobin

HGA homogentisic acid

HGAC high gain adaptive control

hGalR human galanin receptor

Hgb hemoglobin

Hge hemorrhage

HGF hematopoietic growth factor; hepatocyte growth factor; hyperglycemic-glucogenolytic factor

Hg-F fetal hemoglobin

HGFL hepatocyte growth factor-like [protein]

HGF/SF hepatocyte growth factor/scatter factor

HGG herpetic geniculate ganglionitis; human gammaglobulin; hypogammaglobulinemia

HGH, HgH, hGH human gamma globulin; human growth hormone

HGHRF human growth hormone releasing factor

HGI Human Gene Index

HGL heregulin

HGM hog gastric mucosa; human gene mapping; human glucose monitoring

HGMCR human genetic mutant cell repository

HGMD, HGMDB Human Gene Mutation Database

HGMP Human Genome Mapping Project

HGO hepatic glucose output; human glucose output

HGP hepatic glucose production; Human Genome Project; hyperglobulinemic purpura

HGPRT hypoxanthine guanine phosphoribosyl transferase

HGPS hereditary giant platelet syndrome; Hutchinson-Gilford progeria syndrome

hGR human glucocorticoid receptor

hGRH human growth hormone-releasing hormone

HGTS Human Gene Therapy Subcommittee

HGV hepatitis G virus

HH halothane hepatitis; hard-of-hearing; healthy hemophiliac; healthy human; hiatal hernia; Hodgkin-Huxley [model]; holistic health; home help; hydralazine acid-labile hydrazone; hydroxyhexamide; hypergastrinemic hyperchlorhydria; hyperhidrosis; hypogonadotropic hypogonadism; hyporeninemic hypoaldosteronism

H&H hematocrit and hemoglobin

HHA health hazard appraisal; hereditary hemolytic anemia; home health agency;

home health aid; hypothalamo-hypophyseo-adrenal [system]

HHANES Hispanic Health and Nutrition Examination Survey

HHb hypohemoglobinemia; un-ionized hemoglobin

HHC home health care; hypocalciuric hypercalcemia

HHCC home health care classification

HHCS high-altitude hypertrophic cardiomyopathy syndrome

HHD high heparin dose; home dialysis; hypertensive heart disease

HHE health hazard evaluation; hemiconvulsion-hemiplegia-epilepsy [syndrome]; hypotonic hyporesponsive episode

HHG hypertrophic hypersecretory gastropathy; hypogonadotropic hypogonadism

HHH hyperornithinemia, hyperammonemia, homocitrillinuria [syndrome]

HHHH hereditary hemihypotrophy-hemiparesis-hemiathetosis [syndrome]

HHHO hypotonia, hypomentia, hypogonadism, obesity [syndrome]

HHI hereditary hearing impairment

IIIIIE Hearing Handicap Inventory for the Elderly

HHIE-S Hearing Handicap Inventory for the Elderly-Screening Version

HHM humoral hypercalcemia of malignancy

H + Hm compound hypermetropic astigmatism

HHMI Howard Hughes Medical Institutes

HHN handheld nebulizer

HHNC hyperosmolar nonketotic diabetic coma

HHNK hyperglycemic hyperosmoler nonketotic [coma]

HHNS hyperosmolar hyperglycemic nonketotic syndrome

HHP Honolulu Heart Program

HHR hydralazine, hydrochlorothiazide, and reserpine

HHRH hereditary hypophosphatemic rickets with hypercalciuria; hypothalamic hypophysiotropic releasing hormone

HHS [Department of] Health and Human Services; Hearing Handicap Scale; Helsinki Heart Study; hereditary hemolytic syndrome; Honolulu Heart Study; human hypopituitary serum; hyperglycemic hyperosmolar syndrome; hyperkinetic heart syndrome

HHSSA Home Health Services and Staffing Association

HHT head halter traction; hereditary hemorrhagic telangiectasia; heterotopic heart transplantation; homoharringtonine; hydroxyheptadecatrienoic acid

HHV human herpes virus

HI half-scan with interpolation; head injury; health insurance; hearing impaired; heart infusion; hemagglutination inhibition; hepatobiliary imaging; high impulsiveness; histidine; hormone-independent; hormone insensitivity; hospital insurance; humoral immunity; hydroxyindole; hyperglycemic index; hypomelanosis of Ito; hypothermic ischemia

H-I hemagglutination-inhibition

Hi histamine; histidine

HIA Hearing Industries Association; heat infusion agar; hemagglutination inhibition antibody or assay

HIAA Health Insurance Association of America

5-HIAA 5-hydroxyindoleacetic acid

HIB heart infusion broth; hemolytic immune body; *Hemophilus influenzae* type B [vaccine]

Hib *Hemophilus influenzae* type B [vaccine]

HIBAC Health Insurance Benefits Advisory Council

HIC handling-induced convulsions; health insurance claim; Heart Information Center

HICA hydroxyisocaproic acid

HIC-CPR high-impulse compression cardiopulmonary resuscitation

HICH hypertensive intracranial hemorrhage

HiCn cyanomethemoglobin

HI-CPR high-impulse cardiopulmonary resuscitation

HID headache, insomnia, depression [syndrome]; herniated intervertebral disc; human infectious dose; hyperkinetic impulse disorder; hypertension in diabetes

HIDA Health Industry Distributors Association; hepato-iminodiacetic acid (lidofenin) [nuclear medicine scan]; 12-hydroxy-heptadecatrienoic acid

HIE human intestinal epithelium; hyper-IgE [syndrome]; hypoxic-ischemic encephalopathy

HIES hyper-immunoglobulin E [IgE] syndrome

HIF higher integrative functions

HIFBS heat-inactivated fetal bovine serum

HIFC hog instrinsic factor concentrate

HIFCS heat-inactivated fetal calf serum

HiFOS High-Frequency Oscillation Study

HIFU high-intensity focused ultrasound

HIG, hIG human immunoglobulin

HIg hyperimmunoglobulin

HIH hypertensive intracerebral hemorrhage

HIHA high impulsiveness, high anxiety

HiHb hemiglobin (methemoglobin)

HII Health Industries Institute; health information infrastructure; Health Insurance Institute; hemagglutination inhibitor immunoassay

HILA high impulsiveness, low anxiety

HILDA human interleukin in DA [cells]

HIM health information management; hepatitis-infectious mononucleosis; hexose-phosphate isomerase; hyperimmunoglobulin M

HIMA Health Industry Manufacturers Association

HIMC hepatic intramitochondrial crystalloid

HIMP high-dose intravenous methylprednisolone

HIMS healthcare information management system

HIMSS Healthcare Information Management Systems Society

HIMT hemagglutination inhibition morphine test

HIN health information network; Hemophilia in the Netherlands [study]

HI:NC health information: nursing component

HINT healthcare information networks and technologies; hierarchical interpolation; Holland Interuniversity Nifedipine/Metoprolol Trial

Hint Hinton [test]

HIO health insuring organization; hypoiodism

HIOMT hydroxyindole-O-methyl transferase

HIOS high index of suspicion

HIP health illness profile; health insurance plan or program; help for incontinent people; homograft incus prosthesis; hospital insurance program; hydrostatic indifference point

HIPA heparin-induced platelet activation

HIPAA Health Insurance Portability and Accountability Act

HIPC Health Information Policy Council; health insurance purchasing collective; health insurance purchasing cooperative

HIPDM N-trimethyl-n-(2-hydroxyl-3-methyl-5-iodobenzyl)-1,3-propendiamine

HIPE Hospital Inpatient Enquiry

HiPIP high potential iron protein

HIPO hemihypertrophy, intestinal web, preauricular skin tag, and congenital corneal opacity [syndrome]; Hospital Indicator for Physicians Orders

HIPOS Hypertension in Pregnancy: Offspring Study

HiPPI high-performance parallel interface

HiPRF high pulse repetition frequency

HIPS health information processing system; Heparin Delivery with Infusasleeve Catheter Prior to Stent Implantation [study]; Heparin Infusion Prior to Stenting [study]

HIR head injury routine

HIRMIT High-Risk Myocardial Ischemia Trial

HIRS healthcare-specific incident reporting scheme

HIS health information system; Health Interview Survey; Hemodilution in Stroke [study]; histatin; histidine; Hormones in Stroke [study]; hospital information system; Hungarian Isradipine Study; hyperimmune serum

His histidine

HISA [European] Health Information System Architecture

HISAAP Hunter Illawarra Study of Airways and Air Pollution

HISB Health Insurance Standards Board

HISCC Healthcare Information Standards Coordinating Committee

HISKEW Health Information Skeletonized Eligibility Write-off [file, Medicare]

HISPP Healthcare Informatics Standards Planning Panel

HISSG Healthcare Information System Sharing Group; Hospital Information Systems Sharing Group

HIST hospital in-service training

hist histamine, history

HISTLINE History of Medicine Online [NLM database]

Histo histoplasmin skin test

histol histological, histologist, histology

HIT health integration team; hemagglutination inhibition test; heparin-induced thrombocytopenia; High-Density Lipoprotein Cholesterol Intervention Trial; Hirudin for the Improvement of Thrombolysis [study]; histamine inhalation test; hypertrophic infiltrative tendonitis

HITB, HiTB *Hemophilus influenzae* type B

HITF Health Insurance Trust Fund

HIT-SK Hirudin for the Improvement of Thrombolysis with Streptokinase

HITT heparin-induced thrombocytopenia and thrombosis

HITTS heparin-induced thrombosis-thrombocytopenia syndrome

HIU hyperplasia interstitialis uteri

HIV human immunodeficiency virus

HIV1 human immunodeficiency virus type 1

HIV Ag human immunodeficiency virus antigen

HIVAN human immunodeficiency virus-associated nephropathy

HIV-G human immunodeficiency virus-associated gingivitis

HIVRT human immunodeficiency virus [HIV] reverse transcriptase

HJ Howell-Jolly [bodies]

HJR hepatojugular reflex

HK hand to knee; heat-killed; heel-to-knee; hexokinase; human kidney

H-K hand to knee

hK2 human glandular kallikrein 2

HKAFO hip, knee, ankle, and foot orthosis

HKAO hip-knee-ankle orthosis

HKB hybrid knowledge base

HKC human kidney cell

HKLM heat-killed *Listeria monocytogenes*

HKS hyperkinesis syndrome

HL hairline; hairpin loop; hairy leukoplakia; half life; health level; hearing level; hearing loss; heparin lock; hepatic lipase; histiocytic lymphoma; histocompatibility locus; Hodgkin lymphoma; human leukocyte; hydrolethalus [syndrome]; hyperlipidemia; hypermetropia, latent; hypertrichosis lanuginosa

H&L heart and lung [machine]

H/L hydrophil/lipophil [ratio]

Hl hypermetropia, latent

hl hectoliter

HL7 health level 7

HLA histocompatibility leukocyte antigen; histocompatibility locus antigen; homologous leukocyte antibody; human leukocyte antigen; human lymphocyte antigen

HL-A human leukocyte antigen

HLAA human leukocyte antigen A

HLAB human leukocyte antigen B

HLAC human leukocyte antigen C

HLAD human leukocyte antigen D

HLA-LD human lymphocyte antigen-lymphocyte defined

HLA-SD human lymphocyte antigen-serologically defined

HLB hydrophilic-lipophilic balance; hypotonic lysis buffer

HLBI human lymphoblastoid interferon

HLC heat loss center

HLCL human lymphoblastoid cell line

HLD hepatolenticular degeneration; herniated lumbar disk; Hippel-Lindau disease; hypersensitivity lung disease

HLDH heat-stable lactic dehydrogenase

HLDM high-level data model

HLEG hydrolysate lactalbumin Earle glucose

HLF heat-labile factor; hepatic leukemia factor

HLH helix-loop-helix; hemophagocytic lymphohistiocytosis

hLH human luteinizing hormone

HLHS hypoplastic left heart syndrome

HLI human leukocyte interferon

H-L-K heart, liver, and kidneys

HLL hypoplastic left lung

HLLAPI high-level language application programming interface

HLN hilar lymph node; hyperplastic liver nodules

HLP hepatic lipoperoxidation; hind leg paralysis; holoprosencephaly; hyperkeratosis lenticularis perstans; hyperlipoproteinemia

HLQ high-level question
HLR heart-lung resuscitation; high-level resistance
HLS Health Learning System; Hippel-Lindau syndrome
HLT heart-lung transplantation; human lipotropin; human lymphocyte transformation
HLTx heart-lung transplant
HLV hamster leukemia virus; herpes-like virus; hypoplastic left ventricle
HLVS hypoplastic left ventricle syndrome
HM hand movements; health maintenance; heart murmur; hemifacial microsomia; hemodynamic monitoring; Holter monitoring; home management; homosexual male; hospital management; human milk; hydatidiform mole; hyperbaric medicine; hyperimmune mouse
Hm manifest hypermetropia
hm hectometer
HMA health care management alternatives; heteroduplex morbidity assay; human monocyte antigen; hydroxymethionine analog
HMAB human monocyte antigen B
HMAC Health Manpower Advisory Council
HMAS hyperimmune mouse ascites
HMB homatropine methobromide; hydroxymethylbilane
HMBA hexamethylene bisacetamide
HMBS hydroxymethylbilane synthetase
HMC hand-mirror cell; health maintenance cooperative; heroin, morphine, and cocaine; histocompatibility complex, major; hospital management committee; hypertelorism-microtia-clefting [syndrome]
HMCA hydroxymethyl-cyclophenyl adenine
HMCCMP human mammary carcinoma cell membrane proteinase
HMD head-mounted display [computer graphics]; hyaline membrane disease
HMDC health maintenance and diagnostic center
HMDP hydroxymethylenediphosphonate
HME Health Media Education; heat and moisture exchanger; heat, massage, and exercise
HMEF heat and moisture exchanger filter

HMF hydroxymethylfurfural
HMG high-mobility group; human menopausal gonadotropin; 3-hydroxy-3-methylglutaryl
hMG human menopausal gonadotropin
HMG CoA 3-hydroxy-3-methylglutaryl coenzyme A
HMI healed myocardial infarct; hypomelanosis of Ito
HMIS hazardous materials identification system; hospital medical information system
HML human milk lysosome
HMM heavy meromyosin; hexamethylmelamine; hidden Markov model
HMMA 4-hydroxy-3-methoxymandelic acid
HMN hereditary motor neuropathy
H-MNPM [Department of] Health Education and Welfare-Medicus Nursing Process Methodology
HMO health maintenance organization; heart minute output
HMOX heme oxygenase
HMP hexose monophosphate pathway; hot moist packs
HMPA hexamethylphosphoramide
HMPAO hexamethyl-propyleneamine oxine
HM-PAO hexamethyl-propyleneamine-oxime
HMPG hydroxymethoxyphenylglycol
HMPS hexose monophosphate shunt
HMPT hexamethylphosphorotriamide
HMQC heteronuclear multiple-quantum correlation
HMR health maintenance record; health maintenance recommendations; histiocytic medullary reticulosis
HMRI Hospital Medical Records Institute [Canada]
H-mRNA H-chain messenger ribonucleic acid
HMRTE human milk reverse transcriptase enzyme
HMS hexose monophosphate shunt; Household Multipurpose Survey; hypermobility syndrome
HMSA health manpower shortage area
HMSAS hypertrophic muscular subaortic stenosis
HMSN hereditary motor and sensory neuropathy

HMSS Hospital Management Systems Society

HMT hematocrit; histamine-N-methyltransferase; hospital management team

HMTA hexamethylenetetramine

HMU hydroxymethyl-uracil

5-HMU 5-hydroxymethyl uridine

HMW high-molecular-weight

HMWC high-molecular-weight component

HMWGP high-molecular-weight glycoprotein

HMWK high-molecular-weight kininogen

HMX heat, massage, and exercise

HN head and neck; head nurse; hemagglutinin neuraminidase; hematemesis neonatorum; hemorrhage of newborn; hereditary nephritis; high necrosis; hilar node; histamine-containing neuron; home nursing; human nutrition; hypertrophic neuropathy

H&N head and neck

HNA healthcare network architecture; heparin neutralizing activity

HNB human neuroblastoma

HNBD has not been drinking

HNC hypernephroma cell; hyperosmolar nonketotic coma; hypothalamoneurohypophyseal complex

HNF hepatocyte nuclear factor

HNF1A hepatocyte nuclear factor-1-alpha

HNKC hyperosmolar nonketotic coma

HNKDS hyperosmolar nonketotic diabetic state

HNL histiocytic necrotizing lymphadenitis

HNMT histamine N-methyltransferase

HNN hierarchical neural network

HNP hereditary nephritic protein; herniated nucleus pulposus; human neurophysin

HNPCC hereditary nonpolyposis colorectal cancer; Hereditary Non-Polyposis Colorectal Cancer [Database]; human nonpolyposis colorectal cancer

HNPP hereditary neuropathy with liability to pressure palsies

HNR harmonic-to-noise ratio

hnRNA heterogeneous nuclear ribonucleic acid

hnRNP heterogeneous nuclear ribonucleoprotein [RNP]

HNRP heterogenous nuclear ribonucleoprotein

HNRPG heterogenous nuclear ribonucleoprotein peptide G

HNS head and neck surgery; home nursing supervisor

HNSHA hereditary nonspherocytic hemolytic anemia

HNTD highest nontoxic dose

HNV has not voided; health network venture

HO hand orthosis; heterotopic ossification; high oxygen; hip orthosis; history of; Holt-Oram [syndrome]; house officer; hyperbaric oxygen

H/O, h/o history of

Ho horse; [Cook-Medley] hostility scale

HOA hip osteoarthritis; hypertrophic osteoarthropathy

HoaRhLG horse anti-rhesus lymphocyte globulin

HoaTTG horse anti-tetanus toxoid globulin

HOB head of bed

HOC human ovarian cancer; hydroxycorticoid

HOCAP Hypertrophic Obstructive Cardiomyopathy Ablation Pacing [study]

HOCM high-osmolar contrast medium; hypertrophic obstructive cardiomyopathy

HOD hyperbaric oxygen drenching

HOF hepatic outflow

HofF height of fundus

HOGA hyperornithinemia with gyrate atrophy

HOH hard of hearing

HOI hospital onset of infection

HoIg horse immunoglobulin

HOKPP hypokalemic periodic paralysis

HOLON health object library online

HOME Home Observations for Measurement of the Environment

Homeop homeopathy

HOMO highest occupied molecular orbital; homosexual

homo homosexual

HON Health on the Net [Foundation]

HONC hyperosmolar nonketotic coma

HONK hyperosmolar nonketosis

HOOD hereditary onycho-osteodysplasia

HOODS hereditary onycho-osteodysplasia syndrome

HOOE heredopathia ophthalmo-oto-encephalica

HOOP Health Online Outreach Project

HOP high oxygen pressure; holoprosencephaly-polydactyly [syndrome]

HOPE Health Outcomes Prevention Evaluation; Healthcare Options Plan Entitlement; health-oriented physical education; holistic orthogonal parameter estimation; Hospital Outcomes Project for the Elderly; Hypertensive Old People in Edinburgh [study]

HOPG highly oriented pyrolytic graphite

HOPI history of present illness

HOPP hepatic occluded portal pressure

HOPWA housing opportunities for people with AIDS

hor horizontal

HORG health care organization [UMLS]

HOS health opinion survey; high-order spectrum; Holt-Oram syndrome; human osteosarcoma; hypoosmotic swelling [test]

HoS horse serum

Hosp, hosp hospital

HOST healthcare open systems and trials; hybrid open system technology; hypo-osmotic shock treatment

HOT health-oriented telecommunication; human old tuberculin; hyperbaric oxygen therapy; Hypertension Optimal Treatment [study]

HOT MI Hyperbaric Oxygen and Thrombolysis in Myocardial Infarction [study]

HOTS hypercalcemia-osteolysis-T-cell syndrome

HOX homeobox

Ho:YAG holmium:yttrium:aluminum:garnet [laser]

HP halogen phosphorus; handicapped person; haptoglobin; hard palate; Harvard pump; health profession(al); heat production; heel to patella; hemiparkinsonism; hemipelvectomy; hemiplegia; hemoperfusion; *Hemophilus pleuropneumoniae*; heparin; hepatic porphyria; high potency; high power; high pressure; high protein; highly purified; horizontal plane; horsepower; hospital participation; hot pack; house physician; human pituitary; hydrophilic petrolatum; hydrostatic pressure; hydroxypyruvate; hyperparahyroidism; hypersensitivity pneumonitis; hypophoria

H&P history and physical examination

Hp haptoglobin; hematoporphyrin; hemiplegia

HPA Health Care Practice Act; Health Policy Agenda for the American People; health promotion advocates; *Helix pomatia* agglutinin; hemagglutinating penicillin antibody; *Histoplasma capsulatum* polysaccharide antigen; human platelet antigen; humeroscapular periarthritis; hypertrophic pulmonary arthropathy; hypothalamo-pituitary-adrenocortical [system]; hypothalam-opituitary axis

HPAA hydroperoxyarachidonic acid; hydroxyphenylacetic acid; hypothalamo-pituitary-adrenal axis

HPAC high-performance anion-exchange chromatography; hypothalamo-pituitary-adreno-cortical

HPAFT hereditary persistence of alfa-fetoprotein

H-PAGE horizontal polyacrylamide gel

HPAH hydralazine pyruvic acid hydrazone

HPASE high-performance application for science and engineering

HPB hepatobiliary

HPBC hyperpolarizing bipolar cell

HPBF hepatotrophic portal blood factor

HPBL human peripheral blood leukocyte

HPC health professional card; hemangiopericytoma; high-performance computing; hippocampal pyramidal cell; history of present complaint; holoprosencephaly; hydroxypropylcellulose

HPCA human progenitor cell antigen

HPCC health plan purchasing cooperative; high-performance computing and communications

HPCHA high red-cell phosphatidylcholine hemolylic anemia

HPD hearing protective device; hereditary progressive dystonia; high-protein diet; home peritoneal dialysis

HPGe hyperpure germanium

HPDR hypophosphatemic D-resistant rickets

HPE hepatic portoenterostomy; high-permeability edema; history and physical examination; holoprosencephaly; hydrostatic permeability edema

HPES holoprosencephaly

HPETE hydroxyperoxy-eicosotetranoic [acid]

HPF heparin-precipitable fraction; hepatic plasma flow; high-pass filter; high-power field [microscope]; hypocaloric protein feeding

HPFH hereditary persistence of fetal hemoglobin

hPFSH, HPFSH human pituitary follicle-stimulating hormone

hPG, HPG human pituitary gonadotropin

HpGe hyperpure germanium

HPH *Helix pomatia* hemocyanin; hygromycin B phosphotransferase

HPI hepatic perfusion index; history of present illness

HPL human parotid lysozyme; human peripheral lymphocyte; human placental lactogen

hPL human placental lactogen; human platelet lactogen

HPLA hydroxyphenyl lactic acid

HPLAC high-pressure liquid-affinity chromatography

HPLC high-performance liquid chromatography; high-power liquid chromatography; high-pressure liquid chromatography

HPLE hereditary polymorphic light eruption

HPLH hypoplastic left heart

HPM high-performance membrane

HPMC human peripheral mononuclear cell

HPN hepsin; home parenteral nutrition; hypertension

hpn hypertension

HPNAT high-performance networking application team

HPNS high pressure neurological syndrome

HPNSP high performance network service provider

HPO high-presure oxygen; hydroperoxide; hydrophilic ointment; hypertrophic pulmonary osteoarthropathy

HPOA hypertrophic pulmonary osteoarthropathy

HPP hereditary pyropoikilocytosis; history of presenting problems

HPP, hPP hydroxyphenylpyruvate; hydroxypyrozolopyrimidine; human pancreatic polypeptide

HPPA hydroxyphenylpyruvic acid

HPP-CFC high proliferative potential colony-forming cell

HPPD hours per patient day; hydroxyphenylpyruvate dioxygenase

HPPH 5-(4-hydroxyphenyl)-5-phenyl-hydantoin

HPPO high partial pressure of oxygen; hydroxyphenyl pyruvate oxidase

HPQ Health Perceptions Questionnaire

HPR haptoglobin-related gene; health practices research

HPr human prolactin

hPRL human prolactin

HPRP human platelet-rich plasma

HPRT hypoxanthine-guanine phosphoribosyltransferase

HpRz hairpin ribozyme

HPS Hantavirus pulmonary syndrome; Helsinki Policemen Study; hematoxylin, phloxin, and saffron; Hermansky-Pudlak syndrome; high-protein supplement; His-Purkinje system; Hopkins Precursors Study; human platelet suspension; hypertrophic pyloric stenosis; hypothalamic pubertal syndrome

HPSA health professional shortage area

HPSL health professions student loan

HPSS high-performance storage system

HPT histamine provocation test; human placental thyrotropin; hyperparathyroidism; Hypertension Prevention Trial; hypothalamo-pituitary-thyroid [system]

1°HPT primary hyperparathyroidism

2°HPT secondary hyperparathyroidism

HPTH hyperparathyroid hormone

HPTIN human pancreatic trypsin inhibitor

HPTLC high-performance thin-layer chromatography

HPU heater probe unit

HPV *Hemophilus pertussis* vaccine; hepatic portal vein; human papillomavirus; human parvovirus; hypoxic pulmonary vasoconstriction

HPVD hypertensive pulmonary vascular disease

HPV-DE high-passage virus-duck embryo

HPV-DK high-passage virus-dog kidney

HPVG hepatic portal venous gas

HPVM high-performance virtual machine

HPW hypergammaglobulinemic purpura of Waldenström

HP/W health promotion/wellness [program]

HPX high peroxidase [content]; hypophysectomized

HPZ high pressure zone

[3H]QNB (-)[3H]quinuclidinyl benzilate

HR hairpin ribozyme; hazard ratio; heart rate; hematopoietic reconstitution; hemorrhagic retinopathy; hepatorenal; high resolution; higher rate; histamine receptor; histamine release; hormonal response; hospital record; hospital report; hospitalization rate; hyperimmune reaction; hypertensive rat; hypophosphatemic rickets

hr hairless [mouse]; host-range [mutant]; hour

H&R hysterectomy and radiation

HRA health record analyst; health risk appraisal; heart rate audiometry; hereditary renal adysplasia; histamine release activity; Human Resources Administration

HRAE high right atrium electrogram

HRBC horse red blood cell

HRC health reference center; hereditary renal cancer; high-resolution chromatography; horse red cell; human rights committee

h/rCRF human recombinant corticotropin-releasing factor

HRCT, HR-CT high-resolution computed tomography

HRE hepatic reticuloendothelial [cell]; high-resolution electrocardiography; hormone receptor enzyme; hormone response element

HREH high-renin essential hypertension

HREM high-resolution electron microscopy

HRF health-related facility; heart rate fluctuations; histamine-releasing factor; human readable format

HRG histidine-rich glycoprotein

HRGP histidine-rich glycoprotein

HrHRF human recombinant histamine-releasing factor

HRH2 histamine receptor H2

HRIG, HRIg human rabies immunoglobulin

HRL head rotation to the left

HRLA human reovirus-like agent

HRmax maximal heart rate

HRMS health records management system

hRNA heterogeneous ribonucleic acid

HRNB Halstead-Reitan Neuropsychological Battery

HRP high-risk patient; high-risk pregnancy; histidine-rich protein; horseradish peroxidase

HRPD Hamburg Rating Scale for Psychiatric Disorders

hr-PET high-resolution positron emission tomography

HRPT hyperparathyroidism

HRQOL health-related quality of life

HRR Hardy-Rand-Rittler [color vision test]; head rotation to the right; heart rate range

HRRI heart rate retardation index

HRS Hamilton Rating Scale; Hamman-Rich syndrome; Haw River syndrome; health and rehabilitative services; hepatorenal syndrome; high rate of stimulation; hormone receptor site; humeroradial synostosis

HRSA Health Resources and Services Administration

HRS-D Hamilton Rating Scale for Depression; Hirschsprung disease

HRSP high-resolution storage phosphor

HRSUB submaximal heart rate

HRT heart rate; Heidelberg retinal tomography; hormone replacement therapy; Hormone Replacement Trial

HRTE human reverse transcriptase enzyme

HRTEM high-resolution transmission electron microscopy

HRV heart rate variability; human reovirus; human rhinovirus; human rotavirus

HS Haber syndrome; half strength; Hallopeau-Siemens [syndrome]; hamstring; hand surgery; Hartmann solution; head sling; health services; healthy subject; heart sounds; heat-stable; heavy smoker; Hegglin syndrome; heme synthetase; hemorrhagic shock; Henoch-Schönlein [purpura]; heparan sulfate; hereditary spherocytosis; herpes simplex; hidradenitis suppurativa; hippocampal system; home surgeon; homologous serum; horizontally selective; Horner syndrome; horse serum; hospital ship; hospital staff; hospital stay; hours of sleep; house surgeon; human serum; Hurler syndrome; hybrid sign; hypereosinophilic syndrome; hypersensitive site; hypersensitivity; hypertonic saline

hs history; hospitalization

H/S helper-suppressor [ratio]

H&S hemorrhage and shock; hysterectomy and sterilization

HSA Hazardous Substances Act; Health Services Administration; health systems agency; hereditary sideroblastic anemia; horse serum albumin; human serum albumin; hypersomnia-sleep apnea

HSAG N-2-hydroxyethylpiperazine-N-2-ethanesulfonate-saline-albumin-gelatin

HSAM highly selective affinity modification

HSAN hereditary sensory and autonomic neuropathy

HSAP heat-stable alkaline phosphatase

HSAS hydrocephalus due to stenosis of aqueduct of Sylvius; hypertrophic subaortic stenosis

HSC Hand-Schüller-Christian [syndrome]; Health and Safety Commission; health sciences center; health screening center; hematopoietic stem cell; human skin collagenase

HSCD Hand-Schüller-Christian disease

HSCL Hopkins Symptom Check List

HS-CoA reduced coenzyme A

HSCR Hirschsprung disease

HSCS health state classification system; Hypertension-Stroke Cooperative Study

HSCSG Hypertension-Stroke Cooperative Study Group [trial]

HSCT hematopoietic stem cell transplantation

HSD Hallervorden-Spatz disease; honestly significant difference; hydroxysteroid dehydrogenase; hypertonic saline and dextran

H(SD) Holtzman Sprague-Dawley [rat]

HSDB hazardous substances data bank

HSDO health services delivery organization

HSE health, safety, and environment; heat stress element; herpes simplex encephalitis; hemorrhagic shock and encephalopathy

hSEAP human secreted alkaline phosphatase

HSEES Hazardous Substances Emergency Events Surveillance [system]

HSEP heart synchronized evoked potential

HSES hemorrhagic shock-encephalopathy syndrome

HSF heat shock factor; hepatocyte stimulatory factor; histamine sensitizing factor; human serum esterase; hypothalamic secretory factor

HSG herpex simplex genitalis; hysterosalpingogram, hysterosalpingography

hSGF human skeletal growth factor

HSGP human sialoglycoprotein

HSH hypomagnesemia with secondary hypocalcemia

HSHC hydrocortisone hemisuccinate

HSI health service indicator; health supervision index; heat stress index; hue saturation intensity [imaging]; human seminal plasma inhibitor

HSIL high-grade squamous intraepithelial lesion

HSK herpes simplex keratitis

HSL hormone-sensitive lipase

HSLC high-speed liquid chromatography

HSM health system model; hepatosplenomegaly; holosystolic murmur

HSMHA Health Services and Mental Health Administration

HSN hereditary sensory neuropathy; hospital satellite network

HSO health service organization

hSOD human superoxide dismutase

HSP Health Systems Plan; healthcare security policy; heat shock protein; Hemorrhagic Stroke Project; hemostatic screening profile; Henoch-Schönlein purpura; hereditary spastic paraparesis; Hospital Service Plan; human serum prealbumin; human serum protein

hsp heat shock protein [gene]

HS PACS high-speed picture archive and communication system

HS-PG heparan sulfate-proteoglycan

HSPM hippocampal synaptic plasma membrane

HSPN Henoch-Schönlein purpura nephritis

HSQ health status questionnaire; home screening questionnaire

HSQB Health Standards and Quality Bureau

HSQC heteronuclear single-quantum correlation

HSR Harleco synthetic resin; heated serum reagin; homogeneously staining region

HSRC Health Services Research Center; Human Subjects Review Committee

HSRD hypertension secondary to renal disease

HSR&D health services research and development

HS-RDEB recessively inherited dystrophic epidermolysis bullosa of Hallopeau and Siemens

HSRI Health Systems Research Institute
HSRPROJ Health Services Research Project in Progress [NLM database]
HSRS Health-Sickness Rating Scale
HSRV human spuma retrovirus
HSS Hallermann-Streiff syndrome; Hallervorden-Spatz syndrome; Henoch-Schönlein syndrome; high-speed supernatant; hyperstimulation syndrome; hypertrophic subaortic stenosis
HSSCC hereditary site-specific colon cancer
HSSD hospital sterile supply department
HSSU hospital sterile supply unit
HST health sciences and technology
HSTAR health services and technology assessment research
HSTAT Health Science/Technology Assessment Text [NLM database]
HSTF heat shock transcription factor; heat stress transferring factor; human serum thymus factor
HSTM health state transition matrix
HSUS Health Services Utilization Study
HSV herpes simplex virus; high selective vagotomy; hop stunt viroid; hyperviscosity syndrome
HSV-1 herpes simplex virus type 1
HSV-2 herpes simplex virus type 2
HSVE herpes simplex virus encephalitis
HSVTK, HSVtk herpes simplex virus [HSV] thymidine kinase
HSVtk herpes simplex virus thymidine kinase
HSyn heme synthase
HT Hashimoto thyroiditis; head trauma; hearing test; hearing threshold; heart; heart transplantation, heart transplant; hemagglutination titer; hereditary tyrosinemia; high-frequency transduction; high temperature; high tension; high threshold; histologic technician; home treatment; hospital treatment; Hubbard tank; human thrombin; hydrocortisone test; hydrotherapy; hydroxytryptamine; hypermetropia, total; hypertension; hypertensive; hyperthyroidism; hypertransfusion; hypodermic tablet; hypothalamus; hypothyroidism
H&T hospitalization and treatment
³HT tritiated thymidine
5-HT 5-hydroxytryptamine [serotonin]

Ht height of heart; heterozygote; hyperopia, total; hypothalamus
H$_t$ dose equivalent to individual tissues
ht heart; heart tones; height; high tension
HTA health technology assessment; heterophil transplantation antigen; human thymocyte antigen; hydroxytryptamine; hypophysiotropic area
HTACS human thyroid adenyl-cyclase stimulator
ht aer heated aerosol
HT(ASCP) Histologic Technician certified by the American Society of Clinical Pathologists
HTB house tube feeding; human tumor bank
HTC hepatoma cell; hepatoma tissue culture; home telecare; homozygous typing cell
Htc hematocrit
HTCMS home telecare management system
HTCVD hypertensive cardiovascular disease
HTD human therapeutic dose
HTDW heterosexual development of women
HTF heterothyrotropic factor; house tube feeding; HpaII tiny fragment
HTG hypertriglyceridemia
HTGL hepatic triglyceride lipase
HTH helix-turn-helix; homeostatic thymus hormone; hypothalamus
Hth hypothermic
HTHD hypertensive heart disease
HTIG human tetanus immune globulin
HTK heel to knee
HTL hamster tumor line; hearing threshold level; high-L-leucine transport; histotechnologist; human T-cell leukemia; human thymic leukemia
HTLA high-titer, low acidity; human T-lymphocyte antigen
HTL(ASCP) Histotechnologist certified by the American Society of Clinical Pathologists
HTLF human T-cell leukemia virus enhancer factor
HTLV human T-cell leukemia/lymphoma virus; human T-lymphocyte virus; human T-lymphotropic virus
HTLV-III human T-lymphocyte virus type III

HTLV-MA cell membrane antigen associated with the human T-cell leukemia virus

HTLV-I-MA human T-cell leukemia virus-I-associated membrane antigen

HTLVR human T-cell leukemia virus receptor

HTML hypertext markup language

HTMT hybrid technology multi-threaded technology

HTN Hantaan-[like virus]; histatin; hypertension; hypertensive nephropathy

HTO high tibial osteotomy; high turnover osteoporosis; hospital transfer order

HTOR 5-hydroxytryptamine oxygenase regulator

HTP House-Tree-Person [test]; hydroxytryptophan; hypothromboplastinemia

5-HTP 5-hydroxy-L-tryptophan

HtPA hexahydrophthalic anhydride

HTPN home total parenteral nutrition

HTR hemolytic transfusion reaction; histidine transport regulator; 5-hydroxytryptamine receptor

hTR human thyroid receptor

hTRβ human thyroid receptor beta

HTS Hamilton Twin Study; head traumatic syndrome; HeLa tumor suppression; high-throughput screening; human thyroid-stimulating hormone, human thyroid stimulator; hypertonic saline [solution]

hTS human thymidylate synthase

HTSAB human thyroid-stimulating antibody

HTSC home telecare service center

HTSH, hTSH human thyroid-stimulating hormone

HTST high temperature, short time

HTT 5-hydroxytryptamine transformer

HTTP hypertext transfer protocol

HTV herpes-type virus

HTVD hypertensive vascular disease

HTX heterotaxy, X-linked; histrionicotoxin

HU heat unit; hemagglutinating unit; hemolytic unit; Hounsfield unit; human urine, human urinary; hydroxyurea; hyperemia unit

Hu human

HUAA home uterine activity assessment

HUC human uroepithelial cell; hypouricemia

HuCS human-centered system

HuEPO human erythropoietin

HU-FSH human urinary follicle-stimulating hormone

HUGO Human Genome Organization

HUI headache unit index; Health Utilities Index

HUIFM human leukocyte interferon meloy

HuIFN human interferon

HUK human urinary kallikrein

HUM Hilbert uniqueness method

Hum humerus

HUMANE human-oriented universal medical assessment system under network environment

HUP Hospital Utilization Project

HUR hydroxyurea

HURA health in underserved rural areas

HURT hospital utilization review team

HUS heel ultrasonography; hemolytic uremic syndrome; hyaluronidase unit for semen

HuSA human serum albumin

hut histidine utilization [gene]

HUTHAS human thymus antiserum

HUV human umbilical vein

HUVEC human umbilical vein endothelial cell

HV hallux valgus; Hantaan virus; heart volume; hepatic vein; herpesvirus; high voltage; high volume; hospital visit; hyperventilation

hv hypervariable region

H&V hemigastrectomy and vagotomy

HVA homovanillic acid

HVAC heating, ventilating, and air conditioning

HVC Health Visitor's Certificate

HVD Hantavirus [HV] disease; hypertensive vascular disease

HVDRR hypocalcemic vitamin D-resistant rickets

HVE hepatic venous effluence; high-voltage electrophoresis

HVEM herpesvirus [HV] entry mediator

HVG host versus graft [disease]

HVGS high-voltage galvanic stimulation

HVH *Herpesvirus hominis*

HVJ hemagglutinating virus of Japan

HVL, hvl half-value layer

HVLP high volume, low pressure

HVM high-velocity missile

HVPC high-voltage pulsed current

HVPE high-voltage paper electrophoresis

HVPG hepatic venous pressure gradient

HVR hepatic vascular resistance; hypervariable region; hypoxic ventilation response

HVS herpesvirus of Saimiri; herpesvirus sensitivity; high vaginal swab; high-voltage stimulation; high-voltage spine-and-wave [discharge]; hyperventilation syndrome; hyperviscosity syndrome

HVSD hydrogen-detected ventricular septal defect

HVT half-value thickness; herpesvirus of turkeys

HVTEM high-voltage transmission electron microscopy

HVUS hypocomplementemic vasculitis urticaria syndrome

HVWP hepatic vein wedge pressure

HW healing well; heart weight

HWB hot water bottle

HWC Health and Welfare, Canada

HWCD Hans-Weber-Christian disease

HWD heartworm disease

HWE healthy worker effect; hot water extract

HWML health and welfare makeup language

HWP hepatic wedge pressure; hot wet pack

HWS hot water-soluble

HX histiocytosis X; hydrogen exchange; hypophysectomized; hypoxanthine

Hx hallux; history; hypoxanthine

hx hospitalization

HXB hexabrachion

HXIS hard x-ray imaging spectrometry

HXM hexamethylmelamine

HXR hypoxanthine riboside

Hy hypermetropia; hyperopia; hypophysis; hypothenar; hysteria

HYC hycanthone methylsulfonate

Hy-C Hydralazine vs Captopril [trial]

HYCAT Hytrin Community Assessment Trial

HYCONES Hybrid Connectionist Expert System

HYCX hydrocephalus due to congenital stenosis of aqueduct of Sylvius

HYD hydralazine; hydration, hydrated; hydrocortisone; hydrodensitometry; hydroxyurea

hydr hydraulic

hydro hydrotherapy

HYE healthy years equivalent

hyg hygiene, hygienic, hygienist

HYL, Hyl hydroxylysine

HYNON Hypertension Non-Drug treatment [cooperative study]

HYP hydroxyproline; hypnosis

Hyp hydroxyproline; hyperresonance; hypertrophy; hypothalamus

hyp hypophysis, hypophysectomy

HyperGEN Hypertension Genetic Epidemiology Network

hyper-IgE hyperimmunoglobulinemia E

hypn hypertension

hypno hypnosis

Hypo hypodermic, hypodermic injection

hypox hypophysectomized

HYPP hyperkalemic periodic paralysis

HYPPOS Hypertensive Population Survey

HYPREN Hypertension under Prazosin and Enalapril [study]

HypRF hypothalamic releasing factor

Hypro hydroxyproline

hys, hyst hysterectomy; hysteria, hysterical

HYSTENOX Enoxaparin Following Hysterectomy [study]

HyTk hybromycin-thymidine kinase

HYVET Hypertension in the Very Elderly Trial

HZ herpes zoster

Hz hertz

Hz/G hertz/gauss

HZO herpes zoster ophthalmicus

HZV herpes zoster virus

I electric current; impression; incisor [permanent]; independent; index; indicated; induction; inertia; inhalation; inhibition, inhibitor; inosine; insoluble; inspiration, inspired; insulin; intake; intensity; intermittent; internal medicine; intervention; intestine; iodine; ionic strength; ischemia; isoleucine; isotope; nuclear spin quantum number; region of a sarcomere that contains only actin filaments; Roman numeral one

I-131 iodine-131

i electric current; incisor [deciduous]; insoluble; isochromosome; optically inactive

ι see *iota*

IA ibotenic acid; image analysis; immediately available; immune adherence; immunoadsorbent; immunobiologic activity; impedance angle; indolaminergic accumulation; indolic acid; indulin agar; infantile autism; infected area; inferior angle; information assurance; inhibitory antigen; inpatient admission; internal auditory; intra-alveolar; intra-amniotic; intra-aortic; intra-arterial; intra-articular; intra-atrial; intra-auricular; intracellular anchor [segment]; intrinsic activity; irradiation area; isopropyl alcohol

I&A identification and authentication; irrigation and aspiration

Ia immune response gene-associated antigen

IAA imidazoleacetic acid; indoleacetic acid; infectious agent, arthritis; insulin autoantibody; International Antituberculosis Association; interruption of the aortic arch; iodoacetic acid

IAAA inflammatory abdominal aortic aneurysm

IAAR imidazoleacetic acid ribonucleotide

IAB Industrial Accident Board; intra-abdominal; intra-aortic balloon

IABA intra-aortic balloon assistance

IABC, IABCP intra-aortic balloon counter-pulsation

IABM idiopathic aplastic bone marrow

IABP intra-aortic balloon pump

IABS International Association for Biological Standards

IAC image analysis cytometry; ineffective airway clearance; internal auditory canal; interposed abdominal compression; intra-arterial catheter; intra-arterial chemotherapy

IAC CPR interposed abdominal compression cardiopulmonary resuscitation

IACD implantable automatic cardioverter-defibrillator; intra-arterial conduction defect

IACI idiopathic arterial calcification of infancy

IACP intra-aortic counterpulsation

IACS International Academy of Cosmetic Surgery

IACUC institutional animal care and utilization committee

IACV International Association of Cancer Victims and Friends

IAD inactivating dose; instructional advance directive; internal absorbed dose; internal age distribution; intrasact distance

IADH inappropriate antidiuretic hormone

IADHS inappropriate antidiuretic hormone syndrome

IADL instrumental or intermediate activities of daily living

IADR International Association for Dental Research

IADSA, IA-DSA intra-arterial digital subtraction angiography

IAds immunoadsorption

IAEA International Atomic Energy Agency

IAET International Association for Enterostomal Therapy

IAF idiopathic alveolar fibrosis

IAFC International Association of Fire Chiefs

IAFF International Association of Fire Fighters

IAFI infantile amaurotic familial idiocy

IAG International Association of Gerontology; International Academy of Gnathology

IAGP International Association of Geographic Pathology

IAGUS International Association of Genito-Urinary Surgeons

IAH idiopathic adrenal hyperplasia; implantable artificial heart

IAHA idiopathic autoimmune hemolytic anemia; immune adherence hemagglutination

IAHD idiopathic acquired hemolytic disorder

IAHS infection-associated hemophagocytic syndrome; International Association of Hospital Security

IAI intra-abdominal infection; intra-abdominal injury

IAIMS Integrated Advanced Information Management System

IAIS insulin autoimmune syndrome

IαTI inter-alpha trypsin inhibitor

IAM immune adhesion molecule; Institute of Aviation Medicine; internal auditory meatus

i am intra-amniotic

IAMA Infection in Atherosclerosis and Use of Macrolide Antibiotics [study]

IAMM International Association of Medical Museums

IAMS International Association of Microbiological Societies

IAN idiopathic aseptic necrosis; indole acetonitrile

iANP immunoreactive atrial natriuretic peptide

IAO immediately after onset; intermittent aortic occlusion; International Association of Orthodontists

IA OCA oculocutaneous albinism type IA

IAOM International Association of Oral Myology

IAP idiopathic acute pancreatitis; immunosuppressive acidic protein; inosinic acid pyrophosphorylase; Institute of Animal Physiology; intermittent acute porphyria; International Academy of Pathology; International Academy of Proctology; International Atherosclerosis Project; intra-abdominal pressure; intracellular action potential; intracisternal A-type particle; islet-activating protein

IAPB International Association for Prevention of Blindness

IAPG interatrial pressure gradient

IAPM International Academy of Preventive Medicine

IAPP International Association for Preventive Pediatrics; islet amyloid polypeptide

IAPSRS International Association of Psychosocial Rehabilitation Services

IAPV intermittent abdominal pressure ventilation

IAR immediate asthma reaction; inhibitory anal reflex; iodine-azide reaction

IARC International Agency for Research on Cancer

IARF ischemic acute renal failure

IARG International Anticoagulant Review Group [study]

IARS image archival and retrieval system

IARSA idiopathic acquired refractory sideroblastic anemia

IAS immunosuppressive acidic substance; infant apnea syndrome; insulin autoimmune syndrome; interatrial septum; interatrial shunting; internal anal sphincter; International Acquired Immune Deficiency Syndrome Society; intra-amniotic saline

IASA interatrial septal aneurysm

IASD interatrial septal defect; inter-auricular septal defect

IASH isolated asymmetric septal hypertrophy

IASHS Institute for Advanced Study in Human Sexuality

IASL International Association for Study of the Liver

IASP International Association for Study of Pain

IASSH Italian Acute Stroke Study with Hemodilution

IAT instillation abortion time; intrinsic accuracy test; iodine azide test; invasive activity test

IATI inter-alpha-trypsin inhibitor

IATIL inter-alpha-trypsin inhibitor, light chain

IAV intermittent assisted ventilation; intra-arterial vasopressin

IAVM intramedullary arteriovenous malformation

IB idiopathic blepharospasm; immune body; inclusion body; index of body build; infectious bronchitis; Institute of Biology; interface bus; ipratropium bromide

ib in the same place [Lat. *ibidem*]

IBAT intravascular bronchoalveolar tumor

IBB intestinal brush border

IBBBB incomplete bilateral bundle branch block

IBC Institutional Biosafety Committee; iodine-binding capacity; iron-binding capacity; isobutyl cyanoacrylate

IBCA isobutyl-2-cyanoacrylate

IBC-R Injury Behavior Checklist–Revised

IBD identical-by-descent; inflammatory bowel disease; irritable bowel disease

IBDlist Inflammatory Bowel Disease List [database]

IBE International Bureau for Epilepsy

IBED Inter-African Bureau for Epizootic Diseases

IBEN individual behavior [UMLS]

iB-EP immunoreactive beta-endomorphin

IBF immature brown fat; immunoglobulin-binding factor; Insall-Burstein-Freeman [total knee instrumentation]; intestinal blood flow

IBG insoluble bone gelatin

IBI intermittent bladder irrigation; ischemic brain infarction

ibid in the same place [Lat. *ibidem*]

IBIDS ichthyosis-brittle hair-impaired intelligence-decreased fertility-short stature [syndrome]; International Bibliographic Information on Dietary Supplements [NIH database]

IBIS Invasive Bacterial Infection Surveillance [study]

IBK infectious bovine keratoconjunctivitis

IBM inclusion body myositis

IBMP International Board of Medicine and Psychology

IBMX 3-isobutyl-1-methylxanthine

IBNR incurred but not reported

IBO information-bearing object

IB OCA oculocutaneous albinism type IB

IBP insulin-like growth factor binding protein; International Biological Program; intra-aortic balloon pumping; iron-binding protein

IBPMS indirect blood pressure measuring system

IBQ Illness Behavior Questionnaire

IBR infectious bovine rhinotracheitis

IBRO International Brain Research Organization

IBRV infectious bovine rhinotracheitis virus

IBS identical-by-state; imidazole buffered saline; immunoblastic sarcoma; integrated backscatter; Iowa Breakfast Study; irritable bowel syndrome; isobaric solution

IBSA iodinated bovine serum albumin

IBSN infantile bilateral striated necrosis

IBSP integrin-binding sialoprotein

IBT ink blot test

IBU ibuprofen; international benzoate unit

i-Bu isobutyl

IBV infectious bronchitis vaccine; infectious bronchitis virus

IBW ideal body weight

IC icteric, icterus; immune complex; immunoconjugate; immunocytochemistry; immunocytotoxicity; impedance cardiogram; imprinting center; indirect calorimetry; individual counseling; infection control; inferior colliculus; informed consent; inner canthal [distance]; inorganic carbon; inspiratory capacity; inspiratory center; institutional care; integrated circuit; integrated concentration; intensive care; intercostal; intermediate care; intermittent catheterization; intermittent claudication; internal capsule; internal carotid; internal conjugate; interstitial cell; intracapsular; intracardiac; intracarotid; intracavitary; intracellular; intracerebral; intracisternal; intracranial; intracutaneous; irritable colon; islet cells; isovolumic contraction

IC 1/2/3 intermediate care 1/2/3

IC$_{50}$ inhibitory concentration of 50%

ICA immunocytochemical analysis; independent component analysis

ICAA International Council on Alcohol and Addictions; Invalid Children's Aid Association

ICAAC Interscience Conference on Antimicrobial Agents and Chemotherapy

ICAb islet cell antibody

ICAI intelligent computer-aided instruction

ICAM integrated computer-aided manufacturing; intercellular adhesion molecule

ICAMI International Committee Against Mental Illness

ICAO internal carotid artery occlusion

ICARIS Intervention Cardiology Risk Stratification [study]

ICARUS Islet Cell Antibody Register User Study

ICASO International Committee of Acquired Immunodeficiency Syndrome Service Organisations

ICBDMS International Clearinghouse for Birth Defects Monitoring Systems

ICBF inner cortical blood flow

ICBG idiopathic calcification of basal ganglia

ICBM International Consortium for Brain Mapping

ICBP intracellular binding protein

ICBR increased chromosomal breakage rate

ICC immunocompetent cells; immunocytochemistry; Indian childhood cirrhosis; infection control committee; intensive coronary care; intercanthal distance; interchromosomal crossing over; interclass correlation coefficient; intercluster constraint; internal conversion coefficient; International Certification Commission; interventional cardiac center; intracervical device; intraclass correlation coefficient; intracranial cavity

ICCE intracapsular cataract extraction

iCCK immunoreactive cholecystokinin

ICCM idiopathic congestive cardiomyopathy

ICCS International Classification of Clinical Services

ICCR International Committee for Contraceptive Research

ICCU intensive coronary care unit; intermediate coronary care unit

ICD I-cell disease; immune complex disease; impedance cardiogram; implantable cardioverter defibrillator; impulse-control disorder; induced circular dichroism; Institute for Crippled and Disabled; International Center for the Disabled; International Classification of Diseases, Injuries, and Causes of Death; International Statistical Classification of Diseases and Health-related Problems; intrauterine contraceptive device; ischemic coronary disease; isocitrate dehydrogenase; isolated conduction defect

ICDA International Classification of Diseases, Adapted

ICD/BPA International Classification of Diseases as adapted by the British Paediatric Association

ICDC implantable cardioverter-defibrillator catheter

ICD-9-CM International Classification of Diseases-ninth revision-Clinical Modification

ICD-10 International Statistical Classification of Diseases and Health-related Problems, 10th revision

ICDH isocitrate dehydrogenase

ICD-O International Classification of Diseases-Oncology

ICDRC International Contact Dermatitis Research Center

ICDREC International Computer Database for Radiation Accident Case Histories

ICDS Integrated Child Development Scheme; International Cardiac Doppler Society

ICE ice, compression, elevation; ichthyosis-cheek-eyebrow [syndrome]; immunochemical evaluation; integration, codification and evaluation; interleukin converting enzyme; iridocorneal endothelial [syndrome]

ICECA International Committee for Electronic Communication on Acquired Immunodeficiency Syndrome

ICED Index of Co-existent Diseases

ICER inducible cyclic adenosine monophosphate

ICES information collection and evaluation system

ICF immunodeficiency-centromeric instability-facial anomalies [syndrome]; indirect centrifugal flotation; intensive care facility; intercellular fluorescence; interciliary fluid; intermediate-care facility; International Cardiology Foundation; intracellular fluid; intravascular coagulation and fibrinolysis

ICFA incomplete Freund adjuvant; induced complement-fixing antigen

ICFF important clinical field finding

ICF(M)A International Cystic Fibrosis (Mucoviscidosis) Association

ICF-MR intermediate-care facility for the mentally retarded

ICF/MR intensive care facilities for mental retardation

ICG impedance cardiogram; impedance cardiography; indocyanine green; isotope cisternography

ICGC indocyanine-green clearance

ICGN immune-complex glomerulonephritis

ICH idiopathic cortical hyperostosis; infectious canine hepatitis; Institute of Child Health [UK]; intracerebral hematoma; intracranial hemorrhage; intracranial hypertension

ICHD Inter-Society Commission for Heart Disease Resources

ICHPPC International Classification of Health Problems in Primary Care

ICI intracardiac infection

ICi intracisternal

ICIDH International Classification of Impairments, Disabilities, and Handicaps

ICIN Intracoronary Streptokinase Trial of the Interuniversity Cardiology Institute of the Netherlands

iCJD iatrogenic Creutzfeldt-Jakob disease

ICL idiopathic CD4 T-cell lymphocytopenia; implantable contact lens; intracranial lesion; iris-clip lens; isocitrate lyase

ICLA International Committee on Laboratory Animals

ICLAS International Council for Laboratory Animal Science

ICLH Imperial College, London Hospital

ICM inner cell mass; integrated conditional model; intelligent cardiovascular monitor; intercostal margin; International Confederation of Midwives; intracytoplasmic membrane; introduction to clinical medicine; ion conductance modulator; isolated cardiovascular malformation

ICMI Inventory of Childhood Memories and Imaginings

ICMSF International Commission on Microbiological Specifications for Foods

ICN intensive care nursery; International Council of Nurses

ICNa intracellular concentration of sodium

ICNB International Committee on Nomenclature of Bacteria

ICNC intracerebral nuclear cell

ICNND Interdepartmental Committee on Nutrition in National Defense

ICNP International Classification of Nursing Practice

ICNV International Committee on Nomenclature of Viruses

ICO idiopathic cyclic oedema; impedance cardiac output; infection control officer

ICOMS input, constrains, output, and mechanisms

ICOPER International Cooperative Pulmonary Embolism Registry

ICP incubation period; indwelling catheter program; infantile cerebral palsy; infection-control practitioner; infectious cell protein; inflammatory cloacogenic polyp; integrated care pathway or planning; interactive closest point [algorithm]; interdisciplinary care plan; intermittent catheterization protocol; intracranial pressure; intracytoplasmic; intrahepatic cholestasis of pregnancy

ICPA International Commission for the Prevention of Alcoholism

ICPB International Collection of Phytopathogenic Bacteria

ICPEMC International Commission for Protection against Environmental Mutagens and Carcinogens

ICPI Intersociety Committee on Pathology Information

ICP-MS inductively coupled plasma mass spectrometry [or spectrometer]

ICR [distance between] iliac crests; Institute for Cancer Research; Institute for Cancer Research [mouse]; intermittent catheter routine; international consensus report; International Congress of Radiology; intracardiac catheter recording; intracavitary radium; intracorneal ring; intracranial reinforcement; ion cyclotron resonance

ICRC infant care review committee; International Committee of the Red Cross

ICRD Index of Codes for Research Drugs

ICRE International Commission on Radiological Education

ICRETT International Cancer Research Technology Transfer

ICREW International Cancer Research Workshop

ICRF Imperial Cancer Research Fund [UK]

I-CRF immunoreactive corticotropin-releasing factor

ICRF-159 razoxane

ICRP International Commission on Radiological Protection; International Committee on Radiation Protection

ICRS Index Chemicus Registry System

ICRU International Commission on Radiation Units and Measurements

ICS ileocecal sphincter; immotile cilia syndrome; impulse-conducting system; incident command system; integrated case study; intensive care, surgical; intercellular space; intercostal space; intercuspidation splint; International College of Surgeons; International Cytokine Society; intracellular segment; intracranial stimulation; Iohexol Cooperative Study; irritable colon syndrome

ICSA islet cell surface antibody

ICSB International Committee on Systematic Bacteriology

ICSC idiopathic central serous choroidopathy

ICS$_f$ final intercuspidation splint

ICSG International Cooperative Study Group

ICSH International Committee for Standardization in Hematology; interstitial cell-stimulating hormone

ICSI Institute for Clinical Systems Integration; intracytoplasmic sperm injection

ICSK intracoronary streptokinase

ICSO intermittent coronary sinus occlusion

ICSP Interagency Council on Statistical Policy; International Council of Societies of Pathology

ICSS intracranial self-stimulation

ICSTI International Council for Scientific and Technical Information

ICSU International Council of Scientific Unions

ICT icteric, icterus; indirect Coombs test; inflammation of connective tissue; insulin coma therapy; intensive conventional therapy; intermittent cervical traction; interstitial cell tumor; intracardiac thrombus; intracranial tumor; isovolumic contraction time

Ict icterus

iCT immunoreactive calcitonin

ICTMM International Congress on Tropical Medicine and Malaria

ICTS idiopathic carpal tunnel syndrome

ICTV International Committee for the Taxonomy of Viruses

ICTX intermittent cervical traction

ICU infant care unit; immunologic contact urticaria; intensive care unit; intermediate care unit

ICUS intracoronary ultrasound

ICV intracellular volume; intracerebroventricular

icv intracerebroventricular

ICVS International Cardiovascular Society

ICW intensive care ward; intermediate care ward; intracellular water

ICWS integrated clinical workstation

ICx immune complex; inter-cartridge exchange

ID identification; identifier; idiotype; iditol dehydrogenase; immunodeficiency; immunodiffusion; immunoglobulin deficiency; inappropriate disability; inclusion disease; index of discrimination; individual dose; infant death; infectious disease; infective dose; inhibitory dose; initial diagnosis; initial dose; initial dyskinesia; injected dose; inside diameter; interdigitating; interhemispheric disconnection; interstitial disease; intradermal; intraduodenal

I-D intensity-duration

I&D incision and drainage

ID$_{50}$ median infective dose

Id infradentale; interdentale

id the same [Lat. *idem*]

IDA idamycin; iduronidase; image display and analysis; iminodiacetic acid; insulin-degrading activity; iron deficiency anemia

IDAV immunodeficiency-associated virus

IDB image data baser

IDBS infantile diffuse brain sclerosis

IDC idiopathic dilated cardiomyopathy; infiltrating ductal carcinoma; interdigitating cell

IDCI intradiplochromatid interchange

IDCS Idiopathic Dilated Cardiomyopathy Study

IDCT inverse discrete cosine transform

IDD insulin-dependent diabetes; intraluminal duodenal diverticulum; Inventory to Diagnose Depression

IDDF investigational drug data form

IDDM insulin-dependent diabetes mellitus

IDDM-MED insulin-dependent diabetes mellitus-multiple epiphyseal dysplasia [syndrome]

IDDT immune double diffusion test

IDE insulin-degrading enzyme; intelligent drive electronics; investigational device exemption

IDEA Individuals with Disabilities Education Act; Internet Database of Evidence-based Abstracts and Articles
IDEF Integrated [Computer-Aided Manufacturing] Definition
IDF inverse document frequency
IDFT inverse discrete Fourier transform
IDG intermediate dose group
IDH isocitrate dehydrogenase
IDHS Indian Diet Heart Study
IDI immunologically detectable insulin; induction-delivery interval; inter-dentale inferius
I-5DI type I 5'deiodinase
IDIC Internal Dose Information Center
idic isodicentric
IDISA intraoperative digital subtraction angiography
IDK internal derangement of knee
IDL Index to Dental Literature; interface definition language; intermediate density lipoprotein; intermediate differentiation of lymphocytic lymphoma
IDL-C, IDL-c intermediate density lipoprotein-cholesterol complex
IDLH immediate danger to life and health
IDM idiopathic disease of myocardium; immune defense mechanism; indirect method; infant of diabetic mother; intermediate-dose methotrexate; inverse different moment
ID-MS isotope dilution-mass spectrometry
IDN integrated delivery network
iDNA intercalary deoxyribonucleic acid
IDP immunodiffusion procedure; inflammatory demyelinating neuropathy; initial dose period; inosine diphosphate
IDPH idiopathic pulmonary hemosiderosis
IDPN iminodipropionitrile; inflammatory demyelinating polyneuropathy
IDQ Individualized Dementia Questionnaire
IDR intradermal reaction; item discrimination ratio
IDS iduronate sulfatase; immune deficiency state; inhibitor of deoxyribonucleic acid [DNA] synthesis; intraduodenal stimulation; Inventory for Depressive Symptomatology; investigational drug service
IdS interdentale superius

IDSA Infectious Diseases Society of America
IDSAN International Drug Safety Advisory Network
IDS-SR Inventory for Depressive Symptomatology-Systems Review
IDT immune diffusion test; instillation delivery time; interdisciplinary team; intradermal typhoid [vaccine]
IDU idoxuridine; injecting drug use; injection or intravenous drug user; iododeoxyuridine
IDUA iduronidase
IdUA iduronic acid
IDUR idoxuridine
IdUrd idoxuridine
IDUS injecting drug users
IDV intermittent demand ventilation
IDW initial deflection width [respiratory sounds]
IDVC indwelling venous catheter
IDX 4'-iodo-4'-deoxyoxorubicin
Idx cross-reactive idiotype
IE imaging equipment; immunizing unit [Ger. *Immunitäts Einheit*]; immunoelectrophoresis; infective endocarditis; inner ear; intake energy; internal elastica; intraepithelial
ie that is [Lat. *id est*]
I/E inspiratory/expiratory [ratio]; internal/external
I:E inspiratory/expiratory [ratio]
IEA immediate early antigen; immunoelectroadsorption; immunoelectrophoretic analysis; infectious equine anemia; inferior epigastric artery; International Epidemiological Association; intravascular erythrocyte aggregation
IEC injection electrode catheter; inpatient exercise center; International Electrotechnical Commission; intraepithelial carcinoma; ion-exchange chromatography
IECa intraepithelial carcinoma
IED inherited epidermal dysplasia; intermittent explosive disorder
IEE inner enamel epithelium
IEEE Institute of Electrical and Electronics Engineers
IEF International Eye Foundation; isoelectric focusing
IEG immediate early gene
IEI isoelectric interval

IEL internal elastic lamina; intraepithelial lymphocyte
IEM immuno-electron microscopy; inborn error of metabolism
IEMA immunoenzymatic assay
IEMCT individualized epidural morphine conversion tool
IEMG integrated electromyogram; integrated electromyography
IEOP immunoelectro-osmophoresis
IEP immunoelectrophoresis; individualized education program; isoelectric point
IES impact of events scale
IESS Intergroup Ewing Sarcoma Study
IET intrauterine exchange transfusion
IETF Internet Engineering Task Force
IETT immediate exercise treadmill testing
IF idiopathic fibroplasia; idiopathic flushing; immersion foot; immunofluorescence; indirect fluorescence; infrared; inhibiting factor; initiation factor; instantaneous flow; interferon; interior facet; intermediate filament; intermediate frequency; internal fixation; interstitial fluid;interventional fluoroscopy; intrinsic factor; involved field [radiotherapy]
IF1, IF2, IF3 interferon 1, 2, 3
IFA idiopathic fibrosing alveolitis; immunofluorescence assay; immunofluorescent antibody; incomplete Freund's adjuvant; indirect fluorescent antibody; indirect fluorescent assay; International Fertility Association; International Filariasis Association
IFAA International Federation of Associations of Anatomists
IFABP intestinal fatty acid binding protein
IFAP ichthyosis follicularis-atrichia-photophobia [syndrome]
IFAT indirect fluorescent antibody test
IFC intermittent flow centrifugation; intrinsic factor concentrate
IFCC International Federation of Clinical Chemistry
IFCR International Foundation for Cancer Research
IFCS inactivated fetal calf serum
IFDS isolated follicle-stimulating hormone deficiency syndrome
IFE immunofixation electrophoresis; interfollicular epidermis
IFF inner fracture face

IFFH International Foundation for Family Health
IFG inferior frontal gyrus; interferon gamma
IFGO International Federation of Gynecology and Obstetrics
IFGS interstitial fluid and ground substance
IFGT irradiation and fusion gene transfer
IFHP International Federation of Health Professionals
IFHPMSM International Federation for Hygiene, Preventive Medicine, and Social Medicine
IFI immune interferon
IFIP International Federation for Information Processing
IFL immunofluorescence
IFLrA recombinant human leukocyte interferon A
IFM internal fetal monitor
IFMBE International Federation for Medical and Biological Engineering
IFME International Federation for Medical Electronics
IFMP International Federation for Medical Psychotherapy
IFMSA International Federation of Medical Student Associations
IFMSS International Federation of Multiple Sclerosis Societies
IFN interferon
IFNA interferon alpha
If nec if necessary
IFNG interferon gamma
IFNGT interferon gamma transducer
IFP inflammatory fibroid polyp; insulin, compound F [hydrocortisone], prolactin; intermediate filament protein; intimal fibrous proliferation; intrapatellar fat pad
IFPM International Federation of Physical Medicine
IFR infrared; inspiratory flow rate
IFRA indirect fluorescent rabies antibody [test]
IFRP International Fertility Research Program
IFRT involved field radiotherapy
IFS interstitial fluid space
IFSM International Federation of Sports Medicine
IFSP individualized family service plan

IFSSH International Federation of Societies for Surgery of the Hand
IFT immunofluorescence test
IFU interferon unit
IFV interstitial fluid volume; intracellular fluid volume
IG immature granule; immunoglobulin; insulin and glucose; intragastric; irritable gut
Ig immunoglobulin
IGA infantile genetic agranulocytosis
IgA immunoglobulin A
IgA1, IgA2 subclasses of immunoglobulin A
IgAGN immunoglobulin A glomerulonephritis
IgAN immunoglobulin A nephropathy
IGC immature germ cell; intragastric cannula
IGCP intraglomerular capillary pressure
IGD idiopathic growth hormone deficiency; Integrated Genome Database; interglobal distance; isolated gonadotropin deficiency
IgD immunoglobulin D
IgD1, IgD2 subclasses of immunoglobulin D
IGDM infant of mother with gestational diabetes mellitus
IGE idiopathic generalized epilepsy; impaired gas exchange
IgE immunoglobulin E
IgE1 subclass of immunoglobulin E
IGF insulin-like growth factor
IGF-I insulin-like growth factor-I
IGFPB insulin-like growth factor binding protein
IGFBP-3 IGF-binding protein 3
IGFET insulated gate field effect transistor
IGFL integral green fluorescence
IGFR insulin-like growth factor receptor
IgG immunoglobulin G
IgG1, IgG2, IgG3, IgG4 subclasses of immunoglobulin G
IGH immunoreactive growth hormone
IgH immunoglobulin heavy chain
IgHC immunoglobulin heavy chain constant region
IGHD immunoglobin delta heavy chain; isolated growth hormone deficiency
IGHE immunoglobulin epsilon heavy chain

IGHV immunoglobulin heavy chain variable region
IGIF interferon-γ-inducing factor
IGIV immune globulin intravenous
IGKDEL immunoglobulin kappa deleting element
IGL immunoglobulin lambda
IGLJ immunoglobulin lambda light chain J
IGLL immunoglobulin lambda-like
IGM Internet Grateful Med
IgM immunoglobulin M
IgM1 subclass of immunoglobulin M
IgMN immunoglobulin M nephropathy
IGO1 immunoglobulin kappa orphan 1
IGP intestinal glycoprotein
IGR immediate generalized reaction; integrated gastrin response
iGrid international grid
IGS image-guided surgery; inappropriate gonadotropin secretion; internal guide sequence
Igs immunoglobulins
IgSC immunoglobulin-secreting cell
IGSF immunoglobulin superfamily
IGT impaired glucose tolerance
IGTT intravenous glucose tolerance test
IGV intrathoracic gas volume
IH idiopathic hirsutism; idiopathic hypercalciuria; immediate hypersensitivity; incompletely healed; indirect hemagglutination; industrial hygiene; infantile hydrocephalus; infectious hepatitis; inguinal hernia; inhibiting hormone; in hospital; inner half; inpatient hospital; intermittent heparinization; intracranial hematoma; iron hematoxylin
IHA idiopathic hyperaldosteronism; indirect hemagglutination; indirect hemagglutination antibody
IHAC Industrial Health and Advisory Committee
IHAPS interactive health appraisal system
IHBT incompatible hemolytic blood transfusion
IHC idiopathic hemochromatosis; idiopathic hypercalciuria; immunohistochemistry; inner hair cell; intrahepatic cholestasis
IHCA individual health care account; isocapnic hyperventilation with cold air
IHCP Institute of Hospital and Community Psychiatry
IHCM ichthyosis hystrix, Curth-Macklin [type]

IHD in-center hemodialysis; intermittent dialysis; ischemic heart disease

IHDI ischemic heart disease index

IHDP Infant Health and Development Program

IHDPORT Ischemic Heart Disease Patient Outcomes Research Team

IHD SDP Ischemic Heart Disease Shared Decision-Making Program

IHES idiopathic hypereosinophilic syndrome

IHF Industrial Health Foundation; integration host factor; International Hospital Foundation

IHGD isolateral human growth deficiency

IHH idiopathic hypogonadotropic hypogonadism; idiopathic hypothalamic hypogonadism; infectious human hepatitis

IHHS idiopathic hyperkinetic heart syndrome

IHI Institute for Healthcare Improvement

IHIS integrated hospital information system

IHL International Homeopathic League

IHM in-hospital malnutrition

IHN integrated health care network

IHO idiopathic hypertrophic osteo-arthropathy

IHOU in-hospital observation unit

IHP idiopathic hypoparathyroidism; idiopathic hypopituitarism; individualized health plan; inositol hexaphosphate; interhospitalization period; inverted hand position

IHPC intrahepatic cholestasis

IHPH intrahepatic portal hypertension

IHPP Intergovernmental Health Project Policy

IHQL index of health-related quality of life

IHR intrahepatic resistance; intrinsic heart rate

IHRA isocapnic hyperventilation with room air

IHRB Industrial Health Research Board

IHS idiopathic hypereosinophilic syndrome; inactivated horse serum; Indian Health Service; innovative health care system; integrated health system; International Headache Society; International Health Society; intracranial hypotension syndrome

IHSA iodinated human serum albumin

IHSC immunoreactive human skin collagenase

IHSS idiopathic hypertrophic subaortic stenosis

IHT insulin hypoglycemia test; intravenous histamine test; ipsilateral head turning

I5HT intraplatelet serotonin

Ii incision inferius

II icterus index; image intensification or intensifier; Roman numeral two

I&I illness and injuries

IIC ineffective individual coping

IICP increased intracranial pressure

II-para secundipara

IID insulin-independent diabetes

IIDM insulin-independent diabetes mellitus

IIE idiopathic ineffective erythropoiesis

IIF immune interferon; indirect immunofluorescence; isolated intraperitoneal fluid

IIFT intraoperative intraarterial fibrinolytic therapy

IIG imagineering interest group; interactive image-guided [surgery]

IIGR ipsilateral instinctive grasp reaction

IIH idiopathic infantile hypercalcemia

IIHD Israeli Ischemic Heart Disease [study]

III Roman numeral three

III-para tertipara

IIME Institute of International Medical Education

IIMS Interest in Internal Medicine Scale

IIP idiopathic interstitial pneumonia; idiopathic intestinal pseudo-obstruction; increased intracranial pressure

I-123 IPPA I-123 Iodo-Phenylpentadecanoic Acid [Viability Multicenter Study]

IIS intensive immunosuppression; International Institute of Stress

IIT induction of immune tolerance; ineffective iron turnover; interactive image tool

IIUK Intraoperative Intra-Arterial Urokinase [study]

IIVS Institute for In-Vitro Sciences

IJ ileojejunal; internal jugular; intrajejunal; intrajugular

IJCAI International Joint Conference on Artificial Intelligence

IJD inflammatory joint disease

IJP inhibitory junction potential; internal jugular pressure

IJV internal jugular vein

IK immobilized knee; immune body [Ger. *Immunekörper*]; *Infusoria* killing [unit]; interstitial keratitis

IKE Internet key exchange protocol; ion kinetic energy

IKU *Infusoria* killing unit

IL ileum; iliolumbar; incisolingual; independent laboratory; inguinal ligament; inspiratory load; intensity load; interleukin; internal loop; intralumbar

Il promethium [*illinium*]

IL-1 interleukin 1

IL-2 interleukin 2

IL-3 interleukin 3

ILA insulin-like activity; International Leprosy Association

ILa incisolabial

ILAR Institute of Laboratory Animal Research

ILB infant, low birth [weight]; initial lung burden

ILBBB incomplete left bundle branch block

ILBW infant, low birth weight

ILC ichthyosis linearis circumflex; incipient lethal concentration

ILD interstitial lung disease; intraoperative localization device; ischemic leg disease; ischemic limb disease; isolated lactase deficiency

ILDBP interleukin-dependent deoxyribonucleic acid-binding protein

ILE, ILe, Ileu isoleucine

IleRS isoleucyl ribonucleic acid synthetase

ILGF insulin-like growth factor

ILH immunoreactive luteinizing hormone

ILL interlibrary loan; intermediate lymphocytic lymphoma

ILLE inverted [position] with lower limbs extended

ILM insulin-like material; internal limiting membrane

ILMA intubating laryngeal mask airway

ILMS Israel Longitudinal Mortality Study

ILNR intralobar nephrogenic rest

ILo iodine lotion

ILP inadequate luteal phase; insufficiency of luteal phase; interstitial laser photocoagulation; interstitial lymphocytic pneumonia

ILR interleukin receptor; irreversible loss rate

ILRA interleukin receptor alpha

IL1-RA interleukin-1 receptor antagonist

ILRB interleukin receptor beta

ILRCFS Iowa Lipid Research Clinics Family Study

ILS idiopathic leucine sensitivity; idiopathic lymphadenopathy syndrome; increase in life span; infrared liver scanner; intermittent light stimulation; intralobal sequestration

ILSA Italian Longitudinal Study on Aging

ILSI International Life Sciences Institute

ILSS integrated life support system; intraluminal somatostatin

ILT iliotibial tract

ILTV infectious laryngotracheitis virus

ILV independent lung ventilation

ILVEN inflamed linear verrucous epidermal nevus

IM idiopathic myelofibrosis; immunosuppressive method; implementation monitoring; Index Medicus; indomethacin; industrial medicine; infection medium; infectious mononucleosis; information management; inner membrane; innocent murmur; inspiratory muscles; intermediate; intermediate megaloblast; internal malleolus; internal mammary [artery]; internal medicine; intramedullary; intramuscular; invasive mole

im intramuscular

2IM 2-ipomeanol

IMA Industrial Medical Association; inferior mesenteric artery; Interchurch Medical Assistance; internal mammary artery; Irish Medical Association

IMAA iodinated macroaggregated albumin

IMAB internal mammary artery bypass

IMAC image management archiving and communications; information management, archiving, and communication; Intervention in Myocarditis and Acute Cardiomyopathy [study]

IMACS image archiving and communication system; image management and communication system

IMAGE integrated molecular analysis of gene expression; International Metaprolol/Nifedipine Angina Exercise Trial; International Multicenter Angina Exercise [study]; International Multicenter Aprotinin Graft Patency Experience [trial]

IMAGES Intravenous Magnesium Efficacy in Stroke [trial]

IMAI internal mammary artery implant

IMB intermenstrual bleeding

IMBC indirect maximum breathing capacity

IMBI Institute of Medical and Biological Illustrators

IMC indigent medical care; information-memory-concentration [test]; interdigestive migrating contractions; internal mammary chain; internal medicine clinic; International Medical Corps; intestinal mast cell

IMCT Information-Memory-Concentration Test; International Multicentre Trial

IMCU intermediate medical care unit

IMD immunodeficiency; immunologically mediated disease; institution for mentally disabled

ImD$_{50}$ immunizing dose sufficient to protect 50% of the animals in a test group

IMDC intramedullary metatarsal decompression

IMDD idiopathic midline destructive disease

IMDG International Maritime Dangerous Goods [code]

IMDP imidocarb diproprionate

IME independent medical examination; indirect medical education

IMEG innovations in medical education grant

IMEM improved minimum essential medium

IMEP Investigation in Menopausal Women of the Effect of Estradiol and Progesterone on Cardiovascular Risk Factors

IMET isometric endurance test

IMF idiopathic myelofibrosis; immunofluorescence; intermaxillary fixation; intermediate filament; intramaxillary fixation

IMG inferior mesenteric ganglion; internal medicine group [practice]; international medical graduate

IMGG intramuscular gammaglobulin

IMGT International Immuno-Genetics Database

IMH idiopathic myocardial hypertrophy; indirect microhemagglutination [test]

IMHP 1-iodomercuri-2-hydroxypropane

IMHT indirect microhemagglutination test

IMI immunologically measurable insulin; impending myocardial infarction; Imperial Mycological Institute [UK]; inferior myocardial infarction; intermeal interval; intramuscular injection

Imi imipramine

IMIA International Medical Informatics Association

IMIC International Medical Information Center

IMIS Integrative Molecular Information System [database]

IML intermediolateral

IMLA intramural left anterior [artery]

IMLAD intramural left anterior descending [artery]

IMLNS idiopathic minimal lesion nephrotic syndrome

ImLy immune lysis

IMM immunization [database]; inhibitor-containing minimal medium; inner mitochondrial membrane; internal medial malleolus

immat immaturity, immature

IMMC interdigestive migrating motor complex

IMO idiopathic multicentric osteolysis

imoa instantaneous maximum over the array [transformation]

immobil immobilization, immobilize

immun immune, immunity, immunization

IMN internal mammary node

IMP idiopathic myeloid proliferation; impression; incomplete male pseudohermaphroditism; individual Medicaid practitioner; inosine 5'-monophosphate; intramembranous particle; intramuscular compartment pressure; N-isopropyl-p-iodo-amphetamine

Imp impression

imp impacted, impaction

IMPA incisal mandibular plane angle

IMPAC Information for Management, Planning, Analysis and Coordination

IMPACT Immunisation Monitoring Programme Active [Canada]; Initiatives to Mobilize for the Prevention and Control of Tobacco Use; Integrilin to Minimize Platelet Aggregation and Prevent Coronary Thrombosis [trial]; Interdisciplinary Maternal Perinatal Australasian Clinical Trials; International Mexiletine and Placebo Antiarrhythmia Coronary Trial

IMPACT-II Integrilin to Minimize Platelet Aggregation and Coronary Thrombosis [trial]

IMPACT-AMI Integrilin to Minimize Platelet Aggregation and Prevent Coronary Thrombosis–Acute Myocardial Infarction [trial]

IMPACT-Stent Integrilin to Minimize Platelet Aggregation and Coronary Thrombosis in Stenting [trial]

IMPATH interactive microcomputer patient assessment tool for health

IMPC International Myopia Prevention Center

IMPD inosine-5'-monophosphate dehydrogenase

IMPDH inosine-5'-monophosphate dehydrogenase

IMPDHL inosine-5'-monophosphate dehydrogenase-like

IMPG interphotoreceptor matrix proteoglycan

IMPR integrated microscopy resource

IMPRESS Intramural Low Molecular Weight Heparin for Prevention of Restenosis Study

IMPROVED Is Introduction of Mycophenolate Mofetil and Reduction of Cyclosporine Valuable in Renal Dysfunction After Heart Transplantation? [study]

IMPS Inpatient Multidimensional Psychiatric Scale; intact months of patient survival

Impx impacted

IMR individual medical record; infant mortality rate; infant mortality risk; Institute for Medical Research; institution for mentally retarded; integrated microscopy resource

IMS incurred in military service; Indian Medical Service; industrial methylated spirit; information management system; integrated medical services; international metric system

IMS/DL1 information management system/data language one

IMSS in-flight medical support system

IMT indomethacin; induced muscular tension; inspiratory muscle training

IMU Index of Medical Underservice

IMV inferior mesenteric vein; informative morphogenetic variant; intermittent mandatory ventilation; intermittent mechanical ventilation; isophosphamide, methotrexate, and vincristine

IMViC, imvic indole, methyl red, Voges-Proskauer, citrate [test]

IMVP idiopathic mitral valve prolapse

IMVS Institute of Medical and Veterinary Science

IN icterus neonatorum; impetigo neonatorum; incidence; incompatibility number; infundibular nucleus; insulin; integrase; interneuron; interstitial nephritis; intranasal; irritation of nociceptors

In index; indium; inion; insulin; inulin

in inch

in² square inch

in³ cubic inch

INA infectious nucleic acid; inferior nasal artery; International Neurological Association

INAA instrumental neutron activation analysis

INABIS First Internet World Congress for Biomedical Sciences

INAD infantile neuroaxonal dystrophy

INAH isonicotinic acid hydrazide

INB internuclear bridging; ischemic necrosis of bone

inbr inbreeding

INC internodular cortex; inside needle catheter

inc incision; inclusion; incompatibility; incontinent; increase; increased; increment; incurred

INCB International Narcotics Control Board

IncB inclusion body

INCD infantile nuclear cerebral degeneration

IN-CHF Italian Network Congestive Heart Failure

INCL infantile neuronal ceroid lipofuscinosis

incl inclusion or include

INCLEN International Clinical Epidemiology Network

incr increase, increased; increment

incur incurable

IND indomethacin; industrial medicine; investigational new drug

ind indirect; induction

INDANA Individual Data Analysis of Antihypertensive Intervention Trials

indic indication, indicated

indig indigestion
indiv individual
INDO indoleamine-2,3-dioxygenase; indomethacin
INDOR internuclear double resonance
indust industrial
INE infantile necrotizing encephalomyelopathy
INEPT insensitive nuclei enhanced by polarization transfer
INET image network
INF infant, infantile; infection, infective, infected; inferior; infirmary; infundibulum; infusion; interferon
Inf influenza
inf infant, infantile; inferior
INF APC infero-apical
infect infection, infected, infective; inferoapical
Inflamm inflammation, inflammatory
inf mono infectious mononucleosis
InfoMAP information management and assessment process
INFORMM Information Network for Online Retrieval and Medical Management
INFSEC information security
ING isotope nephrogram
ing inguinal
InGP indolglycerophosphate
INH Indian hedgehog homolog; inhalation; isoniazid; isonicotinic acid hydrazide
INHA inhibin alpha
inhal inhalation
INHB inhibin beta
INHBA inhibitin beta A
INHBB inhibitin beta B
INHBC inhibitin beta C
inhib inhibition, inhibiting
INI intranuclear inclusion
inj injection; injury, injured, injurious
INJECT International Joint Efficacy Comparison of Thrombolytics [trial]; International Joint Evaluation of Coronary Thrombolysis [trial]
inject injection
INJR injury or poisoning [UMLS]
INK injury not known
INL International Nursing Library
INLINIS Ireland-Netherlands Lisinopril-Nifedipine Study
INLSD ichthyosis and neutral lipid storage disease

INN International Nonproprietary Names
innerv innervation, innervated
innom innominate
INNOVO Inhaled Nitric Oxide Compared to Ventilatory Support Without Inhaled Nitric Oxide [for neonates with severe respiratory failure] [trial]
INO internuclear ophthalmoplegia; inosine
Ino inosine
INOC isonicotinoyloxycarbonyl
inoc inoculation, inoculated
inorg inorganic
iNOS inducible macrophage-type nitric oxide synthase
Inox inosine, oxidized
INP idiopathic neutropenia
INPAV intermittent negative pressure assisted ventilation
INPEA isopropyl nitrophenylethanolamine
INPH iproniazid phosphate
INPP1 inositol polyphosphate 1-phosphatase
INPV intermittent negative-pressure ventilation
INQ interior nasal quadrant
InQ inquiry mode questionnaire
InQ(R) inquiry mode questionnaire, reliability assessment
INR international normalized ratio
INREM internal roentgen-equivalent, man
INRIA National Institute for Research in Computers and Automation [France] [Institut National de la Recherche Informatique et Automatique]
INROAD In-Stent Restenosis Optimal Angioplasty Device [trial]
INS idiopathic nephrotic syndrome; insulin; insurance
Ins insulin; insurance, insured
ins insertion; insulin; insurance, insured
INSECT intensity normalized stereotaxic environment for classification of tissues
insem insemination
INSIGHT International Nifedipine Study Intervention as a Goal in Hypertension Treatment
insol insoluble
Insp inspiration
INSPIRE increasing participation in cardiac rehabilitation; Intravascular Ultrasound Study Predictor of Restenosis [trial]

INSR insulin receptor
INSRR insulin receptor-related receptor
INSS international neuroblastoma staging system
Inst institute
instab instability
instill instillation
insuf insufflation
insuff insufficient, insufficiency; insufflation
INT interference; intermediate; intermittent; intern, internship; internal; interval; intestinal; intima; p-iodonitrotetrazolium
Int international; intestinal
int internal
INTACT International Nifedipine Trial on Antiatherosclerotic Therapy
INTEG integument
INTEL-SAT international communication satellite
INTERCEPT Incomplete Infarction Trial of European Research Collaborators Evaluating Prognosis Post-Thrombolysis
INTERMAP International Study of Macronutrients and Blood Pressure
intern internal
Internat international
INTERSALT International Study of Salt and Blood Pressure
INTERSEPT International Sepsis Trial
intes intestine
Intest intestine, intestinal
Int/Ext internal/external
INTH intrathecal
INTIMA Infusion of Tissue Plasminogen-Activator in Myocardial Infarction at the Acute Phase [study]
in-TIME Intravenous Lanoteplase for Treating Infarcting Myocardium Early [trial]
Intmd intermediate
Int Med internal medicine
INTOX, Intox intoxication
INTR intermittent
INTRO-AMI Integrilin and Reduced Dose of Thrombolysis in Acute Myocardial Infarction
Int Rot internal rotation
INTRP Inventory of Negative Thoughts in Response to Pain
Int trx intermittent traction
INTRUC Introducing Catheter [study]

intub intubation
INV inferior nasal vein
Inv, inv inversion; involuntary
Inv/Ev inversion/eversion
INVEST International Verapamil SR/Trandolapril [study]
invest investigation
inv ins inverted insertion
INVM isolated noncompaction of left ventricular myocardium
invol involuntary
involv involvement, involved
inv(p+q-) pericentric inversion
inv(p-q+) pericentric inversion
IO incisal opening; inferior oblique; inferior olive; internal os; interorbital; intestinal obstruction; intraocular; intraoperative; intra-osseous
I&O in and out; intake and output
I/O input/output; intake/output
Io ionium; onset of inspiration
IOA inner optic anlage; International Osteopathic Association
IOC International Organizing Committee on Medical Librarianship; intern on call
IOCG intraoperative cholangiogram
IOD injured on duty; integrated optical density; interorbital distance
IOE intraoperative echocardiography
IOFB intraocular foreign body
IOH idiopathic orthostatic hypotension
IOL induction of labor; intraocular lens
IOM inferior orbitomental [line]; Institute of Medicine [National Research Council]; interosseous membrane
IOMP International Organization for Medical Physics
ION ischemic optic neuropathy
IONDT Ischemic Optic Neuropathy Decompression Trial
IOP improving organizational performance; intraocular pressure
IOR index of response
IORT intraoperative radiotherapy
IOS infant observation scale; International Organization for Standardization
IOS RF intact outlet strut resonance frequency
IOT intraocular tension; intraocular transfer; ipsilateral optic tectum
IOTA information overload testing aid
ι Greek letter *iota*

IOU intensive care observation unit; international opacity unit

IOUS intraoperative ultrasound [examination]

IOV inside-out vesicle

IP icterus praecox; imaging plate; immune precipitate; immunoblastic plasma; immunoperoxidase technique; inactivated pepsin; incisoproximal; incisopulpal; incontinentia pigmenti; incubation period; induced potential; induction period; infection prevention; inflation point; infundibular process; infusion pump; inhibition period; inorganic phosphate; inosine phosphorylase; inositol phosphate; inpatient; instantaneous pressure; L'Institut Pasteur; intermediate purity; International Pharmacopoeia; Internet protocol; interpeduncular; interphalangeal; interpupillary; intestinal pseudo-obstruction; intramuscular pressure; intraperitoneal; intrapulmonary; ionization potential; ischemic preconditioning; isoelectric point; isoproterenol

Ip peak of inspiratory effort

ip intraperitoneal

i/p inpatient

IP1 incontinentia pigmenti 1

IP$_1$ inositol-1-phosphate

IP2 incontinentia pigmenti 2

IP$_3$ inositol triphosphate

IPA immunoperoxidase assay; incontinentia pigmenti achromians; independent physician or practice association; independent practice organization; individual practice association; infantile papular acrodermatitis; International Pediatric Association; International Pharmaceutical Association; International Psychoanalytical Association; intrapleural analgesia; isopropyl alcohol

I$_{pa}$ pulse average intensity

IPAA International Psychoanalytical Association

IPAC Information Policy Advisory Committee

IPAG The Influenza and Pneumonia Action Group

IPAP inspiratory positive airway pressure

I-para primipara

IPAT Institute of Personality and Ability Testing; Iowa Pressure Articulation Test

IPB injury-prone behavior; integrated problem-based curriculum

IPBH intraparenchymal brain hemorrhage

IPC intermittent pneumatic compression; International Poliomyelitis Congress; ion pair chromatography; isopropyl carbamate; isopropyl chlorophenyl

IPCD infantile polycystic disease

IPCP interdisciplinary patient care plan

IPCS intrauterine progesterone contraception system

IPD idiopathic Parkinson disease; idiopathic protracted diarrhea; immediate pigment darkening; increase in pupillary diameter; incurable problem drinker; inflammatory pelvic disease; intermittent peritoneal dialysis; intermittent pigment darkening; International Pharmacopeal Database; interocular phase difference; interpupillary distance; Inventory of Psychosocial Development

IPE infectious porcine encephalomyelitis; interstitial pulmonary emphysema

IPEH intravascular papillary endothelial hyperplasia

IPF idiopathic pulmonary fibrosis; infection-potentiating factor; insulin promoter factor; interstitial pulmonary fibrosis

IPFM integral pulse frequency modulation

IPFM/SDC integral pulse frequency modulation/Smith delay compensator

IPG impedance plethysmography; inspiration-phase gas

iPGE immunoreactive prostaglandin E

IPH idiopathic portal hypertension; idiopathic pulmonary hemosiderosis; idiopathic pulmonary hypertension; inflammatory papillary hyperplasia; interphalangeal; intraparenchymal hemorrhage; intraperitoneal hemorrhage

IPHR inverted polypoid hamartoma of the rectum

IPI interpulse interval

IPIA immunoperoxidase infectivity assay

IPITA International Pancreas and Islet Transplant Association

IPJ interphalangeal joint

IPK intractable plantar keratosis

IPKD infantile polycystic kidney disease

IPL inner plexiform layer; intrapleural

IPM impulses per minute; inches per minute; interphotoreceptor matrix

IPMI information processing in medical imaging

IPMS inhibited power motive syndrome

IPN infantile polyarteritis nodosa; infectious pancreatic necrosis [of trout]; intern progress note; interpeduncular nucleus; interstitial pneumonitis

IPNA isopropyl noradrenalin

IPO improved pregnancy outcome

IPOF immediate postoperative fitting

IPOP immediate postoperative prosthesis

IPP independent practice plan; individual patient profile; inflatable penile prosthesis; inorganic pyrophosphate; intermittent positive pressure; intracisternal A particle-promoted polypeptide; intrahepatic partial pressure; intrapericardial pressure

Ipp interpulse potential

IPPA inspection, palpation, percussion, and auscultation; iodophenylpentadecanoic acid

IPPB intermittent positive-pressure breathing

IPPB-I intermittent positive-pressure breathing-inspiration

IPPHS International Primary Pulmonary Hypertension Study

IPPI interruption of pregnancy for psychiatric indication

IPPO intermittent positive-pressure inflation with oxygen

IPPPSH International Prospective Primary Prevention Study in Hypertension

IPPR integrated pancreatic polypeptide response; intermittent positive-pressure respiration

IPPV intermittent positive-pressure ventilation

IPQ intimacy potential quotient

IPR imidozaline preferring receptor; insulin production rate; intraparenchymal resistance; ipratropium

i-Pr isopropyl

IPRD intellectual product [UMLS]

IPRL isolated perfused rat liver or lung

IPRT interpersonal reaction test

IPS idiopathic pain syndrome; idiopathic postprandial syndrome; inches per second; infundibular pulmonary stenosis; initial prognostic score; intensive care unit point system; interpractice system; intrapartum stillbirth; intraperitoneal shock; ischiopubic synchondrosis

ips inches per second

IPSC inhibitory postsynaptic current

IPSC-E Inventory of Psychic and Somatic Complaints in the Elderly

IPsec Internet protocol security

IPSF immediate postsurgical fitting

IPSID immunoproliferative small intestine disease

IPSP inhibitory postsynaptic potential

IPT immunoperoxidase technique; immunoprecipitation; interpersonal psychotherapy; isoproterenol

IPTG isopropyl thiogalactose

iPTH immunoassay for parathyroid hormone; immunoreactive parathyroid hormone

IPTX intermittent pelvic traction

IPU inpatient unit

IPV inactivated poliomyelitis vaccine or virus; infectious pustular vaginitis; infectious pustular vulvovaginitis; interpersonal violence, intimate partner violence; intrapulmonary vein

IPW interphalangeal width

IPZ insulin protamine zinc

IQ institute of quality; intelligence quotient

IQAS internal quality assurance system

IQB individual quick blanch

IQCODE information questionnaire on cognitive decline in the elderly

IQOLA International Quality of Life Assessment [project]

IQR interquartile range

IQ&S iron, quinine, and strychnine

IQW interactive query workstation

IR drop of voltage across a resistor produced by a current; ileal resection; immune response; immunization rate; immunoreactive; immunoreagent; in room; index of response; impedance rheography; individual reaction; inferior rectus [muscle]; inflow resistance; information retrieval; infrared; infrarenal; inside radius; insoluble residue; inspiratory reserve; inspiratory resistance; insulin resistance; internal resistance; internal rotation; interventional radiology; intrarectal; intrarenal; inversion recovery; inverted repeat; irritant reaction; ischemia-reperfusion; isovolumic relaxation

I-R Ito-Reenstierna [reaction]

I/R ischemia/reperfusion

Ir immune response [gene]; iridium

ir immunoreactive; intrarectal; intrarenal

IRA immunoradioassay; immunoregulatory alpha-globulin; inactive renin activity; infarct-related artery

IR-ACTH immunoreactive adrenocorticotropic hormone

IRAD International Registry of Aortic Dissection

IrANP, ir-ANP immunoreactive atrial natriuretic peptide

IR APAP immediate release acetaminophen

IRAS Insulin Resistance Atherosclerosis Study

IR-AVP immunoreactive arginine-vasopressin

IRB immunoreactive bead; institutional review board

IRBBB incomplete right bundle branch block

IRBC immature or infected red blood cell

ir-BNP immunoreactive brain natriuretic enzyme

IRBP intestinal retinol-binding protein

IRC inspiratory reserve capacity; instantaneous resonance curve; International Red Cross; International Research Communications System

IRCA intravascular red cell aggregation

IRCC International Red Cross Committee

IRCU intensive respiratory care unit

IRD infantile Refsum syndrome; isorhythmic dissociation

IRDP insulin-related DNA polymorphism

IRDS idiopathic respiratory distress syndrome; infant respiratory distress syndrome

IRE internal rotation in extension; iron regulatory element; iron-responsive element; isolated rabbit eye

IREBP iron-responsive element binding protein

IRED infrared emission detection; infrared light-emitting diode

IRES internal ribosome entry site; ischemia residua

IRF idiopathic retroperitoneal fibrosis; impulse response function; interferon regulatory factor; internal rotation in flexion

IRFL integral red fluorescence

IRG immunoreactive gastrin; immunoreactive glucagon

IRGH immunoreactive growth hormone

IRGl immunoreactive glucagon

IRH Institute for Research in Hypnosis; Institute of Religion and Health; intrarenal hemorrhage

IRHCS immunoradioassayable human chorionic somatomammotropin

IRhGH immunoreactive human growth hormone

IRhPL immunoreactive human growth hormone

IRI immunoreactive insulin; [near]-infrared intereactance; insulin resistance index

IRIA indirect radioimmunoassay

IRIg insulin-reactive immunoglobulin

IRIS integrated risk information system; interleukin regulation of immune system; International Research Information Service; Isosents for Reperfusion Intervention Study

IRK inwardly rectifying potassium [channel]

IR-LED infrared light emitting diode

IRM innate releasing mechanism; Institute of Rehabilitation Medicine

IRMA immunoradiometric assay; intraretinal microvascular abnormalities

iRNA immune ribonucleic acid; informational ribonucleic acid

ir-NP immunoreactive natriuretic peptide

IROS ipsilateral routing of signal

IRP immunoreactive plasma; immunoreactive proinsulin; incus replacement prosthesis; insulin-releasing polypeptide; interstitial radiation pneumonitis

IRR insulin receptor-related receptor; intrarenal reflux

Irr irradiation; irritation

IRRD Institute for Research in Rheumatic Diseases

irreg irregularity, irregular

irrig irrigation, irrigate

IRS immunoreactive secretion; incident reporting scheme; infrared sensor; infrared spectrophotometry; insulin receptor species; insulin receptor substrate; insulin-related substrate; intergroup rhabdomyosarcoma study; internal resolution site; International Rhinologic Society; Invasive Reperfusion Study; ionizing radiation sensitivity

IRS-1 insulin receptor substrate 1

IRS-2 insulin receptor substrate 2

IRSA idiopathic refractory sideroblastic anemia; iodinated rat serum albumin

IRT immunoreactive trypsin; interresponse time; interstitial radiotherapy

IRTIS Integrated Radiation Therapy Information System

IRTO immunoreactive trypsin output

IRTU integrating regulatory transcription unit

IRU industrial rehabilitation unit; interferon reference unit

IRV inferior radicular vein; inspiratory reserve volume; inverse ratio ventilation

IRW intelligent radiology workstation

IS ileal segment; immediate sensitivity; immune serum; immunosuppression; impingement syndrome; incentive spirometer; index of sexuality; infant size; infantile spasms; information services; information system; infundibular septum; insertion sequence; in situ; insulin secretion; intercellular space; intercostal space; interictal spike; international standards; interstitial space; intracardial shunt; intraspinal; intrasplenic; intrastriatal; intraventricular septum; invalided from service; inversion sequence; ischemic score; isoproterenol

Is incision superius

is in situ; island; islet; isolated

ISA Information Science Abstracts; Instrument Society of America; intracarotid sodium amytal; intrinsic simulating activity; intrinsic sympathomimetic activity; iodinated serum albumin; irregular spiking activity

I$_{sa}$ spatial average intensity [pulse]

ISAAC International Study of Asthma and Allergies in Childhood

ISADH inappropriate secretion of antidiuretic hormone

ISAKEMP Internet Security Association and Key Management Protocol

ISAM indexed sequential access manager; Intravenous Streptokinase in Acute Myocardial Infarction [trial]

I$_{sapa}$ spatial average pulse average

I$_{sapt}$ spatial peak, temporal average intensity [pulse]

ISAR Intracoronary Stenting and Antithrombotic Regimen [trial]

I$_{sata}$ spatial average, temporal average intensity [pulse]

ISB incentive spirometry breathing

ISBI International Society for Burn Injuries

ISBN international standard book number

ISBP International Society for Biochemical Pharmacology

ISBT International Society for Blood Transfusion

ISC immunoglobulin-secreting cells; innerstrand crosslink; information system center; insoluble collagen; International Society of Cardiology; International Society of Chemotherapy; intensive supportive care; intershift coordination; interstitial cell; irreversibly sickled cell

IS&C image save and carry

ISCAB Israeli Coronary Artery Bypass [study]

ISCD International Society of Clinical Densitometry

ISCF interstitial cell fluid

ISCLT International Society for Clinical Laboratory Technology

ISCM International Society of Cybernetic Medicine

ISCN International System for Human Cytogenetic Nomenclature

ISCO immunostimulating complex [vaccine]

ISCOAT Italian Study on Complications of Oral Anticoagulant Therapy

ISCP infection surveillance and control program; International Society of Comparative Pathology

ISCW immunosuppression of streptococcal wall [antigen]

ISD immunosuppressive drug; Information Services Division; inhibited sexual desire; interset distance; interstimulus distance; interventricular septal defect; isosorbide dinitrate

ISDB information source database

ISDN integrated services digital network; isosorbide dinitrate

iSDR inducible stable DNA replication

ISE inhibited sexual excitement; intelligent synthesis environment; International Society of Endocrinology; International Society of Endoscopy; inversion spin-echo pulse sequence; ion-selective electrode

ISEFT ion-sensitive field effect transistor

ISEK International Society of Electromyographic Kinesiology

ISEM immunosorbent electron microscopy

ISF interstitial fluid

ISFC International Society and Federation of Cardiology

ISFV interstitial fluid volume

ISG Ibopamine Study Group [trial]; immune serum globulin

ISGE International Society of Gastroenterology

ISH icteric serum hepatitis; in situ hybridization; internal self helper; International Society of Hematology; International Society of Hypertension; isolated septal hypertrophy

ISHAM International Society for Human and Animal Mycology

ISHT International Society for Heart Transplantation [registry]

ISHTAR Implementing Secure Healthcare Telematics Application

ISI infarct size index; initial slope index; injury severity index; Institute for Scientific Information; insulin sensitivity index; International Sensitivity Index; International Standardized Index; interstimulus interval

ISIH interspike interval histogram

ISIS image selected in vivo spectroscopy; imaging science and information system; information system-imaging system; interactive system for image selection; International Study of Infarct Survival

ISIT interactive simulation and identification tool

ISKDC International Study of Kidney Diseases in Childhood

ISL inner scapular line; interspinous ligament; isoleucine

ISLAND Infant Size Limitation: Acute *N*-Acetylcysteine Defense [trial]

ISM Information Source Map [UMLS]; International Society of Microbiologists; intersegmental muscle

ISMED International Society on Metabolic Eye Disorders

ISMH International Society of Medical Hydrology

ISMHC International Society of Medical Hydrology and Climatology

ISMN isosorbide mononitrate

ISN integrated service network; International Society of Nephrology; International Society of Neurochemistry

ISO International Standards Organization; isoprenaline

iso isoproterenol; isotropic

isol isolation, isolated

isom isometric

ISO-OSI International Standards Organization-Open Systems Interconnection

ISP distance between iliac spines; international standardized profile; Internet service provider; interspace; interstitial pressure; intraspinal; isoproterenol

I_{sp} spatial peak intensity [pulse]

ISPI integrated services protocol instrument

ISPO International Society for Prosthetics and Orthotics

ISPOCD International Study of Postoperative Cognitive Dysfunction

ISPOT International Study of Perioperative Transfusion

I_{sppa} spatial peak pulse average intensity

ISPS International Society of Pediatric Surgery

ISPT interspecies ovum penetration test

isq unchanged [Lat. *in status quo*]

ISR information storage and retrieval; Institute for Sex Research; Institute of Surgical Research; insulin secretion rate; intelligent stroke registry

ISRE interferon-stimulated response element

ISRM International Society of Reproductive Medicine

ISS idiopathic short stature; injury severity score; infantile sialic acid storage [disease]; instructional support services; International Society of Surgery; ion-scattering spectroscopy; ion surface scattering; isotonic saline solution

ISSD infantile sialic acid storage disease

ISSI interview schedule for social interaction; Israeli Study of Surgical Infections

ISSN international standard serial number

IST inappropriate sinus tachycardia; insulin sensitivity test; insulin shock therapy; International Society on Toxicology; International Stroke Trial; Internet Security Team; isometric systolic tension

IS&T Society for Imaging Science and Technology

ISTD International Society of Tropical Dermatology

ISTU isometric strength testing unit
ISU International Society of Urology
I-sub inhibitor substance
ISUP International Society of Urological Pathology
ISW interstitial water
ISWI incisional surgical wound infection
ISY intrasynovial
IT immunological test; immunotherapy; implantation test; individual therapy; information technology; inhalation test; inhalation therapy; injection time; insulin therapy; intensive therapy; intentional tremor; intermittent traction; internal telomere; interstitial tissue; intradermal test; intratesticular; intrathecal; intrathoracic; intratracheal; intratracheal tube; intratuberous; intratumoral; ischial tuberosity; isolation transformer; isomeric transition
I/T information technology; intensity/time
I&T intolerance and toxicity
IT² Internet technology for the twenty-first century
ITA inferior temporal artery; information transmission analysis; internal thoracic artery; International Tuberculosis Association
I$_{ta}$ temporal average intensity [pulse]
ITAM immunoreceptor tyrosine activation motif
ITB iliotibial band
ITC imidazolyl-thioguanine chemotherapy; inferior temporal cortex; Interagency Testing Committee; in the canal [hearing aid]; intrathecal chemotherapy; isothermal titration calorimetry; isothiocyanate
ITc International Table calorie
ITCM information technology for crises management teams
ITCP idiopathic thrombocytopenic purpura
ITCVD ischemic thrombotic cerebrovascular disease
ITD idiopathic torsion dystonia; intensely transfused dialysis; iodothyronine deiodinase
ITE insufficient therapeutic effect; in the ear [hearing aid]; in-training examination; intrapulmonary interstitial emphysema
ITET isotonic endurance test
ITF Interagency Tack Force [Department of Health and Human Services]; interferon

ITFS iliotibial tract friction syndrome; incomplete testicular feminization syndrome
ITG integrin
ITGA integrin alpha
ITGB integrin beta
ITH interstitial hyperthermia
ITh, ith intrathecal
IThP intrathyroidal parathyroid
ITI inter-alpha-trypsin inhibitor; intertrial interval
ITIH2 inter-alpha-trypsin inhibitor, heavy chain 2
ITIL inter-alpha-trypsin inhibitor, light chain
ITIM immunoreceptor tyrosine-based inhibition motif
ITL information technology laboratory
ITLC instant thin-layer chromatography
ITM improved Thayer-Martin [medium]; intermediate transient memory; intrathecal methotrexate; Israel turkey meningoencephalitis
ITMTX intrathecal methotrexate
ITO indium tin oxide
ITOU intensive therapy observation unit
ITP idiopathic thrombocytopenic purpura; immune thrombocytopenia; immunogenic thrombocytopenic purpura; increased torque production; individualized treatment plan; inosine triphosphate; inositol 1,4,5-triphosphate; islet-cell tumor of the pancreas; isotachophoresis
I$_{tp}$ temporal peak intensity [pulse]
ITPA Illinois Test of Psycholinguistic Abilities; inosine triphosphatase
ITPASMT International Tissue Plasminogen Activator/Streptokinase Mortality Trial
ITPK inositol 1,4,5-triphosphate-3-kinase
ITPKA inositol 1,4,5-triphosphate-3-kinase A
ITPKB inositol 1,4,5-triphosphate-3-kinase B
ITPR inositol 1,4,5-triphosphate receptor
ITPV intratracheal pulmonary ventilation
ITQ inferior temporal quadrant
ITR intraocular tension recorder; intratracheal; inverted terminal repeat; isotretinoin
ITS infective toxic shock; insulin-transferrin-selenium; intelligent tutoring [computer] system; International Twin Study; Israeli Thrombolytic Survey
ITSHD isolated thyroid-stimulating hormone deficiency

ITT insulin tolerance test; intent to treat; internal tibial torsion

IT&T information technology and telematics

ITU intensive therapy unit

ITV inferior temporal vein

IU immunizing unit; infection unit; international unit; intrauterine; in utero; 5-iodouracil

iu infectious unit

IUA intrauterine adhesions

IUB International Union of Biochemistry

IUBS International Union of Biological Sciences

IUC idiopathic ulcerative colitis

IUCD intrauterine contraceptive device

IUD intrauterine death; intrauterine device

IUDR, IUdR iodeoxyuridine

IUF isolated ultrafiltration

IUFB intrauterine foreign body

IUG infusion urogram; intrauterine growth

IUGR intrauterine growth rate; intrauterine growth retardation

IUI intrauterine insemination

IUIS International Union of Immunological Societies

IU/l international units per liter

IUM internal urethral meatus; intrauterine [fetus] malnourished; intrauterine membrane

IU/min international units per minute

IUP intrauterine pregnancy; intrauterine pressure

IUPAC International Union of Pure and Applied Chemistry

IUPAP International Union of Pure and Applied Physics

IUPAT intrauterine pregnancy at term

IUPD intrauterine pregnancy delivered

IUPHAR International Union of Pharmacology

IUPS International Union of Physiological Sciences

IUPTB intrauterine pregnancy, term birth

IURES International Union of Reticuloendothelial Societies

IUT intrauterine transfusion

IUVDT International Union against Venereal Diseases and the Treponematoses

IV ichthyosis vulgaris; initial visit; interventricular; intervertebral; intravaginal; intravascular; intravenous; intraventricular; intravertebral; invasive; in vivo; in vitro; iodine value; Roman numeral four; symbol for class 4 controlled substances

iv intravascular; intravenous

IVA interpretative value analysis; intraoperative vascular angiography; isovaleric acid

IVAP in-vivo adhesive platelet

IVB intraventricular block; intravital

IVBAT intravascular bronchioalveolar tumor

IVBC intravascular blood coagulation

IVC inferior vena cava; inspiratory vital capacity; integrated vector control; intravascular coagulation; intravenous cholangiogram, intravenous cholangiography; intraventricular catheter

IVCC intravascular consumption coagulopathy

IVCD intraventricular conduction defect

IVCH intravenous cholangiography

IVCP inferior vena cava pressure

IVCR inferior vena cava reconstruction

IVCT inferior vena cava thrombosis; intravenously enhanced computed tomography

IVCV inferior venocavography

IVD interactive videodisk; intervertebral disc

IVDA/IVDU intravenous drug abuse/abuser; intravenous drug use/user

IVDSA intravenous digital subtraction angiography

IVET in vivo expression technology

IVF interventricular foramen; intervertebral foramen; intravascular fluid; intravenous fluid; in vitro fertilization

IVF-ET in vitro fertilization-embryo transfer

IVGG intravenous gammaglobulin

IVGTT intravenous glucose tolerance test

IVH intravenous hyperalimentation; intraventricular hemorrhage; in vitro hyperploidy

IVI intravenous infusion

IVIG, IVIg, ivIG intravenous immunoglobulin

IVISTAT Intravenous Immunoglobulin or Sulfamethaxazole/Trimethoprim as Additional Therapy for Systemic Vasculitis [study]

IVJC intervertebral joint complex

IVL involucrin

IVM intravascular mass

IVMG intravenous magnesium sulfate
IVMP intravenous methylprednisolone
IVN intravenous nutrition
IVNA in vivo neutron activation [analysis]
IVNAA in vivo neutron activation analysis
IVOTTS Irvine viable organ-tissue transport system
IVOX intravascular oxygenator
IVP intravenous push; intravenous pyelogram, intravenous pyelography; intraventricular pressure
IVPB intravenous piggyback
IVPF isovolume pressure flow curve
IVPSB International Veterinary Pathology Slide Bank
IVR idioventricular rhythm; interactive voice response; intravaginal ring; isolated volume responder
IVRA intravenous regional anesthesia
IVRT isovolumic relaxation time
IVS inappropriate vasopressin secretion; intervening sequence; interventricular septum; intervillous space
IVSA International Veterinary Students Association
IVSCT in vitro skin corrosivity test
IVSD interventricular septal defect
IVT index of vertical transmission; interventional video tomography; intrasound

vibration test; intravenous transfusion; intraventricular; in vitro tetraploidy; isovolumetric time
IVTT in vitro transcription and translation
IVTTT intravenous tolbutamide tolerance test
IVU intravenous urography
IVUS intravascular ultrasound
IVUS/QCA Intravascular Ultrasound Quantitative Coronary Angiography [study]
IVV influenza virus vaccine; intravenous vasopressin
IW inner wall; inpatient ward; input word
IWB indeterminate Western blot [test]; index of well being
IWGMT International Working Group on Mycobacterial Taxonomy
IWHS Iowa Women's Health Study
IWI inferior wall infarction; interwave interval
IWL insensible water loss
IWMI inferior wall myocardial infarct
IWPS info-window presentation system
IWRP Individualized Written Rehabilitation Program
IWS Index of Work Satisfaction
IXDB X Chromosome Integrated Database
IZ infar

J dynamic movement of inertia; electric current density; flux density; joint; joule; journal; juvenile; juxtapulmonary-capillary receptor; magnetic polarization; a polypeptide chain in polymeric immunoglobulins; a reference point following the QRS complex, at the beginning of the ST segment, in electrocardiography; sound intensity

J flux [density]

j jaundice [rat]

JA judgment analysis; juvenile atrophy; juxta-articular

JAI juvenile amaurotic idiocy

JAK Janus kinase

JAK-STAT Janus kinase-signal transducers and activators of transcription

JAMG juvenile autoimmune myasthenia gravis

JAMIA Journal of the American Medical Informatics Association

JaMSPUK Japanese Multicenter Study for Pro-Urokinase

JAN Japanese accepted name

JANS Jenkins Activity Survey

JAS Jenkins Activity Survey; juvenile ankylosing spondylitis

jaund jaundice

JB jugular bulb

JBE Japanese B encephalitis

JBS Johanson-Blizzard syndrome

JC Jakob-Creutzfeldt; joint contracture

J/C joules per coulomb

jc juice

JCA juvenile chronic arthritis

JCAE Joint Committee on Atomic Energy

JCAH Joint Commission on Accreditation of Hospitals

JCAHO Joint Commission on Accreditation of Healthcare Organizations

JCAI Joint Council of Allergy and Immunology

JCC Joint Committee on Contraception

JCD Jakob-Creutzfeldt disease

JCF juvenile calcaneal fracture

JCM Japanese Collection of Microorganisms

JCML juvenile chronic myelogenous leukemia

JCN Jefferson Cancer Network

JCP juvenile chronic polyarthritis

JCQ job contentment questionnaire

jct junction

JCV Jamestown Canyon virus

JD jejunal diverticulitis; juvenile delinquent; juvenile diabetes

JDF Juvenile Diabetes Foundation

JDM juvenile diabetes mellitus

JDMS juvenile dermatomyositis

JE Japanese encephalitis; junctional escape

JEB junctional epidermolysis bullosa

JEE Japanese equine encephalitis

Jej, jej jejunum

JEMBEC agar plates for transporting cultures of gonococci

JER junctional escape rhythm

JEV Japanese encephalitis virus

JF joint fluid; jugular foramen; junctional fold

JFET junction field effect transistor

JFS jugular foramen syndrome

JG, jg juxtaglomerular

JGA juxtaglomerular apparatus

JGC juxtaglomerular cell

JGCT juvenile granulosa cell tumor; juxtaglomerular cell tumor

JGI jejunogastric intussusception; juxtaglomerular granulation index

JGP juvenile general paresis

JH juvenile hormone

J$_H$ heat transfer factor

JHA juvenile hormone analog

JHITA Joint Healthcare Information Technology Association

JHMO Junior Hospital Medical Officer

JHPS Johns Hopkins Precursors Study

JHR Jarisch-Herxheimer reaction

JI jejunoileal; jejunoileitis; jejunoileostomy

JIB jejunoileal bypass

JIH joint interval histogram

JIMI Japanese Intervention Trial in Myocardial Infarction

JIS Japanese industrial standard; juvenile idiopathic scoliosis

JJ jaw jerk; jejunojejunostomy
J/kg joules per kilogram
JLO judgment of line orientation
JLP juvenile laryngeal papilloma
JLRCPS Jerusalem Lipid Research Clinic Prevalence Study
JMD juvenile macular degeneration
JME juvenile myoclonus epilepsy
JMS Juberg-Marsidi syndrome; junior medical student
JN Jamaican neuropathy
Jn junction
JNA Jena Nomina Anatomica
JNC Joint National Committee
JNC-V Fifth Report of the Joint National Committee on Detection, Evaluation and Treatment of High Blood Pressure
JNC-VI Sixth Report of the Joint National Committee on Detection, Evaluation and Treatment of High Blood Pressure
JND just noticeable difference
JNK Jun N-terminal kinase
JNP Jadassohn nevus phakomatosis
jnt joint
JOAG juvenile open-angle glaucoma
JOD juvenile-onset diabetes
JODM juvenile-onset diabetes mellitus
JOR jaw opening response
jour journal
JP Jackson-Pratt [drain]; joining peptide; juvenile periodontitis
JPA juvenile pilocytic astrocytoma
JPB junctional premature beat
JPC junctional premature contraction
JPD juvenile plantar dermatosis
JPEG Joint Photographic Experts Group
JPI Jackson Personality Inventory
JPS joint position sense

JPSTH joint peristimulus histogram
JR Jolly reaction; junctional rhythm
JRA juvenile rheumatoid arthritis
JRC CVT Joint Review Committee on Education in Cardiovascular Technology
JRC DMS Joint Review Committee on Diagnostic Medical Sonography
JRC/EMT Joint Review Committee for Emergency Medical Technicians
JROM joint range of motion
JRT junctional recovery time
JS jejunal segment; Job syndrome; junctional slowing
J/s joules per second
JSAIR Japanese Society of Angiography and Interventional Radiology
JSATO$_2$ jugular vein oxygen saturation
JSDN Japan Standardized Disease Names
JSV Jerry-Slough virus
JT jejunostomy tube
J/T joules per tesla
jt joint
JTPS juvenile tropical pancreatitis syndrome
Ju jugale
JUA joint underwriting association
jug jugular
junct junction
juv juvenile
JV jugular vein; Junin virus
JVC jugular venous catheter
JVD jugular venous distention
JVP jugular vein pulse; jugular venous pressure; jugular venous pulsations
JVPT jugular venous pulse tracing
juxt near [Lat. *juxta*]
JWS Jackson-Weiss syndrome
Jx junction
JXG juvenile xanthogranuloma

K absolute zero; capsular antigen [Ger. *Kapsel*, capsule]; carrying capacity; cathode; coefficient of heat transfer; constant improvement factor [in imaging]; in electroencephalography, a burst of diphasic slow waves in response to stimuli during sleep; electron capture; electrostatic capacity; equilibrium constant; ionization constant; kallikrein inhibiting unit; kanamycin; Kell factor; kelvin; kerma; kidney; Kilham [virus]; killer [cell]; kilo-; kinetic energy; *Klebsiella;* knee; lysine; modulus of compression; the number 1024 in computer core memory; vitamin K

°K degree on the Kelvin scale

K_1 phylloquinone

K4 fourth Korotkoff sound

K5 fifth Korotkoff sound

17-K 17-ketosteroid

k Boltzmann constant; constant; kilo; kilohm

κ see *kappa*

KA alkaline phosphatase; kainic acid; keratoacanthoma; keto acid; ketoacidosis; King-Armstrong [unit]; knowledge acquisition; knowledge aggregate

K/A ketogenic/antiketogenic ratio

Ka cathode

K_a acid ionization constant

kA kiloampere

ka cathode

KAAD kerosene, alcohol, acetic acid, and dioxane

KAAS Keele assessment of auditory style

KABC Kaufman Assessment Battery for Children

KAF conglutinogen-activating factor; killer-assisting factor; kinase activating factor

KAFO knee-ankle-foot orthosis

KAL Kallmann [syndrome]

Kal potassium [Lat. *kalium*]

KAL1 Kallmann gene

KALP Kallmann pseudogene

KAMI Koch Acute Myocardial Infarction [study]

KAMIT Kentucky Acute Myocardial Infarction Trial

KAO knee-ankle orthosis

κ Greek letter *kappa*; magnetic susceptibility

kan kanamycin

kan^r kanamycin resistance

kappa a light chain of human immunoglobulins [chain]

KAPS Kuopio Atherosclerosis Prevention Study

KAPT, K_{ATP} kidney adenosine triphosphate [ATP] [secretory channel]

KAS Katz Adjustment Scales; Kennedy-Alter-Sung [syndrome]

KAT kanamycin acetyltransferase; knowledge acquisition tool; Kuopio Angioplasty Gene Transfer Trial

kat katal

kat/l katals per liter

KAU King-Armstrong unit

KB human oral epidermoid carcinoma cells; Kashin-Bek [disease]; ketone body; kilobyte; Kleihauer-Betke [test]; knee brace; knowledge [data] base

K-B Kleihauer-Betke [test]

Kb kilobit

K_b base ionization constant

kb kilobase; kilobyte

KDB knowledge base dictionary

KBG syndrome of multiple abnormalities designated with the original patient's initials

KBM knowledge base manager

kbp kilobase pair

Kbps kilobits per second

kBq kilobecquerel

KBS Klüver-Bucy syndrome; knowledge-based system

KBTA knowledge-based temporal abstraction

KC cathodal closing; keratoconus; keratoconjunctivitis; knee-to-chest; Kupffer cell

kC kilocoulomb

kc kilocycle

K Cal, Kcal, kcal kilocalorie

KCC cathodal closing contraction; Kulchitzky cell carcinoma

KCCT kaolin-cephalin clotting time
KCD kinostatic change detector
K cell killer cell
KCF key clinical finding
KCG kinetocardiogram
kCi kilocurie
KCO transfer coefficient
kcps kilocycles per second
KCS Kenny-Caffey syndrome; keratoconjunctivitis sicca
kc/s kilocycles per second
KCSS Keio Cooperative Stroke Study
KCT, KCTe cathodal closing tetanus
KD cathodal duration; Kawasaki disease; Kennedy disease; killed; Krabbe disease
K$_d$ dissociation constant; distribution coefficient; partition coefficient
kd, kDa kilodalton
KDA known drug allergies
KDAPPIMT Kawasaki Disease Aneurysm Prevention Protocol and Italian Multicenter Trial
KDB kinase insert domain; knowledge database
KDC kidney disease treatment center
KDD knowledge discovery in databases
KDD-R knowledge discovery in databases using rough sets
KDI knowledge and distributed intelligence
kdn kidney
KDNA kinetoblast deoxyribonucleic acid
KDO ketodeoxyoctonate
KDS Kaufman Developmental Scale; King-Denborough syndrome; knowledge data system; Kocher-Debré-Semelaigne [syndrome]; Kupfer-Detre system
KDT cathodal duration tetanus
kdyn kilodyne
KE Kendall compound E; kethoxal; kinetic energy
K$_e$ exchangeable body potassium
KED Kendrick extrication device
Kera keratitis
KERMA kinetic energy released per unit mass
KERV Kentucky equine respiratory virus
keV kiloelectron volt
KF Kenner-fecal medium; kidney function; Klippel-Feil [syndrome]; knowledge finder
KF, K-F Kayser-Fleischer [rings]

K$_f$ Klenow fragment
kf flocculation rate in antigen-antibody reaction; kilogram force
KFAB kidney-fixing antibody
KFAO knee-foot-ankle orthosis
KFC Ketanserin for Carcinoid [trial]; Ketanserin on Fibroblast Culture [study]
K$_{fc}$ filtration coefficient
KFD Kyasanur forest disease
KFR Kayser-Fleischer ring
KFS Klippel-Feil syndrome
KFSD keratosis follicularis spinulosa decalvans
KG ketoglutarate; knowledge graph
kG kilogauss
kg kilogram
KG-1 Koeffler Golde-1 [cell line]
kg-cal kilocalorie
kg/cm^2 kilogram per square centimeter
KGD ketoglutarate dehydrogenase
KGF keratocyte growth factor
kgf kilogram-force
KGFR keratocyte growth factor receptor
kg/l kilograms per liter
KGM keratinocyte growth medium
kg-m kilogram-meter
kg/m kilograms per meter
kg-m/s^2 kilogram-meter per second squared
Kgn kininogen
kgps kilograms per second
KGS ketogenic steroid
17-KGS 17-ketogenic steroid
KH K-homologous, Krebs-Henseleit [buffer]
K24H potassium, urinary 24-hour
KHB Krebs-Henseleit buffer
KHb potassium hemoglobinate
KHC kinetic hemolysis curve
KHD kinky hair disease
KHF Korean hemorrhagic fever
KHM keratoderma hereditaria mutilans
KHN Knoop hardness number
KHP King's Honorary Physician
KHS King's Honorary Surgeon; kinky hair syndrome; Krebs-Henseleit solution
kHz kilohertz
KI karyopyknotic index; Krönig's isthmus
KIA Kligler iron agar
KIC ketoisocaproate; keto isocaproic acid
KICB killed intracellular bacteria
KID keratitis, ichthyosis, and deafness [syndrome]

KIHD Kuopio Ischemic Heart Disease Risk Factor Study
kilo kilogram
KIMSA Kirsten murine sarcoma
KIMSV, Ki-MSV Kirsten murine sarcoma virus
KIN keratinocytic intraepidermal neoplasia
KINDS Kinmen Neurologic Disorders Survey
KIP key intermediary protein
KiP kilopascal
KIPS key indicators, probes, and scoring method [for evaluating compliance with requirements for accreditation]
KIRA kinase receptor activation
KISS keep it simple and safe; keep it simple, stupid; key integrative social system; Kobe Idiopathic Cardiomyopathy Survival Study; saturated solution of potassium iodide
KIT Kahn Intelligence Test
KIU kallikrein inactivation unit
KIVA keto isovaleric acid
KJ, kj knee jerk
kJ kilojoule
KK knee kick
kkat kilokatal
KKS kallikrein-kinin system
KL Karhunen-Loéve [transform]; kidney lobe; Kit ligand; Klebs-Loeffler [bacillus]; Kleine-Levin [syndrome]
kl kiloliter
KLC Karhunen-Loéve coefficient
Klebs *Klebsiella*
KLH keyhole limpet hemocyanin
KLK kallikrein
KLM killed *Mycobacterium*
KLKR kallikrein
KLS kidneys, liver, and spleen; Kreuzbein lipomatous syndrome
KLT Karhunen-Loéve transform
KM kanamycin
km kilometer
km² square kilometer
K$_m$ Michaelis-Menten constant
KMC K-means clustering analysis
kMc kilomegacycle
K-MCM potassium-containing minimum capacitation medium
kMc/s kilomegacycles per second
KMEF keratin, myosin, epidermin, and fibrin

kmps kilometers per second
KMS kabuki make-up syndrome; knowledge management system; kwashiorkor-marasmus syndrome
K-MSV Kirsten murine sarcoma virus
KMV killed measles virus vaccine
KN knowledge networking
Kn knee; Knudsen number
kN kilonewton
kn knee
K nail Küntscher nail
KNG kininogen
KNN, k-NN K-nearest neighbor
KNRK Kirsten sarcoma virus in normal rat kidney
KNS kinesin
KNSL kinesin-like
KO keep on; keep open; killed organism; knee orthosis; knock out
KOC cathodal opening contraction
KOH potassium hydroxide
KOPS thousand of operations per second
kΩ kilohm
KP Kaufmann-Peterson [base]; keratitic precipitate; keratitis punctata; kidney protein; killed parenteral [vaccine]; *Klebsiella pneumoniae*
kPa kilopascal
kPa·s/l kilopascal seconds per liter
KPB ketophenylbutazone; potassium phosphate buffer
KPC keratoconus posticus circumscriptus
KPE Kelman pharmacoemulsification
KPI kallikrein-protease inhibitor; karyopyknotic index
kpm kilopodometer
KPR key pulse rate
KPS Karnofsky Performance Status
KPT kidney punch test
KPTI Kunitz pancreatic trypsin inhibitor
KPTT kaolin partial thromboplastin time
KPV key process variable; killed parenteral vaccine
KQC key quality characteristics
KQML knowledge query and manipulation language
KR key-ridge; knowledge representation; Kopper Reppart [medium]
Kr krypton
kR kiloroentgen
KRB Krebs-Ringer buffer

KRBG Krebs-Ringer bicarbonate buffer with glucose

KRBS Krebs-Ringer bicarbonate solution

KRIS Kaunas-Rotterdam Intervention Study

KRP Kolmer test with Reiter protein [antigen]; Krebs-Ringer phosphate

KRR knowledge representation and reasoning

KRRS kinetic resonance Raman spectroscopy

KRS knowledge representation syntax

KRT keratin

KS Kabuki [make-up] syndrome; Kallmann syndrome; Kaposi sarcoma; Kartagener syndrome; Kawasaki syndrome; keratan sulfate; ketosteroid; Klinefelter syndrome; Korsakoff syndrome; Kveim-Siltzbach [test]

K-S Kearns-Sayre [syndrome]

17-KS 17-ketosteroid

ks kilosecond

KSC cathodal closing contraction

KSHV Kaposi sarcoma-associated herpesvirus

KS/OI Kaposi sarcoma with opportunistic infection

KSOM Kohonen's self-organizing map

K$_{sp}$ solubility product

KSP Karolinska Scales of Personality; kidney-specific protein

17-KSR 17-ketosteroid reductase

KSS Kearns-Sayre syndrome; Kearns-Sayre-Shy [syndrome]

KSS0 knowledge support system zero

KST cathodal closing tetanus; kallistatin

KT kidney transplant, kidney transplantation

KTA kidney transplant alone

KTI kallikrein-trypsin inhibitor

KTS Klippel-Trenaunay syndrome

KTSA Kahn test of symbol arrangement

KTU knowledge transfer and utilization

KTW, KTWS Klippel-Trenaunay-Weber [syndrome]

KTx kidney transplant

KU kallikrein unit; Karmen unit

Ku kurchatovium; Peltz factor

KUB kidneys and upper bladder; [x-ray examination of the] kidneys, ureters, and bladder

KUMIS Kumamoto University Myocardial Infarction Study

KUN Kunjin [virus]

KUS, kidney, ureter, spleen

KV kanamycin and vancomycin; killed vaccine

kV, kv kilovolt

kVA kilovolt-ampere

kvar kilovar

KVBA kanamycin-vancomycin blood agar

kVcp, kvcp kilovolt constant potential

KVE Kaposi's varicelliform eruption

KVLBA kanamycin-vancomycin laked blood agar

KVO keep vein open

kVp, kvp kilovolt peak

KW Keith-Wagener [ophthalmoscopic finding]; Kimmelstiel-Wilson [syndrome]; Kugelberg-Welander [syndrome]

Kw weighted kappa

K$_w$ dissociation constant of water

kW, kw kilowatt

KWB Keith-Wagener-Barker [hypertension classification]

KWD Kimmelstiel-Wilson disease

kWh, kW-hr, kw-hr kilowatt-hour

K wire Kirschner wire

KWord 32-bit word

KWS Kimmelstiel-Wilson syndrome; Kugelberg-Welander syndrome

K-XRF K x-ray fluorescence

KYCS Kiryat Yovel Community Study

KYN kynurenic acid

KYN-OH kynurenine-3-hydroxylase

KYSMI Kyoto Shiga Myocardial Infarction [study]

KZ ketoconazole

L angular momentum; Avogadro constant; boundary [Lat. *limes*]; coefficient of induction; diffusion length; inductance; *Lactobacillus*; lambda; lambert; latent heat; latex; Latin; leader sequence; left; *Legionella; Leishmania*; length; lente insulin; lethal; leucine; levo-; lidocaine; ligament; light; light sense; lingual; *Listeria;* liter; liver; low; lower; lumbar; luminance; lymph; lymphocyte; outer membrane layer of cell wall of gram-negative bacteria [layer]; pound [Lat. *libra*]; radiance; self-inductance; syphilis [Lat. *lues*]; threshold [Lat. *limen*]

L-variant a defective bacterial variant that can multiply on hypertonic medium

L$_0$ limes zero [*limes nul*]

L$_+$ limes tod

L1, L2, L3, L4, L5 first, second, third, fourth, and fifth lumbar vertebrae

LI, LII, LIII first, second, third stage of syphilis

L/3 lower third

l azimuthal quantum number; left; length; lethal; levorotatory; liter; long; longitudinal; specific latent heat

Λ see *lambda*

λ see *lambda*

LA lactic acid; large amount; laser angioplasty; late abortion; late antigen; latex agglutination; left angle; left arm; left atrium; left auricle; leucine aminopeptidase; leukemia antigen; leukoagglutination; leuprolide acetate; levator ani; Lightwood-Albright [syndrome]; linear addition; linguo-axial; linoleic acid; lobuloalveolar; local anesthesia; local anesthetic; long-acting [drug]; long arm; long axis; low anxiety; Ludwig angina; lupus anticoagulant; lymphocyte antibody

L&A light and accommodation; living and active

LA50 total body surface area of burn that will kill 50% of patients (lethal area)

La labial; lambda; lambert; lanthanum

LAA left atrial appendage; left atrial area; leukemia-associated antigen; leukocyte ascorbic acid

LAAM L-alpha acetyl methadol; levo-alpha-acetylmethadol

LAAO L-amino acid oxidase

LA/Ao left atrial/aortic [ratio]

LAB, lab laboratory

LabBase laboratory database

LABBB left anterior bundle branch block

LABC locally advancing breast cancer

LABE labetalol

LABP laboratory procedure [UMLS]

LABV left atrial ball valve

LabVISE Laboratory Reporting Scheme in Virology and Serology [Australia]

LAC La Crosse [virus]; lactase; left atrial circumflex [artery]; left atrial contraction; linear attenuation coefficient; linguoaxiocervical; long-arm cast; low-amplitude contraction; lung adenocarcinoma cells; lupus anticoagulant

LaC labiocervical

lac laceration; lactation

LACI lacidipine

LACN local area communications network

LACI lipoprotein-associated coagulation inhibitor

lacr lacrimal

LACS long chain acyl-coenzyme A synthetase

lact lactate, lactating, lactation; lactic

lact hyd lactalbumin hydrolysate

LAD lactic acid dehydrogenase; left anterior descending [coronary artery]; left axis deviation; leukocyte adhesion deficiency; ligament augmentation device; linoleic acid depression; lipoamide dehydrogenase; lymphocyte-activating determinant

LADA laboratory animal dander allergy; left acromio-dorso-anterior [position]; left anterior descending artery

LADB left [coronary] descending branch

LADCA left anterior descending coronary artery

LADD lacrimo-auriculo-dento-digital [syndrome]; left anterior descending diagonal [coronary artery]

LADH lactic acid dehydrogenase; liver alcohol dehydrogenase

LAD-MIN left axis deviation, minimal

LADP left acromio-dorso-posterior [position]; left anterior descending arterial pressure

LADS Lors American Data System

LAE left atrial enlargement

LAEDV left atrial volume in end diastole

LAEI left atrial emptying index

LAESV left atrial volume in end systole

LAF laminar air flow; Latin American female; leukocyte-activating factor; lymphocyte-activating factor

LAFB left anterior fascicular block

LAFR laminar air flow room

LAFU laminar air flow unit

LAG labiogingival; leukocyte antigen group; linguo-axiogingival; lymphangiogram; lymphocyte activation gene

LaG labiogingival

LAH lactalbumin hydrolysate; left anterior hemiblock; left atrial hypertrophy; Licentiate of Apothecaries Hall; lithium, aluminum, hydroxide

LAHB left anterior hemiblock

LAHC low affinity-high capacity

LAHT laser-assisted hair transplantation

LAHV leukocyte-associated herpesvirus

LAI latex particle agglutination inhibition; leukocyte adherence inhibition

LaI labioincisal

LAIF leukocyte adherence inhibition factor

LAIT latex agglutination inhibition test

LAK lymphokine-activated killer [cells]

LAL left axillary line; limulus amebocyte lysate; low air loss; lysosomal acid lipase

LaL labiolingual

LALB low air-loss bed

LALI lymphocyte antibody-lymphocytolytic interaction

LALL lymphomatous acute lymphoblastic leukemia

LALR lexically assign, logically refine [computer strategy]

LAM laminectomy; laminin; late ambulatory monitoring; Latin American male; left anterior measurement; left atrial myxoma; linear associative memory; lymphangioleiomyomatosis; lymphocyte adhesion molecule

lam laminectomy

LAMA laminin A

LAMB laminin B; lentigines, atrial myxoma, mucocutaneous myxomas, blue nevi [syndrome]

λ Greek lower case letter *lambda*; craniometric point; decay constant; an immunoglobulin light chain; mean free path; microliter; thermal conductivity; wavelength

LAMBR laminin B receptor

LAMC laminin C

LAMMA laser microprobe mass analyzer

LAMP lysosome-associated membrane protein

LAN local area network; long-acting neuroleptic [agent]

LANC long-arm navicular cast

LANE lidocaine, atropine, naloxone, epinephrine [drugs that may be administered via endotracheal tube]

LANV left atrial neovascularization

LAO left anterior oblique; left atrial overload; Licentiate of the Art of Obstetrics

LAP laboratory accreditation program; laparoscopy; laparotomy; latency-active promoter; left arterial pressure; left atrial pressure; leucine aminopeptidase; leukemia-associated phosphoprotein; leukocyte alkaline phosphatase; liver-enriched transcriptional activator protein; low atmospheric pressure; lyophilized anterior pituitary

lap laparoscopy; laparotomy

lap & dye laparoscopy and injection of dye

LAPIS Late Potentials in Myocardial Infarction Study

LAPSE long-term ambulatory physiologic surveillance

LAPSS Los Angeles Prehospital Stroke Screen

LAPW left atrial posterior wall

LAR laryngology; late asthmatic response; late reaction; left arm recumbent; legally authorized representative; leukocyte antigen-related

lar larynx; left arm reclining

LARA Low-Dose Aspirin Trial on Restenosis after Angioplasty

LARab laryngeal abductor

LARad laryngeal adductor

LARC leukocyte automatic recognition computer

LARD lacrimoauriculoradiodental [syndrome]

LARIS laser atomization resonance ionization spectroscopy

LARS laparoscopic antireflux surgery; laser angioplasty in the treatment of restenosis developing within coronary stents; leucyl-tRNA synthetase

Laryngol laryngology

LAS laboratory automation system; lateral amyotrophic sclerosis; laxative abuse syndrome; left anterior-superior; leucine acetylsalicylate; linear alkylsulfonate; local adaptation syndrome; long arm splint; lower abdominal surgery; lymphadenopathy syndrome; lymphangioscintigraphy

LASA linear-analogue self assessment

LASAF low quantities of acetylsalicylic acid in atrial fibrillation

LASA-P linear-analogue self-assessment-Pristman

LASAR Local Alcohol and Stent Against Restenosis [trial]

LASA-S linear-analogue self-assessment-Selby

LASE laser-assisted spinal endoscopy

LASER light amplification by stimulated emission of radiation

LASH left anterior superior hemiblock

LA SI linearly-additive spatially invariant [image]

LASIK laser-assisted in situ keratomileusis

L-ASP L-asparaginase

LASS labile aggregation stimulating substance

LAST Left Anterior Small Thoracotomy [study]

LASTAK laser transluminal angioplasty catheter

LASTLHY Latin American Study of Lacidipine in Hypertension

LAT latency-associated transcript; lateral; latex agglutination test; left atrial thrombus; less acute mode of transportation; lysolecithin acyltransferase

Lat Latin

lat latent; lateral

lat bend lateral bending

LATCH literature attached to charts

LATE Late Assessment of Thrombolytic Efficacy [trial]

l·atm liter atmosphere

LATP left atrial transmural pressure

LATPT left atrial transesophageal pacing test

LATS long-acting thyroid stimulator

LATS-P long-acting thyroid stimulator-protector

LATu lobulo-alveolar tumor

LAUP laser-assisted uvulopalatoplasty

LAV leafhopper A virus; liquid-assisted ventilation; lymphadenopathy-associated virus

lav lavoratory

LAVA laser angioplasty vs. angioplasty; Leiden Artificial Valves and Anticoagulation [study]

LAVH laparoscopy-assisted vaginal hysterectomy

LAW left atrial wall

LAX, LAx long axis

lax laxative; laxity

LAX-DSS long axis-discrete subaortic stenosis

lax oc laxative of choice

LB lamellar body; large bowel; left breast; left bronchus; left bundle; left buttock; leiomyoblastoma; lipid body; live birth; liver biopsy; loose body; low back [pain]; lung biopsy; Luria-Bertani [medium]

L&B left and below

Lb *Leishmania brasiliensis;* pound force

lb pound [Lat. *libra*]

LBA laser balloon angioplasty; left basal artery

LBB left bundle branch; low back bending

LBBB left bundle branch block

LBBsB left bundle branch system block

LBC lidocaine blood concentration; lymphadenosis benigna cutis

LBCD left border of cardiac dullness

LBCF Laboratory Branch complement fixation [test]

LBD large bile duct; left border of dullness; Lewy body dementia; ligand-binding domain

LBF *Lactobacillus bulgaricus* factor; limb blood flow; liver blood flow

lbf pound force

lbf-ft pound force foot

LBH length, breadth, height

LBI low back injury; low serum-bound iron

lb/in² pounds per square inch

LBL labeled lymphoblast; lymphoblastic lymphoma

LBM last bowel movement; lean body mass; loose bowel movement; lung basement membrane

L-BMAA L-beta-N-methylamino-L-alanine

LBNP lower body negative pressure

LBO large bowel obstruction

LBP lipopolysaccharide-binding protein; low back pain; low blood pressure; lumbar back pain

LBPF long bone or pelvic fracture

LBPP lower body positive pressure

LBPQ Low Back Pain Questionnaire

LBRF louse-borne relapsing fever

LBS low back syndrome; Lübeck Blood [Pressure] Study; lumbar back strain; Lutheran Brotherhood Study

LBSA lipid-bound sialic acid

LBT low back tenderness or trouble

LBTI lima bean trypsin inhibitor

lb tr pound troy

LBV left brachial vein; lung blood volume

LBW lean body weight; low birth weight

LBWI low-birth-weight infant

LBWR lung-body weight ratio

LC Laennec cirrhosis; Langerhans cell; laparoscopic cholecystectomy; large chromophobe; late clamped; lateral canthotomy; lateral cortex; lecithin cholesterol acyltransferase; left circumflex [artery]; lethal concentration; Library of Congress; life care; light chain; linguocervical; lipid cytosomes; liquid chromatography; liquid crystal; liver cirrhosis; living children; locus ceruleus; long chain; low calorie; lower calyceal; lung cancer; lung cell; lymphocyte count

LC$_{50}$ median lethal concentration

LCA Leber congenital amaurosis; left carotid artery; left circumflex artery; left coronary artery; leukocyte common antigen; lithocholic acid; liver cell adenoma; lymphocyte chemotactic activity

LCa low calcium [diet]

LCAH lipoid congenital adrenal hyperplasia

LCAL large-cell anaplastic lymphoma

LCAM liver cell adhesion molecule

L1CAM L1CAM Mutation Database

LCAO linear combination of atomic orbitals

L-CAPS Low-Density Lipoprotein Coronary Atherosclerosis Prospective Study

LCAR late cutaneous anaphylactic reaction

LCAS Lipoprotein and Coronary Atherosclerosis Study

LCAT lecithin cholesterol acyltransferase

LCATA lecithin cholesterol acetyltransferase alpha

LCB Laboratory of Cancer Biology; Leber congenital blindness; left costal border; lymphomatosis cutis benigna

LCBF local cerebral blood flow

LCBI laboratory-confirmed bloodstream infection

LCC lactose coliform count; left circumflex coronary (artery); left common carotid; left coronary cusp; life cycle cost [analysis]; lipid-containing cell; liver cell carcinoma

LCCA late cortical cerebellar atrophy; leukoclastic angiitis

LCCME Liaison Committee on Continuing Medical Education

LCCS lower cervical cesarean section

LCCSCT large-cell calcifying Sertoli cell tumor

LCD lattice corneal dystrophy; liquid crystal diode; liquid crystal display; coal tar solution [liquor carbonis detergens]; localized collagen dystrophy; low-calcium diet

LCDD light chain deposition disease

LCED liquid chromatography with electrochemical detection

LCF least common factor; lymphocyte culture fluid

LCFA, L-cFA long-chain fatty acid

LCFU leukocyte colony-forming unit

LCG Langerhans cell granule

LCGL large-cell granulocytic leukemia

LCGME Liaison Committee on Graduate Medical Education

LCGR lutropin-choriogonadotropin receptor

LCGU local cerebral glucose utilization

LCH Langerhans cell histiocytosis

LCh Licentiate in Surgery

L-CHAD long-chain 3-hydroxyacyl coenzyme A dehydrogenase

LCI length complexity index

LCIS lobular carcinoma in situ

LCL lateral collateral ligament; Levinthal-Coles-Lillie [body]; lower confidence limit; lower control limit; lymphoblastoid cell line; lymphocytic lymphosarcoma; lymphoid cell line

LCLC large-cell lung carcinoma

LCM latent cardiomyopathy; left costal margin; leukocyte-conditioned medium; lowest common multiple; lymphatic choriomeningitis; lymphocytic choriomeningitis

LCME Liaison Committee on Medical Education

LCMG long-chain monoglyceride

L/cm H$_2$O liters per centimeter of water

LCMV lymphocytic choriomeningitis virus

LCN lateral cervical nucleus; left caudate nucleus; lipocalin

LCNB large core needle biopsy

LCO left coronary ostium; low cardiac output

LCOS low cardiac output syndrome

LCP long-chain polysaturated [fatty acid]; lymphocyte cytosol polypeptide

LCPD Legg-Calvé-Perthes disease

LCPS Licentiate of the College of Physicians and Surgeons

LCQ Learning Climate Questionnaire

LCR late cutaneous reaction; lifetime clinical record; ligase chain reaction; locus control region

LCRB locus control region beta

LCRI limit cycle reciprocal interaction

LCRUS Leigh Clinical Research Unit Study

LCrv retroventral lateral cortex

LCS cerebrospinal fluid [Lat. *liquor cerebrospinalis*]; left coronary sinus; Leydig cell stimulation; lichen chronicus simplex; life care service; low constant suction; low continuous suction; lymphocyte culture supernatants

LCSB Liaison Committee for Specialty Boards

LCSG Lung Cancer Study Group

LCSS lethal congenital contracture syndrome

LcSSc limited cutaneous systemic sclerosis

LCSW licensed clinical social worker

LCT liver cell tumor; long-chain triglyceride; lymphocytotoxicity; lymphocytotoxin

LCTA lymphocytotoxic antibody

LCU life change unit

LCV lecithovitellin; leukocytoclastic vasculitis

LCWI left cardiac work index

LCX left circumflex [coronary artery]

LCXB left [coronary] circumflex branch

LD label dictionary; labor and delivery; laboratory data; labyrinthine defect; lactate dehydrogenase; L-dopa (levodopa); laser Doppler; learning disability; learning disorder; left deltoid; Legionnaires' disease; lethal dose; levodopa; light differentiation; limited disease; linear dichroism; linguodistal; linkage disequilibrium; lipodystrophy; liver disease; living donor; loading dose; Lombard-Dowell [agar]; longitudinal diameter; low density; low dose; Lyme disease; lymphocyte-defined; lymphocyte depletion

L-D Leishman-Donovan [body]

L/D light/darkness [ratio]

L&D labor and delivery

LD$_1$ isoenzyme of lactate dehydrogenase found in the heart, erythrocytes, and kidneys

LD$_2$ isoenzyme of lactate dehydrogenase found in the lungs

LD$_3$ isoenzyme of lactate dehydrogenase found in the lungs

LD$_4$ isoenzyme of lactate dehydrogenase found in the liver

LD$_5$ isoenzyme of lactate dehydrogenase found in the liver and muscles

LD$_{50}$ median lethal dose

LD$_{50/30}$ a dose that is lethal for 50% of test subjects within 30 days

LD$_{100}$ lethal dose in all exposed subjects

Ld *Leishmania donovani*

LDA laser Doppler anemometry; left dorso-anterior [fetal position]; linear discriminant analysis; low density area; lymphocyte-dependent antibody

LDAC low-dose cytosine arabinoside

LDAR latex direct agglutination reaction

LDB lamb dysentery bacillus; Legionnaires' disease bacillus

LDC lactose digestion capacity; lymphoid dendritic cell; lysine decarboxylase

L-dC L-deoxycytidine

LDCC lectin-dependent cellular cytotoxicity

LDCI low-dose continuous infusion

LDCMC Lady Davis Carmel Medical Center

LDCT late distal cortical tubule
LDD late dedifferentiation; light-dark discrimination
LDDB London Dysmorphology Database
LDDE low-dose dobutamine echo
LDER lateral-view dual-energy radiography
LD-EYA Lombard-Dowell egg yolk agar
LDF laser Doppler flowmetry; laser Doppler flux, laser Doppler fluxometry; limit dilution factor
LDFA linear discrimination functional analysis
LDG lactic dehydrogenase; limit grid displacement; lingual developmental groove
L-dG L-deoxyguanosine
LDH lactate dehydrogenase; low-dose heparin
LDHA lactic dehydrogenase A
LDHB lactic dehydrogenase-B
LDHC lactic dehydrogenase-C
LDHSPS Low Dose Heparin Stroke Prevention Study
LDL loudness discomfort level; low density lipoprotein
LDLA low-density lipoprotein apheresis
LDL-C, LDL-c low-density lipoprotein [LDL]-cholesterol complex
LDL/HDL low-density lipoproteins, LDL/high-density lipoproteins, HDL [ratio]
LDLP low-density lipoprotein
LDLR, LDL-R low density lipoprotein receptor; low-density lipoprotein [LDL] Receptor Mutation Database
LDM lactate dehydrogenase, muscle; limited dorsal myeloschisis
LDMF latissimus dorsi myocutaneous flap
LD-NEYA Lombard-Dowell neomycin egg yolk agar
L-DOPA, L-dopa levodopa, levo-3, 4-dihydroxyphenylalanine
LDP left dorsoposterior [fetal position]; lumbodorsal pain
LDR labor, delivery, recovery; lifetime data repository; low dose rate
LDRI leukotriene D4 receptor inhibitors
LDRPS labor-delivery-recovery-postpartum suite
LDRS labor-delivery-recovery suite
LDS Licentiate in Dental Surgery; locked door seclusion

LDSc Licentiate in Dental Science
LDT left dorsotransverse [fetal position]
LDUB long double upright brace
LDUH low-dose unfractionated heparin
LDV lactic dehydrogenase virus; large dense-cored vesicle; laser Doppler velocimetry; lateral distant view
LE lactate extraction; law enforcement; left ear; left eye; leukocyte elastase; leukoerythrogenic; life expectancy; live embryo; Long Evans [rat]; low exposure; lower extremity; lupus erythematosus [cell]
LEA lower extremity amputation; lumbar epidural anesthesia
LEAF layman education and activation system
LEAP Lower Extremity Amputation Prevention [program]
LEC leukoencephalitis; long Evans cinnamon [rat]; lower esophageal contractility
LECP low-energy charged particle
LED light-emitting diode; lowest emitting dose; lupus erythematosus disseminatus
LEDC low-energy direct current
LEE locus of enterocyte effacement
LEED low-energy electron diffraction
LEEDS low-energy electron diffraction spectroscopy
LEEP left end-expiratory pressure; loop electrosurgical excision procedure
LEER likelihood equivalent error
LEET Low Energy Endotak Trial
LEF leukokinesis-enhancing factor; lupus erythematosus factor; lymphoid-enhanced binding factor
leg legislation; legal
LeIF leukocyte interferon
LEIS low-energy ion scattering
LEL lower explosive limit; lowest effect level
LEM lateral eye movement; Leibovitz-Emory medium; leukocyte endogenous mediator; light electron microscope; light emission microscopy; low-electrolyte meal
LEMO lowest empty molecular orbital
LEMS Lambert-Eaton myasthenic syndrome
lenit lenitive
LEOPARD lentigines, EKG abnormalities, ocular hypertelorism, pulmonary stenosis, abnormalities of genitalia, retardation of growth, and deafness [syndrome]

LEP laboratory of enteric pathogens; lethal effective phase; lipoprotein electrophoresis; low egg passage; lower esophageal pressure

lep leptotene

L$_{EPN}$ effective perceived noise level

Leq loudness equivalent

LER lysozomal enzyme release

LERG local electroretinogram

LERS learning from examples based on rough sets

LES Lambert-Eaton syndrome; Lawrence Experimental Station [agar]; Life Experiences Survey; lifestyle evaluation system; local excitatory state; Locke egg serum; low excitatory state; lower esophageal sphincter; lupus erythematosus, systemic

les lesion

LESD Letterer-Siwe disease

LESP lower esophageal sphincter pressure

LESS lateral electrical spine stimulation

LESSD lupus erythematosus, specific skin disease

LESTR leukocyte-derived seven-transmembrane domain receptor

LET Losartan Effectiveness and Tolerability [study]; lidocaine, epinephrine, and tetracaine [solution]; linear or low energy transfer

LETD lowest effective toxic dose

LETS large external transformation-sensitive [protein]; Leiden Thrombophilia Study

LEU leucine; leucovorin; leukocyte equivalent unit

Leu leucine

leuc leukocyte

LeuRS leucyl ribonucleic acid synthetase

LEUT leucine transport

LEV Levamisole

LEW Lewis [rat]

l/ext lower extremity

LF labile factor; lactoferrin; laryngofissure; Lassa fever; latex fixation; left foot; left forearm; lethal factor; leukotactic factor; ligamentum flavum; limit of flocculation; low fat [diet]; low flow; low forceps; low frequency

L/F Latin female

Lf limit of flocculation

lf lactoferrin; low frequency

LFA left femoral artery; left frontal craniotomy; left fronto-anterior [fetal position]; leukocyte function associated antigen; leukotactic factor activity; logical framework analysis; low-friction arthroplasty; lymphocyte function-associated antigen

LFB luxol fast blue [stain]

LFBMA lattice function biological movement artifacts

LFC living female child; low fat and cholesterol [diet]

LFD lactose-free diet; large for date [fetus]; late fetal death; lateral facial dysplasia; least fatal dose; low-fat diet; low-fiber diet; low forceps delivery

LFE local frequency estimation

LFER linear free-energy relationship

LFH left femoral hernia

LFHL low-frequency hearing loss

LFL left frontolateral; leukocyte feeder layer; lower flammable limit

LFN lactoferrin

L-[form] a defective bacterial variant that can multiply on hypertonic medium

LFP left frontoposterior [fetal position]

LFPPV low-frequency positive pressure ventilation

LFPS Licentiate of the Faculty of Physicians and Surgeons

LFR lymphoid follicular reticulosis

LFS lateral facet syndrome; Li-Fraumeni syndrome; limbic forebrain structure; liver function series

LFT latex fixation test; latex flocculation test; left fronto-transverse [fetal position]; liver function test; low-frequency tetanus; low-frequency transduction; low-frequency transfer; lung function test

LFU lipid fluidity unit

LFV Lassa fever virus; low-frequency ventilation

LFx linear fracture

LG lactoglobulin; lamellar granule; laryngectomy; left gluteal; Lennox-Gastaut [syndrome]; leucylglycine; linguogingival; lipoglycopeptide; liver graft; low glucose; lymphatic gland

lg large; leg

LGA large for gestational age; left gastric artery

LGALS lecithin, galactoside-binding, soluble

LGB Landry-Guillain-Barré [syndrome]; lateral geniculate body

LGBS Landry-Guillain-Barré syndrome

LGD limb girdle dystrophy

LGE Langat encephalitis

LGF lateral giant fiber

LGH lactogenic hormone

LGI large glucagon immunoreactivity; low gastrointestinal

LGL large granular leukocyte; large granular lymphocyte; Lown-Ganong-Levine [syndrome]

LGL-NK large granular lymphocyte-natural killer

LGM left gluteus medius

LGMD limb-girdle muscular dystrophy

LGN lateral geniculate nucleus; lateral glomerulonephritis

LGP labioglossopharyngeal

LGS Langer-Giedion syndrome; Lennox-Gastaut syndrome; limb girdle syndrome

LGSS low-grade stromal sarcoma

LGT late generalized tuberculosis

LGTI lower genital tract infection

LGV large granular vesicle; lymphogranuloma venereum

LGVHD lethal graft-versus-host disease

LgX lymphogranulomatosis X

LH late healing; lateral habecular [nucleus]; lateral hypothalamic [syndrome]; lateral hypothalamus; left hand; left heart; left hemisphere; left hyperphoria; liver homogenate; loop of Henle; lower half; lues hereditaria; lung homogenate; luteinizing hormone; Lyon hypertensive [rat]

L/H lung-to-heart [ratio]

LHA lateral hypothalamic area; left hepatic artery; low height for age

LHB luteinizing hormone beta chain

LHBV left heart blood volume

LHC Langerhans cell histiocytosis; left heart catheterization; left hypochondrium; light-harvesting complex; Local Health Council

LHCGR luteinizing hormone-choriogonadotropin receptor

LHD lateral head displacement [sperm]

LHe liquid helium

LHEG local healthcare executive group

LHF left heart failure

LHFA lung Hageman factor activator

LHG left hand grip; localized hemolysis in gel

LHI lipid hydrocarbon inclusion

LHIPS Local Heparin Infusion Pre-Stenting [trial]

LHL left hepatic lobe

LHM lysuride hydrogen maleate

LHMP Life Health Monitoring Program

LHN lateral hypothalamic nucleus

LHNCBC Lister Hill National Center for Biomedical Communication

LHON Leber hereditary optic neuropathy

LHP lifetime health plan

LHPZ low high-pressure zone

LHR leukocyte histamine release; lifetime health record; lymph node homing receptor

l-hr lumen-hour

LHRF luteinizing hormone-releasing factor

LHRH, LH-RH luteinizing hormone-releasing hormone

LHRHR luteinizing hormone-releasing hormone receptor

LHS left hand side; left heart strain; left heelstrike; Losartan Hemodynamic Study; library of health sciences; Lung Heart Study; lymphatic/hematopoietic system

LHT left hypertropia; Lifestyle Heart Trial

LHV left hepatic vein

LI labeling index; lactose intolerance; lacunar infarct; lamellar ichthyosis; Langerhans islet; large intestine; *Leptospira icterohaemorrhagica;* linguoincisal; lithogenic index; low impulsiveness

L&I liver and iron

Li a blood group system; labrale inferius; lithium

l-I late inspiratory

LIA Laser Institute of America; left iliac artery; leukemia-associated inhibitory activity; lock-in amplifier; lymphocyte-induced angiogenesis; lysine iron agar

LIAF laser-induced arterial fluorescence; lymphocyte-induced angiogenesis factor

LIAFI late infantile amaurotic familial idiocy

lib a pound [Lat. *libra*]

LIBC latent iron-binding capacity

LIC left internal carotid [artery]; left interventricular coronary [artery]; limiting isorrheic concentration; local intravascular coagulation

Lic licentiate

LICA left internal carotid artery

LICM left intercostal margin

LicMed Licentiate in Medicine
LICS left intercostal space
LID large intraluminal density; late immunoglobulin deficiency; lymphocytic infiltrative disease
LIF laser-induced fluorescence; left iliac fossa; left index finger; leukemia-inhibiting factor; leukocyte inhibitory factor; leukocytosis-inducing factor
LIFE lifestyle intervention, food, and exercise program; Losartan Intervention for Endpoint Reduction in Hypertension [trial]; lung imaging fluorescence endoscope
LIFO last in, first out
LIFR leukemia inhibitory factor receptor
LIFT late intervention following thrombolysis; lymphocyte immunofluorescence test
lig ligament; ligation
LIH left inguinal hernia
LIHA low impulsiveness, high anxiety
LIHFE living with heart failure [questionnaire]
LIHPS Local Delivery of Heparin in Stenting for Suboptimal Result or Threatened Closure Post-Percutaneous Transluminal Coronary Angioplasty Using the Local Med Infusasleeve; local infusion of heparin prior to stenting
LIJ left internal jugular [vein]
LILA low impulsiveness, low anxiety
LIM line isolation monitor
lim limit, limited
LIMA left internal mammary artery
LIME Leeds interactive medical education [UK]
LIMIT Laboratory for Integrated Medical Interface Technology; Leicester Intravenous Magnesium Intervention Trial; low-molecular weight heparin delivered intramurally to inhibit thrombosis and restenosis
LIMIT-AMI Double Blind, Placebo-Controlled, Multicenter Angiographic Trial of Rhumab cd 18 in Acute Myocardial Infarction
LIMITS Liquemin in Myocardial Infarction during Thrombolysis with Saruplase [trial]
LIMM lethal infantile mitochondrial myopathy
LIN linear statistical classifier

LINAC linear accelerator
LINC laboratory instrumentation computer
LINE long interspersed repetitive element
Linim, lin liniment
LIO left inferior oblique
LIP lipase; lipocortin; lithium-induced polydipsia; lymphoid or lymphocytic interstitial pneumonitis
Lip lipoate
LIPB lipase B
LIPD lipase D
LIPID Long-Term Intervention with Pravastatin in Ischemic Disease [trial]
lipoMM lipomyelomeningocele
LIPP laser-induced pressure pulse
LIPS Lescol Intervention Prevention Study
LIQ low inner quadrant
liq liquid [Lat. *liquor*]
liq dr liquid dram
liq oz liquid ounce
liq pt liquid pint
liq qt liquid quart
LIR left iliac region; left inferior rectus
LIRBM liver, iron, red bone marrow
LIS laboratory information system; lateral intercellular space; learning and intelligent system; left intercostal space; library information service; lissencephaly; lobular *in situ*; locked-in syndrome; low intermittent suction; low ionic strength
LISA Lescol in Severe Atherosclerosis [trial]; less invasive surgical approach; Library and Information Science Abstracts
LISP List Processing Language
LISREL linear structural relations
LISS low-ionic-strength saline
LIT Leiden Intervention Trial [with vegetarian diet for coronary atherosclerosis]; liver infusion tryptose; Lopressor Intervention Trial
LITA left internal thoracic artery; Library and Information Technology Association
LITE low-intensity treadmill exercise [protocol]
LIV left innominate vein
liv live, living
LIV-BP leucine, isoleucine, and valine-binding protein
LIVC left inferior vena cava
LIVE Left Ventricular Hypertrophy: Indapamide vs Enalapril [trial]

LIVEN linear inflammatory verrucous epidermal nevus

LJI List of Journals Indexed [in Index Medicus]

LJM limited joint mobility; Lowenstein-Jensen medium

LK lamellar keratoplasty; Landry-Kussmaul [syndrome]; left kidney; lichenoid keratosis; lymphokine

LKKS liver, kidneys, spleen

LKM liver-kidney microsomal [antibody]

LKP lamellar keratoplasty

LKS Landau-Kleffner syndrome; liver, kidneys, spleen

LKSB liver, kidney, spleen, bladder

LKV laked kanamycin vancomycin [agar]

LL large lymphocyte; lateral leminiscus; left lateral; left leg; left lower; left lung; lepromatous [in Ridley-Jopling Hansen disease classification]; lepromatous leprosy; lipoprotein lipase; loudness level; lower [eye]lid; lower limb; lower lip; lower lobe; lumbar length; lymphocytic lymphoma; lymphoid leukemia; lysolecithin

LLA limulus lysate assay

L lat left lateral

LLB left lateral border; long-leg brace

LLBCD left lower border of cardiac dullness

LLC laparoscopic laser cholecystectomy; Lewis lung carcinoma; liquid-liquid chromatography; long-leg cast; lymphocytic leukemia

LLCC long-leg cylinder cast

LLC-MK1 rhesus monkey kidney cells

LLC-MK2 rhesus monkey kidney cells

LLC-MK3 *Cercopithecus* monkey kidney cells

LLC-RK1 rabbit kidney cells

LLD left lateral decubitus [muscle]; leg length discrepancy; long-lasting depolarization

LLE left lower extremity

LLETZ large loop excision of the transformation zone

LLF Laki-Lóránd factor; late-life forgetfulness; left lateral femoral; left lateral flexion

LLI leg length inequality; low-level interface

LLL left lower [eye]lid; left liver lobe; left lower leg; left lower lobe

LLLE lower lid left eye

LLM localized leukocyte mobilization

LLMSE linear least mean square error

LLN lower limit of normal

LLO *Legionella*-like organism

LLP late luteal phase; long-lasting potentiation

LLPV left lower pulmonary vein

LLQ left lower quadrant; low-level question

LLR large local reaction; left lateral rectus [muscle]; left lumbar region; ligation linked [polymerase chain] reaction

LLRE lower lid right eye

LLS lazy leukocyte syndrome; Level of Living Survey; linear least squares; long-leg splint

LLSB left lower scapular border; left lower sternal border

LLSF linear least squares fit

LLT left lateral thigh; lysolecithin

LLV lymphatic leukemia virus

LLV-F lymphatic leukemia virus, Friend associated

LLVP left lateral ventricular preexcitation

LLWC long-leg walking cast

LLX left lower extremity

LLZ left lower zone

LM lactic acid mineral [medium]; lactose malabsorption; laryngeal mask; laryngeal muscle; lateral malleolus; left main [coronary artery]; left marginal [coronary artery]; left median; legal medicine; lemniscus medialis; Licentiate in Medicine; Licentiate in Midwifery; light microscope; light microscopy; light minimum; lincomycin; lingual margin; linguomesial; lipid mobilization; liquid membrane; *Listeria monocytogenes*, localized movement; longitudinal muscle; lower motor [neuron]

L/M Latin male

Lm *Listeria monocytogenes*

lm lower midline; lumen

l/m liters per minute

LMA laryngeal mask airway; left main [coronary] artery; left mentoanterior [fetal position]; limbic midbrain area; liver cell membrane autoantibody

LMB Laurence-Moon-Biedl [syndrome]; left main bronchus; leiomyoblastoma; leukomethylene blue

LMBB Laurence-Moon-Bardet-Biedl [syndrome]

LMBS Laurence-Moon-Biedl syndrome

LMC large motile cell; lateral motor column; left main coronary [artery]; left middle cerebral [artery]; living male child; lymphocyte-mediated cytotoxicity; lymphomyeloid complex

LMCA left main coronary artery; left middle cerebral artery

LMCAD left main coronary artery disease

LMCC Licentiate of the Medical Council of Canada

LMCL left midclavicular line

LMCAO left marginal coronary artery occlusion

LMD lipid-moiety modified derivative; local medical doctor; low molecular weight dextran; lumbar microdiscotomy

LMDS locally multiply damaged sites

LMDX low-molecular-weight dextran

LME left mediolateral episiotomy; leukocyte migration enhancement

LMed&Ch Licentiate in Medicine and Surgery

LMF left middle finger; lymphocyte mitogenic factor

lm/ft² lumens per square foot

LMG lethal midline granuloma

LMH lipid-mobilizing hormone

lmh lumen hour

LMI leukocyte migration inhibition

LMIF leukocyte migration inhibition factor

l/min liters per minute

LML large and medium lymphocytes; left mediolateral; left middle lobe

LMM *Lactobacillus* maintenance medium; lentigo maligna melanoma; light meromyosin

lm/m² lumens per square meter

LMN lower motor neuron

LMNL lower motor neuron lesion

LMO living modified organism; localized molecular orbital

LMP large multifunctional protease; last menstrual period; latent membrane potential; left mentoposterior [fetal position]; lumbar puncture

LMPS lethal multiple pterygium syndrome

LMR left medial rectus [muscle]; localized magnetic resonance; longitudinal medical record; lymphocytic meningopolyradiculitis

LMRCP Licentiate in Midwifery of the Royal College of Physicians

LMS lateral medullary syndrome; least mean square; left main stem [coronary artery]; leiomyosarcoma; Licentiate in Medicine and Surgery

lms lumen-second

LMSSA Licentiate in Medicine and Surgery of the Society of Apothecaries

LMT left main trunk; left mentotransverse [fetal position]; leukocyte migration technique

LMV larva migrans visceralis

LMW low molecular weight

lm/W lumens per watt

LMWD low-molecular-weight dextran

LMWH low molecular weight heparin

LMWP low molecular weight proteinuria

LMWT low molecular weight

LMZ left midzone

LN labionasal; Lesch-Nyhan [syndrome]; lipoid nephrosis; Lisch nodule; low necrosis; lung nodule; lupus nephritis; lymph node; Lyon normotensive [rat]

Ln lymph node

LN₂ liquid nitrogen

L/N letter/numerical [system]

ln natural logarithm

LNAA large neutral amino acid

LNBx lymph node biopsy

LNC lymph node cell

LND lymph node dissection

LNE lymph node enlargement

LNF laparoscopic Nissen fundoplication

LNH large number hypothesis

LNKS low natural killer syndrome

LNL lymph node lymphocyte

LNLS linear-nonlinear least squares

LNM lymph node metastasis

LNMC lymph node mononuclear cell

LNMP last normal menstrual period

LNNB Luria-Nebraska Neuropsychological Battery

LNP large neuronal polypeptide

LNPF lymph node permeability factor

LNS lateral nuclear stratum; Lesch-Nyhan syndrome

LO lateral oblique; linguo-occlusal; lumbar orthosis

5-LO 5-lipooxygenase

LOA leave of absence; Leber optic atrophy; left occipitoanterior [fetal position]

LOC laxative of choice; level of consciousness; liquid organic compound; locus of control; loss of consciousness

lo cal low calorie

lo calc low calcium

LOCAT Lopid Coronary Angiography Trial

LOCF last observation carried forward

lo CHO low carbohydrate

lo chol low cholesterol

LOCM low molecular contrast medium

LOCS laryngoonychocutaneous syndrome

LOD line of duty; log odds ratio [score]

LOF lofexidine

LOFD low outlet forceps delivery

LOG lipoxygenase

LOG, LoG laplacian of gaussian [in imaging]

log logarithm

LOGIC laryngeal and ocular granulations in children of Indian subcontinent [syndrome]

LOH loop of Henle; loss of heterozygosity

LOHF late-onset hepatic failure

LOI level of incompetence; level of injury; limit of impurities; loss of imprinting

LOIH left oblique inguinal hernia

LOINC Logical Observation Identifier of Names and Codes [vocabulary]

lo k low potassium

LOKD late-onset Krabbe disease

LOL left occipitolateral [fetal position]

LOM left otitis media; limitation of motion; loss of motion

LOMC laser optical memory card

LOMIR-MCT-IL Lomir [isradipine] Multicenter Study in Israel

LOMSA left otitis media suppurativa acuta

LOMSC, LOMSCh left otitis media suppurativa chronica

lo Na low sodium

long longitudinal

LONIR Laboratory of Neuro-Imaging Resources

LOP leave on pass; left occipitoposterior [fetal position]

LOPP chlorambucil, vincristine, procarbazine, prednisolone

LOPS length of patient's stay

LOQ lower outer quadrant

LOR long open reading frame; lorazepam; loricrin; loss of righting reflex

Lord lordosis, lordotic

LORF long open reading frame

LOS length of stay; Licentiate in Obstetrical Science; lipo-oligosaccharide; low cardiac output syndrome; lower [o]esophageal sphincter

LOS(P) lower [o]esophageal sphincter (pressure)

LOT lateral olfactory tract; left occipitotransverse [fetal position]; Long-term Outcome after Thrombolysis [study]

lot lotion

LOV large opaque vesicle; loviride

LOWBI low-birth-weight infant

LOX liquid oxygen; lysyl oxidase

LOXL lysyl oxidase-like

LP labile peptide; labile protein; laboratory procedure; lactic peroxidase; lamina propria; laryngopharyngeal; late potential; latent period, latency period; lateral plantar; lateral posterior; lateral pylorus; *Legionella pneumophila;* leukocyte poor; leukocytic pyrogen; levator palati; lichen planus; light perception; lingua plicata; linear predictive [spectral analysis]; linguopulpal; lipoprotein; liver plasma [concentration]; loss of privileges; low potency; low power; low pressure; low protein; lumbar puncture; lumboperitoneal; lung parenchyma; lymphocyte predominant; lymphoid plasma; lymphomatoid papulosis

L/P lactate/pyruvate [ratio]; liver plasma [concentration], lymph/plasma [ratio]

Lp lipoprotein; sound pressure level

L$_p$ pathlength

LPA latex particle agglutination; left pulmonary artery; lipoprotein A; lysophosphatidic acid

Lp(a) lipoprotein A

LPAM L-phenylalanine mustard

LPB, Lp(b) lipoprotein B

LPBP low-profile bioprosthesis

LPC laser photocoagulation; late positive component; leukocyte-poor cell; linear predictive coding; lipocortin; longitudinal primary care [program]; lysophosphatidylcholine

LPCM low-placed conus medullaris

LP/cm line pairs per centimeter

LPCT late proximal cortical tubule

LPD Lovelace Patient Database; low-protein diet; luteal phase defect; lymphoproliferative disease

LPDF lipoprotein-deficient fraction

LPE lipoprotein electrophoresis; lyso-phosphatidylethanolamine

LPF leukocytosis-promoting factor; leukopenia factor; lipopolysaccharide factor; localized plaque formation; low-power field; lymphocytosis-promoting factor

lpf low-power field

LPFB left posterior fascicular block

LPFN low-pass filtered noise

LPFS low-pass filtered signal

LPG left paracolic gutter; lipophosphogly-can

LPH lactase-phlorizin hydrolase; left posterior hemiblock; lipotropic pituitary hormone

LPHAS limb/pelvis-hypoplasia/aplasia syndrome

LPI left posterior-inferior; lysinuric protein intolerance

LPIFB left posteroinferior fascicular block

LPIH left posteroinferior hemiblock

LPK liver pyruvate kinase

LPL lichen planus-like lesion; lipoprotein lipase

LPLA lipoprotein lipase activity

LPM lateral pterygoid muscle; liver plasma membrane

lpm lines per minute; liters per minute

lp/mm line pairs per millimeter

LPN Licensed Practical Nurse

LPO lactoperoxidase; left posterior oblique; light perception only; lipid peroxidation

LPP large plaque parapsoriasis; lateral pterygoid plate

LPPH late postpartum hemorrhage

LPR lactate-pyruvate ratio; late phase reaction

lpro longitudinal prospective [trial]

LPS lateral premotor system; levator palpebrae superioris [muscle]; Lovastatin Pravastatin Study; linear profile scan; lipase; lipopolysaccharide

lps liters per second

LPSR lipopolysaccharide receptor

LPT Language Proficiency Test; lipotropin

LPTP Laboratory Proficiency Test Program [Canada]

LPV left portal view; left pulmonary veins

LPVP left posterior ventricular preexcitation

LPW lateral pharyngeal wall

lpw lumens per watt

LPX, Lp-X lipoprotein-X

LQ longevity quotient; lordosis quotient; lower quadrant

LQT long QT [syndrome]

LQTS long QT syndrome

LR labeled release; laboratory references; laboratory report; labor room; lactated Ringer's [solution]; large reticulocyte; latency reaction; latency relaxation; lateral rectus [muscle]; lateral retinaculum; left rotation; level of risk; light reaction; light reflex; likelihood ratio; limb reduction [defect]; limit of reaction; local recurrence; logistic regression; low renin; lymphocyte recruitment

LR[+] positive likelihood ratio

LR[−] negative likelihood ratio

L-R left to right

L/R left-to-right [ratio]

L&R left and right

Lr lawrencium; Limes reacting dose of diphtheria toxin

LRA local relevance aggregation [algorithm for insulin therapy]; low right atrium

LRC learning resource center; lipid research clinic; lower rib cage

LRC-CDPT Lipid Research Clinics Coronary Drug Project Trial

LRC-CPPT Lipid Research Clinics Coronary Primary Prevention Trial

LRC-MFS Lipid Research Clinics Mortality Follow-Up Study

LRCP Licentiate of the Royal College of Physicians; low-risk chest pain

LRCS Licentiate of the Royal College of Surgeons

LRCSE Licentiate of the Royal College of Surgeons, Edinburgh

LRD living related donor

LRDT living related donor transplant

LRE lamina rara externa; leukemic reticuloendotheliosis; lymphoreticuloendothelial

LREH low renin essential hypertension

LRES long-range evaluation system

LRes limited resuscitation

lretro longitudinal retrospective trial

LRF latex and resorcinol formaldehyde; liver residue factor; luteinizing hormone-releasing factor

LRG leucine-rich glycoprotein

LRH likelihood ratio for heterogeneity; luteinizing hormone-releasing hormone

LRI lamina rara interna; lower respiratory [tract] illness; lower respiratory [tract] infection; lymphocyte reactivity index

LRLT living-related donor transplantation

LRM left radical mastectomy; logistic regression model

LRMP last regular menstrual period

LRN lateral reticular nucleus

LROP lower radicular obstetrical paralysis

LRP lichen ruber planus; lipoprotein receptor-related protein; long-range planning

LRQ lower right quadrant

lr-PET low resolution positron emission tomography

LRR labyrinthine righting reflex; local regional recurrence; lymph return rate

LRS laboratory results; lactated Ringer solution; lateral recess stenosis; lateral recess syndrome; low rate of stimulation; lumboradicular syndrome

LRSF lactating rat serum factor; liver regenerating serum factor

LRSS late respiratory systemic syndrome

LRT lateral reticular nucleus; living related transplant; local radiation therapy; long terminal repeat; Lovastatin Restenosis Trial; lower respiratory tract

LRTI lower respiratory tract illness; lower respiratory tract infection

LRV left renal vein

LS lateral septum; lateral suspensor; leader sequence; left sacrum; left septum; left side; legally separated; Leigh syndrome; leiomyosarcoma; length of stay; Leriche syndrome; Letterer-Siwe [disease]; Licentiate in Surgery; life sciences; light sensitive, light-sensitivity; light sensor; light sleep; Likert score; liminal sensation; linear scleroderma; lipid synthesis; liver and spleen; long sleep; longitudinal section; longitudinal study; Lowe syndrome; low-sodium [diet]; lower strength; lumbar spine; lumbosacral; lung surfactant; lymphosarcoma

L-S Letterer-Siwe [disease]; lipid-saccharide

L/S lactase/sucrase [ratio]; lecithin/ sphingomyelin [ratio]; lipid/saccharide [ratio]; longitudinal section; lumbosacral

L&S liver and spleen

LSA left sacro-anterior [fetal position]; left subclavian artery; leukocyte-specific activity; lichen sclerosus et atrophicus; lymphosarcoma

LS&A lichen sclerosus et atrophicus

LSAH Longitudinal Study of Astronaut Health

LSANA leukocyte-specific antinuclear antibody

LSA/RCS lymphosarcoma-reticulum cell sarcoma

LSB least significant bit; left sternal border; left scapular border; long spike burst; lumbar sympathetic block

LS-BMD lumbar spine bone mineral density

LSC late systolic click; least significant change; left side colon cancer; left subclavian; lichen simplex chronicus; liquid scintillation counting; liquid-solid chromatography; locus subcoeruleus

LSc local scleroderma

LScA left scapulo-anterior [fetal position]

LSCL lymphosarcoma cell leukemia

LScP left scapulo-posterior [fetal position]

LSCS lower segment cesarean section

LSD laryngeal sound discrimination; least significant difference; least significant digit; low-sodium diet; lysergic acid diethylamide

LSD-25 lysergic acid diethylamide

LSDIS large scale distributed information system

LSE least squares error; left sternal edge

LSect longitudinal section

LSEP left somatosensory evoked potential; lumbosacral somatosensory evoked potential

LSER linear solvation energy relationship

LSF linear spread function; lymphocyte-stimulating factor

LSFB least squares forward backward

LSG labial salivary gland; losigamone

LSH lutein-stimulating hormone; lymphocyte-stimulating hormone

LSHTM London School of Hygiene and Tropical Medicine

LSI large-scale integration; life satisfaction index; lumbar spine index

LSK liver, spleen, kidneys

LSKM liver-spleen-kidney-megalia

LSL left sacrolateral [fetal position]; left short leg; lymphosarcoma [cell] leukemia

LSM late systolic murmur; least square mean; least square matching [algorithm]; lymphocyte separation medium; lysergic acid morpholide

LSN large scale networking; left substantia nigra

LSNWG Large Scale Networking Working Group

LSO lateral superior olive; left salpingo-oophorectomy; left superior oblique; lumbosacral orthosis

LSP left sacroposterior [fetal position]; linguistic string project; liver-specific protein; lymphocyte-specific protein

LS PACS low-speed picture archive and communication system

LSp life span

L-Spar asparaginase (Elspar)

LSP-MLP linguistic string project-medical language processor

LSSA lipid-soluble secondary antioxidant

LSR lanthanide shift reagent; lecithin/sphingomyelin ratio; left superior rectus [muscle]; liver/spleen ratio

LSRA low septal right atrium

LSRO Life Sciences Research Office

LSS Life Span Study; life support station; liver-spleen scan; lumbar spinal stenosis; lumbosacral spine

LS-SEDUHS Longitudinal Study on Socio-Economic Differences in Utilization of Health Services

LS-SEHD Longitudinal Study on Socio-Economic Health Differences

LST lateral spinothalamic tract; left sacrotransverse [fetal position]; life-sustaining treatment

LSTAT life support for trauma and transport

LSTL laparoscopic tubal ligation

LSU lactose-saccharose-urea [agar]; life support unit

LSV lateral sacral vein; left subclavian vein; longitudinal sound velocity

LSVC left superior vena cava

LSVT large scale vocabulary test; left saphenous vein thrombophlebitis

LSWA large amplitude slow wave activity

LT heat-labile toxin; laminar tomography; Laplace transform; left; left thigh; less than; lethal time; leukotriene; Levin tube; levothyroxine; light; long-term; low temperature; lumbar traction; lymphocytic thyroiditis; lymphocytotoxin; lymphotoxin; syphilis [lues] test

L-T3 L-triiodothyronine

L-T4 L-thyroxine

lt left; light; low tension

LTA leukotriene A; lipoate transacetylase; lipotechoic acid; local tracheal anesthesia; long-term archives; lost-time accident

L-TAP Lipid Treatment Assessment Project

LTAS lead tetra-acetate Schiff

LTB larparoscopic tubal banding; laryngotracheobronchitis; leukotriene B

LTC large transformed cell; leukotriene C; lidocaine tissue concentration; long-term care; lysed tumor cell

L1TC level 1 trauma center

LTCF long-term care facility

LTCIC, LTC-IC long-term culture-initiating cell

LTCS low transverse cervical section

LTD Laron-type dwarfism; leukotriene D; long-term disability

LTE laryngotracheoesophageal; leukotriene E

LT-ECG long-term electrocardiography

LTF lactotransferrin; lateral tegmental field; lipotropic factor; lymphocyte-transforming factor

LTFU lost to follow-up

LTG lamotrigine; long-term goal; long-term survivor; low-tension glaucoma

LTH lactogenic hormone; local tumor hyperthermia; low temperature holding; luteotropic hormone

LTI lupus-type inclusions

LTK laser thermokeratoplasty; leukocyte tyrosine kinase

lt lat left lateral

LTM long-term memory

LTN lateral telangiectatic nevus

LTNP long-term non-progressor

LTO₂ long-term oxygen therapy

LTOT long-term oxygen therapy

LTP Learning Technologies Project; leukocyte thromboplastin; lipid transfer protein; long-term potentiation; L-tryptophan

LTPP lipothiamide pyrophosphate

LTR location transactivating region; long terminal repeat

LTRA long-term repopulating ability

LTS laboratory tests; long-term survival; long-term survivor

LTST low-temperature stabilization technology

LTT lactose tolerance test; leucine tolerance test; limited treadmill test; lymphocyte transformation test

LTV lung thermal volume

LTW Leydig-cell tumor in Wistar rat

LU left upper [limb]; loudness unit; Lupron; lytic unit

Lu lutetium

L&U lower and upper

LUC large unstained cell; luciferase

LUE left upper extremity

LUF luteinized unruptured follicle

LUFS luteinized unruptured follicle syndrome

LUL left upper eyelid; left upper limb; left upper lobe; left upper lung

lumb lumbar

LUMD lowest usual maintenance dose

LUMO lowest unoccupied molecular orbital

LUMPS liver unit management protocol system

LUO left ureteral orifice

LUOQ left upper outer quadrant

LUP left ureteropelvic

LUPV left upper pulmonary vein

LUQ left upper quadrant

LURD living unrelated donor

LUS laparoscopic ultrasound; lower uterine segment

LUSB left upper scapular border; left upper sternal border

LUT look-up table

LUTO lower urinary tract obstruction

LUV large unilamellar vesicle

LUZ left upper zone

LV laryngeal vestibule; lateral ventricle; lecithovitellin; left ventricle, left ventricular; leucovorin; leukemia virus; live vaccine; live virus; low voltage; low volume; lumbar vertebra; lung volume

Lv brightness or luminance

lv leave

LVA left ventricular aneurysm; left vertebral artery

LVAD left ventricular assist device

LVAS left ventricular assist system

LVBP left ventricular bypass pump

LVC low-viscosity cement

LVCS low vertical cesarean section

LVD left ventricular dysfunction

LVDd left ventricular dimension in end-diastole

LVDI left ventricular dimension

LVDP left ventricular developed pressure; left ventricular diastolic pressure

LVDT linear variable differential transformer

LVDV left ventricular diastolic volume

LVE left ventricular ejection; left ventricular enlargement

LVED left ventricular end-diastole

LVEDA left ventricular end-diastolic area

LVEDC left ventricular end-diastolic circumference

LVEDD left ventricular end-diastolic diameter

LVEDP left ventricular end-diastolic pressure

LVEDV left ventricular end-diastolic volume

LVEF left ventricular ejection fraction

LVEJT left ventricular ejection time

LVEP left ventricular end-diastolic pressure

LVESD left ventricular end-systolic dimension

LVESV left ventricular end-systolic volume

LVET left ventricular ejection time; low volume eye test

LVETI left ventricular ejection time index

LVF left ventricular failure; left ventricular function; left visual field; low-voltage fast; low-voltage foci

LVFP left ventricular filling pressure

LVH large vessel hematocrit; left ventricular hypertrophy

LVI left ventricular insufficiency; left ventricular ischemia

LVID left ventricular internal dimension

LVIV left ventricular infarct volume

LVL left vastus lateralis

LVLG left ventrolateral gluteal

LVM left ventricular mass

LVMF left ventricular minute flow

LVN lateral ventricular nerve; lateral vestibular nucleus; Licensed Visiting Nurse; Licensed Vocational Nurse

LVO left ventricle outflow

LVOH left ventricle outflow [tract] height

LVOT left ventricular outflow tract

LVOTO left ventricular outflow tract obstruction

LVP large volume parenteral [infusion]; left ventricular pressure; levator veli palatini; lysine-vasopressin

LVPFR left ventricular peak filling rate

LVP$_{max}$ maximum left ventricular pressure

LVP$_{min}$ minimum left ventricular pressure

LVPW left ventricular posterior wall

LVQ learning vector quantization

LVR loviride

LVRS lung volume reduction surgery

LVS laryngovideostroboscopy; left ventricular strain

LVSEMI left ventricular subendocardial ischemia

LVSI left ventricular systolic index

LVSO left ventricular systolic output

LVSP left ventricular systolic pressure

LVST lateral vestibulospinal tract

LVSV left ventricular stroke volume

LVSW left ventricular stroke work

LVSWI left ventricular stroke work index

LVT left ventricular tension; levetirazecam; lysine vasotonin

LVV left ventricular volume; Le Veen valve; live varicella vaccine; live varicella virus

LVW left ventricular wall; left ventricular work

LVWI left ventricular work index

LVWM left ventricular wall motion

LVWT left ventricular wall thickness

LW lacerating wound; lateral wall; Lee-White [method]

L&W, L/W living and well

Lw lawrencium

LWA low weight for age

LWBS leaving [hospital] without being seen

LWCT Lee-White clotting time

LWK large white kidney

LWP lateral wall pressure

LWS Lowry-Wood syndrome

LX local irradiation; lower extremity

Lx latex

lx larynx; lower extremity; lux

L-XRF L x-ray fluorescence

LXT left exotopia

LY lactoalbumin and yeastolate [medium]; lymphocyte

Ly a T-cell antigen used for grouping T-lymphocytes into different classes

LYDMA lymphocyte-detected membrane antigen

LYES liver yang exuberance syndrome

LYG lymphomatoid granulomatosis

lym, lymph lymphocyte, lymphocytic

LyNeF lytic nephritic factor

lyo lyophilized

LYP lactose, yeast, and peptone [agar]; lower yield point

LYS, Lys lysine; lysodren; lytes electrolytes

LySLk lymphoma syndrome leukemia

Lyso-PC lysophosphatidyl phosphatidylcholine

LYZ lysozyme

LZM, Lzm lysozyme

M blood factor in the MNS blood group system; chin [Lat. *mentum*]; concentration in moles per liter; death [Lat. *mors*]; dullness [of sound] [Lat. *mutitas*]; macerate; macroglobulin; macroscopic magnetization vector; magnetization; magnification; male; malignant; married; masculine; mass; massage; maternal contribution; matrix; mature; maximum; mean; meatus; median; mediator; medical, medicine; medium; mega; megohm; membrane; memory; mental; mesial; metabolite; metanephrine; metastases; meter; methionine; methotrexate; *Micrococcus*; *Microspora*; minim; minute; mitochondria; mitosis; mix, mixed, mixture; mobility, molar [permanent tooth]; molar [solution]; molarity; mole; molecular; moment of force; monkey; monocyte; month; morgan; morphine; mother; motile; mouse; mucoid [colony]; mucous; multipara; murmur [cardiac]; muscle; muscular response to an electrical stimulation of its motor nerve [wave]; *Mycobacterium*; *Mycoplasma*; myeloma or macroglobulinemia [component]; myopia; strength of pole; thousand [Lat. mille]

M-I first meiotic metaphase

M₁ mitral component [first heart sound]; mitral first [sound]; myeloblast; slight dullness

1M, 2M, 3M, 4M, 5M first, second, third, fourth, fifth metatarsal [head]

M-II second meiotic metaphase

M₂ dose per square meter of body surface; marked dullness; promyelocyte

2-M 2-microglobulin

M₃ absolute dullness; myelocyte at the 3rd stage of maturation

3-M [syndrome] initials for Miller, McKusick, and Malvaux, who first described the syndrome

M/3 middle third

M₄ myelocyte at the 4th stage of maturation

M₅ metamyelocyte

M₆ band form in the 6th stage of myelocyte maturation

M₇ polymorphonuclear neutrophil

M/10 tenth molar solution

M/100 hundredth molar solution

m electron rest mass; electromagnetic moment; magnetic moment; magnetic quantum number; male; mass; median; melting [temperature]; metastable; meter; milli-; minim; minimum; minute; molality; molar [deciduous tooth]; mutated

m² square meter

m³ cubic meter

m₈ spin quantum number

μ see mu

MA malignant arrhythmia; management and administration; mandelic acid; Martin-Albright [syndrome]; masseter; Master of Arts; maternal age; maximum amplitude; mean arterial; mechanical activity; medial amygdaloid [nucleus]; medical assistance; medical audit; medical authorization; mega-ampere; megaloblastic anemia; megestrol acetate; membrane antigen; menstrual age; mental age; mentum anterior [fetal position]; metatarsus adductus; meter-angle; methacrylic acid; microadenoma; microagglutination; microaneurysm; microscopic agglutination; Miller-Abbott [tube]; milliampere; mitochondrial antibody; mitogen activation; mitotic apparatus; mixed agglutination; moderately advanced; monoamine; monoarthritis; monoclonal antibody; movement artifacts; moving average; multiple action; muscle activity; mutagenic activity; myelinated axon

M/A male, altered [animal]; mood and/or affect

MA-104 embryonic rhesus monkey kidney cells

MA-111 embryonic rabbit kidney cells

MA-163 human embryonic thymus cells

MA-184 newborn human foreskin cells

Ma mass of atom

mA, ma milliampere; meter-angle

mÅ milliångström

ma milliampere

MAA macroaggregated albumin; Medical Assistance for the Aged; melanoma-associated antigen; microphthalmia (or anophthalmos) with associated anomalies; moderate aplastic anemia; monoarticular arthritis

MAAC maximum allowable actual charges

MAACL Multiple Affect Adjective Check List

MAAGB Medical Artists Association of Great Britain

MAAP multiple arbitrary amplicon profiling

MAAS Multicenter Anti-Atherosclerosis Study; Multicenter Anti-Atheroma Study

MAB, MAb monoclonal antibody

mAB monoclonal antibody

m-AB m-aminobenzamide

MABIS Munich and Berlin Infarction Study

MABP mean arterial blood pressure

Mabs, mABs, mAbs monoclonal antibodies

MAC MacConkey [broth]; magnetic authentication code; major ambulatory category; malignancy-associated changes; maximum allowable concentration; maximum aerobic capacity; maximum allowable cost; medical alert center; membrane attack complex; midarm circumference; minimum alveolar concentration; minimum antibiotic concentration; mitral anular calcium; modulator of adenylate cyclase; monitored anesthesia care; multiaccess catheter; *Mycobacterium avium* complex

MACAS Marburg Cardiomyopathy Study

MACDP Metropolitan Atlanta Congenital Defects Program

MACE main adverse coronary event; Mayo Asymptomatic Carotid Endarterectomy [trial]

macer maceration

MACH machine activity [UMLS]; Mortality Assessment in Congestive Heart Failure [study]

mAChR muscarinic acetylcholine receptor

MACR mean axillary count rate

macro macrocyte, macrocytic; macroscopic

MACS maximum aortic cusp separation; Multicenter Acquired Immunodeficiency Syndrome (AIDS) Cohort Study; myristoylated alanine-rich protein kinase C

MACTAR McMaster-Toronto arthritis and rehumatism [questionnaire]

MAD major affective disorder; mandibuloacral dysplasia; maximum allowable dose; mean axis direction; median absolute deviation; methylandrostenediol; mind-altering drug; minimum average dose; mitotic arrest defective; mucosal atomization device; myoadenylate deaminase

mAD, MADA muscle adenylate deaminase; myoadenylate deaminase

MADAM Moexipril as Antihypertensive Drug after Menopause [study]

MadCAM mucosal address in cell adhesion molecule

MADD Mothers Against Drunk Driving; multiple acyl-CoA dehydrogenase deficiency

MADDS monoacetyldiaminodiphenylsulfone

MADGE microliter array diagonal gel electrophoresis

MADIT Multicenter Automatic Defibrillator Implantation Trial

MADIT/CES Multicenter Automatic Defibrillator Implantation Trial Cost/Effectiveness Study

MADPA Medicaid Antidiscriminatory Drug Pricing and Patient Benefit Restoration Act

MADRS Medicare Automated Data Retrieval System; Montgomery Asberg Depression Rating Scale

MADT morphology alteration and disintegration test

MADU methylaminodeoxyuridine

MAE mean absolute error; medical air evacuation; moves all extremities; multilingual aphasia examination

MAF macrophage activation factor; macrophage agglutinating factor; maximum atrial fragmentation; minimum audible field; mouse amniotic fluid

MAFD manic affective disorder

MAFF Ministry of Agriculture, Fisheries and Food [UK]

MAFH macroaggregated ferrous hydroxide

MAFI Medic Alert Foundation International

MAG multi-tumor aberrant growth; myelin-associated glycoprotein

Mag magnesium

mag, magn large [Lat. *magnus*]; magnification

mag cit magnesium citrate
MAGF male accessory gland fluid
MAggF macrophage agglutination factor
MAGIC Magnesium in Cardiac Arrest [trial]; Magnesium in Coronaries [trial]; microprobe analysis generalized intensity correction; mouth (or mucosal) and genital ulceration with inflamed cartilage [syndrome]
MAGICA Magnesium in Cardiac Arrhythmia [trial]
MAGP microfibril-associated glycoprotein
MAGPIE Magnesium Sulfate Compared with Placebo in Pre-Eclampsia [study]
MAGUK membrane-associated guanylate kinase
mAH, mA-h milliampere-hours
MAHA microangiopathic hemolytic anemia
MAHH malignancy-associated humoral hypercalcemia
MAHIV, MAHIV medically acquired human immunodeficiency virus [HIV]
MAHST Multicenter Austrian Hemodilution Stroke Trial
MAI microscopic aggregation index; movement assessment of infants; multilevel assessment instrument; *Mycobacterium avium* infection; *Mycobacterium avium intracellulare*
MAIDS mouse acquired immunodeficiency syndrome
MAIESTRO The Michael Reese Hospital–Institute of Technology Expert System for Stroke
MAIN medication-induced, autoimmune, infectious, and neoplastic [diseases associated with antiphospholipid antibodies]
MAJIC Mayo Japan Investigation on Chronic Total Occlusion
MAKA major karyotypic abnormality
MAL midaxillary line
Mal malate; malfunction; malignancy
mal malaise; male; malposition
Mal-BSA maleated bovine serum albumin
MALDI matrix-assisted laser desorption/ionization
MALG Minnesota antilymphoblast globulin
MALiMET Master List of Medical Indexing Terms

MALT male, altered [animal]; mucosa-associated lymphoid tissue; Munich Alcoholism Test
MALTOMA mucosal associated lymphoid tissue lymphoma
MAM metabolically active mass; methylazoxymethanol
mam milliampere-minute; myriameter
M+Am compound myopic astigmatism
6-MAM monoacetyl-morphine
MAMA medical application multimedia authoring; monoclonal anti-malignin antibody
MAM Ac methylazoxymethanol acetate
MAMC mean arm muscle circumference
mA-min, ma-min milliampere-minute
Mammo mammogram, mammography
MAN metropolitan area network
MAN, Man mannose
MAN-6-P mannose-6-phosphate
man manipulate
MANA mannosidase alpha
MANB mannosidase beta
mand mandible, mandibular
MANET mobile ad-hoc network
manifest manifestation
manip manipulation
MANOVA multivariate analysis of variance
MANU manufactured object [UMLS]
MAO Master of the Art of Obstetrics; maximal acid output; monoamine oxidase
MAOA monoamine oxidase A
MAOB monoamine oxidase B
MAOI monoamine oxidase inhibitor
MAOUSSC Model of Assistance and Orientation of a User within a System of Coding
MAP malignant atrophic papulosis; mandibular angle plane; maturation-activated protein; maximal aerobic power; *maximum-a-posteriori;* mean airway pressure; mean aortic pressure; mean arterial pressure; Medical Audit Program; megaloblastic anemia of pregnancy; memory algorithm processor; mercapturic acid pathway; methyl acceptor protein; methylacetoxy-progesterone; methylaminopurine; microtubule-associated protein; minimum audible pressure; mitogen-activated protein; moment angle plotter; monophasic action potential; motor [nerve] action potential;

mouse antibody production; muscle action potential

MAPA muscle adenosine phosphoric acid

MAPC migrating action potential complex

MAPCA major aorto-pulmonary collateral artery

MAPE mean absolute percentage error

MAPF microatomized protein food

MAPHY Metoprolol Atherosclerosis Prevention in Hypertension [study]

MAPI microbial alkaline protease inhibitor; Millon Adolescent Personality Inventory

MAPK mitogen-activated protein kinase

MAPPET Management Strategy and Prognosis of Pulmonary Embolism Trial

MAPREC mutant analysis by polymerase chain reaction and restriction enzyme cleavage

MAPS Make a Picture Story [test]; Micro-AIDS Processing System; Multidimensional Affect and Pain Survey; Multivessel Angioplasty Prognosis Study

MAPT microtubule-associated protein tau

MAPV mean area-peak value

MAR main admissions room; marasmus; marrow; maximal aggregation ratio; medication administration record; minimal angle resolution; mixed antiglobulin reaction; multiple aberration region; multivariate autoregressive [model]

mar margin; marker [chromosome]

MARC machine-readable catalog; machine-readable cataloging; Multicenter Asthma Research Collaboration; multifocal and recurrent choroidopathy

MARCKS myristoylated alanine-rich protein C kinase substrate

MARIAC Magnetic Resonance Image Analysis Research Centre [UK]

MARS magnetic anchor retinal stimulation; medical archival system; methionyl-transfer ribonucleic acid synthetase; mobile autonomous robot software; Monitored Atherosclerosis Regression Study; mouse antirat serum

MARSA methicillin-aminoglycoside-resistant *Staphylococcus aureus*

MART multiplicative algebraic reconstruction technique

mar(X) marker X [chromosome]

MAS macrophage activation syndrome; magic angle spinning; Manifest Anxiety Scale; marker-assisted selection; maximum average score; McCune-Albright syndrome; meconium aspiration syndrome; medical advisory service; medical audit study; mesoatrial shunt; milk-alkali syndrome; milliampere-second; minor axis shortening; mobile arm support; monoclonal antibodies; Morgagni-Adams-Stokes [syndrome]; motion analysis system; motor assessment scale; multi-agent system

mA-s, mas milliampere-second

MASA Medical Association of South Africa; mental retardation-aphasia-shuffling gait-adducted thumbs [syndrome]

masc masculine; mass concentration

MASCIS Multicenter Animal Spinal Cord Injury Study

MASER microwave amplification by stimulated emission of radiation

MASH mobile Army surgical hospital; multiple automated sample harvester

MASK Medical Anatomy Segmentation Kit

MASS Medicine, Angioplasty, or Surgery Study

mass massage

massc mass concentration

MAST military antishock trousers; Michigan Alcohol Screening Test; Managing Anticoagulation Services Trial

mast mastectomy; mastoid

MAST-E Multicentre Acute Stroke Trial–Europe

MAST-I Multicenter Acute Stroke Trial–Italy

MASU mobile Army surgical unit

MAT manual arts therapist; master of arts in technology; mean absorption time; medical assistance team (emergency medicine); methionine adenosyltransferase; microagglutination test; multifocal atrial tachycardia; multiple agent therapy

Mat, mat maternal [origin]; mature

MATCH Matching Alcoholism Treatment to Client Heterogeneity

MatD maternal disomy

MatDp maternal duplication

MATE Medicine vs Angiography for Thrombolytic Exclusions [trial]

mat gf maternal grandfather

mat gm maternal grandmother

MATH Modern Approach to Treatment of Hypertension [study]

MATSA Marek-associated tumor-specific antigen

MATTIS Multicenter Aspirin and Ticlopidine Trials after Intracoronary Stenting

MATTUS Minimal Access Therapy Training Unit Scotland

MAU multi-attribute utility [model]

MAUS Mammography Attitudes and Usage Study

MAUT multi-attribute utility theory

MAV mechanical auditory ventricle; minimal alveolar ventilation; minimum apparent viscosity; movement arm vector; myeloblastosis-associated virus

MAVD mixed aortic valve disease

MAVERIC Midlands Trial of Empirical Amiodarone vs Electrophysiological Guided Intervention and Cardioverter Implant in Ventricular Arrhythmias

MAVIS mobile artery and vein imaging system

MAVR mitral and aortic valve replacement

max maxilla, maxillary; maximum

MaxEP maximum esophageal pressure

MB Bachelor of Medicine [Lat. *Medicinae Baccalaureus*]; buccal margin; General Modeling Bayesian Fitting [program]; isoenzyme of creatine kinase containing M and B subunits; mammillary body; Marsh-Bender [factor]; maximum breathing; medulloblastoma; megabyte; mesiobuccal; methyl bromide; methylene blue; microbiological assay; muscle balance; myocardial band

Mb megabase; megabit; million bases; mouse brain; myoglobin

mb millibar

MBA methylbenzyl alcohol; methyl bovine albumin

MBAC Member of the British Association of Chemists

MBAR myocardial beta adrenergic receptor

mbar millibar

MBAS methylene blue active substance

MBB modified barbiturate buffer

MBBG metabromobenzylguanidine

MBBS British doctoral degree

MBC male breast cancer; maximal bladder capacity; maximal breathing capacity; memory B cell; metastatic breast cancer; methyl-1-(butylcarbamoyl)-2-benzimidazole-carbamate; methylthymol blue complex; microcrystalline bovine collagen; minimum bactericidal concentration; moving blood cells

MB-CK creatine kinase isoenzyme containing M and B subunits

MBCL monocytoid B-cell lymphoma

MbCO carbon monoxide myoglobin

MBD Marchiafava-Bignami disease; Mental Deterioration Battery; methylene blue dye; minimal brain damage; minimal brain dysfunction; Morquio-Brailsford disease

MBDG mesiobuccal developmental groove

MBF medullary blood flow; mesenteric blood flow; muscle blood flow; myocardial blood flow

MBFC medial brachial fascial compartment

MBFLB monaural bifrequency loudness balance

MBG Marburg [disease], mean blood glucose; morphine-benzedrine group [scale]

MBH medial basal hypothalamus

MBH$_2$ reduced methylene blue

MBHI Millon Behavioral Health Inventory

MBHO managed behavioral healthcare organization

MBI Maslach Burnout Inventory; maximum blink index

MBK methyl butyl ketone

MBL Marine Biological Laboratory; menstrual blood loss; minimum bactericidal level

MBLA methylbenzyl linoleic acid; mouse-specific bone-marrow-derived lymphocyte antigen

MBM mineral basal medium

MBNOA Member of the British Naturopathic and Osteopathic Association

MBO management by objective; mesiobucco-occlusal

MBO$_2$ oxymyoglobin

MBP major basic protein; maltose-binding protein; management by policy; mannose-binding protein; mean blood pressure; melitensis, bovine, porcine [antigen from *Brucella bovis, B. melitensis,* and *B. suis*]; mesiobuccopulpal; myelin basic protein

MBPM modified backward Prony method [spectral analysis of heart sounds]

MBPS multigated blood pool scanning

Mbps megabits per second; myeloblastic syndrome

MBq megabecquerel

MBR methylene blue, reduced

MBRT methylene blue reduction time

MBS Martin-Bell syndrome

MBSA methylated bovine serum albumin

MBT mercaptobenzothiazole; mixed bacterial toxin; myeloblastin

MBTA modeling better treatment advice

MBTE meningeal tick-borne encephalitis

MBTH 3-methyl-2-benzothiazoline hydrazone

MBTI Myers-Briggs type indicator

MBVT Munich and Berlin Trial for Sustained Ventricular Tachyarrhythmias

MC mass casualties; mast cell; Master of Surgery [Lat. *Magister Chirurgiae*]; maximum concentration; Medical Corps; medium chain; medullary cavity; medullary cyst; megacoulomb; melanocortin; melanoma cell; menstrual cycle; Merkel cell; mesiocervical; mesocaval; metacarpal; methyl cellulose; microcephaly; microcirculation; microscopic colitis; midcapillary; mineralocorticoid; mini-catheterization; minimal change; mitomycin C; mitotic cycle; mitral commissurotomy; mixed cellularity; mixed cryoglobulinemia; monkey cell; mononuclear cell; mucous cell; myocardial channeling; myocarditis

M/C male, castrated [animal]

M-C mineralocorticoid

M&C morphine and cocaine

Mc megacurie; megacycle

M$_c$ mitral closure

mC millicoulomb

mc millicurie

MCA major coronary artery; Maternity Center Association; medical care administration; methylcholanthrene; microchannel architecture; middle cerebral artery; monoclonal antibody; multichannel analyzer; multiple congenital anomaly

MCAB monoclonal antibody

MCAD medium chain acyl-CoA dehydrogenase

MCAF monocyte chemotactic and activating factor

MCA/MR multiple congenital anomaly/mental retardation [syndrome]

MCAO middle cerebral artery occlusion

MCAR mixed cell agglutination reaction

MCARE managed care

MCAS middle cerebral artery syndrome

MCAT medical college admission test; middle cerebral artery thrombosis; Multimedia Cardiac Angiogram Tool

MCB membranous cytoplasmic body; monochlorobimane

McB McBurney [point]

mCBF mean cerebral blood flow

MCBIT Munich Coronary Bypass Intervention Trial

MCBM muscle capillary basement membrane

MCBR minimum concentration of bilirubin

MCBS Medicare Current Beneficiary Survey [database]

MCBV minimum conditional bias/variance

MCC mean corpuscular hemoglobin concentration; measles control campaign; medial cell column; Medical Council of Canada; medical information communication controller; metacarpal-carpal [joints]; metacerebral cell; metastatic cord compression; microcalcification cluster; microcrystalline collagen; midstream clean catch [urine]; minimum complete-killing concentration; mucocutaneous candidiasis; mutated in colorectal cancer [gene]

MC-C metacarpo-carpal [joint]

MCCA Medicare Catastrophic Care Act; Medicare Catastrophic Coverage Act

MCCD minimum cumulative cardiotoxic dose

MCCI medical care component of the consumer price index; medical cost control initiative

MCCPI medical care component of the consumer price index

MCCU mobile coronary care unit

MCD magnetic circular dichroism; mast-cell degranulation; mean cell diameter; mean of consecutive differences; mean corpuscular diameter; Medicaid competition demonstration; medical concepts dictionary; medullary collecting duct; medullary cystic disease; metacarpal cortical density;

minimal cerebral dysfunction; minimal change disease; multiple carboxylase deficiency; muscle carnitine deficiency

MCDI Minnesota Child Development Inventory

MCDK multicystic dysplastic kidney

MCDNP medullary cystic disease/nephrolithiasis disease

MCDU mercaptolactate-cysteine disulfiduria

MCE medical care evaluation; military clinical engineering; multicystic encephalopathy; multiple cartilaginous exostosis; myocardial contrast echocardiography

MCES medical care evaluation study; multiple cholesterol emboli syndrome

MCF macrophage chemotactic factor; median cleft face; medium corpuscular fragility; method conversion factor; microcomplement fixation; mononuclear cell factor; myocardial contraction force

MCFA medium-chain fatty acid; miniature centrifugal fast analyzer

MCFP mean circulating filling pressure

MCG magnetocardiogram; membrane coating granule; monoclonal gammopathy

mcg microgram

MCGC metacerebral giant cell

MCGF mast cell growth factor

MCH medical college hospital; melanin-concentrating hormone

MCGN mesangiocapillary glomerulonephritis; minimal change glomerulonephritis; mixed cryoglobulinemia with glomerulonephritis; multiple cutaneous leiomyomata; myeloid cell leukemia

MCGNX mesangiocapillary glumerulonephritis, X-linked

MCH Maternal and Child Health; mean corpuscular hemoglobin; muscle contraction headache

MCh Master of Surgery [Lat. *Magister Chirurgiae*]; methacholine

mc-h, mch millicurie-hour

MCHB maternal and child health bureau

MCHC maternal/child health care; mean corpuscular hemoglobin concentration; mean corpuscular hemoglobin count

MChD Master of Dental Surgery

MCHgb mean corpuscular hemoglobin

MChir Master in Surgery [Lat. *Magister Chirurgiae*]

MChOrth Master of Orthopaedic Surgery

MChOtol Master of Otology

MCHR Medical Committee for Human Rights

mc-hr millicurie-hour

MCHS Maternal and Child Health Service

MCI mean cardiac index; methicillin; molecular connectivity index; mucociliary insufficiency; multiple casualty incident; muscle contraction interference

MCi megacurie

mCi millicurie

MCICU medical coronary intensive care unit

MCID minimum clinically important difference

M-CIDI Münich Composite International Diagnostic Interview

MCi-hr millicurie-hour

MCINS minimal change idiopathic nephrotic syndrome

MCK multicystic kidney

MCKD multicystic kidney disease

MCL maximum containment laboratory; medial collateral ligament; midclavicular line; midcostal line; minimal change lesion; mixed culture, leukocyte; modified chest lead; most comfortable loudness; multiple cutaneous leiomyomata; myeloid cell leukemia

MCLNS, MCLS mucocutaneous lymph node syndrome

MCISci Master of Clinical Science

MCM medical core metadata; methylmalonic coenzyme A mutase; minimum capacitation medium; multi-chip module; multicompartmental model

MCMC Markov Chain Monte Carlo [method]

MCMI Millon Clinical Multiaxial Inventory

MCMV murine cytomegalovirus

MCN maternal child nursing; minimal change nephropathy; mixed cell nodular [lymphoma]

MCNS minimal change nephrotic syndrome

MCO managed care organization; medical care organization; multicystic ovary

MCommH Master of Community Health

mcoul millicoulomb

MCOV modified covariance

MCP maximum closure pressure; maximum contraction pattern; malanocortin receptor; medical command physician; melphalan, cyclophosphamide, and prednisone; membrane cofactor protein; metacarpophalangeal; metoclopramide; mitotic-control protein; monocyte chemotactic protein; mucin clot prevention

MCP-1 monocyte chemotactic protein-1

MCPA Member of the College of Pathologists, Australasia

MCPH metacarpophalangeal

MCPJ metacarpophalangeal joint

MCPP metacarpophalangeal pattern profile; metacarpophalangeal profile; metachlorophenylpiperazine

MCPPP metacarpophalangeal pattern profile plot

MCPS Member of the College of Physicians and Surgeons

Mcps megacycles per second

MCQ multiple-choice question

MCR Medical Corps Reserve; melanocortin receptor; message competition ratio; metabolic clearance rate; myotonia congenita, recessive type

MCRA Member of the College of Radiologists, Australasia

MCRE mother-child relationship evaluation

MCRglc cerebral metabolic rate for glucose

MCRI Multifactorial Cardiac Risk Index

MCS malignant carcinoid syndrome; managed care system; massage of the carotid sinus; Meharry Cohort Study; mesocaval shunt; method of constant stimuli; methylcholanthrene [induced] sarcoma; microculture and sensitivity; Miles-Carpenter syndrome; Minnesota Coronary Survey; moisture-control system; multicenter study; multiple chemical sensitivity; multiple combined sclerosis; myocardial contraction state

MC & S microscopy, culture, and sensitivity

mc/s megacycles per second

MCSA Moloney cell surface antigen

MCSD minimum clinically significant difference

MCSDS Marlowe-Crowne Social Desirability Scale

MCSDT Minnesota Coronary Survey Dietary Trial

MCSF, (M)-CSF macrophage colony-stimulating factor

MCSP Member of the Chartered Society of Physiotherapists

mCSP melanoma-specific chondroitin sulfate proteoglycan

MCSPG melanoma-specific chondroitin sulfate proteoglycan

McSPI Multicenter Study of Perioperative Ischemia

MCSW male commercial sex worker

MCT manual cervical traction; mean cell thickness; mean cell threshold; mean circulation time; mean corpuscular thickness; medial canthal tendon; medium-chain triglyceride; medullary carcinoma of thyroid; medullary collecting tubule; microtoxicity test; multiple compressed tablet

MCTC metrizamide computed tomography cisternography

MCTD mixed connective tissue disease

MCTF mononuclear cell tissue factor

MCU malaria control unit; maximum care unit; micturating cystourethrography; motor cortex unit

MCUG micturating cystogram

MCV mean cell volume; mean clinical value; mean contour value; mean corpuscular volume; measles-containing vaccine; median cell volume; molluscum contagiosum virus; motor conduction velocity

MCx main circumflex [artery]

MD Doctor of Medicine [Lat. *Medicinae Doctor*]; magnesium deficiency; main duct; maintenance dose; major depression; malate dehydrogenase; malignant disease; malrotation of duodenum; manic-depressive; Mantoux diameter; Marek disease; maternal deprivation; maximum dose; mean deviation; Meckel diverticulum; mediastinal disease; medical department; Medical Design [brace]; mediodorsal; medium dosage; mendelian dominant gene; Ménière disease; Menkes disease; mental deficiency; mental depression; mesiodistal; Miller-Dieker [syndrome]; Minamata disease; minimum dose; mitral disease, mixed diet; moderate disability; molecular diagnostics; monocular deprivation; movement disorder; multiple deficiency; muscular dystrophy; mutual information; myelo-dysplasia; myocardial damage; myocardial disease; myotonic dystrophy

Md mendelevium

md median

MDA malondialdehyde; manual dilation of anus; methylene dianiline; 3,4-methyl-enedioxyamphetamine; minimal deviation adenocarcinoma; monodehydroascorbate; motor discriminative acuity; multivariant discriminant analysis; right mentoanterior [fetal position] [Lat. *mento-dextra anterior*]

MDa megadalton

MDAD mineral dust airway disease

MDAP Machover Draw-A-Person [test]

MDB medulloblastoma

MDBDF March of Dimes Birth Defect Foundation

MDBK Madin-Darby bovine kidney [cell]

MDC macrophage-derived chemokine; major diagnostic categories; Metoprolol in Dilated Cardiomyopathy [trial]; minimum detectable concentration; monocyte-de-pleted mononuclear cell; Multicenter Dilated Cardiomyopathy [trial]

MDCK Madin-Darby canine kidney

MDCR Miller-Dieker [syndrome] chromosome region

MDD major depressive disorder; mean daily dose; medical data dictionary; monitored drug dictionary

MDDC monocyte-derived dendritic cell

MDDL medical device data language

MDDS Malmö Diet and Disease Study; medical diagnostic decision support [system]

MDE major depressive episode; minimum defibrillation energy; molecular distance edge

MDEBP mean daily erect blood pressure

MDentSc Master of Dental Science

MDEV medical device [UMLS]

MDF mean dominant frequency; myocardial depressant factor

MDFA multiple developmental field anomalies

MDFD map-dot-fingerprint dystrophy

MDG mean diastolic gradient; methyl-adenine deoxyribonucleic acid glycosylase

MDGF macrophage-derived growth factor

MDH malate dehydrogenase; medullary dorsal horn

MDHR maximum determined heart rate

MDHV Marek disease herpesvirus

MDI manic-depressive illness; metered dose inhaler; Michelson Doppler imager; multiple daily injection; multiple document interface; multiple dosage insulin; Multiscore Depression Inventory

MDIA multidimensional interaction analysis

MDI-A metered-dose inhaler with aero-chamber

MDI-DED metered-dose inhaler with delivery enhancement device

MDIPT Multicenter Diltiazem Postinfarction Trial

MDIS medical diagnostic imaging support; medical diagnostic imaging system

MDIT mean disintegration time

MDK midkine

MDL minimum description length; minimum detection limit

MDLIS molecular diagnostic laboratory information system

MDLS Miller-Dieker lissencephaly syndrome

MDM medical decision making; mid-diastolic murmur; minor determinant mix [penicillin]; monocyte-derived macrophage

MDMA methylenedioxymethamphetamine

MD-MPH Doctor of Medicine–Master of Public Health [combined degree in medicine and public health]

MDMU medical devices for military use

mdn median

MDNB mean daily nitrogen balance; meta-dinitrobenzene

MDNCF monocyte-derived neutrophil chemotactic factor

MDO minimum detectable object

MDOPA, mdopa methyldopa

MDP manic-depressive psychosis; maximum diastolic potential; maximum digital pulse; methylene diphosphate; microsomal dipeptidase; muramyldipeptide; muscular dystrophy, progressive; right mentoposterior [fetal position] [Lat. *mento-dextra posterior*]

MDPD maximum daily permissible dose

MD-PhD combined degree in medicine and science

MDPK myotonic dystrophy protein kinase

MDQ memory deviation quotient; Menstrual Distress Questionnaire; minimum detectable quantity

MDR median duration of response; medical device reporting; minimum daily requirement; multidrug resistance

mdr multidrug resistance

MDRD Modification of Diet in Renal Disease [study]

MDRS Mattis Dementia Rating Scale

MDR-TB multidrug-resistant tuberculosis

MDS Master of Dental Surgery; maternal deprivation syndrome; medical data screening; medical data source; medical data system; mesonephric duct system; microdilution system; milk drinker's syndrome; Miller-Dieker syndrome; minimum data set; monophasic damped sine; Mood Disorders Service [database]; multidimensional scaling; myelodysplastic syndrome; myocardial depressant substance

MDS+ minimum data set (plus)

MDSBP mean daily supine blood pressure

MDS-HC ACP minimum data set home care assessment clients protocol

MDSO mentally disturbed sex offender

MDSS medical decision support system

MDT mast [cell] degeneration test; mean dissolution time; median detection threshold; multidisciplinary team; multidrug therapy; right mentotransverse [fetal position] [Lat. *mento-dextra transversa*]

MDTP multidisciplinary treatment plan

MDTR mean diameter-thickness ratio

MDUO myocardial disease of unknown origin

MDV Marek disease virus; mean dye [bolus] velocity; mucosal disease virus; multidose vial

MDW monophasic defibrillation waveform

MDX Medical Internet Exchange

MDY month, date, year

Mdyn megadyne

ME macular edema; malic enzyme; manic episode; maximum effort; maximum entropy; median eminence; medical education; medical examiner; meningoencephalitis; mercaptoethanol; metabolic energy; metabolic equivalent; metabolism; metamyelocyte; microembolism; microenvironment; middle ear; mouse embryo; mouse epithelial [cell]; muscle examination; myalgic encephalomyelitis; myo-electric; myoepithelial

M/E myeloid/erythroid [ratio]

M+E, M&E monitoring and evaluation

2-ME 2-mercaptoethanol

Me menton; methyl

MEA male-enhanced antigen; Medical Exhibition Association; mercaptoethylamine; monoethanolamine; multiple endocrine adenomatosis

3MeA 3-methyladenine

MEA-I multiple endocrine adenomatosis type I

mEAD monophasic action potential early afterdepolarization

MEADOW Method Alternative: Distal Occlusion and Wash-out in Saphenous Vein Graft [study]

MEANS modular electrocardiogram analysis system

meas measurement

MEAP multiphasic environmental assessment procedure

MEB Medical Evaluation Board; muscle-eye-brain [disease]

MeB methylene blue

ME-BH medial eminence of basal hypothalamus

MEBS muscle-eye-brain syndrome

MeBSA methylated bovine serum albumin

MEC median effective concentration; middle ear canal; middle ear cell; minimum effective concentration; mobile examination center

mec meconium

MeCCNU methylchloroethylcyclohexylnitrosourea [semustine]

MECG mixed essential cryoglobulinemia

MECP methyl-CpG-binding protein

MECTA mobile electroconvulsive therapy apparatus

MECY methotrexate and cyclophosphamide

MED median erythrocyte diameter; medical, medication, medicine; medical electronic desktop; Medical Entities Dictionary; minimum effective dose; minimum erythema dose; multiple epiphyseal dysplasia

med medial; median; medication; medicine, medical; medium

MEDAC multiple endocrine deficiency, Addison's disease, and candidiasis [syndrome]

MED-ART Medical Automated Records Technology

MEDAS medical emergency decision assistant system

MedDRA medical dictionary of drug regulatory activities

MEDEVAC, Medevac medical evacuation

MEDEX, Medex extension of physician [Fr. *médicin extension*]

medic military medical corpsman [Lat. *medicus*]

Medi-Cal Medicaid in California

MEDICO Medical International Cooperation

MED-IDDM multiple epiphyseal dysplasia-insulin dependent diabetes mellitus [syndrome]

MEDIGATE Medical Examination Direct Iconic and Graphic Augmented Test Entry

MEDIHC Military Experience Directed Into Health Careers

MedIndEx medical indexing expert

MEDINFO medical informatics

MEDIPP medical district initiated planning program

MEDIPRO medical district-initiated peer review organization

MEDIX medical data interchange

MED-LAN medical center with local area network

MEDLARS Medical Literature Analysis and Retrieval System [NLM information system]

MedLEE Medical Language Extraction and Encoding [system]

MEDLINE MEDLARS Online

MEDPAR medical provider analysis and review

MEdREP Medical Education Reinforcement and Enrichment Program

MEDRIS Medical Records Interface or Input System

MEDS minimum emergency data set

meds medications

MEDScD Doctor of Medical Science

MEDSTATS Medical Statistics Expert System

Med-surg medicine and surgery

MEDSYNDIKATE Synthesis of Distributed Knowledge Acquired from Medical Text

Med Tech medical technology, medical technologist

MED-TEP Medical Treatment Effectiveness Program

MEDTUTOR microcomputer-based tutorial [for MEDLARS]

MEE measured energy expenditure; methylethyl ether; middle ear effusion; multilocus enzyme electrophoresis

MEES medical element engineering and simulation

MEF maximal expiratory flow; middle ear fluid; midexpiratory flow; migration enhancement factor; mouse embryo fibroblast

MEF$_{50}$ mean maximal expiratory flow

MEFR maximal expiratory flow rate

MEFV maximal expiratory flow volume

MEG magnetoencephalogram, magneto-encephalography; megakaryocyte; Megestrol; mercaptoethylguanidine; multifocal eosinophilic granuloma

MeG methylguanine

meg megacycle; megakaryocyte; megaloblast

Meg-CSA megakaryocyte colony-stimulating activity

MEGD minimal euthyroid Graves disease

mEGF mouse epidermal growth factor

Megs maternally expressed genes

MEGX monoethylglycinexylidide

MEHP Metoprolol in Elderly Hypertensive Patients [study]

MEI master encounter index; Medicare economic index

MEII minimum essential information infrastructure

MEK methylethylketone

MEL metabolic equivalent level; mouse erythroleukemia

mel melena; melanoma

MELAS mitochondrial encephalomyopathy-lactic acidosis- and stroke-like symptoms [syndrome]

MEL B melarsoprol

MELC murine erythroleukemia cell

mel-CSPG melanoma-specific chondroitin sulfate proteoglycan

MELODHY Metoprolol Low Dose in Hypertension [study]

MEM macrophage electrophoretic mobility; malic enzyme, minimal Eagle medium; mitochondrial; minimal essential medium

memb membrane, membranous

MEME Metathesaurus Enhancement and Maintenance Environment [UMLS]

MEM-FBS minimal essential medium with fetal bovine serum

MEMR multiple exostoses-mental retardation [syndrome]

MEN meningitis; multiple endocrine neoplasia

men meningeal; meningitis; meniscus; menstruation

MEND Medical Education for National Defense

MEN-I multiple endocrine neoplasia, type I

MENT maximum entropy [algorithm]

ment mental, mentality

MENTOR Medtronic Wiktor Hepamed Stent Trial

MEO malignant external otitis

5-MeODMT 5-methoxy-N,N-dimethyl-tryptamine

MeOH methyl alcohol

MEOS microsomal ethanol oxidizing system

MEP maximum expiratory pressure; mean effective pressure; mepiridine; mitochondrial encephalopathy; motor end-plate; motor evoked potential

mep meperidine

6-MeP 6-mercaptopurine

MEPC miniature end-plate current

6-MeP-dR 6-mercaptopurine deoxyriboside

MEPP miniature end-plate potential

mEQ, mEq, meq milliequivalent

mEq/l milliequivalents per liter

MER mean ejection rate; medical emergency room; methanol extraction residue; murmur/energy ratio

MERB Medical Examination and Review Board

MERCATOR Multicenter European Research Trial with Cilazapril after Angioplasty to Prevent Transluminal Coronary Obstruction and Restenosis

MERG macular electroretinogram

MERIT Medical Records, Images, Texts Information Exchange

MERIT-HF Metoprolol Controlled-release Randomised Intervention Trial in Heart Failure

MERRF myoclonus epilepsy with ragged red fibers [syndrome]

MERRLA myoclonus epilepsy-ragged red fibers-lactic acidosis [syndrome]

MERS Multiagency Electronic Regulatory Submission

MES maintenance electrolyte solution; maximal electroshock; maximal electroshock seizures; Minitran Efficacy Study; myoelectric signal; multiple endocrine syndrome

Mes mesencephalon, mesencephalic

MESA Marshfield Epidemiologic Study Area; myoepithelial sialadenitis

Mesc mescaline

MESCH Multi-Environment Scheme

MESF molecules of equivalent soluble fluorochrome

MeSH Medical Subject Headings

MESNA [sodium 2-]mercaptoethanesulfonate

MESOR midline estimating statistic of rhythm

MesPGN mesangial proliferative glomerulonephritis

MESS mangled extremity severity score

MEST Medical Equipment Technical Society

MESV murine embryonic stem-cell virus

MET maximal exercise test; metabolic equivalent of the task; metastasis, metastatic; methionine; midexpiratory time; modality examination terminal; multistage exercise test

Met methionine

met metallic [chest sounds]

META medical editors trial accounting; medical editors trial amnesty

metab metabolic, metabolism

metas metastasis, metastatic

Met-Enk methionine-enkephalin

METEOR managing end-to-end operations

METH methicillin

Meth methedrine

meth methyl

Met-Hb methemoglobin

MeTHF methyltetrahydrofolic acid

MetMb metmyoglobin

METR miniature electronic temperature recorder

METS metabolic equivalents [of oxygen consumption]

mets metastases

METT maximum exercise tolerance test

MEU maximum expected utility

MEV maximum exercise ventilation; mevalonate; minimal excursionary ventilation; murine erythroblastosis virus

MeV, mev megaelectron volts

MEWD, MEWDS multiple evanescent white dot [syndrome]

MEXIS Metoprolol and Xamoterol Infarction Study

MF magnetic field; mean field; meat free; medium frequency; megafarad; membrane filler; merthiolate-formaldehyde [solution]; metacarpal fusion; microfibril; microfilament; microflocculation; microscopic factor; mid frequency; midcavity forceps; mitochondrial fragments; mitogenic factor; mitomycin-fluorouracil; mitotic figure; mucosal fluid; multifactorial; multiplication factor; mutation frequency; mycosis fungoides; myelin figure; myelofibrosis; myocardial fibrosis; myofibrillar

M&F male and female; mother and father

M:F, M/F male.female [ratio]

Mf maxillofrontale

mF millifarad

mf microfilaria

MFA master of fine arts [degree]; mean field annealing [imaging]; monofluoroacetate; multifocal functional autonomy; multiple factor analysis

MFAQ multidimensional functional assessment questionnaire

MFAT multifocal atrial tachycardia

MFB medial forebrain bundle; metallic foreign body

MFC mean fluorescence channel; medical follow-up clinic; minimal fungicidal concentration

MFCM Master, Faculty of Community Medicine

MFCV muscle fiber conduction velocity

MFD mandibulofacial dysostosis; midforceps delivery; milk-free diet; minimum fatal dose; multiple fractions per day

mfd microfarad

MFG minimum-distance frontal gyrus

MFH malignant fibrous histiocytoma

MFHom Member of the Faculty of Homeopathy

MFI male factor infertility; multi-facility integration

MFID multielectrode flame ionization detector

MFL myofibril

m flac membrana flaccida [Lat.]

MFLOPS, Mflops megaflops [million floating points per second]

MFO medium frequency oscillator; mixed function oxidase

MFOM Master, Faculty of Occupational Medicine

MFP monofluorophosphate; myofascial pain

MFPR multifetal pregnancy reduction

MFR mean flow rate; mucus flow rate

MFS Marfan syndrome; Medicare fee schedule

MFSS Medical Field Service School

MFST Medical Field Service Technician

MFT multifocal atrial tachycardia; muscle function test

MFUN molecular function [UMLS]

MFUS Manitoba Follow-up Study

MFV maximal flow-volume [loop]

MFW multiple fragment wounds

MG maintenance goal; Marcus Gunn [pupil]; margin, mean gradient; medial gastrocnemius [muscle]; membranous glomerulonephritis; menopausal gonadotropin; mesiogingival; methylglucoside; methylguanidine; monoclonal gammopathy; monoglyceride; mucous granule; muscle group; myasthenia gravis; myoglobin

Mg magnesium

M3G morphine-3-glucuronide

m^{7G} 7-methylguanosine

mg milligram

MGA master of general administration; medical gas analyzer; melengestrol acetate; 3-methylglutaconicaciduria

MgATP magnesium adenosine triphosphate

mγ milligamma

MGB medial geniculate body; myoglobin

MGBG methylglyoxal-bis-(guanylhydrazone)

MGC medical genetics center; medical genetics clinic; megacolon; minimal glomerular change

MgC magnocellular neuroendocrine cell

MGCE multifocal giant cell encephalitis

MGCN megalocornea

MGCR meningioma chromosome region

MGCRB Medicare Geographic Classification Review Board

MGD maximal glucose disposal; mixed gonadal dysgenesis; Mouse Genome Database

mg/dl milligrams per deciliter

MGDS Member in General Dental Surgery

MGEIR Mouse Gene Expression Information Resource

MGES multiple gated equilibrium scintigraphy

MGF macrophage growth factor; maternal grandfather

MGG May-Grünwald-Giemsa [staining]; molecular and general genetics; mouse gammaglobulin; multinucleated giant cell

MGGH methylglyoxal guanylhydrazone

MGH Massachusetts General Hospital

mgh milligram-hour

MGI magnetically guided intubation

mg/kg milligrams per kilogram

MGL minor glomerular lesion

Mgl myoglobin

mg/l milligrams per liter

MGM maternal grandmother; meningioma

mgm milligram

MGMA Medical Group Management Association

MGMT methylguanine-deoxyribonucleic acid methyltransferase

MGN medial geniculate nucleus; membranous glomerulonephritis

MGP marginal granulocyte pool; marginating granulocyte pool; membranous glomerulonephropathy; mucin glycoprotein

MGPS hereditary giant platelet syndrome

MGR modified gain ratio; multiple gas rebreathing

mgr milligram

MGS metric gravitational system

MGSA malignant growth stimulatory activity

MGT multiple glomus tumors

MGUS monoclonal gammopathies of undetermined significance

MGW magnesium sulfate, glycerin, and water

mGy milligray

MH malignant histiocytosis; malignant hyperpyrexia; malignant hypertension; malignant hyperthermia; mammotropic hormone; mannoheptulose; marital history; medial hypothalamus; medical history; melanophore-stimulating hormone; menstrual history; mental health; mental hygiene; moist heat; monosymptomatic hypochondriasis; murine hepatitis; mutant hybrid; *Mycobacterium haemophilum;* myohyoid

mH millihenry

MHA major histocompatibility antigen; May-Hegglin anomaly; Mental Health Association; methemalbumin; microangiopathic hemolytic anemia; microhemagglutination; middle hepatic artery; mixed hemadsorption; Mueller-Hinton agar

MHAM multiple hamartoma

MHAQ modified health assessment questionnaire

M-HART Montreal Heart Attack Readjustment Trial

MHA-TP microhemagglutination-*Treponema pallidum*

MHB maximum hospital benefit; Mueller-Hinton base

MHb methemoglobin; myohemoglobin

MHBSS modified Hank balanced salt solution

MHC major histocompatibility complex; mental health care

MHCS Mental Hygiene Consultation Service

MHCU mental health care unit

MHD maintenance hemodialysis; mean hemolytic dose; mental health department; minimum hemolytic dilution; minimum hemolytic dose

MHDP methylene hydroxydiphosphonate

MHDPS Mental Health Demographic Profile System

M-HEART Multi-Hospital Eastern Atlantic Restenosis Trial

MHFT Munich Mild Heart Failure Trial

MHG metropolitan health group

mHg millimeter of mercury

MHHP Minnesota Heart Health Program

MHHS Minnesota Heart Health Survey

MHI malignant histiocytosis of intestine; Mental Health Index; Mental Health Inventory; minor head injury

MHIQ McMaster health index questionnaire

MHL medial hypothalamic lesion

MHLC Multidimensional Health Locus of Control
MHLS metabolic heat load stimulator
MHN massive hepatic necrosis; Mohs hardness number; morbus hemolyticus neonatorum
MHO microsomal heme oxygenase
mho reciprocal ohm, siemens unit [ohm spelled backwards]
MHP hemiplegic migraine; maternal health program; maternal health program; medical center health plan; 1-mercuri-2-hydroxypropane; metropolitan health plan; monosymptomatic hypochondriacal psychosis; multi-skilled health practitioner
MHPA mild hyperphenylalaninemia
MHPG 3-methoxy-4-hydroxyphenyl-glycol
MHR major histocompatibility region; malignant hyperthermia resistance; maternal heart rate; maximal heart rate; methemoglobin reductase
MHRI Mental Health Research Institute
MHS major histocompatibility system; malignant hyperthermia in swine; malignant hyperthermia syndrome; malignant hypothermia susceptibility; Milan hypertensive [rat]; Minnesota Heart Survey; modified hybrid sign; multiple health screening; multihospital system
MHSA microaggregated human serum albumin
MHSS Military Health Services System
MHT mixed hemagglutination test
MIITS Multiphasic Health Testing Services
MHV magnetic heart vector; middle hepatic vein; mouse hepatitis virus
MHW mental health worker
MHx medical history
MHyg Master of Hygiene
MHz megahertz
MI first meiotic metaphase; magnetic-guided intubation; maturation index; medical illustrator; medical informatics; medical inspection; melanophore index; menstruation induction; mental illness; mental institution; mercaptoimidazole; mesioincisal; metabolic index; microinvasion; migration index; migration inhibition; mild irritant; minimally invasive; mitotic index; mitral incompetence; mitral insufficiency; mononucleosis infectiosa; morphology index; motility index; myocardial infarction; myocardial ischemia; myoinositol
mi mile
MIA Medical Library Association; missing in action
MIAMI Metoprolol in Acute Myocardial Infarction [study]
MIAS Mammographic Image Analysis Society
MIAs multi-institutional arrangements; medically indigent adults
MIB management information base; Medical Impairment Bureau; Medical Information Bureau; minimally invasive biopsy
MIBI methoxyisobutyl isonitrile
MIBG metaiodobenzylguanidine
MIBiol Member of the Institute of Biology
MIBI 2-methoxy-2-methylpropyl isonitrile
MIBK methylisobutyl ketone
MIBT methyl isatin-beta-thiosemicarbazone
MIC maternal and infant care; mean inhibitory concentration; medical intensive care; Medical Interfraternity Conference; microscopy, minimal inhibitory concentration; minimal isorrheic concentration; minocycline; model immune complex; mononuclear inflammatory cell, morphologic, immunologic and cytogenic
MICAB minimally invasive coronary artery bypass surgery
MICAM maturation index for colostrum and mature milk
MICC mitogen-induced cellular cytotoxicity
MICCAI medical image analysis, computer-assisted intervention, medical robotics, and visualization
MICG macromolecular insoluble cold globulin
MICN mobile intensive care nursing
MICOL Multicenter Italian Study of Cholesterol
MICR methacholine inhalation challenge response
MICRA Medical Injury Compensation Reform Act
MICRO Medical Information Collecting Robot
micro microcyte, microcytic; microscopic
microbiol microbiology
microCi microcurie

microg microgram

MICRO-HOPE Microalbuminuria, Cardiovascular and Renal Outcomes–Heart Outcomes Prevention Evaluation

MICS Myocardial Infarction Cost Study

MICT mobile intensive care technician

MICU medical intensive care unit; mobile intensive care unit

MICUP management of intensive care unit and patients minimum

MID maximum inhibiting dilution; mesio-incisodistal; midinfarct dementia; minimum infective dose; minimum inhibitory dose; minimum irradiation dose; multi-infarct dementia; multiple indicator dilution; multiple ion detection

MIDA myocardial ischemia dynamic analysis

mid middle

MIDAS medical image display and analysis system; Medical Information Data Analysis System; microphthalmia-dermal aplasia-sclerocornea [syndrome]; Multi-center Isradipine Diuretic Atherosclerosis Study; Myocardial Infarction Data Acquisition System [study]

MIDCAB minimally invasive direct coronary artery bypass [surgery]

MIDI musical instrument digital interface

MIDS Management Information Decision System

midsag midsagittal

MIDSPAN Middle-aged Span-of-Life Study

MIEMIS model for investment and evaluation of medical information system

MIF macrophage inhibitory factor; melanocyte[-stimulating hormone]-inhibiting factor; maximum inspiratory flow or force; merthiolate-iodine-formaldehyde [method]; microimmunofluorescence; midinspiratory flow; midline interhemispheric fusion; migration-inhibiting factor; mixed immunofluorescence; müllerian inhibiting factor

MIFC merthiolate-iodine-formaldehyde concentration

MIFR maximal inspiratory flow rate

MIFT microphthalmia-associated transcription factor

MIG measles immune globulin; Medicare Insured Groups; Mitochondria Interest Group

MIg malaria immunoglobulin; measles immunoglobulin; membrane immunoglobulin

mIg membrane-anchored immunoglobulin [Ig]

mIgM membrane-anchored immunoglobulin M [IdM]

MIGT multiple inert gas elimination technique

MIH Master of Industrial Health; migraine with interval headache; minimal intermittent heparin [dose]

MIHA minor histocompatibility antigen

MII second meiotic metaphase

MIKA minor karyotype abnormalities

MIKE mass-analyzed ion kinetic energy

MILESTONE Multicenter Iloprost European Study on Endangeitis

MILIS Multicenter Investigation of the Limitations of Infarct Size

MILP mitogen-induced lymphocyte proliferation

MILS medication information leaflet for seniors

MILT medical laboratory technician

MILT-AD medical laboratory technician–associate degree

MILT-C medical laboratory technician–certificate

MIM Mendelian Inheritance in Man; Multilateral Initiative in Malaria

MIME multipurpose Internet mail extension

MIMOSA medical image management in an open system architecture

MIMR minimal inhibitor mole ratio

MIMS medical information management system; medical inventory management system; Migraine and Myocardial Ischemia Study

MIN medial interlaminar nucleus; medical information network

min mineral; minim; minimum, minimal; minor; minute

MINA monoisonitrosoacetone

MINIA monkey intranuclear inclusion agent

MINT Myocardial Infarction with Novastan and Tissue Plasminogen Activator Study

MIO minimum identifiable odor; modular input/output

MiO microorchidism
MIOP magnetic iron oxide particle
MIP macrophage inflammatory protein; major intrinsic protein; maximum inspiratory pressure; maximum intensity projection; mean incubation period; mean intravascular pressure; middle interphalangeal [joint]; minimal inspiratory pressure; minimally invasive procedure
MIPA macrophage inflammatory protein alpha
MIPB macrophage inflammatory protein beta
MIPO minimally invasive plate osteosynthesis
MIPP maximum intensity pixel projection
MIPS mean index procedure sum; millions of instructions per second
MIR multiple isomorphous replacement
MIRACL myocardial ischemia reduction with aggressive cholesterol lowering
MIRC microtubuloreticular complex
MIRD medical internal radiation dose
MIRMO Medical Information Resources Management Office
MIRP myocardial infarction rehabilitation program
MIRRACLE Myocardial Infarction Risk Recognition and Conversion of Life-threatening Events into Survival [trial]
MIRS mean index resuscitation sum
MIRSA Multicenter International Randomized Study of Angina Pectoris
MIRU myocardial infarction research unit
MIS management information system; manager of information system; medical information service; medical information system; meiosis-inducing substance; minimally invasive surgery; motor index score; müllerian inhibiting substance
MiSAD Milan Study on Atherosclerosis and Diabetes
MISC multi-interface sensor controlled
misc miscarriage; miscellaneous
MISCHF management to improve survival in congestive heart failure
MISG modified immune serum globulin
MISHAP microcephalus-imperforate anus-syndactyly-hamartoblastoma-abnormal lung lobulation-polydactyly [syndrome]
MISI multiple input single input
MISJ Medical Instrument Society of Japan

MISNES Multicenter Italian Study on Neonatal Electrocardiography [ECG] and Sudden Infant Death Syndrome
MISS medical image sharing system; Medical Interview Satisfaction Scale; minimally invasive spinal surgery; Modified Injury Severity Scale
MIST Management of Influenza in the Southern Hemisphere Trials; Medical Information Service by Telephone; Mibefradil Ischemia Suppression Trial; Multicenter Isradipine Salt Trial
MIT Massachusetts Institute of Technology; male impotence test; marrow iron turnover; melodic intonation therapy; metabolism inhibition test; miracidial immobilization test; mitomycin; monoiodotyrosine
mit mitral
MITF microphthalmia associated with transcription factor
MITI myocardial infarction triage and intervention
MITIS Modular Integrated Transplant Information System
MITO mitomycin
Mito C mitomycin C
MITRA Maximal Individual Therapy in Acute Myocardial Infarction
MITT Myers introduction to type
mIU milli-international unit; one-thousandth of an international unit
MIVD mobile interactive videodisk
mix, mixt mixture
MJ Machado-Joseph [disease]; marijuana; megajoule
mJ, mj millijoule
MJA mechanical joint apparatus
MJAD Machado-Joseph Azorean disease
MJD Machado-Joseph disease; Mseleni joint disease
MJI Moral Judgment Interview
MJRT maximum junctional recovery time
MJT Mead Johnson tube
MK megakaryocyte; monkey kidney; myokinase
Mk monkey
mkat millikatal
mkat/l millikatals per liter
MKB megakaryoblast
MKC monkey kidney cell
MKF MEDLINE Knowledge Finder

m-kg meter-kilogram

MKHS Menkes' kinky hair syndrome

MkK monkey kidney

MkL megakaryoblastic leukemia

MKMD Molecular Knowledge of Metabolic Diseases [database]

MKP monobasic potassium phosphate

MKS, mks meter-kilogram-second

MKSAP medical knowledge self-assessment program

MKT mean kinetic temperature

MKTC monkey kidney tissue culture

MKV killed measles vaccine

ML Licentiate in Medicine; Licentiate in Midwifery; malignant lymphoma; marked latency; maximum likelihood; medial leminiscus; median load; medio-lateral; mesiolingual; middle lobe; midline; molecular layer; motor latency; mucolipidosis; multiple lentiginosis; muscular layer; myeloid leukemia

ML I, II, III, IV mucolipidosis I, II, III, IV

M/L monocyte/lymphocyte [ratio]

M-L Martin-Lewis [medium]

mL millilambert, milliliter

ml milliliter

MLA left mentoanterior [fetal position] [Lat. *mento-laeva anterior*]; Medical Library Association; mesiolabial; monocytic leukemia, acute

mLa millilambert

MLAA Medical Library Assistance Act

MLAB Multilingual Aphasia Battery

MLAEB middle latency auditory evoked potential

MLAEP middle latency auditory evoked potential

MLaI mesiolabioincisal

MLAP mean left atrial pressure

MLaP mesiolabiopulpal

MLB micro-laryngobronchoscopy; monoaural loudness balance

MLb macrolymphoblast

MLBP mechanical low back pain

MLBW moderately low birthweight

MLC minimum lethal concentration; mixed leukocyte culture; mixed ligand chelate; mixed lymphocyte concentration; mixed lymphocyte culture; morphine-like compound; multilamellar cytosome; multileaf collimator; myelomonocytic leukemia, chronic; myosin light chain

MLCCHF Multicenter Lisinopril Captopril Congestive Heart Failure [study]

MLCK myosin light chain kinase

MLCN multilocular cystic nephroma

MLCO Member of the London College of Osteopathy

MLCP myosin light-chain phosphatase

MLCQ Modified Learning Climate Questionnaire

MLCT metal-to-ligand charge transfer

MLD manual lymph drainage; mean luminal diameter; median lethal dose; metachromatic leukodystrophy; minimal lesion disease; minimal luminal diameter; minimum lethal dose

MLD$_{50}$ median lethal dose

ml/dl milliliters per deciliter

MLE maximum likelihood estimation

MLEL malignant lymphoepithelial lesion

MLF medial longitudinal fasciculus; morphine-like factor

MLG mesiolingual groove; mitochondrial lipid glycogen

MLGN minimal lesion glomerulonephritis

ML-H malignant lymphoma, histiocytic

MLI mesiolinguoincisal; mixed lymphocyte interaction

MLL mixed lineage leukemia; multi-level logistic

ml/l milliliters per liter

MLLT1 mixed lineage leukemia translocated to 1

MLLT2 mixed lineage leukemia translocated to 2

MLM map of local minima; medical logic module

MLN manifest latent nystagmus; membranous lupus nephropathy; mesenteric lymph node; motilin

MLNS minimal lesion nephrotic syndrome; mucocutaneous lymph node syndrome

MLO medio-lateral oblique; mesiolinguoocclusal; *Mycoplasma*-like organism

MLP left mentoposterior [fetal position] [Lat. *mento-laeva posterior*]; match list position; medical language processing; mesiolinguopulpal; microsomal lipoprotein; midlevel practitioner

ML-PDL malignant lymphoma, poorly differentiated lymphocytic

MLR mean length response; middle latency response; mineralocorticoid receptor;

mixed lymphocyte reaction; multiple linear regression

MLRD microgastria-limb reduction defects [association]

MLS maximum likelihood estimator; mean lifespan; median life span; median longitudinal section; microphthalmia–linear skin defects [syndrome]; middle lobe syndrome; mouse leukemia virus; myelomonocytic leukemia, subacute

MLSB migrating long spike burst

MLSI multiple line scan imaging

MLT left mentotransverse [fetal position] [Lat. *mento-laeva transversa*]; mean latency time; median lethal time; Medical Laboratory Technician

MLT-AD medical laboratory technician-associate degree

MLT(ASCP) Medical Laboratory Technician certified by the American Society of Clinical Pathologists

MLTC mixed leukocyte-trophoblast culture; mixed lymphocyte tumor cell

MLT-C medical laboratory technician certificate

MLTI mixed lymphocyte target interaction

MLU mean length of utterance

MLV Moloney leukemia virus; multilaminar vesicle; murine leukemia virus

MLVAR amphotropic receptor for murine leukemia virus

MLVDP maximum left ventricular developed pressure

mlx millilux

MM macromolecule; Maëlzels metronome; major medical [insurance]; malignant melanoma; manubrium to malleus; Marshall-Marchetti; Master of Management; mathematical morphology; medial malleolus; mediastinal mass; medical management; megamitochondria; melanoma metastasis; meningococcal meningitis; menstrually-related migraine; metastatic melanoma; methadone maintenance; minimal medium; mismatched; molecular mechanics; morbidity and mortality; mucous membrane; multiple model; multiple myeloma; muscularis mucosae; myeloid metaplasia; myelomeningocele

M&M morbidity and mortality

mM millimolar; millimole; mini-MED-LINE [database]

mm methylmalonyl; millimeter; mucous membrane; muscles

mm² square millimeter

mm³ cubic millimeter

MMA mastitis-metritis-agalactia [syndrome]; medical management analysis; medical materials account; methylmalonic acid; middle meningeal artery; minor morphologic aberration; monomethyladenosine

MMAA mini-microaggregates of albumin

MMAD mass median aerodynamic diameter

MMAP mean maternal arterial blood pressure

MMAS modified motor assessment scale

MMATP methadone maintenance and aftercare treatment program

MMC Materials Microcharacterization Collaboratory; mechanical myocardial channeling; migrating myoelectric complex; minimum medullary concentration; mitomycin C; mucosal mast cell

MMCO Medicaid managed care organization

MMD mass median diameter; minimum morbidostatic dose; moyamoya disease; myotonic muscular dystrophy

MMDB Molecular Modeling Database [NLM]

MME mini mental examination; M-mode echocardiography; mobile medical equipment; mouse mammary epithelium

MMED Master of Medicine

MMEF maximum midexpiratory flow

MMEFR maximum midexpiratory flow rate

MMEP microcephaly–microphthalmia–electrodactyly–prognathism [syndrome]

MMF maxillomandibular fixation; maximum midexpiratory flow; mean maximum flow; Member of the Medical Faculty

MMFR maximum midexpiratory flow rate; maximal midflow rate

MMFV maximum midrespiratory flow volume

MMG mean maternal glucose

MMH monomethylhydrazine

mmHg millimeters of mercury

mmH₂O millimeters of water

MMI macrophage migration inhibition; maximum medical improvement; methylmercaptoimidazole; mucous membrane irritation

MMIF macrophage migration inhibitory factor

MMIH megacystis-microcolon-intestinal hypoperistalsis [syndrome]

MMIHS megacystis-microcolon-intestinal hypoperistalsis syndrome

MMIRG Multicenter Myocardial Ischemia Research Group

MMIS Medicaid management information system

MML medical markup language; Moloney murine leukemia; monomethyllysine; myelomonocytic leukemia

mM/l millimoles per liter

MMLV Moloney murine leukemia virus

MMM see 3-M [syndrome]; microsome-mediated mutagenesis; myelofibrosis with myeloid metaplasia; myelosclerosis with myeloid metaplasia

MMMF man-made mineral fibers

MMMM megalocornea–macrocephaly–motor and mental retardation [syndrome]

MMMSE Modified Mini-Mental Status Exam

MMMT malignant mixed müllerian tumor

MMN morbus maculosus neonatorum; multiple mucosal neuroma

MMNC marrow mononuclear cell

MMNCB multifocal motor neuropathy with conduction block

MMNN multi-modular neural network

MMO methane monooxygenase

MMOA maxillary mandibular odontectomy alveolectomy

M-mode motion mode

MMoL myelomonoblastic leukemia

mmol millimole

mmol/l millimoles per liter

MMP matrix metalloproteinase; muscle mechanical power

MMPI matrix metalloproteinase inhibitor; Minnesota Multiphasic Personality Inventory

MMPNC Medical Maternal Program for Nuclear Casualties

mmpp millimeters partial pressure

MMPR methylmercaptopurine riboside

MMPS Medicare Mortality Predictor System

MMR mass miniature radiography; masseter muscle rigidity; maternal mortality rate; measles-mumps-rubella [vaccine]; megalocornea-mental retardation [syndrome];

mild mental retardation; mobile mass x-ray; mono-methylorutin; myocardial metabolic rate

MMRB mouth-to-mouth rescue breathing

MMS mass mammographic screening; Master of Medical Science; methyl methane sulfonate; Mini-Mental State

MMSA Master of Midwifery, Society of Apothecaries

MMSc Master of Medical Science

MMSE mini-mental status examination

mm/sec millimeters per second

MMSP malignant melanoma of soft parts

mm st muscle strength

MMT alpha-methyl-m-tyrosine; manual muscle test; microcephaly–mesobrachy-dactyly–tracheoesophageal fistula [syndrome]; mouse mammary tumor

MMTA methylmetatyramine

MMTP methadone maintenance treatment program

MMTT Multicenter Myocarditis Treatment Trial

MMTV mouse mammary tumor virus

MMU medical maintenance unit; mercaptomethyl uracil

mmu millimass unit

mμ millimicron

mμc millimicrocurie

mμg millimicrogram

MMuLV Moloney murine leukemia virus

mμs millimicrosecond

μmμ meson

MMV mandatory minute ventilation; mandatory minute volume

MMVD mixed mitral valve disease

MMWR Morbidity and Mortality Weekly Report

MN a blood group in the MNSs blood group system; malignant nephrosclerosis; Master of Nursing; meganewton; melena neonatorum; melanocytic nevus; membranous nephropathy; membranous neuropathy; mesenteric node; metanephrine; midnight; mononuclear; motor neuron; multinodular; myoneural

M&N morning and night

Mn manganese

mN micronewton; millinormal

mn modal number

MNA maximum noise area

MNAP mixed nerve action potential; multineuron acquisition processor

MNB mannosidase beta; murine neuroblastoma

5-MNBA 5-mercapto-2-nitrobenzoic acid

MNBCCS multiple nevoid basal-cell carcinoma syndrome

MNC mononuclear cell

MNCV median nerve conduction velocity; motor nerve conduction velocity

MND minimum necrosing dose; minor neurological dysfunction; modified neck dissection; motor neuron disease

MNER multichannel neural ensemble recording

MNG/CRD/DA multinodular goiter/cystic renal disease/digital anomalies [syndrome]

mng morning

MNGIE myo-, neuro-, gastrointestinal encephalopathy

MNJ myoneural junction

MNK Menkes syndrome

MNL marked neutrophilic leukocytosis; maximum number of lamellae; mononuclear leukocyte

MN/m² meganewtons per square meter

MNMS myonephropathic metabolic syndrome

MNNG N-methyl N'-nitro-N-nitrosoguanidine

MNP mononuclear phagocyte

MNR marrow neutrophil reserve

MNS medial nuclear stratum; Melnick-Needles syndrome; Milan normotensive [rat]; moesin

Mn-SOD manganese-superoxide dismutase

MNSs a blood group system consisting of groups M, N, and MN

MNU N-methyl-N-nitrosourea

MO macroorchidism; manually operated; Master of Obstetrics; Master of Osteopathy; medical officer; mesio-occlusal; metastases, zero; mineral oil; minute output; modelling object; molecular orbital; mono-oxygenase; month; morbid obesity

MO₂ myocardial oxygen [utilization]

Mo Moloney [strain]; molybdenum; monoclonal

M₀ mitral opening

mo mode; month; morgan

MOA monoamine oxidase

MoA mechanism of action

MoAb monoclonal antibody

MOANS Mayo's Older Americans Normative Studies

MOB mobility [scale]

mob, mobil mobility, mobilization

MOBS Moebius syndrome

MOC maximum oxygen consumption; multiple ocular coloboma

MOCHA Multicenter Oral Carvedilol in Heart Failure Assessment

MOD magnetic optic disk; maturity onset diabetes; Medical Officer of the Day; mesio-occlusodistal

mod moderate, moderation; modification

MODED microcephaly-oculo-digito-esophageal-duodenal [syndrome]

MODEM modulator-demodulator

modem modulator/demodulator

MOD/F multiple organ dysfunction/failure

MODM maturity-onset diabetes mellitus

MODS medically oriented data system; multiple-organ dysfunction syndrome

MODY maturity onset diabetes of the young

MOF marine oxidation/fermentation; methotrexate, Oncovin, and fluorouracil; multiple organ failure

MoF moment of force

MOFE multiple organ failure in the elderly

MOFS multiple organ failure syndrome

MOG myelin-oligodendrocyte glycoprotein

MO&G Master of Obstetrics and Gynaecology

MOH Medical Officer of Health; Ministry of Health

MΩ megohm

mΩ milliohm

MOI master object index; maximum oxygen intake; mechanism of injury; multiplicity of infection

MOIVC membranous obstruction of the inferior vena cava

MOL molecular

mol mole, molecular, molecule

molc molar concentration

molfr mole fraction

mol/kg moles per kilogram

mol/l moles per liter

mol/m³ moles per meter cubed

mol/s moles per second
mol wt molecular weight
MOM milk of magnesia; mucoid otitis media
MoM multiples of the median
MOMA methylhydroxymandelic acid
Mo-MLV Moloney murine leukemia virus
MOMO macrosomia-obesity-macrocephaly-ocular abnormalities [syndrome]
MO-MOM mineral oil and milk of magnesia
MOMP major outer membrane protein
MOMS multiple organ malrotation syndrome
Mo-MSV Moloney murine sarcoma virus
MOMX macroorchidism-marker X chromosome [syndrome]
MON Mongolian [gerbil]
MONET multiwavelength optical network
MONICA monitoring trends and determinants in cardiovascular diseases
mono monocyte; mononucleosis
MOOW Medical Officer of the Watch
MOP major organ profile; medical outpatient
8-MOP 8-methoxypsoralen
MOPD microcephalic osteodysplastic primordial dwarfism
MOPFC medial and orbital prefrontal cortex
MOPEG 3-methoxy-4-hydroxyphenylglycol
MOPP mechlorethamine, Oncovin, procarbazine, prednisone
MOPV monovalent oral poliovirus vaccine
Mor, mor morphine
MORAC mixed oligonucleotides primed amplification of complementary deoxyribonucleic acid
MORC Medical Officers Reserve Corps
MORD magnetic optical rotatory dispersion
MORFAN mental retardation–pre- and post-natal overgrowth–remarkable face–acanthosis nigricans [syndrome]
morphol morphology
mort, mortal mortality
MOS mechanism of stroke deducer; medial orbital sulcus; medical outcomes study; microsomal ethanol-oxidizing system; mitral opening snap; Moloney murine sarcoma; myelofibrosis osteosclerosis
mOs milliosmolal

mos mosaic
MOSA Medical Officers of School Association [UK]
MOSES Morbidity and Mortality after Stroke–Eprosartan vs Nitrendipine for Secondary Prevention [study]
MOSF multiple organ system failure
MOSFET metal oxide semiconductor field effect transistor
mOsm milliosmol
mOsm, MOsm milliosmole
mOsm/kg milliosmoles per kilogram
MOST Mode Selection Trial; mother of super twins
MOT mouse ovarian tumor
Mot, mot motor
MOTA Manitoba oculo-tricho-anal [syndrome]
MOTT medical observation type table; mycobacteria other than tuberculosis
MOTSA multiple overlapping thin slab acquisition [technique]
MOU memorandum of understanding
MOUS multiple occurrence of unexplained symptoms
MOV metal-oxide varistor; minimal occlusive volume
MOVC membranous obstruction of inferior vena cava
MOVIES Monongahela Valley Independent Elders Survey
MOX moxalactam
MP macrophage; matrix protein; mean pressure; melphalan and prednisone; melting point; membrane potential; menstrual period; mentum posterior; mercaptopurine; mesial pit; mesiopulpal; metacarpophalangeal; metaphalangeal; metatarsophalangeal; methylphosphonate; methylprednisolone; Mibelli porokeratosis; middle phalanx; moist pack; moment preserving; monophasic; monophosphate; motor potential; mouth piece; mucopolysaccharide; multiparous; multiprogrammable pacemaker; muscle potential; mycoplasmal pneumonia
3-MP 3-mercaptopropionate
6-MP 6-mercaptopurine
8-MP 8-methylpsoralen
mp millipond; melting point
M&P managerial and professional [staff]
MPA master of public administration; mean pulmonary arterial [pressure]; medial

preoptic area; Medical Procurement Agency; medroxyprogesterone acetate; methylprednisolone acetate; microscopic polyarteritis; minor physical anomaly; multiple project assurance

MPa megapascal

M-PACT Mayo-Physician Alliance for Clinical Trials

MPAP mean pulmonary arterial pressure

MPAS mild perioxic acid Schiff [reaction]

M-PATHY Multicenter Pacing Therapy for Hypertrophic Cardiomyopathy; Multicenter Study of Pacing Therapy for Hypertrophic Cardiomyopathy

MPB male pattern baldness; meprobamate

MPC marine protein concentrate; marker for prostatic cancer; maximum permissible concentration; mean plasma concentration; meperidine, promethazine, and chlorpromazine; metallophthalocyanine; metapyrocatechase; minimum mycoplasmacidal concentration

MPCO micropolycystic ovary syndrome

MPCUR maximum permissible concentration of unidentified radionucleotides

MPD main pancreatic duct; maximum permissible dose; mean population doubling; membrane potential difference; minimal perceptible difference; minimal phototoxic dose; multiple personality disorder; myeloproliferative disease; myofascial pain dysfunction

MPDS mandibular pain dysfunction syndrome; medical priority dispatch service; myofascial pain dysfunction syndrome

MPE malignant proliferation of eosinophils; maximum permissible exposure; maximum possible error; Medicaid program evaluation

MPEAK multispeak [speech-coding strategy]

MPEC monopolar electrocoagulation

MPED minimum phototoxic erythema dose

MPEH methylphenylethylhydantoin

MPF maturation promoting factor; mean power frequency; M-phase [mitosis] promoting factor

MPG magnetopneumography; mercaptopropionylglycine; methyl green pyronine; 3-methylpurine deoxyribonucleic acid glycosylase; monthly prescribing guide

MPGM monophosphoglycerate mutase

MPGN membranoproliferative glomerulonephritis

MPGR multiple planar gradient recalled

MPH male pseudohermaphroditism; Master of Public Health; microtiter plate hybridization; milk protein hydrolysate

MPharm Master of Pharmacy

MPHD multiple pituitary hormone deficiencies

mphot milliphot

MPHR maximum predicted heart rate

MPhysA Member of Physiotherapists' Association

MPI mannose phosphate isomerase; master patient index; maximum permitted intake; maximum point of impulse; message-passing interface; multidimensional pain inventory; Multiphasic Personality Inventory; myocardial perfusion imaging

MPI-I/O message passing interface–input/output

MPIP Multicenter Postinfarction Program

MPJ metacarpophalangeal joint

MPKC management problem-knowledge coupler

MPKUCS Maternal Phenylketonuria Collaborative Study

MPL maximum permissible level; melphalan; mesiopulpolingual; myeloproliferative leukemia

MPLa mesiopulpolabial

MPLS multiprotocol label switching

MPLV myeloproliferative leukemia virus

MPM malignant papillary or pleural mesothelioma; medial pterygoid muscle; minor psychiatric morbidity; mortality probability model; multiple primary malignancy; multipurpose meal

MPME (5R,8R)-8-(4-p-methoxy-phenyl)-1-piperazynylmethyl-6-methylergolene

MPMP 10[(1-methyl-3-piperidinyl)-methyl]-1OH-phenothiazine

MPMT Murphy punch maneuver test

MPMV Mason-Pfizer monkey virus

MPN most probable number

MPNST malignant peripheral nerve sheath tumor

MPO maximum power output; minimal perceptible odor; myeloperoxidase

MPOA medial preoptic area

MPOD myeloperoxidase deficiency

MPP massive peritoneal proliferation; massively parallel processor; methyl phenylpyridinium; medical personnel pool; mercaptopyrazide pyrimidine; metacarpophalangeal profile; myelin protein, peripheral

MPPCD Multifactorial Primary Prevention of Cardiovascular Diseases

mppcf millions of particles per cubic foot of air

MPPEC mean peak plasma ethanol concentration

MPPG microphotoelectric plethysmography

MPPH p-tolylphenylhydantoin

MPPN malignant persistent positional nystagmus

MPPT methylprednisolone pulse therapy; mucin-producing pancreatic tumor

MPQ McGill Pain Questionnaire

MPQ-SF McGill Pain Questionnaire–Short Form

MPR mannose 6-phosphate receptor; marrow production rate; massive preretinal retraction; maximum pulse rate; multiplanar reformatting or reconstruction; myeloproliferative reaction

MP-RAGE magnetization-prepared rapid gradient-echo

MPRD cation-dependent mannose 6-phosphate receptor

MPRG Multicenter Postinfarction Research Group

MPRO mental process [UMLS]

MPS meconium plug syndrome; medial premotor system; Member of the Pharmaceutical Society; microbial profile system; mononuclear phagocyte system; Montreal platelet syndrome; movement-produced stimulus; mucopolysaccharide, mucopolysaccharidosis; multiphasic screening; myocardial perfusion scintigraphy; myofascial pain syndrome

m-PSA mutated prostate-specific antigen [PSA]

MPS I mucopolysaccharidosis I

MPS-I-H mucopolysaccharidosis I, Hurler type

MPS-I-S mucopolysaccharidosis I, Scheie type

MPS II mucopolysaccharidosis II

MPS III mucopolysaccharidosis III

MPS IIIA mucopolysaccharidosis III, type A

MPS IIIB mucopolysaccharidosis III, type B

MPS IIIC mucopolysaccharidosis III, type C

MPS IIID mucopolysaccharidosis III, type D

MPS IV mucopolysaccharidosis IV

MPS IVA mucopolysaccharidosis IV, type A

MPS IVB mucopolysaccharidosis IV, type B

MPS V mucopolysaccharidosis V

MPS VI mucopolysaccharidosis VI

MPS-H/I-S mucopolysaccharidosis, Hurler-Scheie type

MPSoSIS mucopolysaccharidosis

MPSS methylprednisolone sodium succinate; Music Performance Stress Survey

MPSV myeloproliferative sarcoma virus

MPsyMed Master of Psychological Medicine

MPT mean peak torque; Michigan Picture Test

MPTP 1-methyl-4-phenyl-1,2,3,6-tetrahydropyridine

MPT-R Michigan Picture Test, Revised

MPU Medical Practitioners Union

MPV main portal vein; mean platelet volume; mitral valve prolapse

MPVP mean pulmonary venous pressure

MPZ myelin protein, zero

mpz millipièce

MQ memory quotient; motor quotient

M-Q move-quality [descriptor]

MQC microbiologic quality control

MQFD medical quality function deployment

MQIS Medicare quality indicator system

MQL Medical Query Language [computer]

MQSPR model-based quantitative structure-property relationship

MR Maddox rods; magnetic resistance; magnetic resonance; mandibular reflex; mannose-resistant; may repeat; measles and rubella; medial raphe; medial rectus [muscle]; medical record; medical release; medium range; megaroentgen; mental retardation; metabolic rate; methemoglobin reductase; methyl red; mineralocorticoid receptor; mitral reflux; mitral regurgitation; modulation rate; mortality rate; mortality ratio; multicentric reticulohistiocytosis; muscle receptor; muscle relaxant; myocardial revascularization

M&R measure and record

M/R measles/rubella [vaccine]

M$_r$ relative molecular mass

mR, mr milliroentgen

m/r mass attenuation coefficient

MRA magnetic resonance angiography; main renal artery; marrow repopulation activity; medical record analysis or analyst; medical records administrator; mesenteric resistance artery; multivariate regression analysis

MRAB machine-readable archives in biomedicine

MRAC model reference adaptive control

mrad millirad

MRAP alpha-2-macroglobulin receptor-associated protein; maximal resting anal pressure; mean right atrial pressure

MRAS main renal artery stenosis

MRB multiply resistant bacteria

MRBC monkey red blood cell; mouse red blood cell

MRBF mean renal blood flow

MRC maximum recycling capacity; Medical Registration Council; Medical Research Council [UK]; Medical Reserve Corps; methylrosaniline chloride

MRCAS medical robotics and computer-assisted surgery

MRC/BHF Medical Research Council, British Heart Foundation Heart Protection Study

MRC CFAS Medical Research Council [UK] Cognitive Function and Ageing Study

MRCNS methicillin-resistant coagulase-negative staphylococci

MRCOA Medical Research Council [UK] Trial in Older Adults

MRCP magnetic resonance cholangio-pancreatography

MRD magnetic resonance diffusion; maximum rate of depolarization; measles-rindenpest-distemper [virus group]; medical records department; minimal reacting dose; minimal renal disease; minimal residual disease

mrd millirutherford

MRDD mentally retarded/developmentally disabled [person]

MRDI medical records document imaging

MRE maximal resistive exercise; maximal respiratory effectiveness

MREI mean rate ejection index

MRFIT Multiple Risk Factor Intervention Trial

mrem millirem

mrep milliroentgen equivalent physical

MRF Markov random field; medical record file; melanocyte-[stimulating hormone]-releasing factor; mesencephalic reticular formation; midbrain reticular formation; mitral regurgitant flow; moderate renal failure; monoclonal rheumatoid factor; müllerian regression factor; muscle regulatory factor

mRF monoclonal rheumatoid factor

MRFC mouse rosette-forming cell

MRFIT Multiple Risk Factor Intervention Trial

MRFT modified rapid fermentation test

MRH melanocyte-stimulating hormone-releasing hormone; multicentric reticulo-histiocytosis

MRHA mannose-resistant hemagglutination

mrhm milliroentgens per hour at one meter

MRI machine-readable identifier; magnetic resonance imaging; medical records information; Medical Research Institute; moderate renal insufficiency

MRIF melanocyte[-stimulating hormone] release-inhibiting factor

MRIH melanocyte[-stimulating hormone] release-inhibiting hormone

MRIPHH Member of the Royal Institute of Public Health and Hygiene

MRISM magnetic resonance imaging simulation

MRK Mayer-Rokitansky-Küster [syndrome]

MR-K mannose-resistant *Klebsiella*-like [hemagglutinin]

MRKH Mayer-Rikitanski-Küster-Hauser [syndrome]

MRL medical records librarian; Medical Research Laboratory

MRM magnetic resonance mammography; modified radical mastectomy

MRMIB Managed Risk Medical Insurance Board

MRMT Minnesota Rate of Manipulation Test

MRN magnetic resonance neurography; malignant renal neoplasm; medical record number

mRNA messenger ribonucleic acid

mRNA/R messenger ribonucleic acid [RNA] receptor

mRNP messenger ribonucleoprotein

MRO master reference oscillator; medical review officer; minimal recognizable odor; muscle receptor organ

MROD Medical Research and Operations Directorate

MRP mean resisting potential; medical reimbursement plan; multidrug resistance-associated protein; mutual recognition process

MR.PET Magnetic Resonance vs Positron Emission Tomography [for detection of myocardial viability] [study]

MRR marrow release rate; maximum relation rate

MRS magnetic resonance spectroscopy; Mania Rating Scale; medical receiving station; medical record summary; Melkersson-Rosenthal syndrome

MRSA methicillin-resistant *Staphylococcus aureus*

MRSD mental retardation-skeletal dysplasia [syndrome]

MRSE methicillin-resistant *Staphylococcus epidermis*

MRSH Member of the Royal Society of Health

MRSI magnetic resonance spectroscopy imaging

MRSX X-linked mental retardation

MRT magnetic resonance tomography; maximum relaxation time; median range score; median reaction time; median recognition threshold; median relapse time; medical records technician; methyltryptophan; milk ring test; muscle response test

MRTS message routing and translation system

MRU mass radiography unit; meningococcal reference unit; minimal reproductive unit; *Mycobacterium* reference unit

MR/UR Medical Review and Utilization Program

MRV minute respiratory volume; mixed respiratory vaccine

MRVI mixed virus respiratory infection

MRVP mean right ventricular pressure; methyl red, Voges-Proskauer [medium]

MRW multi-resolution wavelet

MRX mental retardation, X-linked

MRXA X-linked mental retardation-aphasia syndrome

MRXS mental retardation, X-linked, syndrome

MS Maffuci syndrome; maladjustment score; mandibular series; Marfan syndrome; Marie-Strümpell [syndrome]; mass spectrometry; Master of Science; Master of Surgery; maternal serum; mean square [statistics]; mechanical stimulation; Meckel syndrome; mediastinal shift; medical services; medical staff; medical student; medical supplies; medical survey; Menkes syndrome; menopausal syndrome; mental status; Meretoja syndrome; microscope slide; Microsporida; minimal support; mitral sounds; mitral stenosis; mobile surgical [unit]; modal sensitivity; modified sphygmomanometer; molar solution; Mongolian spot; morphine sulfate; motile sperm; mucosubstance; Münchausen syndrome; multiple sclerosis; muscle shortening; muscle strength; musculoskeletal

3MS modified mini-mental state examination

MS I, II, III, IV medical student–first, second, third, and fourth year

Ms murmurs

ms millisecond; morphine sulfate

m/s meters per second

m/s² meters per second squared

MSA magnetic resonance angiography; major serologic antigen; male-specific antigen; mannitol salt agar; medical savings account; Medical Services Administration; membrane stabilizing action; membrane-stabilizing activity; metropolitan statistical area; molecular shape analysis; mouse serum albumin; multiple system atrophy; muscle sympathetic activity

MSAA multiple sclerosis-associated agent

MSAEFI Monitoring System for Adverse Events Following Immunisation [UK]

MSAFP, MS-AFP maternal serum alpha-fetoprotein

MSAM master of science in administrative medicine

MSAN medical student's admission note

MSAP mean systemic arterial pressure

MSB Master of Science in Bacteriology; mid-small bowel; most significant bit

MSBC maximum specific binding capacity

MSBLA mouse-specific B lymphocyte antigen

MSC major septic complication; marrow stromal cell; Medical Service Corps; Medical Staff Corps; midsystolic click; multi-specialty clinic

MSc Master of Science

MScD Master of Dental Science

MScMed Master of Science in Medicine

MScN Master of Science in Nursing

MSCP mean spherical candle power

MSCU medical special care unit

MSD material safety data; mean square deviation; mild sickle cell disease; most significant digit; multiple sulfatase deficiency; musculoskeletal dynamic [system]

MSDC Mass Spectrometry Data Centre

MSDI Martin Suicide Depression Inventory

MS-DOS Microsoft Disk Operating System

MSDS material safety data sheet

MSE mean squared error; medical screening examination; medical support equipment; mental status examination; mental status expert; muscle-specific enolase

mse mean square error

MSEA Medical Society Executives Association

msec millisecond

m/sec meters per second

MSEL Materials Science and Engineering Laboratory; myasthenic syndrome of Eaton-Lambert

MSEP mean square error of prediction

MSER mean systolic ejection rate

MSES medical school environmental stress

MSF macrophage slowing factor; macrophage spreading factor; malignant senescent forgetfulness [Alzheimer disease]; Médicins sans Frontières [Doctors without Borders]; Mediterranean spotted fever; melanocyte-stimulating factor; modified sham feeding

MSG monosodium L-glutamate

MSGQ medical student graduation questionnaire

MSGV mouse salivary gland virus

MSH medical self-help; melanocyte-stimulating hormone; melanophore-stimulating hormone; message header

MSHA mannose-sensitive hemagglutination; Mine Safety and Health Administration

MSHIF melanocyte-stimulating hormone-inhibiting factor

MSHR melanocyte stimulating hormone receptor

MSHRF melanocyte-stimulating hormone-releasing factor

MSHRH melanocyte-stimulating hormone-releasing hormone

M-SHRSP malignant stroke-prone spontaneously hypertensive rat

MSHSC multiple self-healing squamous carcinoma

MSHT Mount Sinai Hypertension Trial

MSHyg Master of Science in Hygiene

MSI magnetic source imaging; medium-scale integration

MSIM medical systems infrastructure modernization

MSIS multi-state information system

MSK medullary sponge kidney

MSKCC Memorial Sloan-Kettering Cancer Center

MSKP Medical Sciences Knowledge Profile

MSL midsternal line; multiple symmetric lipomatosis

MSLA mouse-specific lymphocyte antigen

MSLR mixed skin cell-leukocyte reaction

MSLS Marinesco-Sjögren-like syndrome

MSLT multiple sleep latency test

MSM medium-size molecule; men who have sex with men; midsystolic murmur; mineral salts medium

MSMAID machine, suction, monitor, airway equipment, intravenous line, drugs [for bronchoscopy]

MSMB microseminoprotein beta

MSMI Multicenter Study of Myocardial Ischemia

MSN main sensory nucleus; Master of Science in Nursing; mildly subnormal

MSO management services organization; medial superior olive; medical staff organization

MSOF multiple systems organ failure

MSOP medical school objectives project

MSP macrophage stimulating protein; maximum squeeze pressure; median sagittal plane; Medicare secondary payer; microseminoprotein; Münchausen syndrome by proxy

msp muscle spasm
MSPB microseminoprotein beta
MSPGN mesangial proliferative glomerulonephritis
MSPH Master of Science in Public Health
MSPhar Master of Science in Pharmacy
MSPN medical student's progress note
MSPQ Modified Somatic Perception Questionnaire
MSPS myocardial stress perfusion scintigraphy
MSQ mental status questionnaire; Minnesota satisfaction questionnaire
MSR macrophage scavenger receptor; Member of the Society of Radiographers; monosynaptic reflex; muscle stretch reflex
MSRPP Multidimensional Scale for Rating Psychiatric Patients
MSRT Minnesota Spatial Relations Test
MSS Marinesco-Sjögren syndrome; Marshall-Smith syndrome; massage; Medical Superintendents' Society; Medicare Statistical System; mental status schedule; minor surgery suite; motion sickness susceptibility; mucus-stimulating substance; multiple sclerosis susceptibility; muscular subaortic stenosis
mss massage
MSSA methicillin-sensitive *Staphylococcus aureus*
MSSE multiple self-healing squamous epithelioma
MSSG multiple sclerosis susceptibility gene
MSSMI Multicenter Study of Silent Myocardial Ischemia
MSSVD Medical Society for the Study of Venereal Diseases
MST maximal stimulation test; mean survival time; mean swell time; mercaptopyruvate sulfurtransferase; myeloproliferative syndrome, transient
M-Step maximization step
MSTh mesothorium
MSTI multiple soft tissue injuries
MSTP Medical Scientist Training Program [NIH]; medical student training program
MSU maple sugar urine; maple syrup urine; medical studies unit; mid-stream urine; monosodium urate; myocardial substrate uptake
MSUD maple syrup urine disease

MSurg Master of Surgery
MSV maximum sustained level of ventilation; mean scale value; mean spatial velocity; Moloney sarcoma virus; murine sarcoma virus
mSv millisievert
MSVC maximal sustained ventilatory capacity
MSW Master of Social Welfare; Master of Social Work; medical social worker; multiple stab wounds
MSWYE modified sea water yeast extract
MT magnetization transfer; malaria therapy; malignant teratoma; mammary tumor; mammilothalamic tract; manual traction; Martin-Thayer [plate, medium]; mastoid tip; maximal therapy; medial thalamus; medial thickness; medical technologist; medical therapy; melatonin; membrana tympani; mesangial thickening; metallothionein; metatarsal; Metathesaurus [UMLS] methoxytryptamine; methyltyrosine; microtome; microtubule; mid-trachea; minimal touch; minimum threshold; Monroe tidal drainage; more than; motor threshold; movement time; multi-input threshold; multiple tics; Muir-Torre [syndrome]; multitest [plate]; mural thrombus or thrombosis; muscles and tendons; muscle test; music therapy; *Mycobacterium tuberculosis*
M-T macroglobulin-trypsin
M&T *Monilia* and *Trichomonas*
Mt megatonne; *Mycobacterium tuberculosis*
mt mitochondrial
3-MT 3-methoxytyramine
MTA malignant teratoma, anaplastic; medical technical assistant; medical technology assessment; metatarsus adductus; multi-threaded architecture; myoclonic twitch activity
mTA meta-tyramine
MTAC mass transfer area coefficient
MTACR multiple tumor-associated chromosome region
MTAD membrana tympana auris dextrae
MTAL medullary thick ascending limb
MTAP methylthioadenosine phosphorylase
MTAS membrana tympana auris sinistrae
MT(ASCP) Medical Technologist certified by the American Society of Clinical Pathologists

MTase methyltransferase

MTB methylthymol blue; Michelin tire baby [syndrome]

Mtb *Mycobacterium tuberculosis*

MTBE meningeal tick-borne encephalitis; methyltertiary butyl ester

MTBF mean time between (or before) failures

MTBM mean time between maintenance

MTBN modifiable temporal belief network

MTC magnetization transfer contrast; mass transfer coefficient; maximum tolerated concentration; maximum toxic concentration; medical test cabinet; medical training center; medullary thyroid carcinoma; metatarsocuneiform [joint]; mitomycin C

MTD maximum tolerated dose; mean total dose; metastatic trophoblastic disease; Midwife Teacher's Diploma; Monroe tidal drainage; multidrug therapy; multiple tic disorder

MTDDA Minnesota Test for Differential Diagnosis of Aphasia

MT-DN multitest, dermatophytes and *Nocardia* [plate]

mtDNA mitochondrial DNA

MTDT modified tone decay test

MTE monophasic truncated exponential

MTET modified treadmill exercise test

MTF maximum terminal flow; medical treatment facility; modulation transfer function

MTg mouse thyroglobulin

MTGA multiple time graphic analysis

MTH mithramycin

MTHF, mTHF 5,10-methylene tetrahydrofolate

5-MTHF 5-methyl-tetrahydrofolate

MTHFR 5,10-methylene tetrahydrofolate reductase

MTI malignant teratoma, intermediate; minimum time interval; model tag image; moving target indicator

MTL mantle zone lymphoma; medial temporal lobe

MTLE mesial temporal lobe epilepsy

MTLP metabolic toxemia of late pregnancy

MTM Thayer-Martin, modified [agar]; myotubular myopathy

MT-M multitest, mycology [plate]

MTMX myotubular myopathy, X-linked

MTO medical technical officer; medical transport officer; methoxyhydroxyphenylalanine

MTOC microtubule organizing center; mitotic organizing center

MTOP Medical Treatment Outcomes Project

MTOS Major Trauma Outcomes Study

MTP maximum tolerated pressure; medial tibial plateau; median time to progression; metacarpophalangeal; metatarsophalangeal; micropayment transfer protocol; microsomal triglyceride transfer protein; microtubule protein

MT1PA metallothionein-1 pseudogene-A

MTPD mean trabecular plate density

MTPJ metatarsophalangeal joint

MTPS mean trabecular plate separation

MTPT mean trabecular plate thickness

MTQ methaqualone

MTR magnetization transfer ratio; Meinicke turbidity reaction; 5-methylthioribose; methyltetrahydrofolate:L-homocysteine S-methyltransferase

MTS Medicare transaction system; magnetization transfer contrast; methotrexate; Mohr-Tranebjaerg syndrome; multicellular tumor spheroid; musculotendinous structure

MTST maximal treadmill stress test

MTT malignant teratoma, trophoblastic; maximal treadmill test; meal tolerance test; mean transit time; methyl-thiazol-diphenyl-tetrazolium; mucous transport time; Myocarditis Treatment Trial

MTU malignant teratoma, undifferentiated; medical therapy unit; methylthiouracil

MTV mammary tumor virus; metatarsus varus; mouse mammary tumor virus

MTX methotrexate

MT-Y multitest yeast [plate]

MU megaunit; mescaline unit; methyluric [acid]; Montevideo unit; motion unsharpness; motor unit; mouse unit

Mu Mache unit

mU milliunit

mu mouse unit

μ Greek letter *mu*; chemical potential; electrophoretic mobility; heavy chain of immunoglobulin M; linear attenuation coefficient; magnetic moment; mean; micro; micrometer; micron; mutation rate; permeability

μ₀ permeability of vacuum

μA microampere

MUA manipulation under anesthesia; middle uterine artery; motor unit activity

MUAP motor unit action potential

μb microbar

μB Bohr magneton

μbar microbar

MUC maximum urinary concentration; mucilage; mucosal ulcerative colitis

muc mucilage; mucous, mucus

μC microcoulomb

μc microcurie

μch microcurie-hour

μC-hr microcurie-hour

μCi microcurie

μCi-hr microcurie-hour

μcoul microcoulomb

MUD minimum urticarial dose

MUE motor unit estimated

μF, μf microfarad

MUFA monounsaturated fatty acids

MUG Massachusetts General Hospital Utility Multi-Programming System [MUMPS] Users Group

μg microgram

MUGA multiple gated acquisition [blood pool scan]

μγ microgamma

MUGEx multigated blood pool image during exercise

μg/kg micrograms per kilogram

μg/l micrograms per liter

MUGR multigated blood pool image at rest

μGy microgray

μH microhenry

μHg micron of mercury

μin microinch

μIU one-millionth of an International Unit

μkat microkatal

μL, μl microliter

mulibrey muscle-liver-brain-eye nanism or dwarfism

mult multiple

Multi-CSF multi-colony-stimulating factor

MultiODA multivariable optimal discriminant analysis

multip multiparous

MuLV, MuLv murine leukemia virus

μM micromole, micromolar

μm micrometer; micromilli-

μmg micromilligram [nanogram]

μmHg micrometer of mercury

μmm micromillimeter [nanometer]

μmol micromole, micromolar

MUMPS Massachusetts General Hospital Utility Multi-Programming System

MuMTv murine mammary tumor virus

μμC micromicrocurie [picocurie]

μμF micromicrofarad [picofarad]

μμg micromicrogram [picogram]

μN nuclear magneton

MUN(WI) Munich Wistar [rat]

MUO myocardiopathy of unknown origin

μΩ microhm

MUP major urinary protein; maximal urethral pressure; motor unit potential

μP microprocessor

μPa micropascal

mUPD maternal uniparental disomy [UPD]

MUPIBAC Mupirocin in Prevention of Relapses of Wegener Granulomatosis by Elimination of Nasal Bacterial *Staphylococcus aureus* Carriage

mUPID maternal uniparental isodisomy [UPID]

μ/μ mass attenuation coefficient

μR, μr microroentgen

MURAD Moscow-Ulm Radiation Accident Clinical History Database

MURC measurable undesirable respiratory contaminants

MURCS Müllerian duct aplasia, cervicothoracic somite dysostosis [association]

MurNAc N-acetylmuramate

MURP Master of Urban and Regional Planning

MUS mouse urologic syndrome; muscinol

μs microsecond

MUSAGE JAMIA 4/2 p. 141

musc muscle, musculature, muscular

MUSCAT MUSIC Criteria for Stent Implantation Using the Controlled Angioplasty Technology Catheter

MUSE medicated uretheral system for erection

μsec microsecond

MUSIC Multicenter Ultrasound During Stent Implantation in Coronary Arteries [study]; Multicenter Ultrasound Stent in

Coronary Artery Disease [study]; Multicentre Ultrasound Study in Coronaries; musculoskeletal intervention center

MUST medical unit, medication use studies; Multicenter Stent Study; Multicenter Stents Ticlodipine [study]; Multicenter Ultrasound Study with Ticlid; self-contained and transportable

MUST-EECP Multicenter Study of Enhanced External Counterpulsation

MUSTIC multisite stimulation in cardiac insufficiency; multisite stimulation in cardiomyopathy

MUSTT Multicentre Unstable Tachycardia Trial; Multicenter Unsustained Tachycardia Trial

MUT mutagen

mut mutation

MUU mouse uterine unit

μU microunit

μV microvolt

μW microwatt

MUWU mouse uterine weight unit

MV maturation value; measles virus; mechanical ventilation; megavolt; methotrexate/vinblastine; microvascular; microvillus; minute ventilation; minute volume; mitral valve; mixed venous; multivessel; veterinary physician [Lat. *Medicus Veterinarius*]

Mv mendelevium

mV, mv millivolt

MVA mechanical ventricular assistance; mevalonic acid; mitral valve area; motor vehicle accident

MV·A megavolt-ampere

mV·A millivolt-ampere

MVAD mechanical ventricular assist device

mval millival

MVB manual ventilation bag; microvascular bleeding; multivesicular body

MVC maximum voluntary contraction; motor vehicle crash; mucin; multivane collimator; muscle vasoconstriction; myocardial vascular capacity

MVD Doctor of Veterinary Medicine; microvascular decompression; mitral valve disease; multivessel coronary disease

MVE maximum velocity envelope; mitral valve echo; mitral valve excursion; Murray Valley encephalitis

MVF mitral valve flow

MVH massive vitreous hemorrhage

MVI multivalvular involvement; multivitamin infusion

MV-IHIS multi-vendor hospital information system

MVK mevalonate kinase

MVL mitral valve leaflet

MVLS mandibular vestibulolingual sulcoplasty

MVM microvillose membrane; minute virus of mice

MVMT movement

MVN medial ventromedial nucleus

MVO maximum venous outflow; mitral valve opening or orifice

MVO2, MVO₂ myocardial oxygen consumption

MVOA mitral valve orifice area

MVP microvascular pressure; mitral valve prolapse; Multivitamin and Probucol [trial]

MVPP mustine, vinblastine, procarbazine, and prednisone

MVPS Medicare Volume Performance Standards; mitral valve prolapse syndrome

MVP-SC mitral valve prolapse-systolic click [syndrome]

MVPT Motor-Free Visual Perception Test

MVR massive vitreous reaction; microvitreoretinal; minimal vascular resistance; mitral valve replacement

MVS mitral valve stenosis; multivendor service

mV·s millivolt-second

MVSR Monthly Viral Statistics Report

MVT multiattribute value theory

mvt movement

MVV maximal voluntary ventilation

MW Mallory-Weiss [syndrome]; masterworker [computing paradigm]; mean weight; megawatt; microwave; Minot-von Willebrand [syndrome]; molecular weight; multiple-window

mW milliwatt

MWA moving window averaging

MWB modified whole blood

mWb milliweber

MWD microwave diathermy; molecular weight data; molecular weight distribution

MWL mental workload

MWP mean wedge pressure

MWS Marden-Walker syndrome; Moersch-Woltman syndrome

MWT myocardial wall thickness

6-MWT 6-minute walk test
MWTA Medical Waste Tracking Act
MX matrix; methylxanthine
Mx maxwell; extension of physician [MEDEX]
MXA morphometric x-ray absorptiometry
MXIP maximum inspiratory pressure
M$_{xy}$ transverse magnetization
My myopia; myxedema
my mayer
MYBC myosin-binding protein C
MYBH myosin-binding protein H
MYBP myosin-binding protein
Myco *Mycobacterium*
Mycol mycology, mycologist
MyD myotonic dystrophy
MYEL myelogram
Myel myelocyte

myel myelin, myelinated
MYF myogenic factor
MyG myasthenia gravis
MYH heavy chain myosin
MYHC heavy chain cardiac myosin
MYHCA heavy chain cardiac myosin alpha
MYL light chain myosin
MyMD myotonic muscular dystrophy
MYO myoglobin
Myop myopia
MYW modified Yule-Walker [autoregressive technique]
MYX myoxoma
MZ mantle zone; meziocillin; monozygotic
M$_z$ longitudinal magnetization
m/z mass-to-charge ratio
MZA monozygotic twins raised apart
MZT monozygotic twins raised together

N asparagine; Avogadro number; blood factor in the MNS blood group system; loudness; nasal; nasion; nausea; negative; neomycin; neper; nerve; neuraminidase; neurology; neuropathy; neutron number; newton; nicotinamide; nifedipine; nitrogen; nodule; normal [solution]; nucleoside; nucleus; number; number in sample; number of molecules; number of neutrons in an atomic nucleus; population size; radiance; refractive index; signal size; spin density

N I-XII, N 1-12 first to twelfth cranial nerves

0.02N fiftieth-normal [solution]

0.1N tenth-normal [solution]

0.5N half-normal [solution]

2N double-normal [solution]

N/2 half-normal [solution]

N/10 tenth-normal [solution]

N/50 fiftieth-normal [solution]

n amount of substance expressed in moles; born [Lat. *natus*]; haploid chromosome number; index of refraction; nano; nerve; neuter; neutron; neutron night; number density; normal, nostril [Lat. *naris*]; number; number of density of molecule; principle quantum number; refractive index; rotational frequency; sample size

2n haploid chromosome; diploid

3n triploid

4n tetraploid

v see *nu*

NA Avogadro constant or number; nalidixic acid; Narcotics Anonymous; network administrator; neuraminidase; neurologic age; neutralizing antibody; neutrophil antibody; nicotinic acid; Nomina Anatomica; non-A [hepatitis virus]; nonadherent; noradrenalin; not admitted; not applicable; not available; nuclear antibody; nucleic acid; nucleus ambiguus; numerical aperture; nurse's aide; nursing assistant; nursing auxiliary

N/A not applicable

Na Avogadro number

nA nanoampere

NAA N-acetyl aspartate; naphthaleneacetic acid; neutral amino acid; neutron activation analysis; neutrophil aggregation activity; nicotinic acid amide; no apparent abnormalities

NAACLS National Accrediting Agency for Clinical Laboratory Sciences

NAACOG Nurses Association of the American College of Obstetricians and Gynecologists

NAA/Cr N-acetyl aspartate/creatine [ratio]

NA-AAF N-acetoxy-N-acetylaminofluorene

NAAP N-acetyl-4-amino-phenazone

NAB novarsenobenzene

NABP National Association of Boards of Pharmacy

NABPLEX National Association of Boards of Pharmacy Licensing Examination

NAC N-acetylcysteine; National Asthma Center; National Audiovisual Center; neuroimaging analysis center; Noise Advisory Council

NACCHO National Association of County and City Health Officials

NACCT North American Congress of Clinical Toxicology

NACDS North American Clinical Dermatological Society

NACED National Advisory Council on the Employment of the Disabled

NAcHPZ 4-*N*-acetyl hydrazinophthalazin-1-one

NACI New Applications for Coronary Interventions [registry]; New Approaches to Coronary Interventions [registry]

NACI DCA New Approaches to Coronary Interventions [registry]: Directional Coronary Atherectomy [study]

nAChR nicotinic acetylcholine receptor

NACHRI National Association of Children's Hospitals and Related Institutions

NACNEP National Advisory Council for Nursing Education and Practice

NACOR National Advisory Committee on Radiation

NACPTAR North American Cerebral Percutaneous Transluminal Angioplasty Registration [study]

Nacq number of acquisitions

NACS neonate adaptive capacity to stimulus

NACSAP National Alliance Concerned with School-Age Parents

NACT National Alliance of Cardiovascular Technologists

NAD neutrophil actin dysfunction; new antigenic determinant; nicotinamide adenine dinucleotide; nicotinic acid dehydrogenase; no abnormal discovery; no active disease; no acute distress; no apparent distress; no appreciable disease; normal axis deviation; not done; nothing abnormal detected

NAD⁺ oxidized nicotinamide adenine dinucleotide [NAD]

NaD sodium dialysate

NADA New Animal Drug Application

NADABA N-adenoxyldiaminobutyric acid

NADG nicotinamide adenine dinucleotide glycohydrolase

NADH reduced nicotinamide adenine dinucleotide

NADL National Association of Dental Laboratories

NaDodSO₄ sodium dedecyl sulfate

NADP nicotinamide adenine dinucleotide phosphate

NADP⁺ oxidized form of nicotinamide adenine dinucleotide phosphate

NADPH reduced nicotinamide adenine dinucleotide phosphate

NADR National Acquired Immunodeficiency Syndrome [AIDS] Demonstration Research; noradrenalin

NAE net acid excretion

NaE, Naₑ exchangeable body sodium

NAEMD National Academy of Emergency Medical Dispatch

NAEMSP National Association of Emergency Medical Services Physicians

NAEMT National Association of Emergency Medical Technicians

NAEP National Asthma Education Program

NAEPP National Asthma Education and Prevention Program

NaERC sodium efflux rate constant

NAF nafcillin; National Amputation Foundation; National Ataxia Foundation; net acid flux

NAFD Nager acrofacial dysostosis

NAFEC National Association of Freestanding Emergency Centers

NAFTA North American Free Trade Agreement

NAG N-acetyl-D-glucosaminidase; narrow-angle glaucoma; nonagglutinable

NAGA N-acetyl-alpha-D-galactosaminidase

NAGO neuraminidase and galactose oxidase

NAGS N-acetylglutamate synthetase

NAH 2-hydroxy-3-naphthoic acid hydrazide

NAHA National Association of Health Authorities

NAHC National Advisory Heart Council

NAHCS National Association of Health Center Schools

NAHDO National Association of Health Data Organizations

NAHG National Association of Humanistic Gerontology

NAHI National Athletic Health Institute

NAHMOR National Association of Health Maintenance Organization Regulators

NAHPA National Association of Hospital Purchasing Agents

NAHQ National Association for Healthcare Quality

NAHSA National Association for Hearing and Speech Action

NAHSE National Association of Health Services Executives

NAHU National Association of Health Underwriters

NAHUC National Association of Health Unit Clerks-Coordinators

NAHV non-A hepatitis virus

NAI net acid input; no accidental injury; no acute inflammation; nonadherence index

NAIC National Association of Insurance Commissioners

NAIP neuronal apoptosis inhibitory protein

NAIR nonadrenergic inhibitory response

Na,K-ATPase sodium-potassium adenosine triphosphatase

NAL nonadherent leukocyte

NALD neonatal adrenoleukodystrophy

NAM N-acetylmuramic acid; natural actomyosin

NAMCIC National Academic Medical Center Information Consortium

NAMCS National Ambulatory Medical Care Survey

NAME National Association of Medical Examiners; nevi, atrial myxoma, myxoid neurofibroma, ephelides [syndrome]

NAMH National Association for Mental Health

NAMI National Alliance for the Mentally Ill

NAMIS Nifedipine Angina Myocardial Infarction Study

NAMN nicotinic acid mononucleotide

NAMP National Alliance for Mental Patients

NAMRU Navy Medical Reserve Unit

NANA N-acetyl neuraminic acid

NANB non-A, non-B [hepatitis]

NANBH non-A, non-B hepatitis

NANBHV non-A, non-B hepatitis virus

NANBNC non-A, non-B, non-C [hepatitis virus]

NANC nonadrenergic noncholinergic

NAND not-and

NANDA North American Nursing Diagnosis Association

NAOO National Association of Optometrists and Opticians

NAOP National Alliance for Optional Parenthood

NAP nasion, point A, pogonion [convexity or concavity of the facial profile]; nerve action potential; network access point; neutrophil-activating peptide; neutrophil alkaline phosphatase; nodular adrenocortical pathology; nucleic acid phosphatase; nucleosome assembly protein

NAPA N-acetyl-p-aminophenol; N-acetyl procainamide

NAPCA National Air Pollution Control Administration

NAPDP National Association of Prepaid Dental Plans

NaPG sodium pregnanediol glucuronide

NAPH naphthyl; National Association of Public Hospitals; National Asthma Education Program; nicotinamide adenine dinucleotide phosphate

NAPHSIS National Association for Public Health Statistics and Information Systems

NAPHT National Association of Patients on Hemodialysis and Transplantation

NAPL nucleosome assembly protein-like

NAPM National Association of Pharmaceutical Manufacturers

NAPN National Association of Physicians' Nurses

NAPNAP National Association of Pediatric Nurse Associates and Practitioners

NAPNES National Association for Practical Nursing Education and Services

NAPPH National Association of Private Psychiatric Hospitals

NAPQI N-acetyl-p-benzoquinone imine

NAPT National Association for the Prevention of Tuberculosis

NAQAP National Association of Quality Assurance Professionals

NAR nasal airway resistance; National Association for Retarded [Children, Citizens]; no action required

NARA Narcotics Addict Rehabilitation Act; National Association of Recovered Alcoholics

NARAL National Abortion Rights Action League

NARC narcotic; National Association for Retarded Children; nucleus arcuatus

NARCF National Association of Residential Care Facilities

narco narcotic, narcotic addict, drug enforcement agent

NARD National Association of Retail Druggists

NARES nonallergic rhinitis-eosinophilia syndrome

NARF National Association of Rehabilitation Facilities

NARIC National Rehabilitation Information Center

NARL no adverse response level

NARMA nonlinear autoregressive moving average [model]

NARMAX nonlinear autoregressive moving average with exogenous [input]

NARMH National Association for Rural Mental Health

NARP neuropathy–ataxia–retinitis pigmentosa [syndrome]

NARS National Acupuncture Research Society

NARSAD National Alliance for Research on Schizophrenia and Depression

NARSD National Alliance for Research on Schizophrenia and Depression

NARX nonlinear autoregressive model with exogenous input

NAS nasal; National Academy of Sciences; National Association of Sanitarians; neonatal airleak syndrome; neuroallergic syndrome; no added salt; non-*albican* species; Normative Aging Study

NASA National Aeronautics and Space Administration

NASBA nucleic acid sequence-based amplification

NASCET North American Symptomatic Carotid Endarterectomy Trial

NASCIS National Acute Spinal Cord Injury Study

NASD National Association of Schools of Dance

NASE National Association for the Study of Epilepsy

NASEAN National Association for State Enrolled Assistant Nurses

NASHS National Adolescent Student Health Survey

NaSIMM National Study of Internal Medicine Manpower

NASM Naval Aviation School of Medicine

NAS-NRC National Academy of Science-National Research Council

NASPE North American Society for Pacing and Electrophysiology

NASS National Accident Sampling System; North American Spine Society

NASW National Association of Social Workers

NAT N-acetyltransferase; natal; neonatal alloimmune thrombocytopenia; no action taken; nonaccidental trauma

Nat native; natural

NaT sodium tartrate

NATCO North American Transplant Coordinator Organization

Natr sodium [Lat. *natrium*]

NATSAL National Survey of Sexual Attitudes and Lifestyles [UK]

NAVAPAM National Association of Veterans Affairs Physician Ambulatory Care Managers

NAVEL naloxone, atropine, Valium, epinephrine, lidocaine

NAZC neutrophil azurocidin

NB nail bed; needle biopsy; neuro-Behçet [syndrome]; neuroblastoma; neurometric battery; new Ballard [score]; newborn; nitrous oxide-barbiturate; normoblast; note well [Lat. *nota bene*]; nutrient broth

nb newborn; note well [Lat. *nota bene*]

NBA neuron-binding activity

NBAC National Bioethics Advisory Committee

NBAT neutral and basic amino acid transporter

NBC network based computing; nonbattle casualty

NBCC nevoid basal cell carcinoma

NBCCS nevoid basal cell carcinoma syndrome

NBCIE nonbullous congential ichthyosiform erythroderma

NBCOT National Board for Certification in Occupational Therapy

NBD neurogenic bladder dysfunction; no brain damage; nucleotide-binding domain

NBF no breast feeding; nucleotide-binding fold

NBI neutrophil bactericidal index; no bone injury; non-battle injury

NBIC neonatal bedside interface controller

NBICU newborn intensive care unit

NBL neuroblastoma

NBM no bowel movement; normal bone marrow; normal bowel movement; nothing by mouth

nBM nucleus basalis of Meynert

nbM newborn mouse

nbMb newborn mouse brain

NBME National Board of Medical Examiners; normal bone marrow extract

NBMPR nitrobenzylmercaptopurine riboside

NBMPR-P nitrobenzylmercaptopurine riboside phosphate

NBN newborn nursery

NBO non-bed occupancy

NBOME National Board of Osteopathic Medicine Examination

NBP needle biopsy of prostate; neoplastic brachial plexopathy; nucleic acid binding protein

NBRT National Board for Respiratory Therapy

NBS N-bromosuccinimide; National Bureau of Standards; neuroblastoma supressor; nevoid basal cell carcinoma syndrome;

Nijmegen breakage syndrome; normal blood serum; normal bowel sounds; normal brain stem; nystagmus blockage syndrome

NBT nitroblue tetrazolium; non-tumor-bearing; normal breast tissue

NBTE nonbacterial thrombotic endocarditis

NBTNF newborn, term, normal, female

NBTNM newborn, term, normal, male

NBT PABA N-benzoyl-L-tyrosyl para-aminobenzoic acid

NBTS National Blood Transfusion Service

n-Bu n-butyl

NBW normal birth weight

NC nasal cannula; nasal clearance; near card; neck complaint; neonatal cholestasis; neural crest; neurocysticercosis; neurologic check; nevus comedonicus; night call; nitrocellulose; no casualty; no change; no charge; no complaints; noise criterion; noncardiac; noncirrhotic; noncontributory; normal cell; normocephalic; normocytoplasmic; nose cone; not completed; not cultured; nucleocapsid; nucleo-cytoplasmic; nurse counsellor; nursing coordinator

N:C, N/C nuclear-cytoplasmic ratio

nC nanocoulomb

nc nanocurie; not counted

NCA National Certification Agency; National Council on Aging; National Council on Alcoholism; neurocirculatory asthenia; neutrophil chemotactic activity; nodulocystic acne; noncontractile area; nonspecific cross-reacting antigen; nuclear cerebral angiogram

NCa normal calcium [dict]

n-CAD negative coronoradiographic documentation

NCADI National Clearinghouse for Alcohol and Drug Information

NCAE National Council for Alcohol Education

NCAH National Commission on Allied Health

NCAI National Coalition for Adult Immunization

NCAM neural cell adhesion molecule

NCAMI National Committee Against Mental Illness

NCAMLP National Certification Agency for Medical Laboratory Personnel

NcAMP nephrogenous cyclic adenosine monophosphate

N-CAP Nifedipine Gastrointestinal Therapeutic System Circadian Anti-Ischemic Program

NC/AT normal cephalic atraumatic

NCBA National Caucus on Black Aged

NCBI National Center for Biotechnology Information [NLM]

NCC National Certifying Corporation; New Computational Challenges Program; National Science Foundation [NSF]; noncoronary cusp; nursing care continuity

ncc noncoronary cusp

NCCAM National Center for Complementary and Alternative Medicine

NCCDC National Center for Chronic Disease Control

NCCEA Neurosensory Center Comprehensive Examination for Aphasia

NCCH National Council of Community Hospitals

NCCIP National Center for Clinical Infant Program

NCCLS National Committee for Clinical Laboratory Standards

NCCLVP National Coordinating Committee on Large Volume Parenterals

NCCMHC National Council for Community Mental Health Centers

NCCN National Comprehensive Cancer Network

NCCPA National Commission on Certification of Physician Assistants

NCCRA National Colorectal Cancer Research Alliance

NCCS National Coalition for Cancer Survivorship

NCCT noncontrast computed tomography

NCCTG North Central Cancer Treatment Group

NCCU newborn convalescent care unit

NCD National Commission on Diabetes; National Council on Drugs; neurocirculatory dystonia; nitrogen clearance delay; normal childhood disorder; not considered disabling

NCDA National Council on Drug Abuse

ncDCIS noncomedo-type ductal carcinoma in situ

NCDS National Child Development Study

NCDV Nebraska calf diarrhea virus

NCE negative contrast echocardiography; new chemical entity; nonconvulsive epilepsy

NCEH National Center for Environmental Health

NCEP National Center for Environmental Protection; National Cholesterol Education Program

NCEPOD National Confidential Enquiry into Peri-Operative Deaths [study]

NCES National Childhood Encephalopathy Study [UK]; Netherlands Cost-Effectiveness Study

NCF neutrophil chemotactic factor

NCFA Narcolepsy and Catalepsy Foundation of America

NCF(C) neutrophil chemotactic factor (complement)

NCH National Claims History [Medicare data file]; nursing care hours

NCHC National Council of Health Centers

NCHCA National Commission for Health Certifying Agencies

NCHCT National Center for Health Care Technology; noncontrast helical computed tomography

NCHD National Claims History Database

NCHECR National Centre in Human Immunodeficiency Virus Epidemiology and Clinical Research [Australia]

NCHGR National Center for Human Genome Research

NCHLS National Council of Health Laboratory Services

NCHPD National Council on Health Planning and Development

NCHS National Center for Health Statistics

NCHSR National Center for Health Services Research

NCI National Cancer Institute; noncriterion ischemic [animal]; nuclear contour index; nursing care integration

nCi nanocurie

NCIB National Collection of Industrial Bacteria

NCIC National Cancer Institute of Canada

NCIC CTG National Cancer Institute of Canada Clinical Trial Group

NCID National Center for Infectious Diseases

NCIH National Council for International Health

NCIRS National Cancer Incidence Reporting System [Canada]; National Centre for Immunisation Research and Surveillance [Australia]

NC-IUB Nomenclature Committee of the International Union of Biochemistry

NCJ needle catheter jejunostomy

NCKHEkg note chemistry and hematology, laboratory values, and electrocardiographic [ECG] findings

NCL neuronal ceroid-lipofuscinosis; nucleolin

NCLEX-RN National Council Licensure Examination for Registered Nurses

NCM nailfold capillary microscopy; nurse case manager

N/cm² newtons per square centimeter

NCMC natural cell-mediated cytotoxicity

NCMH National Committee for Mental Health

NCMHI National Clearinghouse for Mental Health Information

NCMI National Committee Against Mental Illness

NCN National Cardiovascular Network; National Council of Nurses

NCNR National Center for Nursing Research

NCO/CIC National Coordinating Office for Computing, Information, and Communication

NCoR, N-CoR nuclear receptor compressor

NCP noncollagen protein

N-CPAP, n-CPAP nasal continuous positive airway pressure

NCPDP National Council on Prescription Drug Programs

NCPE noncardiac pulmonary edema

NCPI National Clearinghouse for Primary Care Information

NCPIM National Commission to Prevent Infant Mortality

NCPPB National Collection of Plant Pathogenic Bacteria

NCQA National Committee for Quality Assurance

NCR National Research Council; neutrophil chemotactic response; no carbon required; normotensive control rat; nuclear/cytoplasmic ratio

NCRND National Committee for Research in Neurological Diseases

NCRP National Council on Radiation Protection [and Measurements]

NCRR National Center for Research Resources

NCRSP National Congenital Rubella Surveillance Programme [UK]

NCRV National Committee for Radiation Victims

NCS National Collaborative Study; neocarcinostatin; nerve conduction study; newborn calf serum; no concentrated sweets; noncircumferential stenosis; nystagmus compensation syndrome

NCSA National Center for Supercomputer Applications; National Computational Science Alliance

NCSBN National Council of State Boards of Nursing

NCSI number of combined spherical irradiation

NCSN National Council for School Nurses

NCT neural crest tumor

NCTC National Cancer Tissue Culture; National Collection of Type Cultures

NCTR National Center for Toxicological Research

NCV nerve conduction velocity; noncholera vibrio

NCVHS National Committee on Vital and Health Statistics

NCVIA National Childhood Vaccine Injury Act

NCVS nerve conduction velocity study

NCX sodium-calcium exchanger

NCYC National Collection of Yeast Cultures

ND Doctor of Naturopathy; nasal deformity; natural death; Naval Dispensary; neonatal death; neoplastic disease; neurologic deficit; neuropsychological deficit; neurotic depression; neutral density; new drug; Newcastle disease; newly dead; no data; no disease; nondetectable; nondiabetic; nondiagnostic; nondisabling; normal delivery; normal development; Norrie disease; nose drops; not detected, not determined; not diagnosed; not done; nurse's diagnosis; nutritionally deprived

N/D no defects; not done

N&D nodular and diffuse

N$_D$, n$_D$ refractive index

Nd neodymium

n$_D$ refractive index

NDA National Dental Association; New Drug Application; no data available; no detectable activity; no detectable antibody

NDAC not data accepted

NDATUS National Drug and Alcoholism Treatment Unit Survey

NDC National Data Communications; national drug classification; National Drug Code; National Drug Council; Naval Dental Clinic; nicotine dependence center; nondifferentiated cell

NDCD National Drug Code Directory

NDCG Nursing Development Conference Group

NDD no dialysis days

NDDIC National Digestive Disease Information Clearinghouse

NDDG National Diabetes Data Group

NDE near-death experience; nondestructive evaluation; nondiabetic extremity

NDEC nursing diagnosis extension and classification

NDF neutrophil diffraction factor; new dosage form; no diagnostic findings; no disease found

NDFDA nonadecafluoro-n-decanoic acid

NDGA nordihydroguaiaretic acid

NDHPCCB non-dihydropyridine calcium channel blocker

NDHS National Diet-Heart Study

NDI nephrogenic diabetes insipidus

NDIC National Diabetes Information Clearinghouse

NDIR nondispersive infrared analyzer

NDM naturalistic decision making

NDMA nitrosodimethylamine

NDMR nondepolarizing muscle relaxant

nDNA nuclear deoxyribonucleic acid

NDP net dietary protein; nucleoside diphosphate

NDPK nucleoside diphosphate kinase

NDPKA nucleoside diphosphate kinase A

NDPKB nucleoside diphosphate kinase B

NDR neonatal death rate; normal detrusor reflex

NDRF endothelium-derived relaxing factor

NDRI National Disease Research Interchange

NDS Naval Dental School; neurologic deficit score; new drug submission; normal dog serum

NDSB Narcotic Drugs Supervisory Board

NDSSC National Dietary Survey of School Children

NDT neurodevelopmental treatment; noise detection threshold; nondestructive test, nondestructive testing

NDTI National Disease and Therapeutic Index

NDV Newcastle disease virus

Nd/YAG, Nd-YAG neodynium-yttrium-aluminum garnet

NE national emergency; necrotic enteritis; necrotizing enterocolitis; nephropathia epidemica; nerve ending; nerve excitation; neuroendocrine; neuroendocrinology; neuroepithelium; neurological examination; neutrophil elastase; niacin equivalent; no effect; no exposure; nocturnal exacerbation; nonelastic; nonendogenous; norepinephrine; noninvasive evaluation; not elevated; not enlarged; not equal; not evaluated; not examined; nuclear extract; nutcracker esophagus

Ne neon

NEA neoplasm embryonic antigen; no evidence of abnormality

NEAR National Emergency Airway Registry

NEAS nonerythroid alpha spectrin

NEAT Neurohumoral Effects in Acute Myocardial Infarction of Trandolapril [study]; Nordic Enalapril Exercise Trial

NEB nebulin; neuroendocrine body; neuroepithelial body

NEC National Electrical Code; necrotizing enterocolitis; neuroendocrine cell; neuroendocrine convertase; no essential changes; nonesterified cholesterol; not elsewhere classified or classifiable; nursing ethics committee

NECHI Northeastern Consortium for Health Information

NECR noise-effective count rate

NECT non-enhanced computed tomography

NED no evidence of disease; no expiration date; normal equivalent deviation

NEDEL no epidemiologically detectable exposure level

NEE needle electrode examination

NEEE Near East equine encephalomyelitis

NEEP negative end-expiratory pressure

NEET Nordic Enalapril Exercise Trial

NEF nephritic factor

NEFA nonesterified fatty acid

NEFH heavy polypeptide of neurofilament protein

NEFL light polypeptide of neurofilament protein

NEFM medium polypeptide of neurofilament protein

neg negative

NEGF neurite growth-promoting factor

NEHE Nurses for Environmental Health Education

NEI National Eye Institute

NEISS National Electronic Injury Surveillance System

NEJ neuroeffector junction

NEJM New England Journal of Medicine

NEM nemaline; N-ethylmaleimide; no evidence of malignancy

nem nutritional milk unit [Ger. *Nahrungs Einheit Milch*]

NEMA National Eclectic Medical Association

nema nematode

NEMD nonspecific esophageal motor dysfunction

Neo neomycin; neoplasm or neoplastic

neo neoarsphenamine

NEP negative expiratory pressure; nephrology; neutral endopeptidase; no evidence of pathology

nep nephrectomy

NEPA National Environmental Policy Act

Neph nephron; nephritis; nephrosis

NEPHGE nonequilibrated pH gradient electrophoresis

NEQAS National External Quality Assessment Scheme [for blood coagulation] [UK]

NERHL Northeastern Radiological Health Laboratory

NER no evidence of recurrence; nucleotide excision repair

NERD no evidence of recurrent disease

ner nervous

NERO noninvasive evaluation of radiation output

NERSC National Energy Research Supercomputer Center

NES night eating syndrome; not elsewhere specified

NESO Northeastern Society of Orthodontists

NESP Nurse Education Support Program

NEST Nuclear Emergency Search Team

NET nasoendotracheal tube; nerve excitability test; neuroectodermal tumor; neuroendocrine tumor; norepinephrine transporter

NETRHA North-East Thames Regional Health Authority [study]

NETS National Eye Trauma System; Network for Employers for Traffic Safety

NETT National Emphysema Treatment Trial

NEU, Neu neuraminidase

neu neurilemma

neur, neuro, neurol neurology, neurological, neurologist

neuropath neuropathology

neut neuter, neutral; neutrophil

NEVADA Numerical Evaluation of Variance and Dependence Simulation

NEWDILTIL New Diltiazem vs Tildiem [study]

NEXT New European XT Stent Registry

NEXUS National Emergency X-radiography Utilization Study

NEY neomycin egg yolk [agar]

NEYA neomycin egg yolk agar

NF nafcillin; National Formulary; nephritic factor; neurofibromatosis; neurofilament; neutral fraction; neutrophilic factor; noise factor; normal flow; not filtered; not found; nuclear factor; nucleolar frequency [number of nucleoli per 100 nuclei]

nF nanofarad

NF1 neurofibromatosis type I; neurofibromin gene; nuclear factor 1

NF2 neurofibromatosis type II

NFA National Fire Academy; near-fatal asthma; nuclear factor A

NFAIS National Federation of Abstracting and Indexing Services

NFAR no further action required

N-FAS neurogenic fetal akinesia sequence

NFAT, NF-AT nuclear factor of activated T [cells]

NFATp pre-existing subunit of nuclear factor of activated T [cells]

NFB National Foundation for the Blind; nonfermenting bacteria

NFBM normalized fractional brownian motion

NFC National Fertility Center

NFCE near-fatal choking episode

NFD neurofibrillary degeneration

NFDR neurofaciodigitorenal [syndrome]

NFE nonferrous extract

NFH heavy polypeptide of neurofilament protein; nonfamilial hematuria

NFIC National Foundation for Ileitis and Colitis

NFID National Foundation for Infectious Diseases

NFIRS National Fire Incident Reporting System

NFJ Naegeli-Franceschetti-Jadassohn [syndrome]

NFK nuclear factor kappa

NFKB nuclear factor kappa B

NF-κB nuclear factor-κB

NFL nerve fiber layer; neurofilament protein, light polypeptide

NFLD nerve fiber layer defect

NFLPN National Federation of Licensed Practical Nurses

NFM neurofilament protein, medium polypeptide

NFMD National Foundation for Muscular Dystrophy

NFND National Foundation for Neuromuscular Diseases

NFNID National Foundation for Non-Invasive Diagnostics

NFNS, NF-NS neurofibromatosis-Noonan syndrome

NFP natural family planning; no family physician; not-for-profit [hospital]

NFS National Fertility Study; no fracture seen

NFTD normal full term delivery

NFTT neurogenic failure to thrive

NFW nursed fairly well

NFX nuclear factor X

NG nasogastric; neoplastic growth; new growth; nitroglycerin; nodose ganglion; no growth; not given

N/G nasogastric

Ng *Neisseria gonorrhoeae*

ng nanogram

NGA nutrient gelatin agar

NGAST Nimodipine German-Austrian Stroke Trial

NGBE neuraminidase/beta-galactosidase expression

NGC nucleus reticularis gigantocellularis

NGF nerve growth factor

NGFA nerve growth factor alpha

NGFB nerve growth factor beta

NGFG nerve growth factor gamma

NGFIA nerve growth factor-induced clone A

NGFIC nerve growth factor-induced clone C

NGFR nerve growth factor receptor

NGGR nonglucogenic/glucogenic ratio

NGI Next Generation Internet; nuclear globulin inclusions

NGIX next generation Internet exchange points

NGL neutral glycolipid

ng/mL nanograms per milliliter

NGO nongovernmental organization

NGPA nursing grade point average

NGR narrow gauze roll; nasogastric replacement

NGS next generation software; normal goat serum

NGSA nerve growth stimulating activity

NGSF nongenital skin fibroblast

NGT nasogastric tube; nominal group technique; normal glucose tolerance

NGU nongonococcal urethritis

NH natriuretic hormone; Naval Hospital; neonatal hepatitis; neurologically handicapped; nocturnal hypoventilation; nonhuman; nursing home

N(H) proton density

NHA National Health Association; National Hearing Association; National Hemophilia Association; nonspecific hepatocellular abnormality; nursing home administrator

NHAAP National Heart Attack Alert Program

NHAMCS National Hospital Ambulatory Medical Care Survey

NHANES National Health and Nutrition Examination Survey

NHB National Health Board

NHBCD non–heart-beating cadaver donor

NHBE normal human bronchial epithelial [cell]

NHBPCC National High Blood Pressure Coordinating Committee

NHBPEP National High Blood Pressure Education Program

NHC National Health Council; neighborhood health center; neonatal hypocalcemia; nonhistone chromosomal [protein]; nursing home care

NHCP nonhistone chromosomal protein

NHD non-Hodgkin disease; normal hair distribution

NHDC National Hansen's Disease Center

NHDF normal human diploid fibroblast

NHDL non-n-high-density lipoprotein

NHDS National Health Data System; National Hospital Discharge Survey

NHE National Health Expenditure; sodium-hydrogen exchanger

NHEFS National Epidemiologic Follow-up Study

NHF National Health Federation; National Heart Foundation [Australia]; National Hemophilia Foundation; nonimmune hydrops fetalis; normal human fibroblast

NHG normal human globulin

NHGJ normal human gastric juice

NHGRI National Human Genome Research Institute

NHH neurohypophyseal hormone

NHI National Heart Institute; nuclear hepatobiliary imaging

NHIC National Health Information Council [Canada]

NHIF National Head Injury Foundation

NHIS National Health Interview Survey

NHIS-YRB National Health Interview Survey–Your Risk Behavior

NHK normal human kidney

NHL nodular histiocytic lymphoma; non-Hodgkin lymphoma

NHLA National Health Lawyers Association

NHLBI National Heart, Lung and Blood Institute

NHLBI II National Heart, Lung and Blood Institute Type II [coronary intervention study]

NHLBI-ICD National Heart, Lung and Blood Institute Implantable Cardioverter Defibrillator [trial]

NHLBI-PTCA National Heart, Lung and Blood Institute Percutaneous Transluminal Coronary Angioplasty [registry]

NHLBITS National Heart, Lung and Blood Institute Twin Study

NHML non-Hodgkin malignant lymphoma

NHMRC National Health and Medical Research Council [Australia]

NHP National Hypertension Project [Egypt]; nonhemoglobin protein; nonhistone protein; normal human pooled plasma;

Nottingham Health Profile; nursing home placement

NHPC National Health Planning Council

NHPCC hereditary nonpolyposis colon cancer

NHPF National Health Policy Forum

NHPIC National Health Planning Information Center

NHPP nonhomogenous poison processes

NHPPN National Health Professions Placement Network

NHQRA Nursing Home Quality Reform Act

NHR net histocompatibility ratio

NHRA Nursing Home Reform Act

NHRC National Health Research Center

NHS Nance-Horan syndrome; Nasu-Hakola syndrome; National Health Service [UK]; National Hospice Study; natural history; normal horse serum; normal human serum; Nurses' Health Study

NHS-1 First Natural History Study [of congenital heart defects]

NHS-2 Second Natural History Study [of congenital heart defects]

NHSAS National Health Service Audit Staff

NHSC National Health Service Corps

NHS CCC National Health Service Centre for Coding and Classification [UK]

NHSR National Hospital Service Reserve

NHSTD National Health Service Training Division [UK]

NHT nonpenetrating head trauma

NHTSA National Highway Traffic Safety Administration

NHVR normalized hepatic vascular resistance

NI neuraminidase inhibition; neurological improvement; neutralization index; no information; noise index; not identified; not isolated; nucleus intercalatus

NIA National Institute on Aging; nephelometric inhibition assay; niacin; no information available; Nutritional Institute of America

nia niacin

NIAAA National Institute on Alcohol Abuse and Alcoholism

NIADDK National Institute of Arthritis, Diabetes, Digestive and Kidney Diseases

NIAID National Institute of Allergy and Infectious Diseases

NIAMDD National Institute of Arthritis, Metabolism, and Digestive Diseases

NIAMS National Institute of Arthritis, Musculoskeletal and Skin Diseases

NIAP National Information Assurance Partnership

NIB National Institute for the Blind

NIBP noninvasive blood pressure [monitoring]

NIBSC National Institute for Biological Standards and Control

NIC National Informatics Center; network interface card; neurogenic intermittent claudication; neurointensive care; newborn intensive care; nursing interim care; nursing interventions classification

NICD National Information Center on Deafness

NICET National Institute of Certification in Engineering Technologies

NICHCY National Information Center for Children and Youth with Disabilities

NIC-HFH Nephrology Information Center at Henry Ford Hospital

NICHHD National Institute of Child Health and Human Development

NICHSR National Center on Health Services Research

NICOLE Nisolpidine in Coronary Artery Disease in Leuven

NICU neonatal intensive care unit; neurological intensive care unit; neurosurgical intensive care unit; nonimmunologic contact urticaria

NID nidogen; nonimmunological disease

NIDA National Institute of Drug Abuse

NIDD non-insulin-dependent diabetes

NIDDK National Institute of Diabetes and Digestive and Kidney Diseases

NIDDM non-insulin-dependent diabetes mellitus

NIDDY non-insulin-dependent diabetes in the young

NIDM National Institute for Disaster Mobilization

NIDR National Institute of Dental Research

NIDRR National Institute on Disability and Rehabilitation Research

NIDS nonionic detergent soluble

NIDSEC Nursing Information and Data Set Evaluation Center

NIEHS National Institutes of Environmental Health Sciences

NIH neointimal hyperplasia

NIHAS Northern Ireland Health and Activity Survey

NIF negative inspiratory force; neutrophil immobilizing factor; nonintestinal fibroblast

Nig non-immunoglobulin

nig black [Lat. *niger*]

NIGMS National Institute of General Medical Sciences

NIH National Institutes of Health

NIHL noise-induced hearing loss

Ni-Hon-San Nipponese in Honolulu and San Francisco [comparative cardiovascular disease rate in Japanese-Americans living in Honolulu and San Francisco]

NIHR National Institute of Handicapped Research

NIHS National Institute of Hypertension Studies

NII National Information Infrastructure; National Insurance Institute

NIIC National Injury Information Clearinghouse

NII-HIN National Information Infrastructure-Health Information Network

NIIS National Institute of Infant Services

NIL noise interference level

NILT Nursing Intervention Lexicon and Taxonomy

NIMBY not in my backyard

NIMH National Institute of Mental Health

NIMP National Intern Matching Program

NIMR National Institute for Medical Research

NIMS National Infant Mortality Surveillance

NINCDS National Institute of Neurological and Communicative Disorders and Stroke

NINCDS/ADRDA National Institute of Neurological and Communicative Diseases and Stroke/Alzheimer's Disease and Related Disorders Association

NINDB National Institute of Neurological Diseases and Blindness

NINDS National Institute of Neurological Disorders and Stroke

NINDS-TPAST National Institute of Neurological Disorders and Stroke–Tissue Plasminogen Activator Stroke Trial

NIOSH National Institute for Occupational Safety and Health

NIP National Immunization Program; negative inspiratory pressure; nipple; no infection present; no inflammation present nonimmigrant patient

NIPH National Institute of Public Health

NIPPV noninvasive positive pressure ventilation

NIPS neuroleptic-induced Parkinson syndrome

NIPTS noise-induced permanent threshold shift

NIR near infrared; New Intravascular Rigid Stent Trial

nIR non-insulin-resistance

NIRA nitrite reductase; Nursing Incentives Reimbursement Award

NIRD nonimmune renal disease

NIRMP National Intern and Resident Matching Program

NIRNS National Institute for Research in Nuclear Science

NIRS near-infrared spectroscopy; normal inactivated rabbit serum

NIRVANA NIR Primo Stent Vascular Advanced North America [trial]

NIS nationwide impatient sample; near-infrared intracranial spectroscopy; N-iodo-succinimide; no inflammatory signs; nursing information system

NISO National Information Standards Organization

NISSO Netherlands Institute for Social Sexological Research

NIST National Institute of Standards and Technology [Department of Commerce]

NIT National Intelligence Test; Nutrition Intervention Trial

NITD noninsulin-treated disease

nit nitrous

nitro nitroglycerin

NIV nodule-inducing virus; noninvasive ventilation

NIWG Nursing Informatics Workshop Group

NJ nasojejunal

NJPC National Joint Practice Commission

NK Commission on [Anatomical] Nomenclature [Ger. *Nomenklatur Kommission*]; natural killer [cell]; neurokinin; not known

n/k not known

NK2 neurokinin 2

NKA neurokinin A; no known allergies

nkat nanokatal

NKB neurokinin B

NKC nonketotic coma

NKCA natural killer cell activity

NKCF natural killer cytotoxic factor

NKDA no known drug allergies

NKFA no known food allergies

NKH nonketogenic hyperglycemia; nonketotic hyperosmotic

NKHA nonketotic hyperosmolar acidosis

NKHS nonketotic hyperosmolar syndrome; normal Krebs-Henseleit solution

NKN neurokinin

NKNA neurokinin A

NKNAR neurokinin A receptor

NKNB neurokinin B

NKP North Karelia Project

NKSF natural killer cell stimulatory factor

NKTR natural killer triggering receptor

NL natural language; neural lobe; neutral lipid; nodular lymphoma; normal; normal libido, normal limits

nl nanoliter; normal [value]

NLA National Leukemia Association; neuroleptoanesthesia; normal lactase activity

NLANR National Laboratory for Applied Networking Research [National Science Foundation, NSF]

NLB needle liver biopsy

NLD nasolacrimal duct; necrobiosis lipoidica diabeticorum

NLDL normal low-density lipoprotein

NLE neonatal lupus erythematosus

Nle norleucine

NLF nasolabial fold; neonatal lung fibroblast; nonlactose fermentation

NLG natural language generation

NLH nodular lymphoid hyperplasia

NLK neuroleukin

NLL nonlymphoblastic leukemia

NLLS nonlinear least squares

NLM National Library of Medicine; noise level monitor

NLMC nocturnal leg muscle cramp

NLMS National Longitudinal Mortality Study

NLN National League of Nursing; no longer needed; [technologist in] nuclear medicine

NLNE National League for Nursing Education

NLP natural language processing; no light perception; nodular liquefying panniculitis; normal light perception; normal luteal phase

NLS Names Learning Test; National Longitudinal Surveys [database]; neonatal lupus syndrome; Neu-Laxova syndrome; nonlinear least squares; normal lymphocyte supernatant; nuclear localization signal

NLSC National Longitudinal Survey of Children [Canada]

NLSCY National Longitudinal Survey of Children and Youth [Canada]

NLT normal lymphocyte transfer; not later than; not less than; nucleus lateralis tuberis

NLTCS National Long Term Care Survey

NL2SOL nonlinear least square algorithm

NLUS natural language understanding system

NLX naloxone; nephrolithiasis, X-linked

NM near-miss; neomycin; neuromedin; neuromuscular; neuronal mode; neutrophil migration; nictitating membrane; nitrogen mustard; nocturnal myoclonus; nodular melanoma; nonmotile; normetanephrine; not malignant; not measurable, not measured; not mentioned; not motile; nuclear medicine, technologist in nuclear medicine; nurse/midwife

N&M nerves and muscles; night and morning

N/m newtons per meter

N-m newton-meter

N/m² newtons per square meter

N x m newtons by meter

nM nanomolar

nm nanometer; night and morning [Lat. *nocte et mane*]

NMA National Malaria Association; National Medical Association; neurogenic muscular atrophy; *N*-nitroso-*N*-methylalanine

NMAC National Medical Audiovisual Center

NM(ASCP) Technologist in Nuclear Medicine certified by the American Society of Clinical Pathologists

NMB neuromedin B; neuromuscular blockade; neuromuscular blocking; neuromuscular blocker/blocking [drug, agent]

NMBA neuromuscular blocking agent

NMBR neuromedin B receptor

NMC National Medical Care; Naval Medical Center; neuromuscular control; nonmotor condition; nucleus reticularis magnocellularis

NMCC nasal mucociliary clearance

NMCES National Medical Care Expenditure Survey

NMCUES National Medical Care Utilization and Expenditure Survey

NMD neuromyodysplasia; neuronal migration disorder

NMDA N-methyl-D-aspartate

NMDAR N-methyl-D-aspartate receptor

NmDG N-methyl-D-glutamine

NMDS nursing minimum data set

NME National Medical Enterprises; neuromyeloencephalopathy

NMEP neurogenic motor evoked potential

NMES National Medical Expenditure Survey [database]; neuromuscular electrical stimulation

NMF N-methylformamide; National Medical Fellowship; National Migraine Foundation; nonmigrating fraction

NMFI National Master Facility Inventory

NMHCA National Mental Health Consumers' Association

NMI no mental illness; normal male infant

NMIHS National Maternal and Infant Health Survey

NMIS nursing management information system

NMJ neuromuscular junction

NML nodular mixed lymphoma

NMM nodular malignant melanoma

NMMDS nursing management minimum data set

NMN nicotinamide mononucleotide; normetanephrine

NMNRU National Medical Neuropsychiatric Research Unit

nmol nanomole

nmol/L nanomoles per liter

NMOR nemadione oxidoreductase; N-nitrosomorpholine

NMOS N-type metal oxide semiconductor

NMP normal menstrual period; nucleoside monophosphate

NMPCA nonmetric principal component analysis

NMPTP N-methyl-4-phenyl-1,2,3,6-tetrahydropyridine

NMR national medical resources; neonatal mortality rate; nictitating membrane response; nuclear magnetic resonance

NMRD nuclear magnetic relaxation dispersion

NMRDC Naval Medical Research and Development Command

NMRI Naval Medical Research Institute; nuclear magnetic resonance imaging

NMRL Naval Medical Research Laboratory

NMRS nuclear magnetic resonance spectroscopy

NMRU Naval Medical Research Unit

NMS Naval Medical School; neuroleptic malignant syndrome; neuromuscular spindle; normal mouse serum; Norwegian Multicenter Study

N·m/s newton meters per second

NMSC nonmelanoma skin cancer

NMSE normalized mean square error

NMSIDS near-miss sudden infant death syndrome

NMSS National Multiple Sclerosis Society

NMT neuromuscular tension; neuromuscular transmission; N-methyltransferase; N-myristoyltransferase; no more than; nuclear medicine technology or technologist

NMTS neuromuscular tension state; nuclear matrix-targeting signal

NMTCB Nuclear Medicine Technology Certification Board

NMTD nonmetastatic trophoblastic disease

NMU neuromuscular unit; nitrosomethylurea

NN nearest neighbor; neonatal; neural network or net; nevocellular nevus; normal nutrition; normally not notifiable; nourished; nuclear/nuclear [ratio]; nurse's notes

nn nerves; new name [Lat. *nomen novum*]

NNAS neonatal narcotic abstinence syndrome

NNC National Nutrition Consortium

NND neonatal death; New and Nonofficial Drugs; nonspecific nonerosive duodenitis

NNDC National Naval Dental Center

NNDSS National Notifiable Diseases Surveillance Scheme [Australia and New Zealand]

NNE neonatal necrotizing enterocolitis; nonneuronal enolase; normalized noise energy

NNEB National Nursery Examination Board

NNG nonspecific nonerosive gastritis
NNHS National Nursing Home Survey
NNI noise and number index
NNIS National Nosocomial Infection Surveillance
NNIWG National Nursing Informatics Work Group
NNJ neonatal jaundice
NNK neural network Kubicek [equation]
NNLIT North Norwegian Lidocaine Intervention Trial
NN/LM National Network of Libraries of Medicine
NNM neonatal mortality
NNMC National Naval Medical Center
NNMT nicotinamide *N*-methyltransferase; Norwegian Nifedipine Multicenter Trial
NNN Novy-MacNeal-Nicolle [medium]
NNNMU N-nitroso-N-methylurethane
NNO no new orders
n nov new name [Lat. *nomen novum*]
NNP neonatal nurse practitioner; nerve net pulse
NNR New and Nonofficial Remedies
NNRTI nonnucleoside reverse transcriptase inhibitor
NNS neural network Sramek [equation]; nicotine nasal spray; nonneoplastic syndrome
NNT nuclei nervi trigemini; number needed to treat
NNU neonatal unit
NNWI Neonatal Narcotic Withdrawal Index
NO narcotics officer; nitric or nitrous oxide; none obtained; nonobese; nurse's office
No nobelium
No, no number [Lat. *numero*]
NOA National Optometric Association; nitro-L-arginine
NOABX no antibiotics
NOAEL no observed adverse effect level
NOAH New York Online Access to Health
NOAPP National Organization of Adolescent Pregnancy and Parenting
NOBT nonoperative biopsy technique
NOC not otherwise classified; nursing outcomes classification
NOCDQ nursing organizational climate description questionnaire
NOD Naito-Oyanagi disease; National Organization on Disability; nodular melanoma; nonobese diabetic; notify of death
NOE nuclear Overhauser effect

NOEL no observed effect level
NOESY nuclear Overhauser effect spectroscopy
NOF National Osteopathic Foundation; National Osteoporosis Foundation
NOFT nonorganic failure-to-thrive
NOII nonocclusive intestinal ischemia
NOK next of kin
NOL nitric oxide level
nom dub a doubtful name [Lat. *nomen dubium*]
NOMI nonocclusive mesenteric infarction
NONMEM nonlinear mixed effects model
non-REM non-rapid eye movement [sleep]
NOP not otherwise provided for
NOPHN National Organization for Public Health Nursing
NOR Neurologic Outcome Research; noradrenaline; normal; nortriptyline; nucleolar organizer region
NORA Nordic Research on Aging
NORASEPT North American Sepsis Trial
NORC National Opinion Research Center
NORD National Organization for Rare Disorders
NORDIL Nordic Diltiazem [study]
NORDUnet Nordic Countries Network
NOR-EPI norepinephrine
norleu norleucine
NORM naturally occurring radioactive material
norm normal
NORML National Organization for the Reform of Marijuana Laws
NOS network operating system; nitric oxide synthetase; non-organ-specific; not on staff; not otherwise specified
NOs nitric oxide synthetase
NOSAC nonsteroidal anti-inflammatory compound
NOSER Newton's one-step error reconstructor
NOSIC Neurologic Outcome Scale for Infants and Children
NOSIE Nurses' Observation Scale for Inpatient Evaluation
NOSTA Naval Ophthalmic Support and Training Activity
NOT nocturnal oxygen therapy
NOTB National Ophthalmic Treatment Board

NOTT Nocturnal Oxygen Therapy Trial

NOV Novantrone

nov n new name [Lat. *novum nomen*]

NOVS National Office of Vital Statistics

nov sp new species [Lat. *novum species*]

NOWIS North Wurttemberg Infarction Study

NP nasopharynx, nasopharyngeal; natriuretic peptide; near point; necrotizing pancreatitis; neonatal-perinatal; neuritic plague; neuropathology; neuropeptide; neurophysin; neuropsychiatry; new patient; newly presented; Niemann-Pick [disease]; nitrogen-phosphorus; nitrophenol; no pain; no pressure; nonpalpable; nonparalytic; nonpathogenic; nonphagocytic; nonpracticing; normal plasma; normal pressure; nosocomial pneumonia; not perceptible; not performed; not pregnant; not present; nucleoplasmic; nucleoprotein; nucleoside phosphorylase; nurse practitioner; nursed poorly; nursing procedure; proper name [Lat. *nomen proprium*]

N-P need-persistence

Np neper; neptunium; neurophysin

np nucleotide pair

NPA nasopharyngeal aspirate; National Pharmaceutical Association; National Pituitary Agency; near point accommodation; Nurse Practice Act

nPA lanoteplase

NPACI National Partnership for Advanced Computational Infrastructure

NPA-NIHHDP National Pituitary Agency-National Institutes of Health Hormone Distribution Program

NPB nodal premature beat; nonprotein bound

NPBF nonplacental blood flow

NPBV negative pressure body ventilator

NPC nasopharyngeal carcinoma; near point of convergence; neuroparacoccidioidomycosis; nodal premature contractions; nonparenchymal [liver] cell; nonphysician clinician; nonproductive cough; nucleus of posterior commissure

NPCa nasopharyngeal carcinoma

NPCP National Prostatic Cancer Project; non-*Pneumocystis* pneumonia

NP cult nasopharyngeal culture

NPD narcissistic personality disorder; natriuretic plasma dialysate; negative pressure device; Niemann-Pick disease; nitrogen-phosphorus detector; nonpathologic diagnosis; normal protein diet

NPDB National Practitioner Data Bank

NPDC neurofibromatosis-pheochromocytoma-duodenal carcinoid [syndrome]

NPDL nodular poorly differentiated lymphocytic

NPDR nonproliferative diabetic retinopathy

NPE neurogenic pulmonary edema; neuropsychologic examination; no palpable enlargement; normal pelvic examination

NPF nasopharyngeal fiberscope; National Parkinson Foundation; National Pharmaceutical Foundation; National Provider File; National Psoriasis Foundation; neuronal population function; no predisposing factor

NPFT Neurotic Personality Factor Test

NPH nephrophthisis; neutral protamine Hagedorn (insulin) [not used anymore]; normal pressure hydrocephalus; nucleus pulposus herniation

NPHCE national personal health care expenditures

NPHDO Nadroparin Posthospital Discharge in Orthopedy [study]

NPHE natural phenomenon [UMLS]

NP HRF nasal pool histamine-releasing factor

NPHS National Population Health Survey [Canada]; Northwick Park Heart Study

NPhx nasopharynx

NPI Narcissistic Personality Inventory; National Provider Identifier; neuropsychiatric institution; no present illness; nucleoplasmic index

NPIC neurogenic peripheral intermittent claudication

NPII Neonatal Pulmonary Insufficiency Index

NPJT nonparoxysmal atrioventricular junctional tachycardia

NPK neuropeptide K

NPL National Physics Laboratory; neoproteolipid

NPM nonpacemaker [cells]; nothing per mouth

NPN neural Petri net; nonprotein nitrogen

NPO nothing by mouth [Lat. *nulla per os*]; nucleus preopticus

NPO/HS nothing by mouth at bedtime [Lat. *nulla per os hora somni*]

NPOS nurses professional orientation scale

NPP nitrophenylphosphate; normal pool plasma; nucleus tegmenti pedunculopontinus

NPPase nucleotide pyrophosphatase

NPPC Nursing Professional Practice Council

NPPE negative pressure pulmonary edema

NPPH nucleotide pyrophosphohydrolase

NPPNG nonpenicillinase-producing *Neisseria gonorrhoeae*

NP polio nonparalytic poliomyelitis

NPR net protein ratio; normal pulse rate; nucleoside phosphoribosyl

NPRL Navy Prosthetics Research Laboratory

NPS nail-patella syndrome; nasopharyngeal secretion; neonatal progeroid syndrome

NPSA normal pilosebaceous appartus

NPSH nonprotein sulhydryl [group]

NPT neoprecipitin test; nocturnal penile tumescence; normal pressure and temperature; sodium phosphate transport

NPTR National Pediatric Trauma Registry

NPU net protein utilization

NPUI nursing process utilization inventory

NPV negative predictive value; pressure value; negative pressure ventilation; net present value; nuclear polyhidrosis virus; nucleus paraventricularis

NPY neuropeptide Y

NPYR neuropeptide Y receptor

NQA nursing quality assurance

NQMI non–Q-wave myocardial infarction

NQO NAD(P)H:quinone oxidoreductase

4NQO 4-nitroquinoline 1-oxide

NQR nuclear quadruple resonance

NR do not repeat [Lat. *non repetatur*]; nerve root; neural retina; neutral red; noise reduction; no radiation; no reaction; no recurrence; no refill; no report; no respiration; no response; no result; nonmatch resonse; nonreactive; nonrebreathing; nonresponder; nonretarded; normal range; normal reaction; normotensive rat; not readable; not recorded; not reported; not resolved; nurse; nursing [service]; nutrition ratio; Reynold's number

N/R not remarkable

N$_R$ Reynold's number

nr near

NRA nitrate reductase; nucleus retroambigualis

NRB nonrejoining break; nursing reference base

NRBC National Rare Blood Club; normal red blood cell; nucleated red blood cell

NRbc nucleated red blood cell

NRC National Red Cross; National Research Council; National Response Center; normal retinal correspondence; not routine care; Nuclear Regulatory Commission

NRCAM National Resource for Cell Analysis and Modeling

NRCC National Registry in Clinical Chemistry; National Research Council of Canada

NRCL nonrenal clearance

NRDL Naval Radiological Defense Laboratory

NREH normal renin essential hypertension

NREM nonrapid eye movement [sleep]

NREMT National Registry of Emergency Medical Technicians

NREMT-P nationally registered emergency medical technician-paramedic

NREN National Aeronautics and Space Administration [NASA] Research and Education Network

NRF Neurosciences Research Foundation; normal renal function

NRFC nonrosette-forming cell

NRFD not ready for data

NRG nursing resources grouping

NRGC nucleus reticularis gigantocellularis

NRH nodular regenerative hyperplasia

NRHA National Rural Health Association

NRHS National Runners' Health Study

NRI nerve root involvement; nerve root irritation; nonrespiratory infection

NRICR National Registry of Inhospital Cardiopulmonary Resuscitation

NRK normal rat kidney

NRL nucleus reticularis lateralis

NRM National Registry of Microbiologists; normal range of motion; nucleus reticularis magnocellularis

NRMI National Registry of Myocardial Infarction

NRMP National Resident Matching Program

nRNA nuclear ribonucleic acid

nRNP nuclear ribonucleoprotein

NROM normal range of motion

NRP nucleus reticularis parvocellularis

NRPC nucleus reticularis pontis caudalis

NRPG nucleus reticularis paragigantocellularis

NRR net reproduction rate

NRRC National Rotavirus Reference Centre [Australia]

NRRL Northern Regional Research Laboratory

NRS neurobehavioral rating scale; normal rabbit serum; normal reference serum; Norman-Roberts syndrome; numerical rating scale

NRSA National Research Service Award [NIH]

NRSCC National Reference System in Clinical Chemistry

NRSFPS National Reporting System for Family Planning Services

NRT near-real time; networking research team; nicotine replacement therapy

NRTI nucleoside reverse transcriptase inhibitor

NRU neutral red uptake; nursing research unit

NRV nucleus reticularis ventralis

NRVR normalized renal vascular resistance

NS natural science; Neosporin; nephrosclerosis; nephrotic syndrome; nervous system; neurological surgery, neurosurgery; neurosecretion, neurosecretory; neurosyphilis; neurotic score; nodular sclerosis; noise to signal [ratio]; nonsmoker; nonspecific; nonstimulation; nonstructural; nonsymptomatic; Noonan syndrome; normal saline [solution]; normal serum; normal sodium [diet]; Norwegian scabies; no sample; no sequelae; nosocomial sinusitis; no specimen; not seen; not significant; not specified; not sufficient; not symptomatic; nuclear sclerosis; nursing services; Nursing Sister

N/S noise to signal [ratio]; normal saline [solution]

Ns nasospinale; nerves

ns nanosecond; nonspecific; no sequelae; no specimen; not significant; nylon suture

NSA National Stroke Association; Neurological Society of America; normal serum albumin; no salt added; no significant abnormality; no significant anomaly; number of signals averaged

nsa no salt added

NSABP National Surgical Adjuvant Breast and Bowel Project

NSAD no signs of acute disease

NSAE nonsupported arm exercise

NSAI nonsteroidal anti-inflammatory [drug]

NSAIA nonsteroidal anti-inflammatory agent

NSAID nonsteroidal anti-inflammatory drug

NSAM Naval School of Aviation Medicine

NSC neurosecretory cell; no significant change; nonservice connected; nonspecific suppressor cell; normal child with short stature

nsc nonservice connected; no significant change

NSCC National Society for Crippled Children

NSCD nonservice connected disability

NSCLC non-small-cell lung cancer

NSCS night shift call system

NSCT National Society of Cardiovascular Technologists

NSD N-acetylneuraminic acid storage disease; Nairobi sheep disease; neonatal staphylococcal disease; neurosecretory dysfunction; night sleep deprivation; nominal single dose; nominal standard dose; normal standard dose; no significant defect; no significant deficiency; no significant deviation; no significant difference; no significant disease; normal spontaneous delivery

NSE neuron-specific enolase; nonspecific esterase; normal saline enema

nsec nanosecond

NSEP needle and syringe exchange program; nuclease-sensitive element protein

NSERC Natural Sciences and Engineering Research Council

NSF National Science Foundation; nodular subepidermal fibrosis

NSFNET National Science Foundation (NSF) [Computer] Network

NSFTD normal spontaneous full-term delivery

NSG neurosecretory granule

nsg nursing

NSGC National Society of Genetic Counselors

NSGCT nonseminomatous germ cell tumor

NSGCTT nonseminomatous germ-cell tumor of the testis

NSG Hx nursing history

NSGI nonspecific genital infection

NSH National Society for Histotechnology

NSHD nodular sclerosing Hodgkin disease

NSHG National Study of Health and Growth

NSHL non-syndromic hearing loss

NSHPT neonatal severe hyperparathyroidism

NSI negative self-image; no signs of infection/inflammation; non-syncytium-inducing

NSICU neurosurgical intensive care unit

NSIDS near sudden infant death syndrome

NSILA nonsuppressible insulinlike activity

NSILP nonsuppressible insulinlike protein

NSJ nevus sebaceus of Jadassohn

NSIVCD nonspecific intraventricular conduction delay

NSM neurosecretory material; neurosecretory motor neuron; nonantigenic specific mediator; nutrient sporulation medium

N·s/m² newton seconds per square meter

NSMR National Society for Medical Research

NSN nephrotoxic serum nephritis; nicotine-stimulated neurophysin

NSNA National Student Nurse Association

NSND nonsymptomatic and nondisabling

NSO Neosporin ointment; nucleus supraopticus; Nursing Standard Online

NSP neuron specific protein; nonstructural protein; nurse scheduling problem

NSPB National Society for the Prevention of Blindness

NSPH neonatal severe hyperparathyroidism

NSPN neurosurgery progress note

NSPORT nurse-sensitive patient outcome research team

NSQ Neuroticism Scale Questionnaire; not sufficient quantitiy

NSR nasal septal reconstruction; nonspecific reaction; normal sinus rhythm; no sign of recurrence; not seen regularly

NSR/M no sign of recurrence or metastases

NSS Nordic Sleep Survey; normal saline solution; normal size and shape; not statistically significant; nutrition support services

NSSQ Norbeck social support questionnaire

NSSTT nonspecific ST and T [wave]

NST neospinothalamic [tract]; nonshivering thermogenesis; nonstress test; nutritional support team

NSTC National Science and Technology Council

NSTI necrotizing soft tissue infection

NST-ICF nonstationary ionic channel current fluctuations

NSTT nonseminomatous testicular tumor

NSU neurosurgical unit; nonspecific urethritis

NSurg neurosurgery, neurosurgeon

NSV nonspecific vaginitis/vaginosis

NSVD normal spontaneous vaginal delivery

NSVR normalized systemic vascular resistance

NSVT nonsustained ventricular tachycardia

NSX neurosurgical examination

nsy nursery

NT nasotracheal; neotetrazolium; neurotensin; neurotrophic; neutralization test; nicotine tartrate; nontender; nontumoral; normal temperature; normal tissue; normotensive; nortriptyline; not tested; N-terminal [fragment]; nuchal translucency; nucleotidase; nucleotide

5'NT 5'-nucleotidase

Nt amino terminal

nt nucleotide

N&T nose and throat

NTA natural thymocytotoxic autoantibody; nitrilotriacetic acid; Nurse Training Act

NTAB nephrotoxic antibody

NTBR not to be resuscitated

NTC neotetrazolium chloride

NTCC National Type Culture Collection

NTCP noninvasive transcutaneous cardiac pacing; normal tissue complication probability

NTCT negative temperature-coefficient thermistor

NTD neural tube defect; nitroblue tetrazolium dye; noise tone difference; 5'-nucleotidase

NTE neuropathy target esterase; neurotoxic esterase; not to exceed

NTF neurotrophic factor; normal throat flora

NTFOM normal tissue complication-based figure-of-merit

NTG nitroglycerin; nitrosoguanidine; nontoxic goiter; normal triglyceridemia

NTGO nitroglycerin ointment

Nth normothermia

NTHH nontumorous, hypergastrinemic hyperchlorhydria

NTHi nontypable *Haemophilus influenzae*

NTI nonthyroid illness

NTIA National Telecommunications and Information Administration

NTIG nontreated immunoglobulin

NTIS National Technical Information Service

NTKR neurotrophic tyrosine kinase receptor

NTL near-total laryngectomy

NTLI neurotensin-like immunoreactivity

NTM nontuberculous mycobacteria

NTMI nontransmural myocardial infarction

NTN nephrotoxic nephritis

NTON National Transparent Optical Network

NTOS neurogenic thoracic outlet syndrome

NTP National Toxicology Program; nitroprusside; normal temperature and pressure; nucleoside triphosphate

NT&P normal temperature and pressure

NTR negative therapeutic reaction; nitroreductase; nontranslated region; normotensive rat; nutrition

ntr nutriton

NTRC National Toxins Research Center

NTS nasotracheal suction; nephrotoxic serum; neurotensin; nontropical sprue; nucleus tractus solitarius

NTT nearly total thyroidectomy

NTU Navy Toxicology Unit

N-TUL internal tumescent ultrasound liposculpture

NTV nerve tissue vaccine

NTVR normal transvalvular regurgitation

nt wt net weight

NTX naltrexone

NTZ normal transformation zone

NU name unknown

nU nanounit

nu nude [mouse]

ν Greek letter *nu*; degrees of freedom; frequency; kinematic velocity; neutrino

NUAPS National Unstable Angina Pectoris Study

NUC nonspecific ulcerative colitis; sodium urate crystal

Nuc nucleoside

nuc nucleated

NUCARE nursing care research

nucl nucleus

NUD nonnucler dyspepsia; nursing utilization database

NUG necrotizing ulcerative gingivitis

NUI number user identification

nullip nulliparous

νm nanometers

NUMA nonuniform memory access; nuclear mitotic apparatus

numc number concentration

NURB Neville upper reservoir buffer

Nut nutrition

NUV near ultraviolet

NV nausea and vomiting; negative variation; neovascularization; next visit; nonveteran; normal value; not vaccinated; not venereal; not verified; not volatile

Nv naked vision

nv new variant

N&V nausea and vomiting

NVA near visual acuity

NVB neurovascular bundle

NVD nausea, vomiting, and diarrhea; neck vein distention; neovascularization of the disk; neurovesicle dysfunction; nonvalvular disease; normal vaginal delivery; no venereal disease; Newcastle virus disease; number of vessels diseased

N/V/D nausea, vomiting, diarrhea

NVE native valve endocarditis

NVG neovascular glaucoma; night vision goggles; nonventilated group

NVL no visible lesion

NVM neovascular membrane; nonvolatile matter

NVP nevirapine

NVPO National Vaccine Program Office
NVS neurologic vital signs
NVSS normal variant short stature
NVTS normal volunteer telephone screening
NW naked weight; nasal wash
NWB nonweightbearing
NWDA National Wholesale Druggists Association
NWR normotensive Wistar rat
NWTS National Wilms' Tumor Study
NX naloxane
NXG necrobiotic xanthogranuloma
ny, nyst nystagmus

NYC New York City [medium]
NYD not yet diagnosed; not yet discovered
NYHA New York Heart Association
NYHAFC New York Heart Association Functional Class
NYQAS New York Quality Assurance System
NZ normal zone
NZB New Zealand black [mouse]
NZC New Zealand chocolate [mouse]
NZO New Zealand obese [mouse]
NZR New Zealand red [rabbit]
NZW New Zealand white [mouse]

O blood type in the ABO blood group; eye [Lat. *oculus*]; nonmotile strain of microorganisms [Ger. *ohne Hauch*]; objective findings; observed frequency in a contingency table; obstetrics; obvious; occipital electrode placement in electroencephalography; occiput; occlusal; [doctor's] office; often; ohm; old; opening; operator; operon; opium; oral, orally; orange [color]; orderly respirations [anesthesia chart]; ortho-; orthopedics; osteocyte; other; output; ovine; oxygen; pint [Lat. *octarius*]; respirations [anesthesia chart]; zero

O₂ both eyes; diatomic oxygen; molecular oxygen

O₃ ozone

o eye [Lat. *oculus*]; opening; ovary transplant; pint [Lat. *octarius*]; see *omicron*

ō negative; without

Ω see *ohm*

Ω see *omega*

ω see *omega*

OA obstructive apnea; occipital artery; occipito-anterior; occiput anterior; octanoic acid; ocular albinism; [o]esophageal atresia; old age; oleic acid; opiate analgesia; opsonic activity; optic atrophy; oral alimentation; orotic acid; osteoarthritis; osteoarthrosis; ovalbumin; overall assessment; Overeaters Anonymous; oxalic acid

O&A observation and assessment

O₂a oxygen availability

OAA Old Age Assistance; Older Americans Act; Opticians Association of America; oxaloacetic acid

OAAD ovarian ascorbic acid depletion

OAB ABO blood group; old age benefits

OABP organic anion binding protein

OA/BVM oral airway/bag-valve-mask

OACT occupational activity [UMLS]

OAD obstructive airway disease; organic anionic dye

OADC oleate-albumin-dextrose-catalase [medium]

OAE otoacoustic emission

OAF open air factor; osteoclast activating factor

OAFNS oculo-auriculofrontonasal syndrome

OAG open angle glaucoma

OAH ovarian androgenic hyperfunction

OAIS Outcomes and Information Set

OAISO overaction of the ipsilateral superior oblique

OAK Kjer optic atrophy

OALF organic acid labile fluid

OALL ossification of anterior longitudinal ligament

OAM Office of Alternative Medicine [NIH]; outer acrosomal membrane

OAP Office of Adolescent Pregnancy; old age pension, old age pensioner; ophthalmic artery pressure; osteoarthropathy; oxygen at atmospheric pressure; precocious osteoarthrosis

OAPP Office of Adolescent Pregnancy Programs

OAR organ at risk; Ottawa ankle rule

OARS older Americans resources and services; Optimal Atherectomy Restenosis Study

OAS old age security; oral allergy syndrome; osmotically active substance

OASD ocular albinism-sensorineural deafness [syndrome]

OASDHI Old Age, Survivors, Disability and Health Insurance

OASDI Old Age Survivors and Disability Insurance

OASI Old Age and Survivors Insurance

OASIS Older Adults Service and Information System; Organization to Assess Strategies for Ischemic Syndromes

OASP organic acid soluble phosphorus

OAT *O*-acetyltransferase; Ochanomizu Aspirin Trial; Open Artery Trial; ornithine aminotransferase

OATL ornithine aminotransferase-like

OATR organism attribute [UMLS]

OAV oculoauriculovertebral [dysplasia]

OAVS oculo-auriculovertebral syndrome

OAVD oculoauriculovertebral dysplasia

OAW oral airways

OB obese [mouse]; obese, obesity; objective benefit; obliterative bronchiolitis; obstetrics, obstetrician; occult bacteremia; occult bleeding; olfactory bulb; oligoclonal band

O&B opium and belladonna

OBAD optimal biologically active dose

OBB own bed bath; oriented bounding boxes

OBD organic brain disease

OBE Office of Biological Education

OBF organ blood flow

OBG, ObG obstetrics and gynecology, obstetrician-gynecologist

OBGS obstetrical and gynecological surgery

OB-GYN, ob-gyn obstetrics and gynecology, obstetrician-gynecologist

obj objective

obl oblique

ob/ob obese [mouse]

OBP odorant-binding protein; ova, blood, parasites [in stool]

OBR obesity gene receptor

OBRA Omnibus Reconciliation Act

OBS obesity; obstetrical service; organic brain syndrome

Obs observation, observed; obstetrics, obstetrician

obs obsolete

Obst obstetrics, obstetrician

obst, obstr obstruction, obstructed

OB-US obstetrical ultrasound [examination of the fetus]

OC obstetrical conjugate; occlusocervical; oesophageal candidiasis; office call; on call; only child; optic chiasma; oral contraceptive; order communication [system]; original claim; organ culture; outer canthal [distance]; ovarian cancer; oxygen consumed

O&C onset and course

OCA octylcyanoacrylate; oculocutaneous albinism; olivopontocerebellar atrophy; oral contraceptive agent

OCa ovarian carcinoma

OCAD occlusive carotid artery disease

O₂cap oxygen capacity

OCBAS Optimal Coronary Balloon Angioplasty vs Stent [trial]; Optimal Coronary Balloon Angioplasty with Provisional Stenting vs Primary Stent [trial]

OCBF outer cortical blood flow

OCC object-centered coordinate [method]; oculocerebrocutaneous [syndrome]; optimum care committee; oral cholecystography

occ occasional; occiput, occipital; occlusion; occlusive; occupation; occurrence

occas occasional

OCCI oblique clear corneal incision

occip occiput, occipital

occl occlusion, occlusive

OCCPR open chest cardiopulmonary resuscitation

OccTh occupational therapy, occupational therapist

occ ther occupational therapist or therapy

occup occupation, occupational

occup Rx occupational therapy

OCD obsessive compulsive disorder; Office of Child Development; Office of Civil Defense; osteochondritis dissecans; ovarian cholesterol depletion; oxygen cost diagram

OCF occipito-frontal [circumference]

OCG omnicardiogram; oral cholecystogram

OCH oral contraceptive hormone

OCHAMPUS Office of Civilian Health and Medical Programs of the Uniformed Services [database]

OCHS Office of Cooperative Health Statistics

OCIS Oncology Center Information System

OCLC online computer library center

OCM oral contraceptive medication

OCN oculomotor nucleus; oncology certified nurse

OCP octacalcium phosphate; ocular cicatricial pemphigoid; oral case presentation; oral contraceptive pill

OC&P ova, cysts, and parasites

OCPD obsessive compulsive personality disorder

OCPE office of clinical practice evaluation

OCR oculocardiac reflex; oculocerebrorenal [syndrome]; optical character recognition

oCRF ovine corticotropin-releasing factor

OCRG oxycardiorespirography

oCRH ovine corticotropin-releasing hormone

OCRL oculocerebrorenal [syndrome] of Lowe

OCRS oculocerebrorenal syndrome

OCS occipital condyle syndrome; Ondine's curse syndrome; open canalicular system; oral contraceptive steroid; outpatient clinic substation; Oxford Cholesterol Study

OCSD oculocraniosomatic disease

OCSI orthostatic change in shock index

OCSP Oxfordshire Community Stroke Project

OCT object classification test; optimal cutting temperature; oral contraceptive therapy; ornithine carbamoyltransferase; orthotopic cardiac transplantation; oxytocin challenge test

OCTD overlap connective tissue disease

OCU observation care unit

OCV ordinary conversational voice

OD Doctor of Optometry; object dictionary; obtained absorbance; occipital dysplasia; occupational dermatitis; occupational disease; oculodynamic; Ollier disease; on duty; once a day; open drop [anesthesia]; optical density; optimal dose; originally derived; out-of-date; outside diameter; overdose, overdosage; right eye [Lat. *oculus dexter*]

O-D obstacle-dominance

OD-1 Organ Disease 1 [coronary atherosclerosis multicenter study]

OD-2 Organ Disease 2 [cerebrovascular atherosclerosis multicenter study]

O₂D oxygen delivery

ODA office document architecture; open document architecture; right occipitoanterior [fetal position] [Lat. *occipito-dextra anterior*]

ODB opiate-directed behavior

ODBC open database connectivity

ODC oritidine decarboxylase; ornithine decarboxylase; oxygen dissociation curve

Odc ornithine decarboxylase

ODCP ornithine decarboxylase pseudogene

ODD oculodentodigital [dysplasia]; oppositional defiant disorder; osteodental dysplasia

OD'd overdosed [drug]

ODE Office of Device Evaluation [of FDA]; ordinary differential equation

ODED oculo-digito-esophago-duodenal [syndrome]

ODES Oslo Diet and Exercise Study

ODFR oxygen-derived free radical

ODIF office document interchange format

ODISY Online Deaconess Information System

ODM ophthalmodynamometer, ophthalmodynamometry

ODN oligodeoxyribonucleotide

ODOD oculo-dento-osseous dysplasia

Odont odontogenic

ODP offspring of diabetic parents; right occipitoposterior [fetal position] [Lat. *occipito-dextra posterior*]

ODPHP Office of Disease Prevention and Health Promotion

ODQ on direct questioning

ODS organized delivery system; osmotic demyelination syndrome

ODSG ophthalmic Doppler sonogram

ODT oculodynamic tract; right occipitotransverse [fetal position] [Lat. *occipito-dextra transversa*]

ODTS organic dust toxic syndrome

ODU optical density unit

OE on examination; orofacial cleft; orthopedic examination; otitis externa; out-stationed enrollment

O/E observed/expected [ratio]

O&E observation and examination

Oe oersted

OEE osmotic erythrocyte enrichment; outer enamel epithelium

OEF oil immersion field; oxygen extraction fraction

O₂EI oxygen extraction index

OEIS omphalocele, exstrophy, imperforate anus, spinal defects [complex]

OEL occupational exposure limit

OEM opposite ear masked; original electronic manufacturer

OEP operational effectiveness program

OER osmotic erythrocyte [enrichment]; oxygen enhancement ratio

O₂ER oxygen extraction ratio

OERP Office of Education and Regional Programming

OERR order entry and results reporting

OES oral esophageal stethoscope; optical emission spectroscopy

oesoph esophagus [oesophagus]

OET oral endotracheal tube; oral esophageal tube

O₂Ext oxygen extraction
OF occipitofrontal; opacity factor; open field [test]; optical fundus; orbital fracture; orbitofrontal; osmotic fragility; osteitis fibrosa; oxidation-fermentation
O/F oxidation-fermentation
OFA oncofetal antigen
OFAGE orthogonal field alternation gel electrophoresis
OFBM oxidation-fermentation basal medium
OFC occipitofrontal circumference; optical flow constraint [equation]; orbitofacial cleft; osteitis fibrosa cystica
OFCTAD occipito-facio-cervico-thoraco-abdomino-digital dysplasia
OFD object-film distance; occipital frontal diameter; oro-facial-digital [syndrome]
ofd object-film distance
Off official
OFHA occipitofrontal headache
OFM orofacial malformation
OFNE oxygenated fluorocarbon emulsion [delivery system]
OFTT organic failure to thrive
OFUN organism function [UMLS]
OG obstetrics and gynecology; occlusogingival; 1-O-octyl-beta-D-glucopyranoside; oligodendrocyte; optic ganglion; orange green; orogastric
O&G obstetrics and gynecology
OGC oculogyric crisis
OGD [o]esophago-gastro-duodenoscopy
OGDH oxoglutarate dehydrogenase
OGF ovarian growth factor; oxygen gain factor
OGH ovine growth hormone
OGI oxygen-glucose index
OGJ [o]esophagogastric junction
OGS oxygenic steroid
OGTT oral glucose tolerance test
OGZN organization [UMLS]
OH hydroxycorticosteroid; obstructive hypopnea; occipital horn; occupational health; occupational history; oligomer hybridization; open heart [surgery]; osteopathic hospital; out of hospital; outpatient hospital
17-OH 17-hydroxycorticosteroid
OHA oral hypoglycemic agents
OHAHA ophthalmoplegia-hypotonia-ataxia-hypacusis-athetosis [syndrome]

OHB₁₂ hydroxycobalamin
O₂Hb oxyhemoglobin
OHC occupational health center; outer hair cell; Oxford Haemophilia Centre
5-OHC 5-hydroxycysteine
OHCA out-of-hospital cardiac arrest
OH-Cbl hydroxycobalamin
OHCC hydroxycalciferol; out-of-home child care
OHCOB hydroxycobalamin
OHCS hydroxycorticosteroid
OHD hydroxylase deficiency; hydroxyvitamin D; Office of Human Development; Ondine-Hirschsprung disease; organic heart disease
25-OH-D 25-hydroxyvitamin D
OHDA hydroxydopamine
16-OH-DHAS 16-alpha-hydroxydehydro-epiandrosterone sulfate
8-OH-DPAT 8-hydroxy-2-(di-n-propylamino)tetralin
OHDS Office of Human Development Services
OHE other hospital employee
OHF Omsk hemorrhagic fever
OHFA hydroxy fatty acid
OHFT overhead frame trapeze
OHI Occupational Health Institute; operative hypertension indicator; oral hygiene index; Oral Hygiene Instruction
OHIAA hydroxyindoleacetic acid
OHIPD Office of Health Information Programs Development
OHI-S Oral Hygiene Instruction-Simplified
OHL oral hairy leukoplakia
OHMO Office of Health Maintenance Organizations
OHN occupational health nurse
OHP hydroxyprogesterone; hydroxyproline; occupational health plan; Oregon Health Plan; oxygen under high pressure
17-OHP 17-hydroxyprogesterone
OHPCC Office of High Performance Computing and Communications
OHR occupational health research; Office of Health Research
OHS obesity hypoventilation syndrome; occipital Horn syndrome; occupational health and safety; occupational health service; ocular histoplasmosis syndrome; open heart surgery; Oslo Hypertension Study; ovarian hyperstimulation syndrome

OHSD hydroxysteroid dehydrogenase

OHSS ovarian hyperstimulation syndrome

OHT ocular hypertension; orthotopic heart transplantation; Oslo Heart Trial

OHTA Office of Health Technology Assessment

5-OHU 5-hydroxyuracil

OI obturator internus; occasional insomnia; opportunistic infection; opsonic index; orgasmic impairment; orientation inventory; orthoiodohippurate; osteogenesis imperfecta; oubain insensitivity; oxygen intake

O-I outer and inner

OIC osteogenesis imperfecta congenita

OID object identifier; optimal immunomodulating dose; Organism Identification Number; oxygen insufflation device

OIF observed intrinsic frequency; oil immersion field; Osteogenesis Imperfecta Foundation

OIG Office of the Inspector General

OIH Office of International Health; orthoiodohippurate; ovulation-inducing hormone

OILD occupational immunologic lung disease

oint ointment

OIP organizing interstitial pneumonia

OIR Office of Information Resources; Office of International Research

OIS organ injury scale; Oslo Ischemia Study; outpatient information system

OIT organic integrity test

OJ orange juice

OKC odontogenic keratocyst

OKN optokinetic nystagmus

OKR Ottawa knee rules

OKT ornithine ketoacid amino-transferase

OL open label(ed)

ol left eye [Lat. *oculus laevus*]

OLA left occipitoanterior [fetal position] [Lat. *occipito-laeva anterior*]; oligonucleotide ligation assay

OLAP online analytical processing

OLAS oligoisoadenylate synthetase

OLB olfactory bulb; open liver biopsy; open lung biopsy

OLBx open lung biopsy

OLD obstructive lung disease; orthochromatic leukodystrophy

OLDMEDLINE Old MEDLARS Online [NLM database of 1960-1965 citations]

OLE object linking and embedding

olf olfactory

OLFR olfactory receptor

OLH ovine lactogenic hormone

oLH ovine luteinizing hormone

OLIDS open loop insulin delivery system

OLMC online medical control

OLP left occipitoposterior [fetal position] [Lat. *occipito-laeva posterior*]

OLR otology, laryngology, and rhinology

OLRx orthotopic liver transplantation

ol res oleoresin

OLS ordinary least square; oubain-like substance

OLT left occipitotransverse [fetal position] [Lat. *occipito-laeva transversa*]; orthotopic liver transplantation

OM obtuse marginal [artery]; obtuse mental; occipitomental; occupational medicine; ocular movement; oculomotor; Osborne Mendel [rat]; osteomalacia; osteomyelitis; osteopathic manipulation; otitis media; outer membrane; ovulation method

OMA object management architecture

OMAC otitis media, acute catarrhal

OMAS occupational maladjustment syndrome

OMB Office of Management and Budget

OMC office of managed care; orientation-memory-concentration [test]

OMCH Office of Maternal and Child Health

OMCT Orientation-Memory-Concentration Test

OMD ocular muscle dystrophy; oculomandibulodyscephaly; organic mental disorder; oromandibular dystonia

OME office of medical examiner; otitis media with effusions

Ω Greek capital letter *omega*

Ω ohm

Ω^{-1} ohm-1, siemens

ω Greek lower case letter *omega*; angular velocity

OMERACT Outcome Measures in Rheumatoid Arthritis Clinical Trial

OMFAQ older Americans resources and services (OARS) multidimensional functional assessment questionnaire

OMG object management group; oligodendrocyte-myelin glycoprotein; osteopathic medical school graduate

OMGE Organisation Mondiale de Gastro-Enterologie

OMGP oligodendrocyte-myelin glycoprotein

OMH Office of Mental Health

OMI office of medical investigator; old myocardial infarction

OMIA Online Mendelian Inheritance in Animals [database]

o Greek letter *omicron*

OMIM Online Mendelian Inheritance in Man [database]

OML orbitomental line

OMN oculomotor nerve

OMNI Organizing Medical Networked Information [UK]

OMP olfactory marker protein; oligonucleoside methylphosphonate; ornithine monophosphate; orotidine-5′-monophosphatase; outer membrane protein

OMPA octamethyl pyrophosphoramide; otitis media, purulent, acute

OmpA, ompA outer membrane protein A

OMPC, OMPCh otitis media, purulent, chronic

OmpF, ompF outer membrane protein F

OMR Office of Research and Methodology; oligomycin-resistant; online medical record

OMS organic mental syndrome; otomandibular syndrome

OM&S osteopathic medicine and surgery

OMSA otitis media, suppurative, acute

OMSC otitis media secretory (or suppurative) chronic

OMT object modeling technique; ocular microtremor; O-methyltransferase; ophthalmic medical technician or technologist; osteopathic manipulative therapy

OMVC open mitral valve commissurotomy

ON occipitonuchal; office nurse; olfactory nucleus; onlay; optic nerve; orthopedic nurse; osteonecrosis; osteonectin; overnight

ONC oncogene; oncology; open network communication; Orthopaedic Nursing Certificate; over-the-needle catheter

OND Ophthalmic Nursing Diploma; orbitonasal dislocation; other neurological disorders

ONG optic nerve glioma

ONMRS onychotrichodysplasia-neutropenia-mental retardation syndrome

ONP operating nursing procedure; ortho-nitrophenyl

ONPG o-nitrophenyl-beta-D-galactopyranoside

ONS Oncology Nursing Society

ONTG oral nitroglycerin

ONTR orders not to resuscitate

OO object-oriented; oophorectomy

O&O on and off

OOA object-oriented analysis; outer optic anlage

OOB out of bed

OODB object-oriented database

OODBMS object-oriented database management system

OOG optic oculography

OOH out-of-hospital

OOH/CA out-of-hospital cardiac arrest

OOHRT object-oriented health care terminology respository

OOLR ophthalmology, otology, laryngology, and rhinology

OOM, oom oogonial metaphase

OOP object-oriented programming

OOR out-of-room

OORR orbicularis oculi reflex response

OOSS Outpatient Ophthalmic Surgery Society

OOW out of wedlock

OOWS objective opiate withdrawal scale

OP occipitoparietal; occipitoposterior; occiput posterior; octapeptide; olfactory peduncle; opening pressure; operation, operative; operative procedure; ophthalmology; opponens pollicis; organophosphorus; oropharynx; orthostatic proteinuria; osmotic pressure; osteoporosis; outpatient; ovine prolactin

O&P ova and parasites

O/P outpatient

Op ophthalmology; opisthocranion

op operation; operator

OPA oligonucleoside phosphoramidate; open procurement agency; optic atrophy; organ procurement agency; outcome and process assessment

OPALS Ontario Prehospital Advanced Life Support [study]

op-amp operational amplifier

OPB outpatient basis

OPC oculopalatocerebral [syndrome]; oligonucleotide purification cartridge; outpatient clinic; overall performance category

OPCA olivopontocerebellar atrophy

OPCAB off-pump coronary artery bypass

OPCD olivopontocerebellar degeneration

OPCOS oligomenorrheic polycystic ovary syndrome

OPCRIT operational criteria

OPCS Office of Population Censuses and Surveys [UK]

OPD obstetric prediabetic; optical path difference; otopalatodigital [syndrome]; outpatient department; outpatient dispensary; p-phenylenediamine

O'p-DDD mitotane

OpDent operative dentistry

OPDG ocular plethysmodynamography

OPDS otopalatodigital syndrome

OPG ocular pneumoplethysmography; orthopantomogram; oxypolygelatin

opg opening

OPH obliterative pulmonary hypertension; ophthalmia; organic phosphate

OPH, Oph ophthalmology; ophthalmoscopy, ophthalmoscope

Oph A ophthalmic artery

OPHC Office of Prepaid Health Care

OphD Doctor of Ophthalmology

Ophth ophthalmology

OPI oculoparalytic illusion; Omnibus Personality Inventory

OPIDN organophosphorus-induced delayed neuropathy

OPIM other potentially infectious material

OPK object processing kernal; optokinetic

OPL other party liability; outer plexiform layer; ovine placental lactogen

OPLL ossification of posterior longitudinal ligament

OPM occult primary malignancy; Office of Personnel Management; ophthalmoplegic migraine

OPMD oculopharyngeal muscular dystrophy

OPMSS Olestra Postmarketing Surveillance Study

OPN ophthalmic nurse; osteopontin

OPO Organ Procurement Organization

OPP osmotic pressure of plasma; oxygen partial pressure

opp opposite

OPPA vincristine, procarbazine, prednisone, Adriamycin

OPPG oculopneumoplethysmography

OPRD opiate receptor delta

OPRK opiate receptor kappa

OPRR Office for Protection from Research Risks

OPRT orotate phosphoribosyltransferase

OPRTase orotate phosphoribosyltransferase

OPS operations; optical position sensor; osteoporosis-pseudolipoma syndrome; outpatient service; outpatient surgery

OPSA ovarian papillary serous adenocarcinoma

OpScan optical scanning

OPSI overwhelming postsplenectomy infection

OPSR Office of Professional Standards Review

OPT oligonucleoside phosphorothioate; o-phthaldialdehyde; outpatient; outpatient treatment

opt best [Lat. *optimus*]; optics, optician

OPTHD optimal hemodialysis

OPTICUS Optimization with Intracoronary Ultrasound to Reduce Stent Restenosis [trial]

OPTIMAAL Optimal Trial in Myocardial Infarction with Angiotensin II Antagonist Losartan

OPTIME Outcomes of a Prospective Trial of Intravenous Milrinone for Exacerbations [of chronic heart failure]

OPTIME CHF Outcomes of a Prospective Trial of Intravenous Milrinone for Exacerbations of Chronic Heart Failure

OPTN organ procurement and transplant network

OPUS Orbofiban in Patients with Unstable Coronary Syndromes [study]

OPV oral polio vaccine

OPWL opiate withdrawal

OQAQ Overview Quality Assessment Questionnaire

OR a logical binary relation that is true if any argument is true, and false otherwise; [o]estrogen receptor; odds ratio; oil retention [enema]; oligomer of resveratrol; open reduction; operating room; optic radiation; oral rehydration; orosomucoid; orthopedic; orthopedic research; oubain-resistant

O-R oxidation-reduction

O$_R$ rate of outflow

Or orbitale

ORA opiate receptor agonist

ORACLE Overview of the Role of Antibiotics in Curtailing Labor and Early Delivery [trial]

ORALABX oral antibiotics

ORANS Oak Ridge Analytical System

ORB object request broker

ORBIT Oral Glycoprotein IIb/IIIa Receptor Blockade to Inhibit Thrombosis [trial]

ORBC ox red blood cell

ORC oculo-reno-cerebellar [syndrome]; origin recognition complex

ORCA open record for care

orch orchitis

ORCHIDS Office Records Charts Information Data System

ORD optical rotatory dispersion; oral radiation death

ORDS Office of Research, Demonstration, and Statistics

ORE oil retention enema

OREF Orthopedic Research and Education Foundation

ORF open reading frame

OR&F open reduction and fixation

orf open reading frame

Org, org organic

ORGM organism [UMLS]

ORH order header

ORIF open reduction with internal fixation

oriT origin of transfer

OrJ orange juice

ORL otorhinolaryngology

ORLS Oxford Record Linkage Study

ORM object relational mapping; orosomucoid; other regulated material; oxygen ratio monitor

ORMC oxygen ratio monitor controller

ORN operating room nurse; orthopedic nurse

Orn ornithine

ORNL Oak Ridge National Laboratory

ORO oil red O

OR$_O$ observed odds ratio

OROS oral osmotic

ORP oxidation-reduction potential

ORPM orthorhythmic pacemaker

ORR objective response rate

ORS olfactory reference syndrome; oral rehydration solution; oral surgery, oral surgeon; Orthopaedic Research Society; orthopedic surgeon, orthopedic surgery; oxygen radical scavengers

ORSA osteoclast resorption stimulating activity; oxacillin-resistant *Staphylococcus aureus*

ORT object relations technique; operating room technician; oral rehydration therapy

OR$_T$ true odds ratio

orth, ortho orthopedics, orthopedic

ORW Osler-Rendu-Weber [syndrome]

ORYX outcome research yields excellence

OS left eye [Lat. *oculus sinister*]; occipitosacral; occupational safety; office surgery; oligosaccharide; Omenn syndrome; opening snap; operating system; Opitz syndrome; oral surgery; ordinal scale; organ-specific; orthopedic surgeon, orthopedic surgery; Osgood-Schlatter [disease]; osteogenic sarcoma; osteosarcoma; osteosclerosis; oubain sensitivity; overall survival; oxygen saturation

Os osmium

OSA obstructive sleep apnea; Office of Services to the Aging; Optical Society of America; ovarian sectional area

OSACA Osaka Follow-Up Study for Ultrasonographic Assessment of Carotid Atherosclerosis

OSAS obstructive sleep apnea syndrome

osc oscillation

OSCAR Olive Oil, Safflower Oil, Canola Oil and Rapeseed Oil [dietary study]; online survey, certification and reporting system

OSCC oral squamous cell carcinoma

OSCE objective structured clinical examination

OS-CS osteopathia striata-cranial sclerosis [syndrome]

OSDAT Oslo Study Diet and Antismoking Trial

OS-EM ordered-subsequent expectation maximization

OSF organ system failure; osteoclast-stimulating factor; outer spiral fiber; overgrowth stimulating factor

OSHA Occupational Safety and Health Adminstration

OSH Act Occupational Safety and Health Act of 1970

OSI open systems interconnection [reference model]

OSIRIS Open Study of Infants at High Risk or with Respiratory Insufficiency: the Role of Surfactant; Optimization Study of Infarct Reperfusion Investigated by ST-Monitoring

OSLER objectively structured long examination record

OSM ovine submaxillary mucin; oxygen saturation meter

osm osmole; osmosis, osmotic

OSMED otospondylometaphyseal dysplasia

Osm/kg osmoles per kilogram

Osm/l osmoles per liter

osmol osmole

O-SP O-specific polysaccharide

OSQL object structure query language

OSRC osteosarcoma

OSRD Office of Scientific Research and Development

OSS over-the-shoulder strap

oss osseous

OST object sorting test; Office of Science and Technology; Ottawa Stroke Trial

osteo osteoarthritis; osteomyelitis; osteopathy

OSTI Optimal Stent Implantation [trial]

OSTP Office of Science and Technology Policy

OSUK Ophthalmological Society of the United Kingdom

OT objective test; oblique talus; occlusion time; occupational therapist, occupational therapy; ocular tension; office therapy; old term (in anatomy); old tuberculin; olfactory threshold; optic tract; orientation test ; original tuberculin; ornithine transcarbamylase; orotracheal; orthopedic treatment; otolaryngology; otology; oxytocin; oxytryptamine

Ot otolaryngology

OTA occupational therapy assistant; Office of Technology Assessment; ornithine transaminase; orthotoluidine arsenite

OTC ornithine transcarbamylase; oval target cell; over-the-counter; oxytetracycline

OTCD ornithine carbomoyltransferase deficiency

OTD oculotrichodysplasia; oral temperature device; organ tolerance dose

OTE optically transparent electrode

OTF octamer-binding transcription factor; optical transfer function; oral transfer factor; outpatient treatment file [database]

OTFC oral transmucosal fenatyl citrate

OTI ovomucoid trypsin inhibitor

OTM orthotoluidine manganese sulfate

OTO otology; otorhinolaryngology

Otol otology, otologist

OTPS other than personal services

OTR Ovarian Tumor Registry; Occupational Therapist, Registered

OTReg Occupational Therapist, Registered

OTS n-octadecyltrichlorosilane; occipital temporal sulcus; optical tracking system; orotracheal suction

OTSMD Ornithine Transcarbomylase Structure and Mutation Database

OTT orotracheal tube

OTU olfactory tubercle; operational taxonomic unit

OTW over the wire

OTZ oxathiozolidine

OU observation unit; Oppenheimer-Urbach [syndrome]

ou both eyes together [Lat. *oculi unitas*]

OUB oubain

OUBR oubain resistance

OULQ outer upper left quadrant

OUME operative unit of medical herpetology

OURQ outer upper right quadrant

OURS Oxford University Research Study; oxygen utilization rate study

OUS overuse syndrome

OUTCLAS Outpatient Coronary Low-profile Angioplasty Study

OUTI other urinary tract infections

OV oculovestibular; office visit; osteoid volume; outflow volume; ovalbumin; ovary; overventilation; ovulation

Ov ovary

ov ovum

OVA ovalbumin

ova ovariectomy

OVC ovarian cancer

OVD occlusal vertical dimension; ophthalmological viscosurgical device

OvDF ovarian dysfunction

OVLT organum vasculosum of the lamina terminalis

OVX ovariectomized

OW outcome washing; once weekly; open wedge; outer wall; oval window

O/W oil in water

OWI Office of Worksite Initiatives
OWR Osler-Weber-Rendu [syndrome]; ovarian wedge resection
OWS outerwear syndrome
OX optic chiasma; oxacillin; oxalate; oxide; orthopedic examination; oxytocin
Ox oxygen
OXA oxaprotiline
OXCHECK Oxford and Collaborators Health Check [trial]
OxLDL oxidized low-density lipoprotein
OXMIS Oxford Myocardial Infarction Incidence Study

8oxoA 8-oxoadenine
8oxoG 8-oxoguanine
OXP oxypressin
OXPHOS oxidative phosphorylation
OXT oxytocin
OXTR oxytocin receptor
OXY oxytocin
OXY, oxy oxygen
OYE old yellow enzyme
OYS Oslo Youth study
oz ounce
oz ap, oz apoth apothecaries' ounce (US)
oz t, oz tr troy ounce (UK)

P an electrocardiographic wave corresponding to a wave of depolarization crossing the atria; by weight [Lat. *pondere*]; father [Lat. *pater*]; near [Lat. *proximum*]; near point [Lat. *punctum proximum*]; pain; parietal electrode placement in electroencephalography; parity; part; partial pressure; *Pasteurella*; paternal; patient; penicillin; percent; percussion; perforation; permeability; peta-; pharmacopeia; phenophthalein; phenylalanine; phosphate group; phosphorus; physiology; pig; pint; placebo; plan; plasma; *Plasmodium*; *Pneumocystis*; point; poise; poison, poisoning; polarity; polarization; pole; polymyxin; pons; population; porcelain; porcine; porphyrin; position; positive; posterior; postpartum; power; precipitin; precursor; prednisone; premolar; presbyopia; pressure; primary; primipara; probability; product; progesterone; prolactin; proline; properdin; propionate; protein; *Proteus*; proximal; *Pseudomonas*; psychiatry; pulmonary; pulse; pupil; radiant power; significance probability [value]; sound power; weight [Lat. *pondus*]

P₁, P-one first parental generation
P₂ pulmonic second sound
P₃ proximal third
P-50 oxygen half-saturation pressure
p atomic orbital with angular momentum quantum number 1; freeze preservation; the frequency of the more common allele of a pair; momentum; papilla; phosphate; pico-; pint; pond; pressure; probability; proton; pupil; short arm of chromosome; sound pressure
p after; pulse
p- para
p24 HIV antigen
Π see *pi*
π see *pi*
ψ see *psi*

φ see *phi*
PA panic attack; pantothenic acid; paralysis agitans; paranoia; passive aggressive; pathology; patient's advocate; peak amplitude; performance assessment; periarteritis; peridural artery; periodic acid; periodontal abscess; pernicious anemia; perpetual asymmetry; phakic-aphakic; phenylalkylamine; phosphatidic acid; phenylalanine; phosphoarginine; photoallergy; phthalic anhydride; physical abuse; physician advisor; physician assistant; pituitary-adrenal; plasma adsorption; plasma aldosterone; plasminogen activator; platelet adhesiveness; platelet aggregation; platelet-associated; polyamine; polyarteritis; polyarthritis; post-aural; posteroanterior; prealbumin; predictive accuracy; pregnancy-associated; presents again; pressure augmentation [respiration]; primary aldosteronism; primary amenorrhea; primary anemia; prior to admission; proactivator; proanthocyanidin; procainamide; professional association; prolonged action; propionic acid; prostate antigen; protective antigen; proteolytic action; prothrombin activity; protrusio acetabuli; pseudoaneurysm; *Pseudomonas aeruginosa;* psychoanalysis; psychogenic aspermia; pulmonary arterial [pressure]; pulmonary artery; pulmonary atresia; pulpoaxial; puromycin aminonucleoside; pyruvic acid; pyrrolizidine alkaloid; yearly [Lat. *per annum*]
Pₐ alveolar pressure; atrial pressure; paternal allele
PA3 Atrial Pacing Peri-Ablation for Paroxysmal Atrial Fibrillation [trial]
P-A posteroanterior
P&A percussion and auscultation
Pa acellular pertussis [vaccine]; pascal; pathologist, pathology; protactinium; *Pseudomonas aeruginosa;* pulmonary arterial [pressure]
Pₐ partial pressure of arterial fluid
pA picoampere
pa through the anus [Lat. *per anum*]; yearly [Lat. *per annum*]
PAA partial agonist activity; phenylacetic acid; phosphonoacetic acid; physical abilities analysis; plasma angiotensinase activity;

polyacrylamide; polyamino acid; pyridine acetic acid

pAAM polyacrylamide

PAAS panic and anticipatory anxiety scale

PAB para-aminobenzoate; performance assessment battery; pharmacologic autonomic block; poly(A)-binding [protein]; premature atrial beat; purple agar base

Pab abdominal pressure

PABA para-aminobenzoic acid

PABD predeposit autologous blood donation

PABP pulmonary artery balloon pump

PABV percutaneous aortic balloon valvuloplasty

PAC P1 artificial chromosome; papular acrodermatitis of childhood; parent-adult-child; pericarditis-arthropathy-camptodactyly [syndrome]; phenacetin, aspirin, and caffeine; physical activity [scale]; plasma aldosterone concentration; platelet-associated complement; Policy Advisory Committee; preadmission certification; premature atrial contraction; product of ambulatory care; pulmonary artery catheterization

pac pachytene

PACAP pituitary adenylate cyclase activating polypeptide

PAC-A-TACH Pacemaker Atrial Tachycardia [trial]

PACC primary ambulatory care center; promoting aphasics' communicative competence

PACCO Pulmonary Artery Catheterization and Clinical Outcomes [study]

PACCS Prospective Army Coronary Calcium Study

PACE Pacing and Clinical Electrophysiology; paired basic amino acid cleaving enzyme; Patient Care Expert [artificial intelligence nursing decision support]; people with arthritis can exercise [program]; personalized aerobics for cardiovascular enhancement; population-adjusted clinical epidemiology; Prevention with Low-dose Aspirin of Cardiovascular Diseases in the Elderly [study]; primary ambulatory care and education; Program of All-inclusive Care for the Elderly; pulmonary angiotensin I converting enzyme

PACI Partnership for Advanced Computational Infrastructure

PACIFIC potential angina class improvement from intramyocardial channels

PACK Prevention of Atherosclerotic Complications with Ketanserin [study]

PA$_{CO}$ mean alveolar gas volume

PA$_{CO_2}$ partial pressure of carbon dioxide in alveolar gas

Pa$_{CO2}$ partial pressure of carbon dioxide in arterial blood

PACP pulmonary alveolar-capillary permeability; pulmonary artery counterpulsation

PACS picture archiving and communication system; postoperative atrial fibrillation in cardiac surgery

PACS DB picture archiving and communication system data base

PACST Putney Auditory Comprehension Screening Test

PACT papillary carcinoma of thyroid; Philadelphia Association of Clinical Trials; Plasminogen Activator Angioplasty Compatibility Trial; Plasminogen Activator Coronary Angioplasty Trial; precordial acceleration tracing; Prehospital Application of Coronary Thrombolysis [study]; prepaid accountable care term; prescription analyses and cost; Prospective Acute Coronary Syndrome Trial; Pro-urokinase in Acute Coronary Thrombosis [study]

PACU postanesthetic care unit

PACWP pulmonary arterial capillary wedge pressure

PAD pain and distress; patient surface axis depth; percutaneous abscess drainage; percutaneous automated discectomy; peripheral artery disease; phenacetin, aspirin, and desoxyephedrine; photon absorption densitometry; practitioners accessing data; primary affective disorder; psychoaffective disorder; public-access defibrillation; pulmonary artery diastolic; pulsatile assist device

PAD-I Public Access Defibrillation I [trial]

PADL personal activities of daily living

PADP pulmonary artery diastolic pressure

PADS patient archiving and documentation system

PADUA progressive augmentation by dilating the urethra anterior

PAE paradoxical air embolism; postanoxic encephalopathy; post-antibiotic effect; progressive assistive exercise

paed pediatrics, pediatric [*paediatrics, paediatric*]

PAEDP pulmonary artery end-diastolic pressure

PAEP progestagen-associated endometrial protein

PAES popliteal artery entrapment syndrome

PAF paroxysmal atrial fibrillation; peroxisomal assembly factor; phosphodiesterase-activating factor; plain abdominal film; platelet-activating factor; platelet-aggregating factor; pollen adherence factor; premenstrual assessment form; progressive autonomic failure; pulmonary arteriovenous fistula

PA&F percussion, auscultation, and fremitus

PAFA priority based assessment of foot additives

PAF-A platelet-activating factor of anaphylaxis

PAFAC Prevention of Atrial Fibrillation After Cardioversion [study]

PAFAMS Pan-American Federation of Associations of Medical Schools

PAFD percutaneous abscess and fluid drainage; pulmonary artery filling defect

PAFI platelet-aggregation factor inhibitor

PAFIT Paroxysmal Atrial Fibrillation Italian Trial

PAFIB paroxysmal atrial fibrillation

PAFP pre-Achilles fat pad

PAFT Propafenone Atrial Fibrillation Trial

PAG periaqueductal gray [matter]; polyacrylamide gel; pregnancy-associated globulin; proliferation-associated gene; pulmonary arteriography

pAg protein A-gold [technique]

PAGA proliferation-associated gene A

PAGE perfluorocarbon-associated gas exchange; polyacrylamide gel electrophoresis

PAGIF polyacrylamide gel isoelectric focusing

PAGMK primary African green monkey kidney

PAGOD pulmonary hypoplasia-hypoplasia of pulmonary artery-agonadism-omphalocele/diaphragmatic defect-dextrocardia [syndrome]

PAH para-aminohippurate; phenylalanine hydroxylase; Phenylalanine Hydroxylase Locus Database; polycyclic aromatic hydrocarbon; predicted adult height [by Bayley-Pinneau]; pulmonary alveolar hypoventilation; pulmonary artery hypertension; pulmonary artery hypotension

PAHA para-aminohippuric acid; procainamide-hydroxylamine

PAHO Pan-American Health Organization

PAHVC pulmonary alveolar hypoxic vasoconstrictor

PAI patient assessment instrument; plasminogen activator inhibitor; platelet accumulation index

PAI-1 plasminogen-activator inhibitor-1

PAIC procedures, alternatives, indications, and complications

PAICS phosphoribosylaminoimidazole carboxylase

PAID problem areas in diabetes [scale]

PAIDS paralyzed academic investigator's disease syndrome; pediatric acquired immunodeficiency syndrome

PAIg platelet-associated immunoglobulin

PAIgG platelet-associated immunoglobulin G

PAIMS Plasminogen Activator Italian Multicenter Study

PAIN pyoderma gangrenosum, aphthous stomatitis, inflammatory eye disease, erythema nodosum [disorders associated with inflammatory bowel disease]

PAIRS Pain and Impairment Relationship Scale

PAIS partial androgen insensitivity syndrome; phosphoribosylaminoimidazole synthetase; Pravastatin in Acute Ischemic Syndromes [study]; psychosocial adjustment to illness scale

PAIS-SR psychosocial adjustment to illness scale-self reported

PAIVS Pulmonary Atresia with Intact Ventricular Septum [collaborative study]

PAJ paralysis agitans juvenilis

PAK pancreas after kidney [transplantation]

PAL pathology laboratory; peptidyl-alpha-hydroxyglycine alpha-amidating lysine phase alteration plane; posterior assisted levitation [cataract surgery]; posterior axillary line; product of activated lymphocytes; pyogenic abscess of the liver

pal palate

PALA N-(phosphonacetyl)-L-aspartate
PALP placental alkaline phosphatase
palp palpation, palpate
palpi palpitation
PALS parietolateral lymphocyte sheath; pediatric advanced life support; prison-acquired lymphoproliferative syndrome
PAM pancreatic acinar mass; penicillin aluminum monostearate; peptidylglycine alpha-amidating monooxygenase; phenylalaline mustard; physical agent modality; p-methoxyamphetamine; postauricular myogenic; potassium-aggravated myotonia; pralidoxime; pre-arrest morbidity [index]; pregnancy-associated α-macroglobulin; primary amebic meningoencephalitis; principles of ambulatory medicine; professions allied to medicine; pulmonary alveolar macrophage; pulmonary alveolar microlithiasis; pulse amplitude modulation; pyridine aldoxime methiodide
PAMC pterygoarthromyodysplasia congenital
PAMD primary adrenocortical micronodular dysplasia
PAME preanesthesia medical examination; primary amebic meningoencephalitis
PAMI Primary Angioplasty in Myocardial Infarction [trial]
PAMIE physical and mental impairment of function evaluation
PAMI-No SOS Primary Angioplasty in Myocardial Infarction with No Surgery on Site
PAMP pulmonary artery mean pressure
PAMR progressively automated medical record
PAN periarteritis nodosa; periodic alternating nystagmus; peroxyacylnitrate; polyarteritis nodosa; positional alcohol nystagmus; puromycin aminonucleoside
pan pancreas, pancreatic, pancreatectomy
Panc pancreas or pancreatic
P-ANCA perinuclear anti-neutrophilic cytoplasmic antibody
PAND primary adrenocortical nodular dysplasia
PANDA Paediatric Asthma Education of a New Multidose Dry Powder Inhaler [study]
PANDAS pediatric autoimmune neuropsychiatric disorders associated with streptococcal infection

PANE pediatric ambulance needs evaluation
PANI polyanilide
PANS puromycin aminonucleoside
PANSS Positive and Negative Syndrome Scale
PAO peak acid output; peripheral airway obstruction; plasma amine oxidase; polyamine oxidase; pulmonary artery occlusion; pustulotic arthroosteitis
PAo airway opening pressure; ascending aortic pressure; pulmonary artery occlusion pressure
PAO$_2$ alveolar oxygen partial pressure
PaO$_2$ partial arterial oxygen tension
PaO$_2$/FiO$_2$ arterial oxygen tension/fraction of inspired oxygen ratio
PAOD peripheral arterial occlusive disease; peripheral arteriosclerotic occlusive disease
Pao, max peak airway pressure
PAOP, PaOP pulmonary artery occlusion pressure
PAP pancreatitis-associated protein; Papanicolaou [test]; papaverine; passive-aggressive personality; patient assessment program; peak airway pressure; phosphoadenosine phosphate; peroxidase antibody to peroxidase; peroxidase-antiperoxidase [method]; placental acid/alkaline phosphatase; poly A polymerase; positive airway pressure; primary atypical pneumonia; prostatic acid phosphatase; pseudoallergic reaction; pulmonary alveolar proteinosis; pulmonary artery pressure; purified alternate pathway
Pap Papanicolaou test
pap papilla
PAPF platelet adhesiveness plasma factor
papova papilloma-polyoma-vacuolating agent [virus]
PAPP para-aminopropiophenone; pregnancy-associated plasma protein
PAPPA pregnancy-associated plasma protein A
PAPPC pregnancy-associated plasma protein C
PAPS 3'-phosphoadenosine-5'-phosphosulfate; primary antiphospholipid antibody syndrome
Paps papillomas
Pap sm Papanicolaou smear

PAPUFA physiologically active poly-unsaturated fatty acid

pa-pv pulmonary arterial pressure-pulmonary venous pressure

PAPVC partial anomalous pulmonary venous connection

PAPVD partial anomalous pulmonary venous drainage

PAPVR partial anomalous pulmonary venous return

PAQ patient asked questions; Personal Attitudes Questionnaire

PAR participating provider; passive avoidance reaction; percentage abnormal results; perennial allergic rhinitis; photosynthetically active radiation; Physical Activity Recall [Questionnaire]; physiological aging rate; plain abdominal radiograph; platelet aggregation receptor; platelet aggregate ratio; Policy, Action, and Rational Drug Use [WHO]; population-attributable risk; postanesthesia recovery; postanesthesia [recovery] room; posterior wall or aortic root; primary angioplasty research; Program for Alcohol Recovery; proximal alveolar region; pseudoautosomal region; pulmonary arteriolar resistance

par paraffin; paralysis

PAR% population-attributable risk percent

PARA, Para, para number of pregnancies producing viable offspring

para paraplegic; parathyroid, parathyroidectomy

para 0 nullipara

para I primipara

para II secundipara

para III tripara

para IV quadripara

PARADIGM Platelet Aggregation Receptor Antagonist Dose Investigation for Perfusion Gain in Myocardial Infarction [study]

PARADISE Platelet IIb/IIIa Antagonism for the Reduction of Acute Coronary Events Dose Investigation and Safety Evaluation [study]

PARAGON Platelet IIb/IIIa Antagonist for the Reduction of Acute Coronary Syndrome Events in a Global Organization Network [study]

parasit parasitology; parasite, parasitic

parasym parasympathetic

PARAT Prevention of Arterial Restenosis Angiographic Trial

PARC Palo Alto Research Center

parent parenteral\

pArg poly-L-arginine

PARIS Peripheral Artery Radiation Investigational Study; Persantine Aspirin Reinfarction Study

PARK Postangioplasty Restenosis Ketanserin [study]; Prevention of Angioplasty Reocclusion with Ketanserin

parox paroxysm, paroxysmal

PARP poly(adenosine diphosphate ribose) polymerase

PARR postanesthesia recovery room

PARS Personal Adjustment and Role Skills Scale

PART Prevention of Atherosclerosis with Ramipril Therapy [trial]; Probucol Angioplasty Restenosis Trial

PART-1 Predictors of Atherosclerosis Risk and Thrombosis [trial]

PART-2 Predictors of Atherosclerosis Risk and Thrombosis [trial]

PARTNER Peripheral Arterial Disease Response to Taprostene with New Established Response Criteria [trial]

PARTY prevent alcohol and risk-related trauma in youth

PARU postanesthetic recovery unit

ParVox Parallel Volume Rendering System for Scientific Visualization [trial]

PAS para aminosalicylate; Paragon Elective or Acute Stent [trial]; Parent Attitude Scale; patient administration system; patient appointments and scheduling; periodic acid-Schiff [reaction]; peripheral anterior synechia; persistent atrial standstill; Personality Assessment Scale; photoacoustic spectroscopy; phosphatase acid serum; physician-assisted suicide; Polish Amiodarone Study; posterior airway space; pre-admission screening; pregnancy advisory service; premature atrial stimulus; professional activity study; progressive accumulated stress; pulmonary arterial stenosis; pulmonary artery systolic

Pas pascal-second

Pa x s pascals per second

PASA para-aminosalicylic acid; primary acquired sideroblastic anemia; proximal articular set angle

PASARR pre-admission screening and resident review

PASAT Paced Auditory Serial Addition Task

PASB protein-associated strand breaks

PAS-C para-aminosalicylic acid crystallized with ascorbic acid

PASD after diastase digestion

PASE Pacemaker Selection in the Elderly [trial]; physical activity scale for the elderly [evaluation]

PASG pneumatic antishock garment

PASH periodic acid-Schiff hematoxylin

PASM periodic acid-silver methenamine

PASP pancreas-specific protein; pulmonary artery systolic pressure

PASS Piracetam in Acute Stroke Study; Postarthroplasty Screening Study [for deep venous thrombosis]; Practical Applicability of Saruplase Study; Prehospital Applicability of Saruplase Study

pass passive

pass ROM passive range of motion

PASSOR Physiatric Association for Spine, Sports, and Occupational Rehabilitation

PAST periodic acid-Schiff technique

Past *Pasteurella*

PASTA Percutaneous Ambulatory Stent Trial; Primary Angioplasty vs Stent Implantation in Acute Myocardial Infarction [trial]

PASVR pulmonary anomalous superior venous return

PASW personal assistance service worker

PAT Pain Apperception Test; paroxysmal atrial tachycardia; patient; patient domain; penetrating abdominal trauma; phenylaminotetrazole; physical abilities test; picric acid turbidity; platelet aggregation test; Polish Amiodarone Trial; polyamine acetyltransferase; preadmission assessment team/test; preadmission testing; predictive ability test; pregnancy at term; psychoacoustic test

pat patella; patent; paternal origin; patient

PATAF Prevention of Arterial Thromboembolism in Nonvalvular Atrial Fibrillation [study]; Primary Prevention of Arterial Thromboembolic Processes in Atrial Fibrillation [trial]

PATCH planned approach to community health

PatDp paternal duplication

PATE Pravastatin Anti-atherosclerosis Trial in the Elderly; psychodynamic and therapeutic education; pulmonary artery thromboembolism

PATENT Pro-Urokinase and Tissue Plasminogen Activator Enhancement of Thrombolysis [trial]

PATG patient group [UMLS]

PATH pathologic function [UMLS]; pathology, pathological; pituitary adrenotropic hormone; physicians at teaching hospitals

path pathogenesis, pathogenic; pathology, pathological

PATHS Prevention and Treatment of Hypertension Study

Patm atmospheric pressure

PATS Poststroke Antihypertensive Treatment Study; Prehospital Administration of Tissue Plasminogen Activator Study

PAT-SED pseudoachondroplastic dysplasia

PA-T-SP periodic acid-thiocarbo-hydrazide-silver proteinate

PAU phenol-acetic acid-urea

PAUP phylogenic analysis using parsimony

PAUSE Popliteal Artery Ultrasound Examination [study]

PAV percutaneous aortic valvuloplasty; poikiloderma atrophicans vasculare; posterior arch vein; proportional assist ventilation

Pav airway pressure

pavex passive vascular exercise

PAVF pulmonary arteriovenous fistula

PAVM pulmonary arteriovenous malformation

PAVNRT paroxysmal atrioventricular nodal reciprocal tachycardia

pAVP plasma arginine vasopressin

PA-VSD pulmonary atresia with ventricular septal defect

PAW peripheral airways; pulmonary artery wedge

Paw mean airway pressure

PAWP pulmonary arterial wedge pressure

PAWS primary withdrawal syndrome

PAX paired box homeotic [family]

PAZ prednisone/azathioprine

PB British pharmacopeia [*Pharmacopoeia Britannica*]; paraffin bath; Paul-Bunnell [antibody]; periodic breathing; peripheral blood; peroneus brevis; phenobarbital; phenoxybenzamine phonetically balanced; pinealoblastoma; polymyxin B; premature beat; pressure breathing; protein binding; punch biopsy

Pb body [surface] pressure; lead [Lat. *plumbum*]; phenobarbital; presbyopia

P_B barometric pressure

P&B pain & burning; phenobarbital and belladonna

PBA polyclonal B-cell activity; pressure breathing assist; prolactin-binding assay; prune belly anomaly; pulpobuccoaxial

PBAL protected bronchoalveolar lavage

PBB polybrominated biphenyl

Pb-B lead in blood

PBBs polybrominated biphenyls

PBC perfusion balloon catheter; peripheral blood cell; point of basal convergence; pre-bed care; primary biliary cirrhosis; progestin-binding complement

PBCC point biserial correlation coefficient

PBCH polymorphic B-cell hyperplasia

PBCL polymorphic B-cell lymphoma

PBCRA progressive bifocal chorioretinal atrophy

PBD postburn day

PBE tuberculin from *Mycobacterium tuberculosis bovis* [Ger. *Perlsucht Bacillen-emulsion*]

PBF peripheral blood flow; placental blood flow; predominant breast feeding; pulmonary blood flow

PBFE peroxisomal bifunctional enzyme

PBFe protein-bound iron

PBG porphobilinogen; progabide

PBGD porphobilinogen deaminase

PBGS, PBG-S porphobilinogen synthase

PBH profiling by hybridization; pulling boat hands; pyrenabutyric acid hydrazide

PBHB poly-beta-hydroxybutyrate

PBI parental bonding instrument; penile pressure/brachial pressure index; protein-bound iodine

PbI lead intoxication

PBIgG platelet surface bound immunoglobulin G

PBK phosphorylase B kinase

PBL peripheral blood leukocyte; peripheral blood lymphocyte; problem-based learning

PBLC peripheral blood lymphocyte count; premature birth living child; problem-based learning curriculum

PBLM problem-based learning module

PBLT peripheral blood lymphocyte transformation

PBM peak bone mass; peripheral basement membrane; peripheral blood mononuclear [cell]; placental basement membrane

PBMC peripheral blood mononuclear cell; pharmaceutical benefit management company

PBMNC peripheral blood mononuclear cell

PBMV pulmonary blood mixing volume

PBN alpha-phenyl-n-tert-butylnitrone; paralytic brachial neuritis; peripheral benign neoplasm; polymyxin B sulfate, bacitracin, and neomycin

PBNA partial body neutron activation

PBO penicillin in beeswax and oil; placebo

PBP penicillin-binding protein; platelet basic protein; porphyrin biosynthesis pathway; prostate-binding protein; pseudobulbar palsy; pulsatile bypass pump

PBPC progressive bulbar palsy of childhood

PBPI penile-brachial pulse index

PBPK physiologically based pharmacokinetic [model]

PBPND progressive bulbar palsy with neural deafness

PBPV percutaneous balloon pulmonary valvuloplasty

PBRN practice-based research network

PBS perfusion-pressure breakthrough syndrome; phenobarbital sodium; phosphate-buffered saline; planar bone scan; primer binding site; protected brush specimen; prune belly syndrome; pulmonary branch stenosis

PBSA phosphate buffered saline [solution]

PBSC peripheral blood stem cell

PBSP prognostically bad signs during pregnancy

PBT Paul-Bunnell test; phenacetin breath test; piebald trait; profile-based therapy

PBT₄ protein-bound thyroxine

PBV predicted blood volume; pulmonary blood volume

PBW posterior bite wing

PBZ personal breathing zone; phenylbuta-zone; phenoxybenzamine; pyribenzamine
PC avoirdupois weight [Lat. *pondus civile*]; pacinian corpuscle; packed cells; paper chromatography; paracortex; paramyotonia congenita; parent cell; particulate compo-nent; partition coefficient; penicillin; pen-tose cycle; peritoneal cell; personal care; personal computer; pharmacology; phase contrast; pheochromocytoma; phosphate cycle; phosphatidylcholine; phosphocre-atine; phosphorylcholine; photoconduc-tion; physicians' corporation; pill counter; piriform cortex; placebo-controlled; plasma concentration; plasma cortisol; plasma-cytoma; plasmin complex; plastocyanin; platelet concentrate; platelet count; pneu-motaxic center; polycarbonate; polycen-tric; polyposis coli; poor condition; poor coordination; portacaval; portal cirrhosis; postcoital; posterior cervical; posterior chamber; posterior commissure; posterior cortex; potential complications; precondi-tioned; preconditioning; precordial; prenatal care; present complaint; primary closure; principal component; printed circuit; pro-collagen; productive cough; professional corporation; prohormone convertase; prosta-tic carcinoma; protein C; protein convertase; proximal colon; pseudocyst; pubococcygeus [muscle]; pulmonary capillary; pulmonary circulation; pulmonary compliance; pul-monic closure; Purkinje cell; pyloric canal; pyruvate carboxylase
pc parsec; percent; picocurie
p/c presenting complaint
PC1 first principal component
PCA para-chloramphetamine; parietal cell antibody; passive cutaneous anaphylaxis; patient care assistant/aide; patient care audit; patient-controlled analgesia; perchlo-ric acid; percutaneous carotid angiography; personal care assistant; Physicians Cor-poration of America; polyclonal antibody; porous coated anatomic [prosthesis]; porta-caval anastomosis; posterior cerebral artery; posterior communicating aneurysm/artery; precoronary care area; prehospital cardiac arrest; President's Council on Aging; prin-cipal components analysis; procoagulant activity; program component area; prosta-tic carcinoma; pyrrolidine carboxylic acid

PCAD Patent Citation Analysis Database; progression of coronary artery disease
PCASSO patient-centered access to secure system online
PCAST President's Committee of Advi-sors on Science and Technology
PCASYS pattern-level classification auto-mation system
PCB paracervical block; polychlorinated biphenyl; portacaval bypass; postcoital bleeding; procarbazine
PcB near point of convergence to the in-tercentral base line [*punctum convergens basalis*]
PC-BMP phosphorylcholine-m-binding myeloma protein
PCC Pasteur Culture Collection; percuta-neous cecostomy; pheochromocytoma; phosphate carrier compound; plasma cate-cholamine concentration; platinum-con-taining compound; pneumatosis cystoides coli; Poison Control Center; precoronary care; premature chromosome condensa-tion; primary care clinic or center; primary care continuum; primary care curriculum; protein C cofactor
PCc periscopic concave
pcc premature chromosome condensation
PCCC pediatric critical care center
PCCF protein C cofactor
PCCM pediatric critical care medicine; primary care case management; primary care case manager
PCCU post-coronary care unit
PCD pacer-cardioverter-defibrillator; pap-illary collecting duct; paraneoplastic cere-bellar degeneration; paroxysmal cerebral dysrhythmia; percutaneous catheter drain-age; pervasive developmental disorder; phosphate-citrate-dextrose; plasma cell dyscrasia; polycystic disease; posterior corneal deposits; premature centromere di-vision; primary ciliary dyskinesia; pro-grammed cell death; prolonged contractile duration; pterin-4a-carbinolamine dehy-dratase; pulmonary clearance delay
PCDC plasma clot diffusion chamber
PCDF polychorinated dibenzofuran
PCE patient care encounter; physical ca-pacity evaluation; pseudocholinesterase
PCEA patient-controlled epidural anes-thesia

PCES patient care evaluation study

PCF peripheral circulatory failure; pharyngoconjunctival fever; platelet complement fixation; posterior cranial fossa

pcf pounds per cubic feet

PCG pneumocardiogram; postcentral gyrus; preconditioned conjugate gradient [algorithm]

PCFIA particle concentration of fluorescence immunoassay

PCFT platelet complement fixation test

PCG pancreatico-cholangiography; paracervical ganglion; phonocardiogram; preventive care group; primate chorionic gonadotropin; pubococcygeus [muscle]

PCH paroxysmal cold hemoglobinuria; patient care hours; polycyclic hydrocarbon

PCHE pseudocholinesterase

PCHI Partners Community Health Care

P²C² HIV Pediatric Pulmonary and Cardiovascular Complications of Human Immunodeficiency Virus Infection [study]; Pediatric Pulmonary and Cardiac Complications of Vertically Transmitted HIV Infection [study]

PCHLS continuous heterogenous lumped systems

PCI patient classification index; pneumatosis cystoides intestinales; prophylactic cranial irradiation; protein C inhibitor

P/CI physical and chemical indicators

pCi picocurie

PCIC Poison Control Information Center

PC-IRV pressure-controlled inverted ratio ventilation

PCIS Patient-Care Information System; point-of-care information system; postcardiac injury syndrome

PCK phosphoenolpyruvate carboxykinase; polycystic kidney

PCKD polycystic kidney disease

PCL pacing cycle length; packaging cell line; persistent corpus luteum; plasma cell leukemia; posterior chamber lens; posterior cruciate ligament; primary care loan; proximal collateral ligament

PCLI plasma cell labeling index

PCM paracoccidioidomycosis; patient care management; patient care manager; patient classification system; primary cutaneous melanoma; process control monitor; protein-calorie malnutrition; protein carboxymethylase

PCMB parachloromercuribenzoate

PCMO Principal Clinical Medical Officer

PCMR Pediatric Cardiomyopathy Registry

PCMS patient care management system

PCMs patient care management categories

PCMT pacemaker circus movement tachycardia; protein carboxyl methyltransferase

PCN parent-child nursing; penicillin; primary care network; primary care nursing

PCNA proliferating cell nuclear antigen

PCNB pentachloronitrobenzene

PCNL percutaneous nephrostolithotomy

PCNV postchemotherapy nausea and vomiting; Provisional Committee on Nomenclature of Viruses

PCO parametric clinical observation; patient complains of; polycystic ovary; posterior capsular opacification; predicted cardiac output

P_CO partial pressure of carbon monoxide

P_CO2, pCO_2 partial pressure of carbon dioxide

PCOC Primary Care Organization Consortium

PCOD polycystic ovarian disease

PCOM posterior communicating [artery]

PCON Primary Care Organization Network

PCOS polycystic ovary syndrome

PCP parachlorophenate; patient care plan; pentachlorophenol; 1-(1-phenylcyclohexyl)piperidine; peripheral coronary pressure; persistent cough and phlegm; phencyclidine; *Pneumocystis carinii* pneumonia; postoperative constrictive pericarditis; primary care physician; primary care provider; prochlorperazine; procollagen peptide; prolylcarboxypeptidase; pulmnary capillary pressure; pulse cytophotometry

PCPA para-chlorophenylalanine

PCPB procarboxypeptide B

PCPL pulmonary capillary protein leakage

pcpn precipitation

PCQ polychloroquaterphenyl

PCR patient contact record; perinatal clinical record; phosphocreatinine; plasma clearance rate; polymerase chain reaction; post-compression remodeling; prehospital care report; principal component regression; protein catabolism rate

PCr phosphocreatine

P_{Cr} plasma creatinine

pcr protein catabolic rate

PCR/SSCP polymerase chain reaction-single stranded conformation polymorphism

PCRV polycythemia rubra vera

PCS palliative care service; patient care system; patient classification system; patient-controlled sedation; patterns of care study; pelvic congestion syndrome; pharmacogenic confusional syndrome; portacaval shunt; post-cardiac surgery; postcardiotomy syndrome; postcholecystectomy syndrome; postconcussion syndrome; premature centromere separation; Prevention of Coronary Atherosclerosis Study; primary cancer site; prolonged crush syndrome; proportional counter spectrometry; proximal coronary sinus; pseudotumor cerebri syndrome

pcs preconscious

PCS/ADS patient care system/application development system

PCSM percutaneous stone manipulation

PCSS Perth Community Stroke Study

PCSW personal care service worker

PCT peripheral carcinoid tumor; plasma clotting time; plasmacrit test; plasmacytoma; polychlorinated triphenyl; polychlorinated triphenyl; porphyria cutanea tarda; portacaval transposition; positron computed tomography; postcoital test; progesterone challenge test; prothrombin consumption time; proximal convoluted tubule

pct percent

PCTI penetrating cardiac trauma index

PCU pain control unit; palliative care unit; primary care unit; progressive care unit; patient care unit; pulmonary care unit

PCV packed cell volume; polycythemia vera; postcapillary venule; pressure-control ventilation

PCVC percutaneous central venous catheter

PCV-M polycythemia vera with myeloid metaplasia

PCW pericanalicular web; personal care worker; primary capillary wedge; pulmonary capillary wedge; purified cell walls

PCWP pulmonary capillary wedge pressure

PCx patient's cardex; periscopic convex

PCZ procarbazine; prochlorperazine

PD Doctor of Pharmacy; Dublin Pharmacopoeia; interpupillary distance; Paget disease; pancreatic duct; panic disorder; papilla diameter; paralyzing dose; Parkinson disease; parkinsonian dementia; paroxysmal discharge; pars distalis; patent ductus; patient day; pediatric, pediatrics; percentage difference; percutaneous discectomy; percutaneous drain; peritoneal dialysis; personality disorder; pharmacodynamics; phenyldichlorarsine; phosphate dehydrogenase; phosphate dextrose; photodiode; photosensitivity dermatitis; Pick disease; plasma defect; poorly differentiated; postdischarge; posterior descending; posterior division; postnasal drainage; postural drainage; potential difference; pregnanediol; present disease; pressor dose; prism diopter; problem drinker; program director; progression of disease; progressive disease; proliferative disease; protein degradation; protein diet; proton density; psychotic depression; pulmonary disease; pulpodistal; pulse duration, pulsed diastolic; pulsed Doppler [wave]; pupil diameter; pupillary distance; pyloric dilator; pyrimidine dimer

P/D proximal-to-distal [vessel]

2-PD two-point discrimination

Pd palladium; pediatrics

P_d diastolic pressure

PDA patent ductus arteriosus; patient distress alarm; personal digital assistant; posterior descending artery; pulmonary disease anemia

PdA pediatric allergy

PDAB para-dimethylaminobenzaldehyde

PD-AB-SAAP pulsed diastolic autologous blood selective aortic arch perfusion

PDAP Palmer drug abuse program

PD/AR photosensitivity dermatitis and actinic reticuloid syndrome

PDAY pathological determinants of atherosclerosis in youth

PDAY/RFEHA Pathobiological Determinants of Atherosclerosis in Youth/Risk Factors in Early Human Atherogenesis [study]

PDB Paget disease of bone; paradichlorobenzene; patient's database; phosphorus-dissolving bacteria; preventive dental [health] behavior; Protein Databank

PDC parkinsonism dementia complex; pediatric cardiology; penta-decylcatechol; phosducin; physical dependence capacity; plasma dioxin concentration; preliminary diagnostic clinic; private diagnostic clinic
PdC pediatric cardiology
PDCA plan-do-check-act
PDCD primary degenerative cerebral disease
PD-CSE pulsed Doppler cross-sectional echocardiography
PDD pervasive developmental disorder; platinum diamminodichloride [cisplatin]; primary degenerative dementia; primary degenerative disorder; pervasive developmental disorder; pyridoxine-deficient diet
PDDD primary degenerative/deformative disorder
PD DNA pyrimidine dimer DNA
PDDNOS pervasive developmental disorder not otherwise specified
PDDR pseudovitamin D-dependent rickets
PDE paroxysmal dyspnea on exertion; partial differential equation; peritoneal dialysis effluent; phosphodiesterase; progressive dialysis encephalopathy; pulsed Doppler echocardiography
PdE pediatric endocrinology
PDEA phosphodiesterase
PDEB phosphodiesterase beta
PDECG platelet-derived endothelial growth [factor]
PD-ECGF platelet-derived endothelial cell growth factor
PDEG phosphodiesterase gamma
PDF parameterized diastolic filling; Parkinson's Disease Foundation; peritoneal dialysis fluid; Portable Document Format; probability density function; pyruvate dehydrogenase
pdf probability density function
PDG parkinsonism-dementia complex of Guam; Pharmacopoeial Discussion Group; phosphogluconate dehydrogenase
PDGA pteroyldiglutamic acid
PDGF platelet-derived growth factor
PDGF-A platelet-derived growth factor A
PDGF-B platelet-derived growth factor B
PDGFR platelet-derived growth factor receptor
PDGFRB platelet-derived growth factor receptor beta

PDGS partial form of DiGeorge syndrome
PD-GXT postdischarge graded exercise test
PDH past dental history; phosphate dehydrogenase; position-of-the-dynamometer-handle [test]; progressive disseminated histoplasmosis; pyruvate dehydrogenase
PDHA pyruvate dehydrogenase alpha
PDHa pyruvate dehydrogenase in active form
PDHB pyruvate dehydrogenase beta
PDHC pyruvate dehydrogenase complex
PdHO pediatric hematology-oncology
PDI pain disability index; periodontal disease index; plan-do integration; psychomotor development index
Pdi transdiaphragmatic pressure
Pdi$_{max}$ maximum transdiaphragmatic pressure
PDIE phosphodiesterase
P-diol pregnanediol
PDIS participatory design of information system
PDK primary duck kidney
PDL pancreatic duct ligation; periodontal ligament; poorly differentiated lymphocyte; population doubling level; progressive diffuse leukoencephalopathy
pdl poundal; pudendal
PDLC poorly differentiated lung cancer
PDLD poorly differentiated lymphocytic-diffuse
PDLL poorly differentiated lymphocytic lymphoma
PDLN poorly differentiated lymphocytic-nodular
PDM point distribution model
PDMS patient data management system; pharmacokinetic drug monitoring service; polydimethylsiloxane
PDN prednisone; private duty nurse
pDNA plasmid deoxyribonucleic acid
PdNEO pediatric neonatology
PdNEP pediatric nephrology
PDP parallel distributed processing; pattern disruption point; peak diastolic pressure; piperidinopyrimidine; platelet-derived plasma; postural drainage and chest percussion; primer-dependent deoxynucleic acid polymerase; Product Development Protocol; programmed data processor
PDPD prolonged-dwell peritoneal dialysis

PDPDM protein-deficient pancreatic diabetes mellitus

PDPH postdural puncture headache

PDPI primer-dependent deoxynucleic acid polymerase index

PDQ Personality Diagnostic Questionnaire; physician's data query; Premenstrual Distress Questionnaire; prescreening developmental questionnaire; protocol data query

PDR pediatric radiology; peripheral diabetic retinopathy; *Physicians' Desk Reference*; postdelivery room; primary drug resistance; proliferative diabetic retinopathy

PdR pediatric radiology

pdr powder

PDRB Permanent Diability Rating Board

PDRT Portland Digit Recognition

PDS pain-dysfunction syndrome; paroxysmal depolarizing shift; patient data system; Patient-Doctor Society; pediatric surgery; penile Doppler study; perfusion defect size; peritoneal dialysis system; plasma-derived serum; polydioxanone sutures; post determination software; predialyzed serum; proteodermatan sulfate

PdS pediatric surgery

PDSG pigment dispersion syndrome glaucoma

PDSIP Physician-delivered Smoking Intervention Project

PDSRS Panic Disorder Self-Rating Scale

PDT photodynamic therapy; population doubling time

PDTC pyrrolidine dithiocarbamate

PDUF pulsed Doppler ultrasonic flowmeter

PDUFA Prescription Drug User Fee Act

PDUR Predischarge Utilization Review

PDV peak disatolic velocity; plasma-derived vaccine

PDVT proximal deep vein thrombosis

PDW platelet distribution width

PDWA proliferative disease without atypia

PDWHF platelet-derived wound-healing factor

PDYN prodynorphin

PE Edinburgh Pharmacopoeia; pancreatic extract; paper electrophoresis; partial epilepsy; peak error; pelvic examination; penile erection; pericardial effusion; peritoneal exudate; pharyngoesophageal; phase-encoded; phenylethylamine; phenylephrine; phenytoin equivalent; phosphatidyl ethanolamine; photographic effect; phycoerythrin; physical education; physical engineering; physical examination; physical exercise; physician extender; physiological ecology; pigmented epithelium; pilocarpine-epinephrine; placental extract; plant engineering; plasma exchange; platinum etoposide; pleural effusion; point of entry; polyethylene; potential energy; powdered extract; preeclampsia; preexcitation; present evaluation; pressure equalization; presumptive eligibility; prior to exposure; probable error; processing element; professional engineer; program evaluation; pseudoexfoliation; pulmonary edema; pulmonary embolism; pyrogenic exotoxin

Pe pressure on expiration

PEA patient-controlled epidural anesthesia; pelvic examination under anesthesia; phenylethyl alcohol; phenylethylamine; polysaccharide egg antigen; pulseless electrical activity

PEACH Physiologic Evaluation After Coronary Hyperemia [trial]

PEAP positive end-airway pressure

PEAR phase encoded artifact reduction

PEARLA pupils equal and react to light and accommodation

PEAS patient education and activation system

PEBG phenethylbiguanide

PEBP patient escorted by police

PEC patient evaluation center; pelvic cramps; peritoneal exudate cell; perivascular epithelioid cell; probability of error in classification; pulmonary ejection click; pyrogenic exotoxin C

PECAM platelet-endothelial cell adhesion molecule

PECS patient evaluation and conference system; pediatrics evaluation in community setting

PECT positron emission computed tomography

PECTE Pulmonary Embolism Colfarit Trial in the Elderly

PECVD plasma-enhanced chemical vapor deposition

PED palmoplantar ectodermal dysplasia; patient examined by doctor; pediatric emergency department; pink-eyed dilution

PED, ped pediatrics
PEDF pigment epithelium-derived factor
PeDS Pediatric Drug Surveillance
PEE phosphate-eliminating enzyme
PEEK polyetheretherketone
PEEP/CPAP positive end-expiratory pressure/continuous positive airway pressure
PEEPrs resistive positive end-respiratory pressure
PEER peer review effectiveness evaluation research
PEF peak expiratory flow; pharyngoepiglottic fold; Psychiatric Evaluation Form; pulmonary edema fluid
PEFR peak expiratory flow rate
PEFV partial expiratory flow volume
PEG Patient Evaluation Grid; percutaneous endoscopic gastrostomy; pneumoencephalogram, pneumoencephalography; polyethylene glycol
PEGASUS Percutaneous Endarterectomy, the Goal of Atherectomy Successfully Guided by Ultrasound [trial]
Pegs paternally expressed genes
PEG-SOD polyethylene glycol superoxide desmutase
PEHO progressive encephalopathy-edema-hypsarrhythmia-optic atrophy syndrome
PEHPC periodic examination and health promotion center
PEI Patient Exit Interview; phosphate excretion index; physical efficiency index; polyethyleneimine
PEIRS pathology expert interpretative reporting system
PEJ percutaneous endoscopic jejunostomy
PEK punctate epithelial kerotopathy
PEL peritoneal exudate lymphocyte; permissible exposure limit
PELA peripheral excimer laser angioplasty
PELCA percutaneous excimer laser coronary angioplasty
PEM pediatric emergency medicine; peritoneal exudate macrophage; polymorphic epithelial mucin; prescription event monitoring; precordial electrocardiographic monitoring; primary enrichment medium; probable error of measurement; protein energy malnutrition; pulmonary endothelial membrane
PEMA phenylethylmalonamide
PE$_{max}$ maximum expiratory pressure

PEMF pulsed electromagnetic field
PEN pharmacy equivalent name; practitioners entering notes
Pen penicillin
PEN&PAD practitioners entering notes and practitioners accessing data [system]
PENK proenkephalin
PENT phenylethanolamine N-methyltransferase
Pent pentothal
PEO progressive external ophthalmoplegia
PEP patient education program; Pediatric Education for Paramedics [course]; peptidase; phospho(enol)pyruvate; peer evaluation program; phosphoenolpyruvate; pigmentation, edema, and plasma cell dyscrasia [syndrome]; polyestradiol phosphate; pore-forming protein; positive expiratory pressure; postencephalitic parkinsonism; postexposure prophylaxis; pre-ejection period; protein electrophoresis; Psychiatric Evaluation Profile
Pep peptidase
PEPA peptidase A; prospective evaluation of prognosis in angina
PEPB peptidase B
PEPC peptidase C
PEPc corrected pre-ejection period
PEPCK phosphoenolpyruvate carboxykinase
PEPD peptidase D
PEPE peptidase E
PEPI pre-ejection period index; Postmenopausal Estrogen-Progestin Intervention [trial]
PEPP positive expiratory pressure plateau; Pregnancy Exposures and Pre-eclampsia Prevention [project]
PEPS peptidase S
PER peak ejection rate; periodogram; protein efficiency ratio
per perineal; periodicity, periodic
perCP peridinin chlorophyll protein
percus percussion
Perf perfusion or perfusionist
perf perforation
PERFEXT Perfusion, Performance, Exercise Trial
PERG pattern electroretinogram
PERI Psychiatric Epidemiology Research Interview

periap periapical
Perio periodontics
PERK prospective evaluation of radial keratotomy [protocol]
PERLA pupils equal, react to light and accommodation
PERM Prospective Evaluation of Perfusion Markers [study]
PerNET peripheral neuroectodermal tumor
perp perpendicular
PERRLA pupils equal, round, and reactive to light and accommodation
PERS Patient Evaluation Rating Scale; pediatric emergency rating scale
PERT phenol-enhanced reassociation technique; program evaluation review technique
PES Patient Escort Service; perceived stress scale; photoelectron spectroscopy; physical examination syndrome; physicians' equity services; polyethylene sulfonate; postextrasystolic; preepiglottic space; preexcitation syndrome; primary empty sella [syndrome]; programmed electrical stimulation; pseudoepileptic seizures; pseudoexfoliation syndrome; pseudoexfoliative syndrome; psychiatric emergency services
Pes esophageal pressure
PESDA perfluorocarbon-exposed sonicated dextrose albumin
PESP postextrasystolic potentiation
PESS problem, etiology, signs and symptoms
Pess pessary
PET paraffin-embedded tissue; peak ejection time; peritoneal equilibrium test; polyethylene terphthalate; polyethylene tube; poor exercise tolerance; positron emission tomography; preeclamptic toxemia; pressure equilization tube; progressive exercise test; psychiatric emergency team
PET$_{CO2}$ end-tidal pressure of carbon dioxide
PETH pink-eyed, tan-hooded [rat]
PETN pentaerythritol tetranitrate
petr petroleum
PETQI patient education total quality improvement
PETSc portable extensible toolkit for scientific computation
PETT pendular eye-tracking test; positron emission transverse tomography

PEU plasma equivalent unit
PEV peak expiratory velocity; positive effect variegation
pev peak electron volts
PEW pulmonary extravascular water
PEWV pulmonary extravascular water volume
PEx physical examination
Pex peak exercise
PF pair feeding; peak flow; peak frequency; pemphigus foliaceus; perfusion fluid; pericardial fluid; periosteal fibroblast; peritoneal fluid; permeability factor; personality factor; picture-frustration [study]; plantar flexion; plasma factor; plasmapheresis; platelet factor; pleural fluid; power factor; primary fibrinolysin; prostatic fluid; pterygoid fossa; pulmonary factor; pulmonary function; Purkinje fiber; purpura fulminans; push fluids; pyrozafurin
P-F picture-frustration [test]
P$_f$ final pressure
PF$_{1-4}$ platelet factors 1 to 4
Pf *Plasmodium falciparum*
pF picofarad
PFA arteria femoris profunda; p-fluorophenylalanine; phosphonotormate
PFAS performic acid-Schiff [reaction]
PFB perflubron; proportion of fed bugs [Chagas disease]
PFC pair-fed control [mice]; patient-focused care; pelvic flexion contracture; perfluorocarbon; perfluorochemical; pericardial fluid culture; persistent fetal circulation; plaque-forming cell
pFc noncovalently bonded dimer of the C-terminal immunoglobulin of the Fc fragment
PFD polyostotic fibrous dysplasia; pseudoinflammatory fundus disease
PFDA perfluoro-decanoic acid
PFE pelvic floor exercise
PFFD proximal focal femoral deficiency
PFG peak flow gauge; pulsed-field gel electrophoresis
PFGE pulsed field gel electrophoresis
PFGS phosphoribosyl formylglycinamide synthetase
PFIB perfluoroisobutylene
PFIC progressive familial intrahepatic cholestasis
PFJ patellofemoral joint

PFK phosphofructokinase; 6-phospho-fructo-2-kinase

PFKF 6-phosphofructo-2-kinase, fibroblast type

PFKL phosphofructokinase, liver type; 6-phosphofructo-2-kinase, liver type

PFKM phosphofructokinase, muscle type

PFKP phosphofructokinase, platelet type; 6-phosphofructo-2-kinase, platelet type

PFKX 6-phosphofructo-2-kinase X

PFL profibrinolysin

pflops pentaflops [floating points per second]

PFM peak flow meter

PFN partially functional neutrophil; profilin; proximal femoral nail

PFO patent foramen ovale

PFOB perfluorocytylbromide

PFP peripheral facial paralysis; plain film pelvis [x-ray]; platelet-free plasma; pulmonary fibroproliferation

PFPS patellofemoral pain syndrome

PFQ personality factor questionnaire

PFR parotid flow rate; particulate filter respirator; peak flow rate

PFRC predicted functional residual capacity

PFS patellofemoral syndrome; primary fibromyalgia syndrome; protein-free supernatant; pulmonary function score

PFSH past, family and social history

PFT pancreatic function test; parafascicular thalamotomy; posterior fossa tumor; prednisone, fluorouracil, and taxomifen; pulmonary function test

PFTBE progressive form of tick-borne encephalitis

PFU plaque-forming unit; pock-forming unit

PFUO prolonged fever of unknown origin

PFV physiologic full value

PG parallel group; paregoric; parotid gland; pentagastrin; pepsinogen; peptidoglycan; Pharmacopoeia Germanica; phosphate glutamate; phosphatidylglycerol; phosphogluconate; pigment granule; pituitary gonadotropin; plasma glucose; plasma triglyceride; polyfalacturonate; post graft; postgraduate; practice guideline; pregnanediol glucuronide; pregnant; progesterone; prolyl hydrolase; propyl gallate; propylene glycol; Prospect Hill [virus];

prostaglandin; proteoglycan; pyoderma gangrenosum

2PG 2-phosphoglycerate

3PG 3-phosphoglycerate

Pg nasopharyngeal electrode placement in electroencephalography; gastric pressure; pogonion; pregnancy, pregnant

pg parthenogenic; picogram; pregnant

PGA pepsinogen A; phosphoglyceric acid; polyglandular autoimmune [syndrome]; polyglycolic acid; prostaglandin A; pteroylglutamic acid

PGA$_{1-3}$ prostaglandins A$_1$ to A$_3$

PGAM monophosphoglycerate mutase

PGAP pilot geriatric arthritis program

PGAS persisting galactorrhea-amenorrhea syndrome; polyglandular autoimmune syndrome

PGB porphobilinogen; prostaglandin B

PGC progastricin; primordial germ cell

PGCL [nucleus] paragigantocellularis lateralis

PGD phosphogluconate dehydrogenase; phosphoglyceraldehyde dehydrogenase; prostaglandin D

PGD$_2$ prostaglandin D$_2$

6-PGD 6-phosphogluconate dehydrogenase

PGDH phosphogluconate dehydrogenase

PGDR plasma glucose disappearance rate

PGE platelet granule extract; posterior gastroenterostomy

PGE, PGE$_1$, PGE$_2$ prostaglandins E, E$_1$, E$_2$

PGF phylogenetic footprint

PGF, PGF$_1$, PGF$_2$ prostaglandins F, F$_1$, F$_2$

PGFT phosphoribosylglycinamide formyltransferase

PG prostaglandin G

PGG polyclonal gamma globulin

PGG$_2$ prostaglandin G$_2$

PGH pituitary growth hormone; porcine growth hormone; prostaglandin H

PGH$_2$ prostaglandin H$_2$

PGHS prostaglandin G/H synthase

PGI phosphoglucose isomerase; potassium, glucose, and insulin; prostaglandin I

PGI$_2$ prostaglandin I$_2$

PGK phosphoglycerate kinase

PGL persistent generalized lymphadenopathy; phosphoglycolipid; 6-phosphogluconolactonase

PGlyM phosphoglyceromutase

PGM phosphoglucomutase; phosphoglycerate mutase
PGMA phosphoglycerate mutase A
PGMB phosphoglycerate mutase B
pg/mL picograms per milliliter
PGN proliferative glomerulonephritis
PGNA prompt gamma neutron activation
PGO ponto-geniculo-occipital [spike]
PGP phosphoglyceroyl phosphatase; postgamma proteinuria; prepaid group practice; progressive general paralysis
PGR progesterone receptor; psychogalvanic response
PgR progesterone receptor
PGS peristent gross splenomegaly; Pettigrew syndrome; plant growth substance; polar grid system; postsurgical gastroparesis syndrome; prostaglandin synthetase
PGSI prostaglandin synthetase inhibitor
PGSR phosphogalvanic skin response
PGT preimplantation genetic testing
PGTR plasma glucose tolerance rate
PGTT prednisolone glucose tolerance test
PGU peripheral glucose uptake; postgonococcal urethritis
PGUT phosphogalactose uridyl transferase
PGV proximal gastric vagotomy
PGWB psychological general well-being [index]
PGX prostacyclin
PGY postgraduate year
PGYE peptone, glucose yeast extract
PH Pallister-Hall [syndrome]; parathyroid hormone; partial hepatectomy; partial hysterectomy; passive hemagglutination; past history; patient's history; persistent hepatitis; personal history; pharmacopeia; pharmacy, pharmacist, or pharmaceutical; physical history; porphyria hepatica; posterior heel; posterior hypothalamus; prehospital; previous history; primary hyperoxaluria; primary hyperparathyroidism; prostatic hypertrophy; pseudohermaphroditism; public health; pulmonary hypertension; pulmonary hypoplasia
Ph phantom; pharmacopeia; phenyl; Philadelphia [chromosome]; phosphate
PH1 primary hyperoxaluria type 1
Ph¹ Philadelphia chromosome
pH hydrogen ion concentration
pH₁ isoelectric point
ph phial; phot

PHA passive hemagglutination [test]; peripheral hyperalimentation; phenylalanine; phytohemagglutinin; phytohemagglutinin antigen; pseudohypoaldosteronism; public health agency; Public Health Association; pulse-height analyzer
pH$_A$ arterial blood hydrogen tension
pH$_a$ arterial hydrogen ion concentration
PHAC phaclofen
PHAF peripheral hyperalimentation formula
PHAL phytohemagglutinin-stimulated lymphocyte
phal phalangeal
PHA-LCM phytohemagglutinin-stimulated leukocyte conditioned medium
PHA-NSP passive hemagglutination to nonstructural protein
PHAP phytohemagglutinin protein
PHAR pharmacologic substance [UMLS]
phar pharmaceutical; pharmacy; pharynx
PHARM Pharmacist in Heart Failure: Assessment, Recommendation and Monitoring [study]
Pharm B Bachelor of Pharmacy [Lat. *Pharmaciae Baccalaureus*]
Phar C pharmaceutical chemist
Pharm pharmacy
Pharm D Doctor of Pharmacy [Lat. *Pharmaciae Doctor*]
Pharm M Master of Pharmacy [Lat. *Pharmaciae Magister*]
pharm pharmacist; pharmacology; pharmacopeia; pharmacy
PHASE prehospital arrest survival evaluation
PHAVER pterygia-heart defects-autosomal recessive inheritance-vertebral defects-ear anomalies-radial defects [syndrome]
PHB polyhydroxybutyrate; preventive health behavior; prohibitin
PhB, Phb Pharmacopoeia Britannica
PHBB propylhydroxybenzyl benzimidazole
PHBQ Physicians' Humanistic Behaviors Questionnaire
PHC personal health costs; posthospital care; premolar hypodontia, hyperhidrosis, [premature] canities [syndrome]; primary health care; primary hepatic carcinoma; proliferative helper cell; public health center
PhC pharmaceutical chemist
Ph¹ᶜ Philadelphia chromosome

PHCC primary hepatocellular carcinoma

PHCP prehospital care provider

PHD pathological habit disorder; personal health data; post-heparin plasma diamine oxidase; potentially harmful drug

PhD Doctor of Pharmacy [Lat. *Pharmaciae Doctor*]; Doctor of Philosophy [Lat. *Philosophiae Doctor*]

PHE periodic health examination; phenylephrine

Phe phenylalanine

PhEEM photoemission electron microscopy

PHEI prevention and health evaluation informatics

pHEMA polyhydroxyethyl methacrylate

PHEN phenomenon or process [UMLS]

Phen phentermine

Pheo pheochromocytoma; pheophytin

PHF paired helical filament; personal hygiene facility

PHFB psyllium husk fiber bar

PHFG primary human fetal glia

PhG Graduate in Pharmacy; Pharmacopoeia Germanica

phgly phenylglycine

PHHI persistent hyperinsulinemic hypoglycemia of infancy

PHHP Pawtucket Heart Health Program

PHI passive hemagglutination inhibition; past history of illness; phosphohexose isomerase; physiological hyaluronidase inhibitor; prehospital index

PhI Pharmacopoeia Internationalis

pHi intramucosal hydrogen ion concentration

φ Greek letter *phi*; magnetic flux; osmotic coefficient

PHICOG Philadelphia Cooperative Group

PHIHM prehospital invasive hemodynamic monitoring

PHIM posthypoxic intention myoclonus

PhIS pharmacy information system

PHK phosphohexokinase; phosphorylase kinase; postmortem human kidney

PHKA phosphorylase kinase, alpha

PHKB phosphorylase kinase, beta

PHKD phosphorylase kinase, delta

PHKG phosphorylase kinase, gamma

PHL public health laboratory

PHLA postheparin lipolytic activity

PHLOP polymerase-halt-mediated linkage of primers

PHLS Public Health Laboratory Service

PHM peptide histidine methionine; peptidylglycine alpha-hydroxylating monooxygenase; posterior hyaloid membrane; pulmonary hyaline membrane

PhM Master of Pharmacy [Lat. *Pharmaciae Magister*]; pharyngeal muscle

PhmG Graduate in Pharmacy

PHN paroxysmal noctural hemoglobinuria; passive Heymann nephritis; postherpetic neuralgia; public health nursing; public health nurse

PHO physician-hospital organization

PH₂O partial pressure of water vapor

phos phosphate

PHOX paired mesoderm homeobox [gene]

PHP panhypopituitarism; postheparin phospholipase; prehospital program; prepaid health plan; primary hyperparathyroidism; pseudohypoparathyroidism

pHPPA p-hydrophenylpyruvic acid

p-HPPO p-hydroxyphenyl pyruvate oxidase

PHPT primary hyperparathyroidism; pseudohypoparathyroidism

pHPT primary hyperparathyroidism

PHPV persistent hyperplastic primary vitreous

PHR parent-held record; peak heart rate; photoreactivity

PHS Physicians' Health Study; pooled human serum; posthypnotic suggestion; pseudoprogeria-Hallermann-Streiff [syndrome]; Public Health Service

PHSC pleuripotent hemopoietic stem cell; powdered human stratum corneum

pH-stat apparatus for maintaining the pH of a solution

PHT phenytoin; portal hypertension; pressure half-time; primary hyperthyroidism; pulmonary hypertension

PhTD Doctor of Physical Therapy

PHTLS prehospital trauma life support

PHV peak height velocity; Prospect Hill virus

PHX pulmonary histiocytosis X

Phx past history; pharynx

PHY pharyngitis; physical; physiology

PHYLLIS Plaque Hypertension Lipid-Lowering Italian Study

PHYS physiologic function [UMLS]; physiology

PhyS physiologic saline [solution]

phys physical; physician
Phys Ed physical education
physio physiology; physiotherapy
Phys Med physical medicine
PHYS-SPEC physician's specialty
PhysPRC Physician's Payment Review Commission
Phys Ther physical therapist or therapy
PI class I protein; first meiotic prophase; isoelectric point; pacing impulse; package insert; pain intensity; pancreatic insufficiency; parainfluenza; pars intermedia; patient's interest; performance intensity; perinatal injury; periodontal index; permeability index; personal injury; personality inventory; Pharmacopoeia Internationalis; phosphatidylinositol; physically impaired; physiologic index; pineal body; plaque index; plasmin inhibitor; pneumatosis intestinalis; poison ivy; ponderal index; postictal immobility; postinfection; postinfluenza; postinjury; postinoculation; preinduction [examination]; premature infant; prematurity index; preparatory interval; present illness; primary infarction; primary infection; principal investigator; product information; proinsulin; prolactin inhibitor; propidium iodide; protamine insulin; protease inhibitor; proximal intestine; pulmonary incompetence; pulmonary index; pulmonary infarction; pulsatility index
P&I pneumonia and influenza
P$_I$ inspiratory pressure
Pi, P$_i$ inorganic phosphate
Pi parental generation; pressure in inspiration; protease inhibitor
pI isoelectric point
p-I postinspiratory
pi post-injection
II Greek capital letter *pi*
π Greek lower case letter *pi;* the ratio of circumference to diameter, 3.1415926536
PIA photoelectric intravenous angiography; plasma insulin activity; preinfarction angina; Psychiatric Institute of America; *R*-phenylisopropyladenosine
PIAF pharmacologic intervention in atrial fibrillation; prognosis in atrial fibrillation
PIAT Peabody Individual Achievement Test
PIAVA polydactyly-imperforate anus-vertebral anomalies [syndrome]

PIBC percutaneous intraaortic balloon counterpulsation [catheter]
PIBIDS, PIBI(D)S photosensitivity–ichthyosis–brittle hair–impaired intelligence–(possibly decreased fertility)–short stature syndrome
PIC pacing in cardiomyopathy; peripherally-inserted indwelling central catheter; Personality Inventory for Children; pre-injury condition; polymorphism information content
PICA percutaneous transluminal coronary angioplasty; Porch Index of Communicative Abilities; posterior inferior cerebellar artery; posterior inferior communicating artery
PICC percutaneous indwelling central venous catheter; peripherally inserted central catheter
PICD primary irritant contact dermatitis
PICFS postinfective chronic fatigue syndrome
PICNIC Pediatric Investigators Collaborative Network on Infections in Canada
PICO Pimobendan in Congestive Heart Failure [study]; population, intervention, comparison and outcome
PICS Pacing in Cardiomyopathy Study
PICSO pressure-controlled intermittent coronary sinus occlusion
PICSS Patent Foramen Ovale in Cryptogenic Stroke Study
PICTURE Post-intracoronary Treatment Ultrasound Results Evaluation [study]
PICU pediatric intensive care unit; pulmonary intensive care unit
PID pain intensity difference [score]; patient identity; pelvic inflammatory disease; photoionization detector; picture image directory; plasma iron disappearance; postinertia dyskinesia; preimplantation diagnosis; prolapsed/protruded intervertebral disk
PIDRA portable insulin dosageregulating apparatus
PIDS primary immunodeficiency syndrome
PIDT plasma iron disappearance time
PIE postinfectious encephalomyelitis preimplantation embryo; prosthetic infectious endocarditis; pulmonary infiltration with eosinophilia; pulmonary interstitial emphysema

PIF paratoid isoelectric focusing variant protein; peak inspiratory flow; photoinhibition factor; proinsulin-free; prolactin-inhibiting factor; prolactin release-inhibiting factor; proliferation-inhibiting factor; prostatic interstitial fluid

PIFG poor intrauterine fetal growth

PIFR peak inspiratory flow rate

PIFT platelet immunofluorescence test

PIG Polaris Investigator Group; polymeric immunoglobulin

PIGA phosphatidylinositol glycan A

pigm pigment, pigmented

PIGR polymeric immunoglobulin receptor

PIH periventricular-intraventricular hemorrhage; phenyl isopropylhydrazine; pregnancy-induced hypertension; prolactin-inhibiting hormone

PII plasma inorganic iodine; primary irritation index

PIIgG surface IgG

PIIP portable insulin infusion pump

PIIS posterior inferior iliac spine

P$_{ij}$ propagation delay

PI3K, PI-3K phosphatidylinositol-3′-kinase

PIL patient information leaflet

PILBD paucity of interlobular bile ducts

PILL Pennebaker Inventory of Limbic Languidness

PILOT Polish Intramural Low Molecular Weight Heparin Outpatient Stent Trial; Preliminary Investigation of Local Therapy [using porous percutaneous transluminal coronary angioplasty balloons]

PILP postinfarction late potential

PILS Pilsen Longitudinal Study

πm pi meson

PIM penicillamine-induced myasthenia

PI$_{max}$ maximum inspiratory pressure at residual volume

PIMI predictive index for myocardial infarction; psychophysiological interventions in myocardial ischemia

PIMS patient information management system

PIN patient information network; personal identification number; product identification number; prostatic intraepithelial neoplasia

Pin inflow pressure

PINN proposed international nonproprietary name

PINV postimperative negative variation

PIO$_2$ partial pressure of inspired oxygen

PION posterior ischemic optic neuropathy

PIOPED Prospective Investigation of Pulmonary Embolism Diagnosis [data base]

PIP paralytic infantile paralysis; peak inflation pressure, peak inspiratory pressure; periodic interim payment; piperacillin; postinfusion phlebitis; pressure inversion point; primary injury prevention; prolactin-inducible protein; proximal interphalangeal [joint]; Psychotic Inpatient Profile; psychosis, intermittent hyponatremia, polydipsia [syndrome]; posterior interphalangeal; probable intrauterine pregnancy

PIP$_2$ phosphatidylinositol 4,5-biphosphate or diphosphate

PI-P phosphatidylinositol-4-phosphate

PIPE persistent interstitial pulmonary emphysema

PIPIDA p-isopropylacetanilido imidodiacetic acid

PIPJ proximal interphalangeal joint

PI-PP phosphatidylinositol-4,5-biphosphate

PIPS patient information protocol system

PIQ Performance Intelligence Quotient

PIR postinhibition rebound; Protein Identification Registry; protein identification resource; Protein Information Resource [protein sequence database]

PIRI plasma immunoreactive insulin

PIRS plasma immunoreactive secretion; postinfarction risk stratification

PIRTS patient identification for rotational therapy system

PIS pharmacy information system; preinfarction syndrome; primary immunodeficiency syndrome; Primary Index Score; Provisional International Standard

pIs isoelectric point

PISA proximal isovelocity surface area

PISA-PED Prospective Investigative Study of Acute Pulmonary Embolism Diagnosis

PISCES percutaneously inserted spinal cord electrical stimulation

PISI pediatric illness severity index

PIT pacing-induced tachycardia; patella inhibition test; pericranial injection therapy; picture identification test; pitocin; pitressin; plasma iron turnover

pit pituitary

PITAC President's Information Technology Advisory Committee
PITC phenylisothiocyanate
PITR plasma iron turnover rate
PIU polymerase-inducing unit; programmed instruction unit
PIV parainfluenza virus; polydactyly-imperforate anus-vertebral anomalies [syndrome]; projective image visualization
PIVD protruded intervertebral disk
PIVH peripheral intravenous hyperalimentation; periventricular-intraventricular hemorrhage
PIVKA protein induced by vitamin K absence or antagonism
P/I/X patients, indicators, external bodies
PIXE particle-induced x-ray emission; proton-induced x-ray emission
Pixel picture element
PIXI paternally imprinted X inactivation
PJ pancreatic juice; Peutz-Jeghers [syndrome]
PJB premature junctional beat
PJC premature junctional contractions
pJC Jamestown Canyon virus plasmid
PJM positive joint mobilization
PJP pancreatic juice protein
PJS peritonojugular shunt; Peutz-Jeghers syndrome
PJT paroxysmal junctional tachycardia
PK penetrating keratoplasty; pericardial knock; pharmacokinetics; pig kidney; Prausnitz-Küstner [reaction]; protein kinase; psychokinesis; pyruvate kinase
Pk peak [rate]
pK negative logarithm of the dissociation constant; plasma potassium
pK' apparent value of a pK; negative logarithm of the dissociation constant of an acid
pk peck
PKA protein kinase A
PkA prekallikrein activator
pK$_a$ negative logarithm of the acid ionization constant
PKAR protein kinase activation ratio
PKase protein kinase
PKB protein kinase B
PKC problem-knowledge coupler; protein kinase C
PKCA protein kinase C alpha
PKCB protein kinase C beta

PKCE protein kinase C epsilon
PKCG protein kinase C gamma
PKCSH protein kinase C heavy chain
PKCSL protein kinase C light chain
PKCZ protein kinase C zeta
PKD polycystic kidney disease; proliferative kidney disease
PKD-1 polycystic kidney disease gene-1
PKD-2 polycystic kidney disease gene-2
PKF phagocytosis and killing function
PKI potato kallikrein inhibitor
PKK plasma prekallikrein
PKL pyruvate kinase, liver type
PKM protein kinase M; pyruvate kinase, muscle
PKN parkinsonism
pkn pseudoknot
PKP penetrating keratoplasty
PK/PD pharmacokinetic/pharmacodynamic [model]
PKR phased knee rehabilitation; Prausnitz-Küstner reaction
Pk/Rr peak respiratory rate
PKS protein kinase sequence
PKT pancreas-kidney transplantation; Prausnitz-Küstner test
PKU phenylketonuria
PKV killed poliomyelitis vaccine
pkV peak kilovoltage
PL palmaris longus; pancreatic lipase; perception of light; peroneus longus; phospholipase; phospholipid; photoluminescence; placebo; placental lactogen; plantar; plasmalemma; plastic surgery; platelet lactogen; polarized light; posterolateral; preleukemia; programming language; prolactin; prolymphocytic leukemia; pulpolingual; Purkinje layer
Pl poiseuille
P$_L$ transpulmonary pressure
pl picoliter; placenta; plasma; platelet
PL/I programming language I (one)
PLA peripheral laser angioplasty; phenyl lactate; phospholipase A; phospholipid antibody; placebo therapy; plasminogen activator; platelet antigen; polylactic acid; potentially lethal arrhythmia; procaine/lactic acid; Product License Application; pulp linguoaxial
P$_{La}$ left atrial pressure
PLa pulpolabial
Pla left atrial pressure

PLA2 phospholipase A2

PLAC Pravastatin Limitation in Atherosclerosis in the Coronary Arteries [study]

PLAC-2 Pravastatin, Lipids and Atherosclerosis in the Carotid Arteries [study]

PLAP placental alkaline phosphatase

PLAT plasminogen activator, tissue-type

Plat platelet

PLAU plasminogen activator, urinary

PLAUR plasminogen activator receptor, urokinase type

PLB parietal lobe battery; phospholamban; phospholipase B; porous layer bead

PLC phospholipase C; pityriasis lichenoides chronica; primary liver cancer; proinsulin-like component; protein-lipid complex; pseudolymphocytic choriomeningitis

PLCC primary liver cell cancer

PLCO postoperative low cardiac output

PLCx posterolateral circumflex branch [of coronary artery]

PLD peripheral light detection; phospholipase D; platelet defect; polycystic liver disease; posterior latissimus dorsi [muscle]; potentially lethal damage

PLDH plasma lactic dehydrogenase

PLDR potentially lethal damage repair

PLE paraneoplastic limbic encephalopathy; protein-losing enteropathy; pseudolupus erythematosus

PLED periodic lateral epileptiform discharge

PLES parallel-line equal space

PLET polymyxin, lysosome, EDTA, thallous acetate [in heart infusion agar]

PLEVA pityriasis lichenoides et varioliformis acuta

PLEXES Pacing Lead Explant with Excimer Sheath [study]

PLF perilymphatic fistula; posterior lung fiber

PLFS perilymphatic fistula syndrome

PLG plasminogen; L-propyl-L-leucyl-glucinamide

PlGF placental growth factor

PLGL plasminogen-like

P-LGV psittacosis-lymphogranuloma venereum

PLH placental lactogenic hormone

PLHP personalized lifetime health plan

PLI professional liability insurance

PLIF posterior lumbar interbody fusion

PLISSIT permission to be sexual, limited information, specific suggestions, intensive therapy

PLL peripheral light loss; phase-locked loop; poly-L-lysine; posterior longitudinal ligament; potential loss of life; pressure length loop; prolymphocytic leukemia

PLM percent labeled mitoses; periodic leg movement; plasma level monitoring; polarized light microscopy; Prevention of Mortality with Low-molecular Weight Heparin in Medical Patients [study]

PLMS periodic limb movements during sleep

PLMV posterior leaf mitral valve

PLN peripheral lymph node; phospholamban

PLNA percutaneous lung needle aspiration

PLND pelvic lymph node dissection

PLNT plant

PLO polycystic lipomembranous osteodysplasia

PLOD procollagen-lysine 2-oxoglutarate 5-dioxygenase

PLOSA Physiologic Low-Stress Angioplasty [trial]

PLP phospholipid; plasma leukapheresis; polypeptide; polystyrene latex particles; posterior lobe of pituitary [gland]; proteolipid protein; pyridoxal phosphate

PLPH post-lumbar puncture headache

PLR pupillary light reflex

PLS Papillon-Lefèvre syndrome; partial least square; polydactyly-luxation syndrome; Postsurgery Logiparin Study; preleukemic syndrome; primary lateral sclerosis; prostaglandin-like substance; pulmonary leukostasis syndrome

PLSA posterolateral segment [coronary] artery

PLSD protected least significant difference

PLSR partial least-square regression

PLST progressively lowered stress threshold

Pl Surg plastic surgeon or surgery

PLT pancreatic lymphocytic infiltration; platelet; primed lymphocyte test; primed lymphocyte typing; psittacosis-lymphogranuloma venereum-trachoma [group]

PLTC Partnership for Long Term Care

PLTP phospholipid transfer protein

plumb lead [Lat. *plumbum*]
PLUT Plutchnik [geriatric rating scale]
PLV partial liquid ventilation; poliomyelitis live vaccine; panleukopenia virus; phenylalanine, lysine, and vasopressin; posterior left ventricle
P_{LV} left ventricular pressure
PLVP peak left ventricular pressure
PLW Prader-Labhart-Willi [syndrome]
PLWA person living with acquired immune deficiency syndrome
PLWS Prader-Labhart-Willi syndrome
plx plexus
PLZ phenelzine
PLZF promyelocytic leukemia zinc finger
PM after death (Lat. *post mortem*); after noon [Lat. *post meridiem*]; mean pressure; pacemaker; pantomography; papillary muscle; papular mucinosis; partial meniscectomy; patient management; pectoralis major [muscle]; perinatal mortality; peritoneal macrophage; petit mal epilepsy [Fr. *petit mal*]; photomultiplier; physical medicine; plasma membrane; platelet membrane; platelet microsome; pneumomediastinum; poliomyelitis; polymorph, polymorphonuclear; polymyositis; poor metabolizer; porokeratosis of Mibelli; posterior mitral; postmenstrual; postmortem; premarketing [approval]; premenstrual; premolar; premotor; presystolic murmur; pretibial myxedema; preventive medicine; primary motivation; Prony method [spectral analysis of heart sounds]; prophylactic mastectomy; prostatic massage; protein methylesterase; protocol management; pterygoid muscle; pubertal macromastia; pulmonary macrophage; pulpomesial; purple membrane
Pm promethium
pM picomolar
pm picometer
PMA index of prevalence and severity of gingivitis, where P = papillary gingiva, M = marginal gingiva, and A = attached gingiva; papillary, marginal, attached [gingiva]; paramethoxyamphetamine; Pharmaceutical Manufacturers Association; phenylmercuric acetate; phorbol myristate acetate; phosphomolybdic acid; premarket approval; primary mental abilities; progressive muscular atrophy; pyridylmercuric acetate

$P+_{max}$ peak positive pressure
$P-_{min}$ peak negative pressure
PMB papillomacular bundle; para-hydroxymercuribenzoate; polychrome methylene blue; polymorphonuclear basophil; polymyxin B; postmenopausal bleeding
PMC paramyotonia congenita; patient management category; percutaneous myocardial channeling; phenylmercuric chloride; physical medicine clinic; pleural mesothelial click; premature mitral closure; probability of misclassification; pseudomembranous colitis
PMCC product-moment correlation coefficient [Pearson]
PMCH pro-melanin-concentrating hormone
PMCHL pro-melanin-concentrating hormone-like
PMC-RIS patient management category-relative intensity score
PMCS patient management computer stimulation
PMD Pelizaeus-Merzbacher disease; posterior mandibular depth; primary myocardial disease; private medicine doctor; primary physician; programmed multiple development; progressive muscular dystrophy
PMDD premenstrual dysphoric disorder
PM/DM polymyositis/dermatomyositis
PMDS persistent müllerian duct syndrome; primary myelodysplastic syndrome
PME pelvic muscle exercise; periodic monitoring examination; phosphomonoester; polymorphonuclear eosinophil; progressive multifocal encephalopathy; progressive myoclonus epilepsy
PMEA 9-(2-phosphomethoxyethyl) adenine
PMEL Pacific Marine Environmental Laboratory
PMF platelet membrane fluidity; progressive massive fibrosis; proton motive force; pterygomaxillary fossa
pmf proton motive force
PMG primary medical group
PMGCT primary mediastinal germ-cell tumor
PMH past medical history; posteromedial hypothalamus
PMHAB Provincial Mental Health Advisory Board [Canada]

PMHR predicted maximum heart rate

PMHx past medical history

PMI pain management inventory; past medical illness; patient medication instruction; perioperative myocardial infarction; photon migration imaging; point of maximal impulse; point of maximal intensity; posterior myocardial infarction; postmyocardial infarction; present medical illness; previous medical illness

PMIA N-(1-pyrenamethyl)-iodoacetamide

PMIS postmyocardial infarction syndrome; PSRO Management Information System

PML peripheral motor latency; polymorphonuclear leukocyte; posterior mitral leaflet; progressive multifocal leukodystrophy; progressive multifocal leukoencephalopathy; prolapsing mitral leaflet; promyelocytic leukemia; pulmonary microlithiasis

PMLD Pelizaeus-Merzbacher-like disease

PMLE polymorphous light eruption

PMM pentamethylmelamine; protoplast maintenance medium

PMMA polymethylmethacrylate

PMMIS Program Management and Medical Information System [Medicare]

PMN polymorphonuclear; polymorphonuclear neutrophil; polymorphonucleotide

PMNC percentage of multinucleated cells; peripheral blood mononuclear cell

PMNG polymorphonuclear granulocyte

PMNL peripheral blood monocytes and polymorphonuclear leukocytes; polymorphonuclear leukocyte

PMNN polymorphonuclear neutrophil

PMNR periadenitis mucosa necrotica recurrens

PMNSG Pravastatin Multinational Study Group

PMO postmenopausal osteoporosis; Principal Medical Officer

pmol picomole

pmol/L picomols per liter

PMP pain management program; patient management problems; patient management program; patient medication profile; peripheral myelin protein; peroxisomal membrane protein; persistent mentoposterior [fetal position]; previous menstrual period

PMPM, pmpm per member per month

PMPS postmastectomy pain syndrome

PMPY per member per year

PMQ phytylmenaquinone

PMR paper medical record; patient metarecord; percutaneous myocardial revascularization; perinatal mortality rate; periodic medical review; physical medicine and rehabilitation; polymyalgia rheumatica; primidone; prior medical record; progressive muscular relaxation; proportionate morbidity/mortality ratio; proton magnetic resonance

PM&R physical medicine and rehabilitation

PMRG Pimobendan Multicenter Research Group; Postmastectomy Rehabilitation Group

PMRS physical medicine and rehabilitation service

^{31}**p-MRS** magnetic resonance spectroscopy with phosphorus 31

PMS patient management system; perimenstrual syndrome; periodic movements during sleep; phenazine methosulfate; polydactyly-myopia syndrome; postmarketing surveillance; postmenstrual stress; postmiotic segregation; postmitochondrial supernatant; Pravastatin Multinational Study; pregnant mare serum; premenstrual syndrome, premenstrual symptoms; psychotic motor syndrome

PMSC pediatric medical special care; pluripotent myeloid stem cell

PMSF phenylmethylsulfonyl fluoride

PMSG pregnant mare serum gonadotropin

PMT parent management training; phenol O-methyltransferase; photomultiplier tube; Porteus maze test; premenstrual tension; pyridoxyl-methyl-tryptophan

PMTS premenstrual tension syndrome

PMTT pulmonary mean transit time

PMV paramyxovirus; percutaneous mitral balloon valvotomy; prolapse of mitral valve

PMVI peak myocardial video intensity

PMVL, pMVL posterior mitral valve leaflet

PMW pacemaker wires; patient management workstation

PMX paired mesoderm homeobox [gene]

PN papillary necrosis; parenteral nutrition; penicillin; perceived noise; percussion note; periarteritis nodosa; perinatal; peripheral nerve; peripheral neuropathy; Petri net; phrenic nerve; plaque neutralization; pneumonia; polyarteritis nodosa; polyneuritis; polyneuropathy; polynuclear; positional nystagmus; posterior nares; postnatal; practical nurse; predicted normal; primary nurse; progress note; protease nexin; psychiatry and neurology; psychoneurotic; pyelonephritis; pyridine nucleotide

P/N positive/negative

P&N psychiatry and neurology

P-5'-N pyridine-5'-nucleosidase

P_{N2} partial pressure of nitrogen

Pn pneumatic; pneumonia

pn pain

PNA Paris Nomina Anatomica; peanut agglutinin; pentosenucleic acid

P_{Na} plasma sodium

pNA p-nitroaniline

pNa plasma sodium

PNAvQ positive-negative ambivalent quotient

PNB p-nitrobiphenyl; perineal needle biopsy; peripheral nerve block; premature nodal beat

PNBT p-nitroblue tetrazolium

PNC penicillin; peripheral nucleated cell; pneumotaxic center; premature nodal contracture; primitive neuroendothelial cell

Pnc pneumococcus

PNCA proliferating nuclear cell antigen

PND paroxysmal nocturnal dyspnea; partial neck dissection; postnasal drainage; postnasal drip; postnatal death; principal neutralizing determinant; purulent nasal drainage

PNdb perceived noise decibel

PNE peripheral neuroepithelioma; plasma norepinephrine; pneumoencephalography; pseudomembranous necrotizing enterocolitis

PNEM paraneoplastic encephalomyelitis

PNET peripheral neuroepithelioma; primitive neuroectodermal tumor

PNEU, pneu, pneum pneumonia

PNF proprioceptive neuromuscular facilitation

PNG penicillin G

PNH paroxysmal nocturnal hemoglobinuria; polynuclear hydrocarbon

PNHA Physicians National Housestaff Association

PNI peripheral nerve injury; postnatal infection; prognostic nutritional index

PNID Peer Nomination Inventory for Depression

PNK polynucleotide kinase; pyridoxine kinase

PNK(H) pyridoxine kinase, high

PNK(L) pyridoxine kinase, low

PNL peripheral nerve lesion; polymorphonuclear neutrophilic leukocyte

PNLA percutaneous needle lung aspiration

PNM perinatal mortality; peripheral dysostosis, nasal hypoplasia, and mental retardation [syndrome]; peripheral nerve myelin

PNMK pyridine nucleoside monophosphate kinase

PNMR postnatal mortality risk

PNMT phenyl-ethanolamine-N-methyl-transferase

PNN polynomial neural network; probabilistic neural network

PNO Principal Nursing Officer

p-NO_2 p-nitrosochloramphenicol

PNP pancreatic polypeptide; para-nitrophenol; peak negative pressure; pediatric nurse practitioner; peripheral neuropathy; pneumoperitoneum; polyneuropathy; predictive value of negative results; psychogenic nocturnal polydipsia; purine nucleoside phosphorylase

P-NP para-nitrophenol

PNPase polynucleotide phosphorylase

PNPB positive-negative pressure breathing

PNPP para-nitrophenylphosphate

PNPR positive-negative pressure respiration

PNS paraneoplastic syndrome; parasympathetic nervous system; partial nonprogressive stroke; peripheral nerve stimulation; peripheral nervous system; posterior nasal spine; practical nursing student

PNT partial nodular transformation; patient; picture naming task

Pnt patient

Pnthx pneumothorax

PNU protein nitrogen unit

PNUT portable nursing unit terminal

PNVX pneumococcal vaccine

Pnx pneumothorax

PNZ posterior necrotic zone

PO parieto-occipital; parietal operculum; period of onset; perioperative; posterior; postoperative; predominant organism; pulse oximetry

P₀ open probability; opening pressure

PO₂, P_{O2}, pO2 partial pressure of oxygen

Po porion

p/o postoperative

POA pancreatic oncofetal antigen; phalangeal osteoarthritis; preoptic area; primary optic atrophy

POADS postaxial acrofacial dysostosis syndrome

POAG primary open-angle glaucoma

POA-HA preoptic anterior hypothalamic area

POB penicillin, oil, beeswax; phenoxybenzamine; place of birth

POBA plain old balloon angioplasty

POBJ physical object [UMLS]

POC particulate organic carbon; point of care; polyolefin copolymer; postoperative care; probability of chance; product of conception; proopiomelanocortin

POCS projection onto convex sets

POD peroxidase; place of death; podiatry; polycystic ovary disease; pool of doctors; postoperative day; pouch of Douglas

PODx preoperative diagnosis

POE pediatric orthopedic examination; physician order entry; point of entry; polyoxyethylene; postoperative endophthalmitis; proof of eligibility

POEA polyoxyethylene amine

POEMS Patient-Oriented Evidence that Matters; polyneuropathy, organomegaly, endocrinopathy, M protein, skin changes [syndrome]

POF pattern of failure; position of function; premature ovarian failure; primary or premature ovarian failure; pyruvate oxidation factor

PofE portal of entry

POFX X-linked premature ovarian failure

POG pediatric oncology group; polymyositis ossificans generalisata

Pog pogonion

POGO percentage of glottic opening

pOH hydroxide ion concentration in a solution

POHI physically or otherwise health-impaired

POHS presumed ocular histoplasmosis syndrome

POI Personal Orientation Inventory; piece of information

poik poikilocyte, poikilocytosis

POIS Parkland On-Line Information Systems

pois poison, poisoning, poisoned

POL physician's office laboratory; physicians' online; polymerase

Pol polymerase

pol polish, polishing

POLA polymerase alpha

pol-GIK Polish Glucose-Insulin-Kalium [study]

polio poliomyelitis

POLIP polyneuropathy-ophthalmoplegia-leukoencephalopathy-intestinal pseudo-obstruction [syndrome]

POLISH Polish [investigators to evaluate the effect of amiodarone on mortality after myocardial infarction]

Pol-MONICA Polish Monitoring Trends and Determinants in Cardiovascular Diseases [study]

POLONIA Polish-American Local Lovenox NIR Stent Assessment [study]

Poly polymorphonuclear

poly-A, poly(A) polyadenylic acid

poly-C, poly(C) polycytidylic acid

poly-dA, poly(dA) polydeoxyadenylic acid

poly-G, poly(G) polyguanylic acid

poly-I, poly(I) polyinosinic acid

poly-IC, poly-I:C copolymer of polyinosinic and polycytidylic acids

polys polymorphonuclear leukocytes

poly-T, poly(T) polythymidylic acid

poly-U, poly(U) polyuridylic acid

POM pain on motion; prescription only medicine

POMC proopiomelanocortin

POMONA pregnancy and postpartum, osteoporosis, mastectomy rehabilitation, osteoarthritis, nerve pain, athletic injuries

POMP phase-offset multiplanar [pulse sequence in magnetic resonance imaging]; principal outer material protein

POMR problem-oriented medical record

POMS Profile of Mood States

POMT phenol *O*-methyltransferase

PON paraoxonase; particulate organic nitrogen

pond by weight [Lat. *pondere*]; heavy [Lat. *ponderosus*]

POP diphosphate group; pain on palpation; paroxypropione; persistent occipitoposterior [fetal position]; pituitary opioid peptide; plasma osmotic pressure; plaster of Paris; polymyositis ossificans progressiva; point-of-presence

Pop popliteal; population

POPG population group [UMLS]

POPLINE Population Information Online

poplit popliteal

POPOP 1,4-bis-(5-phenoxazol-2-yl) benzene

POPS patient outcome plans; postoperative pacing study

pops points of presence

POR patient-oriented research; physician of record; postocclusive oscillatory response; prevalence odds ratio; problem-oriented record

PORC porphyria, Chester type

PORH postoperative reactive hyperemia

PORP partial ossicular replacement prosthesis

PORT Patient Outcomes Research Teams [study]; postoperative respiratory therapy

POS periosteal osteosarcoma; physician order set; point of service; polycystic ovary syndrome; provider of services; psychoorganic syndrome

pos position; positive

POSC problem-oriented system of charting

POSCH Program on Surgical Control of Hyperlipidemia

POSM patient-operated selector mechanism

pOsm plasma osmolality

POSS persistent object storage system; proximal over-shoulder strap

POSSUM Pictures of Standard Syndromes and Undiagnosed Malformations; Physiological and Operative Severity Score for the Enumeration of Morbidity and Mortality [study]

POST posterior; Predictors and Outcomes of Stent Thrombosis [study]

Post, post posterior

POST-CARG postcoronary artery bypass graft

postgangl postganglionic

POST LAT posterolateral

postop, post-op postoperative

Post Pit posterior pituitary [gland]

POT periostitis ossificans toxica; postoperative treatment; precursor onset time

pot potassium; potential

potass potassium

POU placenta, ovary, and uterus

Pout outflow pressure

POV physician order verification

PoV portal vein

PO$_2$v venous oxygen pressure

POW Powassan [encephalitis]

powd powder

POX point of exit

PP diphosphate group; emphysema [pink puffers]; near point of accommodation [Lat. *punctum proximum*]; pacesetter potential; palmoplantar; pancreatic polypeptide; paradoxical pulse; paraplatin; parietal pericardium; parietal pulse; partial pressure; perfusion pressure; peritoneal pseudomyxoma; persisting proteinuria; Peyer patches; photoplethysmography; pinprick; placental protein; placenta previa; planned parenthood; plasma pepsinogen; plasmapheresis; plasma protein; plaster of Paris; polypropylene; polystyrene agglutination plate; population planning; posterior papillary; posterior pituitary; postpartum; postprandial; precocious puberty; preferred provider; primapara; primary provider; primer protein; private practice; proactivator plasminogen; protein phosphatase; protoporphyria; protoporphyrin; proximal phalanx; pseudomyxoma peritonei; pterygoid process; pulmonary pressure; pulse pressure; pulsus paradoxus; purulent pericarditis; pyrophosphatase; pyrophosphate

P-P prothrombin proconvertin

P-5'-P pyridoxal-5'-phosphate

PP$_1$ free pyrophosphate

Pp plateau pressure

pp near point of accommodation [Lat. *punctum proximum*]; postprandial; postpartum

PPA palpation, percussion, auscultation; pepsin A; phenylpropanolamine; phenylpyruvic acid; Pittsburgh pneumonia agent;

plasmid profile analysis; polyphosphoric acid; posterior margin of pulmonary artery; posterior pulmonary artery; postpartum amenorrhea; postpill amenorrhea; preferred provider arrangement; primary progressive aphasia; pure pulmonary atresia

PP&A palpation, percussion, and auscultation

PP2A protein phosphatase 2A

Ppa pulmonary artery pressure

PPACK L-propyl-p-phenylalanyl-chloromethylketone

PPAR peroxisome proliferator activated receptor

PPAS peripheral pulmonary artery stenosis

Ppaw pulmonary artery wedge pressure

PPB plasmatic protein binding; plateletpoor blood; pneumococcal pneumonia and bacteremia; positive pressure breathing

PPb postparotid basic protein

ppb parts per billion

PPBP pro-platelet basic protein

PPBS postprandial blood sugar

PPC patient-physician communication; pentose phosphate cycle; peripheral posterior curve; plasma protein concentration; plasma prothrombin conversion; pneumopericardium; posterior parietal cortex; progressive patient care; proximal palmar crease

PPCA plasma prothrombin conversion accelerator; proserum prothrombin conversion accelerator

PPCD polymorphous posterior corneal dystropy

PPCE postproline cleaving enzyme

PPCF peripartum cardiac failure; plasma prothrombin conversion factor

PPCM postpartum cardiomyopathy

PPCRA pigmented paravenous chorioretinal atrophy

PPD packs per day; paraphenylenediamine; percussion and postural drainage; permanent partial disability; phenyldiphenyloxadiazole; postpartum day; primary physical dependence; progressive perceptive deafness; purified protein derivative; Siebert purified protein derivative of tuberculin

PPDS phonologic programming deficit syndrome

PPD-S purified protein derivative-standard

PPE palmoplantar erythrodysesthesia; personal protective equipment; polyphosphoric ester; porcine pancreatic elastase; pulmonary permeability edema

PPES palmar-plantar erythrodysesthesia syndrome

PPET patient-physician encounter table

PPF pellagra preventive factor; phagocytosis promoting factor; phosphonoformate; plasma protein fraction

PPFA Planned Parenthood Federation of America

PPG phonopneumography; photoelectric plethysmography; photoplethysmography; platelet proteoglycan; portal pressure gradient

ppg picopicogram

PPGA postpill galactorrhea-amenorrhea

PPGB protective protein of beta-galactosidase

PPGF polypeptide growth factor

PPGP prepaid group practice

ppGpp 3'-pyrophosphoryl-guanosine-5'-diphosphate

PPH past pertinent history; persistent pulmonary hypertension; phosphopyruvate hydratase; postpartum hemorrhage; primary prevention of hypertension; primary pulmonary hypertension; protocollagen proline hydroxylase

pphm parts per hundred million

PPHN persistent pulmonary hypertension of the newborn

PPHP pseudopseudohypoparathyroidism

ppht parts per hundred thousand

PPI partial permanent impairment; patient package insert; present pain intensity; proton-pump inhibitor; purified porcine insulin

PPi, PP$_i$ inorganic pyrophosphate

PPIase peptidyl-prolyl isomerase

PPID peak pain intensity difference [score]

PPIE prolonged postictal encephalopathy

PPK palmoplantar keratosis; prekallikrein

PPL penicilloyl polylysine; posterior pulmonary leaflet

Ppl intrapleural pressure; pleural pressure

PPLO pleuropneumonia-like organism

PPM permanent pacemaker; phosphopentomutase; physician practice management; pigmented pupillary membrane; posterior papillary muscle; pulse position modulated

ppm parts per million; pulses per minute

PPMA progressive postmyelitis muscular atrophy

PPMD Provincial Performance Management Database [Canada]

PPMS Performax's Personal Matrix System

PPN partial parenteral nutrition; parameterized Petri net; pedunculopontine nucleus

PPNA peak phrenic nerve activity

PPNAD primary pigmented nodular adrenocortical disease

PPNG penicillinase-producing *Neisseria gonorrhoeae*

PPO platelet peroxidase; preferred provider option; preferred provider organization; protoporphyrin oxidase

P&PO principles and practice of oncology

PPP pain perception profile; palatopharyngoplasty; palmoplantar pustulosis; pentose phosphate pathway; peripheral pulse present; photostimulable phosphor plate; Pickford projective pictures; platelet-poor plasma; pluripotent progenitor; point-to-point protocol; polyphoretic phosphate; porcine pancreatic polypeptide; portal perfusion pressure; Prospective Pravastatin Pooling [project]; protein phosphatase; purified placental protein

PPPA protein phosphatase alpha

PPPBL peripheral pulses palpable both legs

PPPD pylorus-preserving pancreatoduodenectomy

PPPI primary private practice insurance

PPPP porokeratosis punctata palmaris et plantaris

PPP/SLIP point-to-point protocol/serial line internet protocol

PPR patient-provider relationship; percentage of predicted recovery; physician-patient relation; physician payment reform; posterior primary ramus; Price precipitation reaction

PPr paraprosthetic

PPRC Physician Payment Review Commission

PPRF paramedian pontine reticular formation; postpartum renal failure

PPROM preterm premature rupture of fetal membranes

PPRP polyadenosine diphosphate-ribose polymerase

PPRWP poor precordial R-wave progression

PPS Paris Prospective Study; Personal Preference Scale; physician, patient and society [course]; polyvalent pneumococcal polysaccharide; popliteal pterygium syndrome; postpartum sterilization; postperfusion syndrome; postpericardiotomy syndrome; postpolio syndrome; postpump syndrome; primary acquired preleukemic syndrome; prospective payment system; prospective pricing system; protein plasma substitute; pulse per second

PPSC play performance scale for children

PPSH pseudovaginal perineoscrotal hypospadias

PPSTH population poststimulus time histogram

PPT parietal pleural tissue; partial prothrombin time; peak-to-peak threshold; Pfeiffer-Palm-Teller [syndrome]; plant protease test; polypurine tract; postpartum thyroiditis; preprotachykinin; pressure pain threshold; pulmonary platelet trapping; pulmonary physical therapy

ppt parts per trillion; precipitation, precipitate; prepared

pptd precipitated

PPTL postpartum tubul ligation

PPTS pyridinium p-toluenesulfonate

PPV pneumococcal polysaccharide vaccine; porcine parvovirus; positive predictive value; positive pressure ventilation; progressive pneumonia virus; pulmonary plasma volume

PPVr regional pulmonary plasma volume

PPVT Peabody Picture Vocabulary Test

PPVT-R Peabody Picture Vocabulary Test, Revised

Ppw pulmonary wedge pressure

PPY pancreatic polypeptide

PQ paraquat; parent questionnaire; permeability quotient; physician's questionnaire; plastoquinone; pronator quadratus; pyrimethamine-quinine

PQOL Perceived Quality of Life [scale]

PQRST Probucol Quantitative Regression Swedish Trial; provocative and palliative factors, quality of pain, radiation of pain, severity of pain, timing of pain [pain characteristics in low back pain syndrome]

PR by way of the rectum [Lat. *per rectum*]; far point [of accommodation] [Lat. *punctum remotum*]; palindromic rheumatism; parallax and refraction; partial reinforcement; partial remission; partial response; particulate respirator; peer review; perfusion rate; peripheral resistance; per rectum; phenol red; photoreaction; physical rehabilitation; pityriasis rosea; police report; posterior root; postmyalgia rheumatica; postural reflex; potency ratio; preference record; pregnancy; pregnancy rate; preretinal; pressoreceptor; pressure; prevention; Preyer reflex; proctology; production rate; profile; progesterone receptor; progressive relaxation; progressive resistance; progress report; prolactin; prolonged remission; propranolol; prosthion; protein; public relations; pulmonary regurgitation; pulmonary rehabilitation; pulse rate; pulse repetition; pyramidal response

P-R the time between the P wave and the beginning of the QRS complex in electrocardiography [interval]

P&R pelvic and rectal [examination]; pulse and respiration

Pr praseodymium; prednisolone; presbyopia; primary; prism; production, productivity; production rate [of steroid hormones]; prolactin; propyl

pr far point of accommodation [Lat. *punctum remotum*]; pair; per rectum; prism

PRA panel-reactive antibody; phosphoribosylamine; physician recognition award; plasma renin activity; progesterone receptor assay

prac, pract practice, practitioner

PRACTICAL Placebo-Controlled Randomized ACE Inhibition Comparative Trial in Cardiac Infarction and Left Ventricular Function

PRAGMATIC pregnancy, rheumatoid arthritis, acromegaly, glucose metabolism disorders, mechanical injury, amyloid, thyroid disease, infectious disease, crystals in gout or pseudogout [disorders associated with carpal tunnel syndrome]

PRAGUE Primary Angioplasty After Transfer of Patients from General Community Hospitals to Catheterization Units with or without Emergency Thrombolytic Infusion [study]

PrA-HPA protein A hemolytic plaque assay

PRAISE Prospective Randomized Amlodipine Survival Evaluation

PRAMS pregnancy risk assessment monitoring system

PRANN prediction recurrent artificial neural network

PRAS pre-reduced anaerobically sterilized [medium]; pseudo-renal artery syndrome

PRB basic proline-rich protein; Prosthetics Research Board

pRB, pRb retinoblastoma protein

PRBC packed red blood cells; placental residual blood volume

pRB-P phosphorylated form of retinoblastoma protein

PRBS pseudorandom binary sequence

PRBV placental residual blood volume

PRC packed red cells; peer review committee; phase response curve; plasma renin concentration; professional review committee

PRCA pure red cell aplasia

pRCA posterior right coronary artery

PRCCT prospective randomized controlled clinical trial

PRD partial reaction of degeneration; patient reference dosier; physician relations department; Pitt-Rogers-Danks [syndrome]; postradiation dysplasia

PRDP Provincial Resource Directory Project [Canada]

PRDS Pitt-Rogers-Danks syndrome

PRE photoreacting enzyme; physician's report of examination; pigmented retinal epithelium; preliminary evaluation; preplacement examination; progressive resistive exercise; prospective randomized evaluation; proton relaxation enhancement

pre preliminary; preparation or prepare; pretreatment

pre-AIDS pre-acquired immune deficiency syndrome

pre-amp preliminary amplifier

PRECEDE predisposing, reinforcing, and enabling causes in educational diagnosis and evaluation [model]

precip precipitate, precipitated, precipitation

PRECISE Prospective Randomized Evaluation of Carvedilol in Symptoms and Exercise [trial]

PRED prednisone

PREDICT Prospective Randomized Evaluation of Diltiazem CD Trial

PREFACE Pravastatin-Related Effects Following Angioplasty on Coronary Endothelium [study]

prefd preferred

PREFER patient randomization to either femoral or radial catheterization

preg, pregn pregnancy, pregnant

prelim preliminary

prem premature, prematurity

PreMACE prednisone, methotrexate, Adriamycin, cyclophosphamide, etoposide

PREMIS Prehospital Myocardial Infarction Study

pre-mRNA precursor messenger ribonucleic acid

preop, pre-op preoperative

PREP pattern reversal electrical potential; phosphoribosylpyrophosphate; Physician Review and Enhancement Program

prep, prepd prepare, prepared

Pres resistive pressure

PRESEP Pediatric Rural Emergency System and Education Project

preserv preserve, preserved, preservation

PRESERVE Prospective Randomized Enalapril Study Evaluating Regression of Ventricular Enlargement

PRESS Percutaneous Retroperitoneal Spleno-renal Shunt [study]

press pressure

prev prevention, preventive; previous

PREVENT Program in Ex Vivo Vein Graft Engineering via Transfection; Proliferation Reduction Using Vascular Energy Trial; Prospective Randomized Evaluation of the Vascular Effects of Norvasc Trial

PREVMEDU preventive medicine unit

PRF partial reinforcement; patient report form; perforin; plasma recognition factor; pontine reticular formation; postrepetition frequency [Doppler]; progressive renal failure; prolactin releasing factor; pulse repetition frequency

pRF polyclonal rheumatoid factor

PRFLE Prospective Randomized Flosequinan Longevity Evaluation

PRFM premature rupture of fetal membranes

PRG phleborheography; purge

PRGS phosphoribosylglycineamide synthetase

PRH past relevant history; postrepetition frequency [Doppler]; prolactin releasing hormone

PrH propositus hypoglossi

PRHCIT The Project for Rural Health Communication and Information Technologies [Australia]

PRHHP Puerto Rico Heart Health Program

PRI Pain Rating Index; patient review instrument; phosphate reabsorption index; phosphoribose isomerase; placental ribonuclease inhibitor

PRIAS Packard radioimmunoassay system

PRICE protection, relative rest, ice, compression, elevation

PRICEMM protection, relative rest, ice, compression, elevation, modalities, medication

PRICES protection, rest, ice, compression, elevation, support [primary treatment of tendinitis and overuse injury]; physician modalities, rehabilitation, injections, cross-training, evaluation, salicylates [secondary treatment of tendinitis and overuse injury]

PRIDE Parents Resource Institute for Drug Education; Platelet Aggregation and Receptor Occupancy with Integrilin–A Dynamic Evaluation [study]; Primary Implantable Defibrillator [study]

PRIH prolactin release-inhibiting hormone

PRIM primase

PRIME Prematriculation Program in Medical Education; Promotion of Reperfusion by Inhibition of Thrombin During Myocardial Infarction Evaluation [study]; Promotion of Reperfusion in Myocardial Infarction Evolution [study]; Prospective Randomized Ibopamine Mortality Evaluation [study]; Prospective Randomized Study of Ibopamine on Mortality and Efficacy in Heart Failure

PRIME-MD Primary Care Evaluation of Mental Disorders

PRIMEROSE probabilistic rule based on rough sets

PRIMEX primary care extender

PRIMI Prourokinase in Myocardial Infarction [trial]

primip primipara

PRINCE prevention of radiocontrast-induced nephropathy evaluation

PRIND prolonged reversible ischemic neurologic deficit

PRINS primed in situ [labeling]

PRI(S) pain rating intensity score

PRISAM Primary Stenting for Acute Myocardial Infarction [trial]

PRISM pediatric risk of mortality; Platelet Receptor Inhibition in Ischemic Syndrome Management [study]

PRISM-PLUS Platelet Receptor Inhibition in Ischemic Syndrome Management in Patients Limited by Unstable Signs and Symptoms [study]

PRISMS Prevention of Relapses and Disability by Interferon Beta-1a Subcutaneously in Multiple Sclerosis [study]

PRIST paper radioimmunosorbent test

PRISTINE Praxilene in Stroke Treatment in Northern Europe [study]

PRK photorefractive keratectomy; primary rabbit kidney

PRKAR protein kinase, cyclic adenosine monophosphate-dependent, regulatory

PRKAR1A protein kinase, cyclic adenosine monophosphate-dependent, regulatory, type 1 alpha

PRKC protein kinase C

PRKCA protein kinase C alpha

PRL, Prl prolactin

PRLR prolactin receptor

PRM phosphoribomutase; photoreceptor membrane; premature rupture of membranes; Primary Reference Material; primidone; protamine

PrM preventive medicine

PRMSE percent root-mean square error

PRN pertactin; Physicians Research Network; polyradiculoneuropathy; prion; protectin

PRNP prion protein

PRNT plaque reduction neutralization test

PRO peer review organization; physician review organization; Professional Review Organization; pronation; protein

Pro proline; prophylactic; prothrombin

pro protein

PROACT Prolyse in Acute Cerebral Thrombolysis Trial; Prourokinase in Acute Cerebral Thromboembolism [trial]; Prourokinase in Acute Thromboembolic Stroke [trial]

ProACT professionally advanced care team

prob probable

PROBE Prospective, Randomized, Open Blinded Endpoint Trial; Prospective, Randomized, Open Trial with Blinded Endpoint Evaluation

PROC protein C

proc proceedings, procedure; process

PROCAM Prospective Cardiovascular Münster Study

PROC GLM general linear model procedure

proct, procto proctology, proctologist, proctoscopy

prod production, product

PROFET Prevention of Falls in the Elderly Trial

prog progress, progressive

progn prognosis

PROGRESS Perindopril Protection Against Recurrent Stroke Study

PROH propyl-4-hydrolase

PROHB propyl-4-hydrolase, beta

PROLOG Precursor to EPILOG [study]; programming in logic

prolong prolongation, prolonged

PROM passive range of motion; premature rupture of fetal membranes; prolonged rupture of fetal membranes; programmable read only memory; prosthetic range of motion

PROMIS Problem-Oriented Medical Information System

PROMISE Prospective Randomized Milrinone Survival Evaluation [study]

PROMPTOR-FM probabilistic method of prompting for test ordering in family medicine

pron pronator, pronation

PROP propranolol

ProPAC Prospective Payment Assessment Commission

PRO-PBP pro-platelet basic protein

proph prophylactic, prophylaxis

ProPO prophenoloxidase

ProRS propyl transfer ribonucleic acid synthase [RNAse]

PROS Pediatric Research in Office Settings [network]; protein S

pros prostate, prostatic

PROSIT proteinuria screening and intervention

PROSP protein S pseudogene

PROSPECT Proscar Safety Plus Efficacy Canadian Two-Year Study

PROSPER Prospective Study of Pravastatin in the Elderly at Risk

PROSTATE Physicians for Rational Ordering and Screening Tests and Therapeutic Effectiveness

prosth prosthesis, prosthetic

PROTECT Perindopril Regression of Vascular Thickening European Community Trial; Prospective Reinfarction in the Thrombolytic Era: Cardizem-CD Trial

PROTO protoporphyrin; protoporphyrinogen

prov provisional

PROVED Prospective Randomized Study of Ventricular Failure and the Efficacy of Digoxin

prox proximal

PRP photolyase regulatory protein; physiologic rest position; pityriasis rubra pilaris; platelet-rich plasma; polyribosyl ribitol phosphate; postural rest position; pressure rate product; primary Raynaud phenomenon; progressive rubella panencephalitis; proliferative retinopathy photocoagulation; proline-rich protein; Psychotic Reaction Profile; pulse repetition period

PrP, Prp prion protein

PRPH peripherin

PRPP phosphoribosyl pyrophosphate

PRPS prostatic secretory protein

PRQ personal resources questionnaire

PRR proton relaxation rate; pulse repetition rate

PrR progesterone receptor

PRRB Provider Reimbursement Review Board

PRRE pupils round, regular, and equal

PRRF paramedian pontine reticular formation

PR-RSV Prague Rous sarcoma virus

PRS Personality Rating Scale; Pierre Robin syndrome; plasma renin substrate; Prieto syndrome; proctorectosigmoidoscopy

PRSIS Prospective Rate Setting Information System

PRT patient record tree; *Penicillium roqueforti* toxin; pharmaceutical research and testing; phosphoribosyl transferase; pivot repeatability test; postoperative respiratory therapy; prospective randomized trial

PRTH pituitary resistance to thyroid hormone

PRTH-C prothrombin time control

PRTN proteinase

PRTS Partington syndrome

PRU peripheral resistance unit

PRUJ proximal radioulnar joint

PRV polycythemia rubra vera; pseudorabies virus; posterior right ventricle

PRVC pressure-regulated volume control [respiration]

PRVEP pattern reversal visual evoked potential

PRW polymerized ragweed

PRX pseudoexfoliation

Prx prognosis

prx proximal

PRZF pyrazofurin

PS pacemaker syndrome; paired stimulation; paradoxical sleep; paraspinal; parasympathetic; Parkinson syndrome; parotid sialography; partial saturation; partial seizure; pathological stage; patient's serum; pediatric surgery; performing scale [intelligence quotient, IQ]; performance status; periodic syndrome; pferdestärke (German for horsepower); phosphate saline [buffer]; phosphatidyl serine; photosensitivity, photosensitization; photosynthesis; phrenic stimulation; physical status; physiologic saline; plastic surgery; polysaccharide; polystyrene; population sample; Porter-Silber [chromogen]; prescription; precursor state; presenilin; presenting symptom; pressure support; procedural sedation; prostatic secretion; proteasome; protein synthesis; protamine sulfate; protein S; Proteus syndrome; psychiatric; pulmonary stenosis; pyloric stenosis

P/S polisher-stimulator; polyunsaturated/saturated [fatty acid ratio]

P&S paracentesis and suction

Ps prescription; *Pseudomonas;* psoriasis

P$_s$ systolic pressure

ps per second; picosecond

PSA parasternal short axis; pleomorphic salivary gland adenoma; polyethylene sulfonic acid; polysaccharide adhesin;

posterior spinal artery; primary sampling unit; professional services agreement; progressive spinal ataxia; prolonged sleep apnea; prostate specific antigen; protein S alpha; pseudoaneurysm; psoriatic arthritis

PS/A polysaccharide adhesin

Psa systemic blood pressure

PSAAMI Primary Stenting vs Angioplasty in Acute Myocardial Infarction [trial]

PSAC President's Science Advisory Committee

PSACH pseudoachondrodysplasia

PSAD prostate-specific antigen density

PSAG pelvic sonoangiography

PSAGN poststreptococcal acute glomerulonephritis

PSAn psychoanalysis

PSAP primary public safety answering point; prosaposin; pulmonary surfactant apoprotein

P/SAT pediatric severity assessment

PSB protected specimen brush; protein S beta

PSbetaG pregnancy-specific beta-1-glycoprotein

PSBG pregnancy-specific beta-1-glycoprotein

PSC patient services coordination; peripheral stem cell; Porter-Silber chromogen; posterior subcapsular cataract; primary sclerosing cholangitis; professional service corporation; prospective studies collaboration; proteasome component; pulse synchronized contractions

PS-CF pancreatic-sufficient cystic fibrosis

PsChE pseudocholinesterase

PSCI Primary Self Concept Inventory

Psci pressure at slow component intercept

PSCT peripheral stem cell transplantation

PSD particle size distribution; peptone, starch, and dextrose; periodic synchronous discharge; phase-sensitive detector; poststenosis dilation; post-stroke depression; postsynaptic density; power spectrum density

PSDA Patient Self-Determination Act; psychoactive substance abuse and dependence

PSDES primary symptomatic diffuse esophageal spasm

PSE paradoxical systolic expansion; penicillin-sensitive enzyme; portal systemic encephalopathy; Present State Examination; purified spleen extract

psec picosecond

PSEK progressive symmetrical erythrokeratoderma

PSEP post-sexual exposure prophylaxis

PSF peak scatter factor; peptide supply factor; point spread function; prostacyclin stabilizing factor; pseudosarcomatous fasciitis

PSG peak systolic gradient; phosphate, saline, and glucose; polysomnogram; presystolic gallop; pregnancy-specific glycoprotein; programmable sound generator

PSHV pulmonary syndrome hantavirus

PSGN poststreptococcal glomerulonephritis

PSH past surgical history; postspinal headache

PsHD pseudoheart disease

PSI pneumonia severity index; posterior sagittal index; problem solving information; prostaglandin synthetic inhibitor; psychological services index; psychosomatic inventory

psi pounds per square inch

ψ Greek letter *psi*; wave function

psia pounds per square inch absolute

PSICU pediatric surgical intensive care unit

pSIDS partially unexplained sudden infant death syndrome

PSIFT platelet suspension immunofluorescence test

PSIL preferred frequency speech interference level

PSIS posterior sacroiliac spine

PSK protein serine kinase

PSL parasternal line; photostimulable luminescence; potassium, sodium chloride, and sodium lactate [solution]; prednisolone

PSM patient-specific mortality; personal status monitor; postmitochondrial supernatant; presystolic murmur

psm patient-specific mortality

PSMA prostate-specific membrane antigen; proximal spinal muscular atrophy

PSMed psychosomatic medicine

PSMF protein-sparing modified fast

PSMT psychiatric services management team

PSMS physical self-maintenance scale

PSN provider service network
PSNR peak signal to noise ratio
PSO proximal subungual onychomycosis
PSOM probabilistic self-organizing map
PSP pancreatic spasmolytic peptide; paralytic shellfish poisoning; parathyroid secretory protein; peak systolic pressure; periodic short pulse; phenolsulfonphthalein; phosphoserine phosphatase; photostimulable phosphor plate; positive spike pattern; posterior spinal process; postsynaptic potential; prednisone sodium phosphate; primary spontaneous pneumothorax; progressive supranuclear palsy; prostatic secretory protein; pseudopregnancy; pulmonary surfactant apoprotein
PSPS secretory pancreatic stone protein
PSQ Parent Symptom Questionnaire; Patient Satisfaction Questionnaire
PsqO$_2$ subcutaneous tissue oximetry
PSR pain sensitivity range; perspective surface rendering; portal systemic resistance; proliferative sickle retinopathy; pulmonary stretch receptor
PSRC Plastic Surgery Research Council
PSRO Professional Standards Review Organization
PSS painful shoulder syndrome; patient scheduling system; patient stimulation stack; physiologic saline solution; porcine stress syndrome; primary Sjögren syndrome; progressive systemic scleroderma; progressive systemic sclerosis; psoriasis severity scale; Psychiatric Status Schedule; pure sensory stroke
pSS perceived stress scale; primary Sjögren syndrome
PSSS perceived stress support scale
PST pancreatic suppression test; paroxysmal supraventricular tachycardia; penicillin, streptomycin, and tetracycline; penoscrotal transposition; peristimulus time; phenolsulfotransferase; platelet survival time; poststenotic; poststimulus time; prefrontal sonic treatment; protein-sparing therapy; proximal straight tubule
PSTAF Pilsicainide Suppression Trial of Atrial Fibrillation
PSTI pancreatic secretory trypsin inhibitor
PSTV potato spindle tuber virus
PSU patient service unit; photosynthetic unit; primary sampling unit

PSurg plastic surgery
PSV pressure-support ventilation
pSV simian vacuolating virus plasmid
PSVER pattern shift visual evoked response
PSVT paroxysmal supraventricular tachycardia
PSW primary surgical ward; positive sharp wave; psychiatric social worker
PSWT psychiatric social work training
PSX pseudoexfoliation
Psy psychiatry; psychology
psych psychology, psychological
PSYCHE Psychiatry Educator [computer-assisted instruction]
psychiat psychiatry, psychiatric
psychoan psychoanalysis, psychoanalytical
psychol psychology, psychological
psychopath psychopathology, psychopathological
psychosom psychosomatic
psychother psychotherapy
psy-path psychopathic
Ps-ZES pseudo-Zollinger-Ellison syndrome
PT pain threshold; pancreatic transplantation; parathormone; parathyroid; paroxysmal tachycardia; part time; patient; pericardial tamponade; permanent and total; phage type; pharmacy and therapeutics; phenytoin; phosphorothioate; photophobia; phototoxicity; physical therapy, physical therapist; physical training; physiotherapy; pine tar; plasma thromboplastin; pneumothorax; polyvalent tolerance; position tracking; posterior tibial [artery pulse]; posttetanic; posttransfusion; posttransplantation; posttraumatic; premature termination [of pregnancy]; preoperative therapy; preterm; primary tumor; propylthiouracil; protamine; prothrombin time; proton density; pulmonary tuberculosis; psychotherapy; pulmonary thrombosis; pyramidal tract; temporal plane
P&T permanent and total [disability]; pharmacy and therapeutics
Pt patient; platinum
pt part; patient; pint; point
PTA pancreatic transplantation alone; parallel tubular arrays; parathyroid adenoma; peak twitch amplitude; percutaneous transluminal angioplasty; peroxidase-labeled

antibody; persistent truncus arteriosus; phosphotungstic acid; physical therapy assistant; plasma thromboplastin antecedent; posttraumatic amnesia; pretreatment anxiety; prior to admission; prior to arrival; prothrombin activity

PTAF platelet activating factor

PTAFR platelet activating factor receptor

PTAH phosphotungstic acid hematoxylin

PTAP purified diphtheria toxoid precipitated by aluminum phosphate

PTAT pure tone average threshold

PTB patellar tendon bearing; polypyrimidine tract binding; prior to birth

PTb pulmonary tuberculosis

PTBA percutaneous transluminal balloon angioplasty

PTBD percutaneous transhepatic biliary drainage; percutaneous transluminal balloon dilatation

PTBE pyretic tick-borne encephalitis

PTBNA protected transbronchial needle aspirate

PTBPD posttraumatic borderline personality disorder

PTBS posttraumatic brain syndrome

PTBW peak torque to body weight

PTC papillary thyroid carcinoma; percutaneous transhepatic cholangiography; phase transfer catalyst; phenothiocarbazine; phenylthiocarbamide; phenylthiocarbamoyl; plasma thromboplastin component; posttetanic count; premature termination codon; premature tricuspid closure; prior to conception; prothrombin complex; pseudotumor cerebri

PTCA percutaneous transluminal coronary angioplasty; pyrrole-2,3,5-tricarboxylic acid

PT(C)A percutaneous transluminal (coronary] angioplasty

PtcCO$_2$ transcutaneous partial pressure of carbon dioxide

PTCDA perylene-tetracarboxylic dianhydride

PTCER pulmonary transcapillary escape rate

PtcO$_2$ transcutaneous oxygen tension

PTCR percutaneous transluminal coronary recanalization or revascularization

PTCRA percutaneous transluminal coronary rotational ablation

PTD percutaneous transluminal dilatation; permanent total disability; personality trait disorder; preterm delivery; prior to delivery

PTDS posttraumatic distress syndrome

PTE parathyroid extract; posttraumatic epilepsy; pretibial edema; proximal tibial epiphysis; pulmonary thromboembolism

PTED pulmonary thromboembolic disease

PteGlu pteroylglutamic acid

PTEN pentaerythritol tetranitrate

pter end of short arm of chromosome

PTF patient treatment file; plasma thromboplastin factor; posterior talofibular [ligament]; proximal tubular fragment

PTFA prothrombin time fixing agent

PTFE polytetrafluoroethylene

PTFNA percutaneous transthoracic fine-needle aspiration

PTFS posttraumatic fibromyalgia syndrome

PTG parathyroid gland; prostaglandin

PTGE prostaglandin E

PTGER prostaglandin E receptor

PTH parathormone; parathyroid; parathyroid hormone; percutaneous transhepatic drainage; phenylthiohydantoin; plasma thromboplastin component; posttransfusion hepatitis

PTHC percutaneous transhepatic cholangiography

PTHL parathyroid hormone-like

PTHLP parathyroid-hormone-like protein

PTHR parathyroid hormone receptor

PTHRP, PTHrP parathyroid-hormone-related peptide; parathyroid-hormone-related protein

PTHS parathyroid hormone secretion [rate]

PTI pancreatic trypsin inhibitor; penetrating trauma index; persistent tolerant infection; Pictorial Test of Intelligence; placental thrombin inhibitor; pulsatility transmission index

PTK phosphotyrosine kinase; phototherapeutic keratectomy; protein-tyrosine kinase

PTL peritoneal telencephalic leukoencephalomyopathy; pharyngotracheal lumen; plasma thyroxine level posterior tricuspid leaflet; preterm labor

PTLA pharyngeal tracheal lumen airway

PTLC precipitation thin-layer chromatography

PTLD posttransplanatation lymphoproliferative disorder; prescribed tumor lethal dose

PTM posterior trabecular meshwork; post-transfusion mononucleosis; post-traumatic meningitis; prothymosin; pulse time modulation

Ptm pterygomaxillary [fissure]

PTMA phenyltrimethylammonium; prothymosin alpha

PTMDF pupils, tension, media, disc, fundus

PTMPY per thousand members per year

PTMR percutaneous transluminal myocardial revascularization

PTMS parathymosin

PTN pain transmission neuron; pleiotrophin; posterior tibial nerve

pTNM TNM (see p. 383) staging of tumors as determined by correlation of clinical, pathologic, and residual findings

PTO Klemperer's tuberculin [Ger. *Perlsucht Tuberculin Original*]

PTP pancreatic thread protein; pediatric telephone protocol; percutaneous transhepatic portography; phosphotyrosine phosphatase; physical treatment planning; posterior tibial pulse; posttetanic potential; posttransfusion purpura; pretest probability; previously treated patient; protein-tyrosine phosphatase; proximal tubular pressure

Ptp transpulmonary pressure

PTPC protein-tyrosine phosphatase C

PTPG protein-tyrosine phosphatase gamma

PTPI posttraumatic pulmonary insufficiency

PTPM post-traumatic progressive myelopathy

PTPN protein-tyrosine phosphatase, nonreceptor

PTPRA protein-tyrosine phosphatase receptor alpha

PTPRB protein-tyrosine phosphatase receptor beta

PTPRF protein-tyrosine phosphatase receptor F

PTPRG protein-tyrosine phosphatase receptor gamma

PTPS postthrombophlebitis syndrome; 6-pyruvoyl tetrahydropterin synthase

PTPT protein-tyrosine phosphatase, T-cell

PTQ parent-teacher questionnaire

PTR patellar tendon reflex; patient termination record; patient to return; peripheral total resistance; plasma transfusion reaction; prothrombin time ratio; psychotic trigger reaction

PTr porcine trypsin

Ptr intratracheal pressure

PTRA percutaneous transluminal renal angioplasty

PT Rep patient's representative

PTRIA polystyrene-tube radioimmunoassay

Ptrx pelvic traction

PTS para-toluenesulfonic acid; pediatric trauma score; postthrombotic syndrome; posttraumatic syndrome; Pressure and Tension Scale; prior to surgery; 6-pyruvoyl tetrahydropterin synthase

Pts, pts patients

PTSD posttraumatic stress disorder

PTSH poststimulus time histogram

PTSM Plant, Technology and Safety Management

PTSS posttraumatic stress syndrome

PTT partial thromboplastin time; particle transport time; posterior tibial tendon (transfer); protein truncation test; prothrombin time; pulmonary transit time; pulse transmission time

ptt partial thromboplastin time

PTTI penetrating thoracic trauma index

PTU propylthiouracil

PTV planning target volume; posterior tibial vein

PTV₂ planning target volume 2

PTVT planning target volute tool

PTX pentoxifylline; picrotoxinin; pneumothorax

PTx parathyroidectomy; pelvic traction

Ptx pneumothorax

PTXT pointer to text

PTZ pentylenetetrazol

PU palindromic unit; passed urine; patient unit; pepsin unit; peptic ulcer; polyurethane; pregnancy urine; 6-propyluracil; prostatic urethra

Pu plutonium; purine; purple

PUA patient unit assistant

pub public

PUBS percutaneous umbilical blood sampling; purple urine bag syndrome

PUC pediatric urine collector; premature uterine contractions

PUD peptic ulcer disease; pudendal

PuD pulmonary disease

PUF pure ultrafiltration
PUFA polyunsaturated fatty acid
PUH pregnancy urine hormones
PUI platelet uptake index
PUJO pelvi-ureteric junction obstruction
PUL percutaneous ultrasonic lithotripsy
PUL, pul, pulm pulmonary
PULHEMS physique, upper extremity, lower extremity, hearing and ears, eyes and vision, mental capacity, emotional stability [profile]
PULSES physical condition, upper limb function, lower limb function, sensory component, excretory function, mental and status (or support factors in revised version) [profile]
PUM peanut-reactive urinary mucin
PUMF public use microdata file
PUMP putative metalloproteinase
PUMS patient utility measurement set; permanently unfit for military service
PUN plasma urea nitrogen
PUO pyrexia of unknown origin
PUP previously untreated patient
pUPID paternal uniparental isodisomy
PUPPP pruritic urticarial papules and plaques of pregnancy
PUR polyurethrane
Pur purple
pur purulent
purg purgative
PurR purine repressor
PURSUIT Platelet IIb/IIIa Underpinning the Receptor for Suppression of Unstable Ischemia Trial
PUT provocative use test; putamen
PUU puumala [virus]
PUV posterior urethral valve
PUVA psoralen ultraviolet A-range
PV pancreatic vein; papillomavirus; paraventricular; paravertebral; pemphigus vulgaris; peripheral vascular; peripheral vein; peripheral vessel; pityriasis versicolor; plasma viscosity; plasma volume; polio vaccine; poliovirus; polycythemia vera; polyoma virus; polyvinyl; portal vein; postvasectomy; postvoiding; predictive value; pressure velocity; process variable; pulmonary valve; pulmonary vein
P-V pressure-volume [curve]
P&V pyloroplasty and vagotomy
Pv *Proteus vulgaris*; venous pressure

P$_V$ ventricular pressure
PVA Paralyzed Veterans of America; peripheral venous alimentation; polyvinyl acetate; polyvinyl alcohol; pressure volume area
PV$_a$ pulmonary venous atrial
PVAc polyvinyl acetate
PVAd polyvinyladenine
PVALB parvalbumin
PVB cis-platinum, vinblastine, bleomycin; paravertebral block; premature ventricular beat
PVC peripheral venous catheterization; permanent visual circuit; persistent vaginal cornification; polyvinyl chloride; postvoiding cystogram; predicted vital capacity; premature ventricular contraction; primary visual cortex; pulmonary venous confluence; pulmonary venous congestion
PVCM paradoxical vocal cord motion
PV$_{CO2}$ partial pressure of carbon dioxide in mixed venous blood
PVD patient very disturbed; peripheral vascular disease; portal vein dilation; posterior vitreous detachment; postural vertical dimension; premature ventricular depolarization; pulmonary vascular disease
PVDF polyvinylidene difluoride; polyvinyl diisopropyl fluoride
PVE partial volume effect; premature ventricular extrasystole; prosthetic valve endocarditis
PV-ECF plasma volume/extracellular fluid [ratio]
P-VEP pattern visual evoked potential
PVF peripheral visual field; portal venous flow; primary ventricular fibrillation
PVFS postviral fatigue syndrome
PVG pulmonary valve gradient
PVH paraventricular hyperintensity; pulmonary venous hypertension
PVI patient video interview; peripheral vascular insufficiency; perivascular infiltration; positron volume imaging
PVK penicillin V potassium
PVL perivalvular leakage; permanent vision loss
PVM pneumonia virus of mice; proteins, vitamins, and minerals
PVMed preventive medicine
PVN paraventricular nucleus; predictive value negative

PVNPS post-Viet Nam psychiatric syndrome

PVNS pigmented villonodular synovitis

PVO pulmonary venous obstruction

PV$_{O2}$ partial oxygen pressure in mixed venous blood

PVOD pulmonary vascular obstructive disease; pulmonary veno-occlusive disease

PVP penicillin V potassium; peripheral vein plasma; peripheral venous pressure; polyvinylpyrrolidone; portal venous pressure; predictive value of positive results; pulmonary venous pressure

PVP-I polyvinylpyrrolidone-iodine

PVR peripheral vascular resistance; perspective volume rendering; poliovirus receptor; postvoiding residual; pulmonary valve replacement or repair; pulmonary vascular resistance; pulse volume recording

PVRI pulmonary vascular resistance index

PVS percussion, vibration, suction; persistent vegetative state; persistent viral syndrome; Plummer-Vinson syndrome; poliovirus susceptibility; polyvinyl sponge; premature ventricular systole; programmed ventricular stimulation; pulmonary valvular stenosis

PV$_s$ pulmonary venous systolic

PVT paroxysmal ventricular tachycardia; periventricular thalamic [nucleus]; portal vein thrombosis; pressure, volume, and temperature; private patient; psychomotor vigilance task

PVW posterior vaginal wall

PVX potato virus X

PVY potato virus Y

pvz pulverization

PW peristaltic wave; plantar wart; posterior wall [of the heart]; pressure wave; psychological warfare; pulmonary wedge [pressure]; pulsed wave

Pw progesterone withdrawal; whole cell pertussis [vaccine]

PWA people with AIDS

PWB partial weight bearing

PWBC peripheral white blood cell

PWBRT prophylactic whole brain radiation therapy

PWC peak work capacity; physical work capacity

PWCA pure white cell aplasia

PWCR Prader-Willi chromosome region

PWD printed wiring board

pwd powder

PWDS postweaning diarrhea syndrome

PWDU pulse wave Doppler ultrasound

PWE posterior wall excursion

PWI posterior wall infarct

PWLV posterior wall of left ventricle

PWM pokeweed mitogen; pulse with modulation

pw-MW pre-whitening [of data] multiple window

PWP patient word processing; pulmonary wedge pressure

PWS port wine stain; physician's workstation; Prader-Willi syndrome

PWS/AS Prader-Willi/Angelman syndromes

PWT physician waiting time; posterior wall thickness; pseudo-Winger transform

pwt pennyweight

PWV pulse wave velocity

PX pancreatectomized; peroxidase; physical examination

Px past history; peroxidase; physical examination; pneumothorax; prognosis

px pancreas, pancreatic

PXA pleomorphic xanthoastrocytoma

PXE pseudoxanthoma elasticum

PXM projection x-ray microscopy; pseudoexfoliation material

PXMP peroxysomal membrane protein

PXS pseudoexfoliation syndrome

PXT piroxantrone

P$_{xy}$ propagation delay

Py phosphopyridoxal; polyoma [virus]; pyridine; pyridoxal

PYA psychoanalysis

PyC pyogenic culture

PYCR pyrroline-5-carboxylate reductase

PYE peptone yeast extract

PYG peptone-yeast extract-glucose [broth]

PYGM peptone-yeast-glucose-maltose [broth]

PYLL potential years of life lost

PYM psychosomatic

PyNPase pyridine nucleoside phosphorylase

PYP pyrophosphate

Pyr pyridine; pyruvate

PyrP pyridoxal phosphate

PZ pancreozymin; phthalazinone; pregnancy zone; proliferative zone; protamine zinc

Pz 4-phenylazobenzylycarbonyl; parietal midline electrode placement in electroencephalography

pz pièze

PZA pyrazinamide

PZ-CCK pabcreozymin-cholecystokinin

PZE piezoelectric

PZI protamine zinc insulin

PZP pregnancy zone protein

PZQ praziquantel

PZT lead zirconate titanate

Q̇ cardiac output

Q coulomb [electric quantity]; electric charge; flow; 1,4-glucan branching enzyme; glutamine; heat; qualitative; quality; quantity; quart; quartile; Queensland [fever]; query [fever]; question; quinacrine; quinidine; quinone; quotient; radiant energy; reactive power; reaction energy; temperative coefficient; see QRS [wave]

Q$_{10}$ temperature coefficient

q electric charge; long arm of chromosome; quart; quintal

QA quality assessment; quality assurance

QAAA quantitative amino acid analysis

QAC quaternary ammonium compound; quinacrine

QACC quality assurance coordination committee

QAF quality adjustment factor

QAHCS Quality of Australian Health Care Study

QA&I quality assessment and improvement

QALD quality-adjusted life days

QALE quality-adjusted life expectancy

QALPACS quality patient care scale

QALY quality-adjusted life year

QAM quality assurance monitoring

QAP quality assurance program or professional; quinine, atabrine, and pamaquine

QA/QC quality assurance and quality control

QAR quantitative autoradiography

QARANC Queen Alexandra's Royal Army Nursing Corps

QARNNS Queen Alexandra's Royal Naval Nursing Service

QAS quality assurance standard

QAUR quality assurance and utilization review

QB whole blood

Q$_B$ total body clearance

Q$_b$ blood flow

QBC query by case

QBIC query by image content

QBV whole blood volume

QC quality characteristics; quality control; quantum computing; quinine colchicine

Qc pulmonary capillary blood flow

QCA quantitative coronary arteriography or angiography

QCIM Quarterly Cumulative Index Medicus

Q$_{CO_2}$ carbon dioxide evolution by a tissue

QCP quality care program

QCS Quebec Cardiovascular Study; Quick Confusion Scale

QCT quantitative computed tomography

QD Qi deficiency

QDPR quinoid dihydropteridine reductase

QED quantum electrodynamics

QEE quadriceps extension exercise

QEEG, qEEG quantitative electroencephalography

QEF quail embryo fibroblasts

QENF quantifying examination of neurologic function

QEONS Queen Elizabeth's Overseas Nursery Service

QEW quick early warning

QF quality factor; query fever; quick freeze; relative biological effectiveness

QFCM quantitative fluorescence cytometry

QFES Quality Feedback Expert System

Q fever query fever

QHDS Queen's Honorary Dental Surgeon

QHFT Quinapril Heart Failure Trial

QHNS Queen's Honorary Nursing Sister

QHP Queen's Honorary Physician

QHS Queen's Honorary Surgeon

QI quality improvement; quality indicator; Quetelet Index

QIDN Queen's Institute of District Nursing

QIN quality improvement network

QIP quality improvement project

QISMC Quality Improvement System for Managed Care

QJ quadriceps jerk

QL quality of life

Q-LES-Q Quality of Life Enjoyment and Satisfaction Questionnaire

QLQ quality of life questionnaire

QLQ-C quality of life questionnaire-cancer

QLS Quality of Life Scale; quasielastic light-scattering spectroscopy

QM quality management; quinacrine mustard

qm every morning [Lat. *quaque mane*]

QMAN query manager

QMB qualified Medicare beneficiary

QMF quadrature mirror filter

QMI Q-wave myocardial infarction

QMP Quality Management Program

QMR Quick Medical Reference

QMR-DT Quick Medical Reference–Decision Theoretic

QMR-KAT Quick Medical Reference–Knowledge Acquisition Tool

QMRP qualified mental retardation professional

QMT quantitative muscle test

QMWS quasi-morphine withdrawal syndrome

QN, qn quantitative

qn every night [Lat. *quaque nocte*]

QNB quinuclidinyl benzilate

QNS Queen's Nursing Sister

qns quantity not sufficient

QO$_2$ flow of oxygen

Qo oxygen consumption

Q$_{O_2}$ oxygen quotient; oxygen utilization

Q$_o$ flow at origin

qod every other day [Lat. *quaque altera die*]

qoh every other hour [Lat. *quaque altera hora*]

QOLHS Quality of Life Hypertension Study

qon every other night [Lat. *quaque altera nocte*]

QOL quality of life

QOLI quality of life index

QOLI-P quality of life index-Padilla

QLOQ quality of life questionnaire

QoS quality of service

QP quanti-Pirquet [reaction]

Qp pulmonary blood flow

QPC quadratic phase coupling; quality of patient care

Qpc pulmonary capillary blood flow

QPEEG quantitative pharmaco-electroencephalography

Qp:Qs pulmonary-to-systemic flow ratio; pulmonic-to-systemic flow ratio

QR quality review; quieting response; quinaldine red; quinone reductase

qr quadriradial; quarter

QRB Quality Review Bulletin

Q$_{rbc}$ flow of red blood cells

QRM quality and resource management

QRNG quinoline-resistant *Neisseria gonorrhoeae*

QRP quick response program

QRS in electrocardiography, the complex consisting of Q, R, and S waves, corresponding to depolarization of ventricles [complex]; in electrocardiography, the loop traced by QRS vectors, representing ventricular depolarization [interval]

QRS-ST the junction between the QRS complex and the ST segment in the electrocardiogram [junction]

QRS-T the angle between the QRS and T vectors in vectorcardiography [angle]

qRT-PCR quantitative reverse transcriptase [RT] polymerase chain reaction [PCR]

QRZ wheal reaction time [Ger. *Qaddel Reaktion Zeit*]

QS question screening; quiet sleep

Qs systemic blood flow

Q$_s$ systemic blood flow

QSAR quantitative structure-activity relationship

QSART quantitative sudomotor axon reflex testing

QSM quality assurance and safety of medicine

QSPR quantitative structure-property relationship

QSPV quasistatic pressure volume

Q$_S$Q$_T$ shunted blood to total blood flow [ratio]

QSS quantitative sacroiliac scintigraphy

QST quantitative sensory test

QT cardiac output; Quick test

Q-T in electrocardiography, the time from the beginning of the QRS complex to the end of the T wave [interval]

qt quantity; quart; quiet

QTc Q-T interval corrected for heart rate

Q-Tc corrected Q-T [interval]

qter end of long arm of chromosome

QTL quantitative trait locus

Q-TWIST quality-adjusted time without symptoms of disease and subjective toxic effects of treatment

Quad quadratic [potential]

quad quadrant; quadriceps; quadriplegic

QUADS Quinapril Australian Dosing Study

QUAL qualitative attribute [UMLS]

qual quality, qualitative

QUALYs quality-adjusted life years

QUAN quantitative attribute [UMLS]

quant quantity, quantitative

quar quarintine

QUART quadrantectomy, axillary dissection, radiotherapy

QUASAR Quinapril Anti-Ischemia and Symptoms of Angina Reduction [trial]

QUEST Quality, Utilization, Effectiveness, Statistically Tabulated

QUESTT Question the child, Use pain rating scale, Evaluate behavior and physiologic changes, Secure parents' involvement, Take cause of pain into account, Take action and evaluate results [pain assessment in children]

QUEXTA Quantitative Exercise Testing and Angiography [study]

QUICHA quantitative inhalation challenge apparatus

QUIET Quinapril Ischemic Event Trial

QUIN quinolinic acid

quint fifth

QUIS Questionnaire on User Interface Satisfaction

quot quotient

quotid daily, quotidian [Lat. *quotidie*]

QUS quantitative ultrasound

qv which see [Lat. *quod vide*]

QWB quality of well-being [questionnaire, scale, or index]

QYD Qi and Yin deficiency

R arginine; Behnken unit; Broadbent registration point; a conjugative plasmid responsible for resistance to various elements; any chemical group (particularly an alfyl group); electrical resistance; far point [Lat. *remotum*]; in electrocardiography, the first positive deflection during the QRS complex [wave]; gas constant; organic radical; race; racemic; radioactive; radiology; radius; ramus; Rankine [scale]; rapid accelerator; rate; ratio; reaction; Réaumur [scale]; receptor; rectal; rectified; red; registered trademark; regression coefficient; regular; regular insulin; regulator [gene]; rejection factor; relapse; relaxation; release [factor]; remission; remote; reperfusion; repressor; residue; resistance; respiration; respiratory exchange ratio; response; responder; rest; restricted; reverse [banding]; rhythm; ribose; *Rickettsia*; right; Rinne [test]; roentgen; rough [colony]; rub

R′ in electrocardiography, the second positive deflection during the QRS complex

R+ Rinne test positive

R1 first repeat

R2 second repeat

+R Rinne test positive

–R Rinne test negative

°R degree on the Rankine scale; degree on the Réaumur scale

R1, R2, R3, etc. years of resident study

r correlation coefficient; density; radius; ratio; recombinant; regional; ribose; ribosomal; ring chromosome; roentgen; sample correlation coefficient

r² coefficient of determination

ρ see *rho*

RA radioactive; ragocyte; ragweed antigen; rapidly adapting [receptors]; reactive arthritis; reciprocal asymmetrical; refractory anemia; refractory ascites; renal artery; renin-angiotensin; repeat action; residual air; retinoic acid; rheumatoid arthritis; right angle; right arm; right atrium; right auricle; rotation angiography; Roy adaptation [model]

R$_A$ airway resistance

Ra access resistance; radial; radium; radius

rA riboadenylate

RAA renin-angiotensin-aldosterone [system]

RAAMC Royal Australian Army Medical Corps

RAAMI Randomized Angiographic Trial of Alteplase in Myocardial Infarction; Rapid Administration of Alteplase in Myocardial Infarction [trial]

RAAS Randomized Angiotensin II Receptor Antagonist, Angiotensin-Converting Enzyme Inhibitor Study; renin-angiotensin-aldosterone system

rAAV recombinant adeno-associated virus

RAB remote afterloading brachytherapy

RABA rabbit antibladder antibody

Rab rabbit

RAC Recombinant Deoxyribonucleic Acid [DNA] Advisory Committee; research appraisal checklist

rac racemate, racemic

RACE ramipril angiotensin-converting enzyme [ACE]; Ramipril Cardioprotective Evaluation [trial]; rapid amplification of complementary deoxyribonucleic acid ends; Rapid Assessment of Cardiac Enzymes; rate control vs electrical cardioversion

RACGP Royal Australian College of General Practitioners

RACT research activity [UMLS]

RACV relative autonomic conduction velocity

RAD radial artery catheter; radiation absorbed dose; radical; radiography or radiographic; reactive airways disease; right atrium diameter; right axis deviation; roentgen administered dose

Rad radiology; radiotherapy; radium

rad radiation absorbed dose; radial; radian; radical; radius; root [Lat. *radix*]

RADA rosin amine-D-acetate

RADAI rheumatoid arthritis disease activity index

RADAR rapid assessment of disease activity in rheumatology

RADC Royal Army Dental Corps

RADES randomly amplified differentially expressed sequence

RADES-PCR randomly amplified differentially expressed sequence polymerase chain reaction [PCR]

RADIANCE Randomized Assessment of Digoxin on Inhibitors of Angiotensin-Converting Enzyme [ACE] [study]

RADIO radiotherapy

radiol radiology

RADIUS Routine Antenatal Diagnostic Imaging with Ultrasound [trial]

RadLV radiation leukemia virus

RADP right acromiodorsoposterior

RADS reactive airways dysfunction syndrome; retrospective assessment of drug safety

rad/s rad per second; radian per second

rad ther radiation therapy

RADTS rabbit antidog thymus serum

RADTT radiation therapy technologist

RAE right atrial enlargement

RAEB refractory anemia with excess blasts

RAEBIT, RAEB-T refractory anemia with excess blasts in transformation

RAEM refractory anemia with excess myeloblasts

RAF repetitive atrial firing; rheumatoid arthritis factor

RAFMS Royal Air Force Medical Services

RAFT Recurrent Atrial Fibrillation Trial; Rythmol-SR Atrial Fibrillation Trial

RAFW right atrial free wall

RAG radioautography; ragweed; recombinase activating gene

RAGE rapid gradient echo; receptor for advanced glycosylation end-products

Ragg rheumatoid agglutinin

RAH regressing atypical histiocytosis; right atrial hypertrophy

RAHM randomly amplified hybridization microsatellite

RAHO rabbit antibody to human ovary

RAHTG rabbit antihuman thymocyte globulin

RAI radioactive iodine; radioactive isotope; resident assessment instrument; resting ankle index; right atrial inversion; right atrial involvement

RAID radioimmunodetection; redundant array of inexpensive disks

RAIS reflection-absorption infrared spectroscopy

RAITI right atrial inversion time index

RAIU radioactive iodine uptake

RALES Randomized Aldactone Evaluation Study

RALPH renal-anal-lung-polydactylyhamartoblastoma [syndrome]

RALT routine admission laboratory tests

RAM random-access memory; rapid alternating movements; rectus abdominis muscle; rectus abdominis myocutaneous [flap]; reduced acquisition matrix; research aviation medicine; resource allocation methodology; right anterior measurement

RAMC Royal Army Medical Corps

RAM-FAST reduced acquisition matrix-Fourier acquired steady state

RaMI Ravenna Myocardial Infarction [trial]

RAMIT Ravenna Myocardial Infarction Trial

RAMM remote-access multidimensional microscopy

RAMP radioactive antigen microprecipitin; rate modulated pacing; right atrial mean pressure

RAMPO randomly amplified microsatellite polymorphism

RAMT rabbit antimouse thymocyte; right atrial mobile thrombi

RAN random number; remote area nurse [Australia]; resident's admission notes

RANA rheumatoid arthritis nuclear antigen

rANP rat atrial natriuretic peptide

RANTES regulated on activation, T-cell expressed and secreted

RANTTAS Randomized Trial of Tirilazad in Acute Stroke

RAO right anterior oblique

RaONC radiation oncology

RAP rapid atrial pacing; recurrent abdominal pain; regression-associated protein; renal artery pressure; resident assessment protocol; rheumatoid arthritis precipitin; ribonucleic acid [RNA] arbitrarily primed; right atrial pressure

RAPD randomly amplified polymorphic deoxyribonucleic acid [DNA]; relative afferent pupillary defect

RAPDDIP randomly amplified polymorphic deoxyribonucleic acid [DNA] for the diploid cases

RAPDHAP randomly amplified polymorphic deoxyribonucleic acid [DNA] for the haploid cases

RAPID Recombinant Plasminogen Activator Angiographic Phase II International Dose Finding Study; Regional Arizona Prehospital Infarction Diagnosis [study]

RAPK reticulate acropigmentation of Kitamura

RAPM refractory anemia with partial myeloblastosis

RAPO rabbit antibody to pig ovary

RAP-PCR ribonucleic acid [RNA] arbitrarily primed polymerase chain reaction [PCR]

RAPPORT ReoPro in Acute Myocardial Infarction and Primary Percutaneous Transluminal Coronary Angioplasty Organization and Randomized Trial

RAPS Renfrew and Paisley Study; resident assessment protocols

RAPs radiologists, anesthesiologists, and pathologists

RAPT Ridogrel vs Aspirin Potency Trial

RAR rapidly adapting receptor; rat insulin receptor; retinoic acid receptor; right arm reclining; right arm recumbent

RARA retinoic acid receptor alpha

RARB retinoic acid receptor beta

RARE rapid acquisition with relaxation enhancement; retinoic acid response element

RARG retinoic acid receptor gamma

RARLS rabbit anti-rat lymphocyte serum

RARS refractory anemia with ring sideroblasts

RARTS rabbit anti-rat thymocyte serum

RAS rapid atrial stimulation; recurrent aphthous stomatitis; reflex activating stimulus; reliability, availability, serviceability; renal artery stenosis; renin-angiotensin system; residency application service; reticular activating system; rheumatoid arthritis serum

RA-S refractory anemia with ringed sideroblasts

ras retrovirus-associated DNA sequence

RASE rapid acquisition spin echo

RASS rheumatoid arthritis and Sjögren syndrome

RAST radioallergosorbent test

RAT repeat action tablet; rheumatoid arthritis test

RATG rabbit antithymocyte globulin

RATHAS rat thymus antiserum

RATMAP Rat Genome Database

rAT-P recombinant antitrypsin Pittsburgh

RATx radiation therapy

RAU radioactive uptake

RAV Rous-associated virus

RAVC retrograde atrioventricular conduction; Royal Army Veterinary Corps

RAVES Reduced Anticoagulation in Saphenous Vein Graft Stent [trial]; Reduced Anticoagulation Vein Graft Study

RAVLT Rey Auditory Verbal Learning Test

RAW right atrial wall

Raw airway resistance

R_{AW} airway resistance

RAWTS ribonucleic acid amplification with transcript sequencing

RAZ razoxane

RB radiation burn; rating board; rebreathing; reticulate body; retinoblastoma; right bronchus; right bundle

RB1 The RB1 Gene Mutation Database

Rb retinoblastoma

RBA relative binding affinity; rescue breathing apparatus; right basilar artery; right brachial artery; rose bengal antigen

RBAC role-based access control

RBAP repetitive bursts of action potential

RbAP retinoblastoma-associated protein

RBAS rostral basilar artery syndrome

RBB right bundle branch

RBBB right bundle-branch block

RBBP retinoblastoma binding protein

RBBsB right bundle-branch system block

RBBx right breast biopsy

RBC red blood count

rbc red blood cell

RBCD right border cardiac dullness

rBCG recombinant bacille Calmette-Guérin [vaccine]

RBCM red blood cell mass

RBCV red blood cell volume

RBD recurrent brief depression; relative biological dose; RNA binding domain; right border of dullness

RBE relative biological effectiveness

RBF radial basis function; regional blood flow; regional bone mass; renal blood flow

RBG red blue green [Doppler]

RBI radiographic baseline

RBI-EM rescaled block-iterative expectation maximization [algorithm]

Rb Imp rubber base impression

RBL rat basophilic leukemia; Reid baseline; retinoblastoma-like

RBM ribonucleic acid [RNA] binding motif

RBN retrobulbar neuritis

RBNA Royal British Nurses Association

RBNN recurrent backpropagation neural network

RBOW rupture of the bag of waters

RBP retinol-binding protein; riboflavin-binding protein

RBPC cellular retinol-binding protein

RBPI intestinal retinol-binding protein

rBPI recombinant bactericidal/permeability [protein]

RBRVS resource-based relative value scale

RBS random blood sugar; Roberts syndrome; Rutherford backscattering

RbSA rabbit serum albumin

RBST rubber-band straightening transform

RBT resistive breathing training

RBTN rhombotin

RBTNL rhombotin-like

RBV right brachial vein

RBW relative body weight

RBZ rubidazone

RC an electronic circuit containing a resistor and capacitor in series; radiocarpal; reaction center; recrystallization; red cell; red cell casts; red corpuscle; Red Cross; referred care; regenerated cellulose; rehabilitation counseling; residential care; respiration ceases; respiratory care; respiratory center; respiratory compensation; rest cure; retention catheter; retrograde cystogram; rib cage; root canal; routine cholecystography

R&C resistance and capacitance

Rc conditioned response; receptor

RCA red cell agglutination; relative chemotactic activity; renal cell carcinoma; replication-competent adenovirus; replication-competent alphavirus; right coronary artery

RCAMC Royal Canadian Army Medical Corps

rCBF regional cerebral blood flow

rCBV regional cerebral blood volume

RCC radiological control center; rape crisis center; ratio of cost to charges; receptor-chemoeffector complex; red cell cast; red cell count; regulator of chromosome condensation; renal cell carcinoma; reverse cumulative curve; right common carotid; right coronary cusp

RCCM Regional Committee for Community Medicine

RCCP renal cell carcinoma, papillary

RCCS remote clinical communications system

RCCT randomized controlled clinical trial

RCD relative cardiac dullness; robust change detection [algorithm in insulin therapy]

RCDA recurrent chronic dissecting aneurysm

RCDP rhizomelic chondrodysplasia punctata

RCDR relative corrected death rate

RCE reasonable compensation equivalent

RCF red cell ferritin; red cell folate; relative centrifugal field/force; ristocetin cofactor

RCG radioelectrocardiography

RCGP Royal College of General Practitioners

RCH rectocolic hemorrhage

RCHF right congestive heart failure

RCHMS Regional Committee for Hospital Medical Services

RCI respiratory control index

RCIA red cell immune adherence

RCIRF radiologic contrast-induced renal failure

RCIT red cell iron turnover

RCITR red cell iron turnover rate

RCL renal clearance

RCM radial contour model; radiographic contrast medium; red cell mass; reinforced clostridial medium; remacemide; remote center of motion; replacement culture medium; right costal margin; Royal College of Midwives

rCMR regional cerebral metabolism rate

rCMRGlc, rCMRglc regional cerebral metabolic rate for glucose

rCMRO$_2$ regional cerebral metabolic rate for oxygen

RCN right caudate nucleus; Royal College of Nursing

RCO right coronary ostium

RCoF ristocetin cofactor

RCOG Royal College of Obstetricians and Gynaecologists

RCP red cell protoporphyrin; retrocorneal pigmentation; riboflavin carrier protein; Royal College of Physicians

rCP regional cerebral perfusion

rcp reciprocal translocation

RCPath Royal College of Pathologists

RCPG respiratory center pattern generator

RCPH red cell peroxide hemolysis

RCPP recurrent coronary prevention program

RCPSGlas Royal College of Physicians and Surgeons, Glasgow

RCR relative consumption rate; replication-competent recombinant; replication-competent retrovirus; respiratory control ratio

RCRA Resource Conservation and Recovery Act

rCRF recombinant corticotropin-releasing factor

RCS rabbit aorta-contracting substance; real-time control system; red cell suspension; reference coordinate system; renal collector system; reticulum cell sarcoma; right coronary sinus; Royal College of Science; Royal College of Surgeons

RCSE Royal College of Surgeons, Edinburgh

RCSSS resource coordination system for surgical service

RCT radiotherapy and chemotherapy; randomized clinical trial; randomized controlled trial; registered care technologist; retrograde conduction time; root canal therapy; Rorschach content test; rotator cuff tear

rct a marker showing the ability of virulent strains to replicate at 40°C, while vaccine strain shows no replication

RCTE randomized clinical trial evaluator

RCU respiratory care unit

RCV recoverin; red cell volume

RCVS Royal College of Veterinary Surgeons

RD radial deviation; radiology department; rate difference; Raynaud disease; reaction of degeneration; registered dietitian; Reiter disease; related donor; renal disease; resistance determinant; respiratory disease; retinal degeneration; retinal detachment; Reye disease; rheumatoid disease; right deltoid; Riley-Day [syndrome]; Rolland-Desbuquois [syndrome]; rubber dam; ruminal drinking; ruptured disk

Rd rate of disappearance

rd rutherford

R&D research and development

RDA recommended daily allowance; recommended dietary allowance; Registered Dental Assistant; right dorsoanterior [fetal position]

RDB random double-blind [trial]

RDBMS relational database management system

RDBP RD [gene] binding protein

RDB-X random double-blind crossover

RDC research diagnostic criteria

RDCRD Rare Disease Clinical Research Database

RDDA recommended daily dietary allowance

RDDB Rare Disease Database

RDDP ribonucleic acid-dependent deoxynucleic acid polymerase

RDE receptor-destroying enzyme

RDEB recessively inherited dystrophic epidermolysis bullosa

RDE$_D$ radiation dose required

RDES remote data entry system

RDFC recurring digital fibroma of childhood

RDH Registered Dental Hygienist

RDHBF regional distribution of hepatic blood flow

RDI recommended daily intake; respiratory disturbance index; rupture-delivery interval

RDLBBB rate-dependent left bundle-branch block

RDM readmission

RDMS registered diagnostic medical sonographer

rDNA recombinant deoxyribonucleic acid [DNA]

RDOG radiology diagnostic oncology group

RDP right dorsoposterior [fetal position]

RDQ respiratory disease questionnaire

RDR research data repository

RDRP ribonucleic acid [RNA]-dependent ribonucleic acid polymerase

RDRS rapid disability rating scale

RDS Raskin Depression Scale; respiratory distress syndrome; reticuloendothelial depressing substance; rhodanese; slow retinal degeneration

RDT randomized discontinuation trial; retinal damage threshold; routine dialysis therapy

RDV rice dwarf virus

RDW red blood cell distribution width index

RDX radixin

RE radium emanation; readmission; rectal examination; reference emitter; reflux esophagitis; regional enteritis; renal and electrolyte; resistive exercise; resting energy; restriction endonuclease; reticuloendothelial; retinol equivalent; right ear; right eye

R_E respiratory exchange ratio

R&E research and education

Re rhenium

R_o Reynold number

REA radiation emergency area; radioenzymatic assay; renal anastomosis; restriction endonuclease analysis; right ear advantage

rea rearrangement

REAB refractory anemia with excess of blasts

REACH research on endothelin antagonism in chronic heart failure; resource utilization in congestive heart failure [studies]

REACT rapid early action in coronary treatment

REAC/TS Radiation Emergency Assistance Center/Training Site

readm readmission

REALM rapid estimate of adult literacy in medicine

REAP restriction endonuclease analysis of plasmid

REAR renal, ear, anal, and radial [malformation syndrome]

REAS reasonably expected as safe; retained, excluded antrum syndrome

REAT radiological emergency assistance team

REB roentgen-equivalent biological

REC receptor; recombination, recombinant [chromosome]

rec fresh [Lat. *recens*]; recessive; recombinant chromosome; record; recovery; recurrence, recurrent

RECA recombination protein A

RECAP retrosynthetic combinatorial analysis procedure

R_{ECF} extracellular fluid resistance

RECG radioelectrocardiography

recip recipient; reciprocal

RECIT Représentation du Contenu Informationel de Testes Médicaux

recon the smallest unit of DNA capable of recombination [recombination + Gr. *on* quantum]

recond reconditioned, reconditioning

RECPAM recursive partition and amalgamation

recumb recumbent

RECREATE Rescue of Closed Arteries Treated by Stent for Threatened or Abrupt Closure [study]

recryst recrystallization

rect rectal; rectification, rectified; rectum; rectus [muscle]

Rec Ther recreational therapy

recur recurrence, recurrent

RED radiation experience data; rapid erythrocyte degeneration; repeat expansion detection

red reduction

REDAP rural emergency department approved for pediatrics

RED-LIP Reduction of Lipid Metabolism [study]

redox oxidation-reduction

REDS Retrovirus Epidemiology Donor Study

REDUCE Randomized Double-blind Unfractionated Heparin and Placebo-Controlled Multicenter Trial; Restenosis Reduction by Cutting Balloon Evaluation [study]

REE rapid extinction effect; rare earth element; resting energy expenditure

REEDS retention of tears, ectrodactyly, ectodermal dysplasia, and strange hair, skin and teeth [syndrome]

REEG radioelectroencephalography

R-EEG resting electroencephalography

ReEND reproductive endocrinology

REEP right end-expiratory pressure

reev re-evaluate

reex re-examine

REF ejection fraction at rest; rat embryo fibroblast; referred; refused; renal erythropoietic factor; right ventricular ejection fraction

ref reference; reflex

Ref-1 redox factor 1

Ref Doc referring doctor

REFI regional ejection fraction image

ref ind refractive index

refl reflex

REFLECT-1 Randomized Evaluation of Flosequinan on Exercise Tolerance–Initial Efficacy Trial

REFLECT-2 Randomized Evaluation of Flosequinan on Exercise Tolerance–Dose Response Study

REFLEX Randomized Evaluation of Flosequinan on Exercise Tolerance [study]; Restenosis Rates with Flexible GFX Stents [study]

Ref Phys referring physician

REFRAD released from active duty

REFSA Randomized European Femoral Stent vs Angioplasty Trial

REG radiation exposure guide; radioencephalogram, radioencephalography

Reg registered

reg region; regular

regen regenerated, regenerating, regeneration

REGRESS Regression Growth Evaluation Statin Study

reg rhy regular rhythm

REGU regulation [UMLS]

regurg regurgitation

REH renin essential hypertension

rehab rehabilitation, rehabilitated

REIN Ramipril Effect in Nephropathy [study]

REL rate of energy loss; recommended exposure limit; resting expiratory level

rel relative

RELACS Reikjavik experimental light-activated cell sorter

RELANCA relation between antineutrophil cytoplasm autoantibody [ANCA] levels and relapses of ANCA-associated glomerulonephritis and vasculitis

RELAY relayed correlation spectroscopy

RELE resistive exercise of lower extremities

RELP restriction fragment length polymorphism

RelTox Relational Toxicology [Project]

RELV restriction fragment length variant

REM rapid eye movement; recent-event memory; reticular erythematous mucinosis; return electrode monitor; roentgen-equivalent-man

Rem roentgen-equivalent-man

rem removal

REMA repetitive excess mixed anhydride

REMAB radiation-equivalent-manikin absorption

REMAIN remission-maintenance [therapy for systemic vasculitis]

REMATCH Randomized Evaluation of Mechanical Assistance in the Treatment of Congestive Heart Failure [study]

REMCAL radiation-equivalent-manikin calibration

remit remittent

REMO regional emergency medical organization

REMP roentgen-equivalent-man period

REMPAN radiation emergency medical preparedness

REMS rapid eye movement sleep

REMT trigger signal rapid eye movements

REN renal; renin

RENAAL Reduction of Endpoints in Noninsulin-dependent Diabetes Mellitus with Angiotensin II Antagonist Losartan [trial]

RENEWAL Randomized Trial of Endoluminal Reconstruction Using the NIR Stent or WAIL Stent in Angioplasty of Long Segment Disease

REO respiratory enteric orphan [virus]

REP reepithelialization; replication protein; rest-exercise program; restriction endonuclease profile; retrograde pyelogram; Rochester Epidemiology Project; roentgen equivalent-physical

rep replication; roentgen equivalent-physical

REPA replication protein A

REPAIR Reperfusion in Acute Infarction, Rotterdam [study]

repol repolarization

REPR reproductive

REPS reactive extensor postural synergy

rept let it be repeated

req request, requested

RER renal excretion rate; respiratory exchange ratio; rough endoplasmic reticulum

RERC Rehabilitation Engineering Research Center

RERF Radiation Effects Research Foundation

RES radionuclide esophageal scintigraphy; Reproducibility Echocardiography Study; Rotterdam Elderly Study; reticuloendothelial system

res research; resection; resident; residue; resistance

RESAC Real-Time Expert System for Advice and Control

RESCUE Randomized Evaluation of Salvage Angioplasty with Combined Utilization of Endpoints [trial]

RESIST Restenosis after Intravascular Ultrasound-guided Stenting [study]

RESNA Rehabilitation Engineering Society of North America

RESOLVD, RESOLVED Randomized Evaluation of Strategies for Left Ventricular Dysfunction [study]

resp respiration, respiratory; response

Resp Ther respiratory therapy

REST Raynaud's phenomenon, esophageal motor dysfunction, sclerodactyly, and telangiectasia [syndrome]; regressive electroshock therapy; Restenosis Stent Trial

RESTORE Randomized Efficacy Study of Tirofiban for Outcomes and Restenosis [trial]

RESTT respiratory therapy technician

resusc resuscitation

RET reticular; reticulocyte; retina; retention; retained; right esotropia

ret rad equivalent therapeutic

RETA Registry for the Endovascular Treatment of Aneurysms

retard retardation, retarded

ret cath retention catheter

retic reticulocyte

REV reticuloendotheliosis virus

ReV regulator of virion

rev reverse; review; revolution

re-x reexamination

Rex regulator x

RF radial fiber; radiofrequency; receptive field; regurgitant fraction; Reitland-Franklin [unit]; relative flow; relative fluorescence; release factor; renal failure; replacement fluid; replication factor; replicative form; resistance factor; resonant frequency; respiratory failure; respiratory frequency; reticular formation; retroperitoneal fibromatosis; rheumatic fever; rheumatoid factor; riboflavin; risk factor; root canal filling; rosette formation

R^F rate of flow

Rf respiratory frequency; rutherfordium

R$_f$ in paper or thin-layer chromatography, the distance that a spot of a substance has moved from the point of application

rf radiofrequency; rapid filling

rFVIII recombinant factor VIII

RFA resident functional atlas; right femoral artery; right frontoanterior [fetal position]

RFB retained foreign body

RFC replication factor C; request for comments; retrograde femoral catheter; rosette-forming cell

RFDS Royal Flying Doctors Service [Australia]

RFE relative fluorescence efficiency

RFFIT rapid fluorescent focus inhibition test

rFGF1 recombinant fibroblast growth factor 1 [acidic]

rFGF2 recombinant fibroblast growth factor 2 [basic]

RFH right femoral hernia

RFI radiofrequency interference; recurrence-free interval; renal failure index request for information

RFIED round femoral inferior epiphysis dysplasia

RFL right frontolateral [fetal position]

RFLA rheumatoid-factor-like activity

RFLP restriction fragment length polymorphism

RFLS rheumatoid-factor-like substance

Rfm rifampin

RFP recurrent facial paralysis; request for proposal; right frontoposterior [fetal position]

RF-PMR radiofrequency-percutaneous myocardial revascularization [revascularization with radiofrequency energy generator]

RFPS (Glasgow) Royal Faculty of Physicians and Surgeons of Glasgow

RFR rapid fluid resuscitation; refraction
RFS relapse-free survival; renal function study; rotating frame spectroscopy
RFT respiratory function test; rod-and-frame test; right frontotransverse [fetal position]
RFV right femoral vein
RFW rapid filling wave
RG right gluteal
rG regular gene
RGB red-green-blue [imaging]
RGBMT renal glomerular basement membrane thickness
RGC radio-gas chromatography; remnant gastric cancer; retinal ganglion cell; right giant cell
RGD range-gated Doppler; refractional geometric distortions [imaging]
RGE relative gas expansion
RGEA right gastroepiploic artery
RGH rat growth hormone
RGI recovery from growth inhibition
RGM right gluteus medius
rGM-CSF recombinant granulocytemacrophage colony-stimulating factor
RGN refinement grouper number; Registered General Nurse
RGO reciprocating gait orthosis
RGP retrograde pyelography
RGR relative growth rate
RGS Rieger syndrome
RGU regional glucose utilization
RH radiant heat; radiation hybrid; radiological health; reactive hyperemia; recurrent herpes; regulatory hormone; rehabilitation; relative humidity; releasing hormone; renal hemolysis; retinal hemorrhage; right hand; right heart; right hemisphere; right hyperphoria; room humidifier
Rh rhesus [factor]; rhinion; rhodamine; rhodium
Rh+ rhesus positive
Rh– rhesus negative
rh rheumatic
r/h roentgens per hour
RHA Regional Health Authority; relative highest avidity; right hepatic artery
RhA rheumatoid arthritis
RHB right heart bypass
RHBF reactive hyperemia blood flow
RHBs Regional Hospital Boards

RHC rad homolog in *Cerevisiae;* resin hemoperfusion column; respiration has ceased; right heart catheterization; right hypochondrium
RHCSA Regional Hospitals Consultants' and Specialists' Association
RHD radiological health data; relative hepatic dullness; renal hypertensive disease; rheumatic heart disease
rhDNase recombinant human deoxyribonuclease [DNAse]
RHE retinohepatoendocrinologic [syndrome]
RHEED reflection high-energy electron diffraction
rheo rheology
rheu, rheum rheumatic, rheumatoid
RHF right heart failure
Rh F rheumatic fever
RHG right hand grip
rhG-CSF recombinant human granulocyte colony-stimulating factor
rhGM-CSF recombinant human granulocyte macrophage colony-stimulating factor
RHI Rural Health Initiative
rhIGF recombinant human insulin-like growth factor [IGF]
rhIL recombinant human interleukin
RHIN regional health information network
Rhin rhinology
rhino rhinoplasty
RHJSC Regional Hospital Junior Staff Committee
RHL recurrent herpes labialis; right hepatic lobe
RHLN right hilar lymph node
rhm roentgens per hour at 1 meter
RHMAP radiation hybrid mapping program
RhMK rhesus monkey kidney
RhMk rhesus monkey
RhMkK rhesus monkey kidney
RHMV right heart mixing volume
RHN Rockwell hardness number
RHO rhodopsin; right heeloff
ρ Greek letter *rho*; correlation coefficient; electric charge density; electrical resistivity; mass density; reactivity
RHOM rhombosine
RHR renal hypertensive rat; resting heart rate
r/hr roentgens per hour

RHRV relative heart rate variability
RHS Ramsay Hunt syndrome; Rapp-Hodgkin syndrome; reciprocal hindlimb-scratching [syndrome]; Richner-Hanhart syndrome; right hand side; right heelstrike
RHSIG Rehabilitation Hospitals Special Interest Group
RHT renal homotransplantation
RHTC rural health training center
rH-TNF recombinant human tumor necrosis factor
rh-tPA recombinant tissue plasminogen activator
rhTPO recombinant human thrombopoietin
RHU registered health underwriter; rheumatology
rHuEpo recombinant human erythropoietin
rHuTNF recombinant human tumor-necrosing factor
RHV right hepatic vein
rHV recombinant hirudin variant
RI radiation intensity; radioactive isotope; radioimmunology; recession index; recombinant inbred [strain]; refractive index; regenerative index; regional ileitis; regional information system; regular insulin; relative intensity; release inhibition; remission induction; renal index; renal insufficiency; replicative intermediate; resistive index; respiratory illness; respiratory index; response interval; retroactive inhibition; retroactive interference; ribosome; rosette index (or inhibition)
R$_I$ intracellular resistivity
r$_i$ intraclass correlation coefficient
RIA radioimmunoassay; reversible ischemic attack
RIA-DA radioimmunoassay double antibody [test]
RIAS Roter Interactional Analysis System
Rib riboflavin; ribose
RIBA recombinant immunoblot assay
ribotyping ribonucleic acid [RNA]-typing
RIBS Rutherford ion backscattering
RIC right internal carotid [artery]; right interventricular coronary [artery]; Royal Institute of Chemistry
RICE rest, ice, compression, and elevation
R$_{ICF}$ intracellular fluid resistance
RICM right intercostal margin
RiCoF ristocetin cofactor

RICP recurrent intrahepatic cholestasis of pregnancy
RICU respiratory intensive care unit
RID radial immunodiffusion; reduced interference distribution; remission-inducing drug; ruptured intervertebral disc
RIDDOR Reporting of Injuries, Diseases, and Dangerous Occurrences Regulations [UK]
RIDL retrograde intrarenal lithotripsy
RIE reactive ion etching
RIF radiological interface; release-inhibiting factor; rifampin; right iliac fossa; rosette-inhibiting factor
RIFA radioiodinated fatty acid
RIFC rat intrinsic factor concentrate
RIFLE risk factor and life expectancy
rIFN recombinant interferon
RIG rabies immune globulin; rat insuloma gene
RIGH rabies immune globulin, human
RIGHT [Ce]rivastatin Gemfibrozil Hyperlipidemia Treatment [study]
RIH right inguinal hernia
RIHD radiation-induced heart disease
RIHSA radioactive iodinated human serum albumin
rIL recombinant interleukin
RILT rabbit ileal loop test
RIM radioisotope medicine; recurrent induced malaria; relative-intensity measure
RIMA reverse inhibitor of monoamino oxidase A; right internal mammary artery
riMLF rostral interstitial median longitudinal fasciculus
RIMR Rockefeller Institute for Medical Research
RIMS resonance ionization mass spectrometry
RIN radioisotope nephrography; rat insulinoma
R$_{in}$ input resistance
RINB Reitan-Indiana Neuropsychological Battery
RIND reversible ischemic neurologic deficit
RINN recommended international nonproprietary name
RIO right inferior oblique
RIP radioimmunoprecipitation; reflex inhibiting pattern; repeat-induced point [mutation]; respiratory inductance plethysmography

RIPA radioimmunoprecipitation assay

RIPH Royal Institute of Public Health

RIPHH Royal Institute of Public Health and Hygiene

RIPP resistive-intermittent positive pressure

RIR relative incidence rates; right interior rectus [muscle]

RIRB radioiodinated rose bengal

RIRL retrograde intrarenal lipotripsy

RIRS retrograde intrarenal surgery

RIS radiology information system; rapid immunofluorescence staining; relative intensity score; resonance ionization spectroscopy

RISA radioactive iodinated serum albumin; radioimmunosorbent assay

RISC Radiology Information System Consortium; reduced instruction set chip [microprocessor]; Research on Instability in Coronary Artery Disease [study]

RISK Risk Intervention Skills Study

RISL recessive least square lattice

RIST radioimmunosorbent test

RIT radioimmune trypsin; radioiodinated triolein; radioiodine treatment; rosette inhibition titer

RITA Randomised Intervention Treatment of Angina [UK]; right internal thoracic artery

RITC rhodamine isothiocyanate

RITED Italian Registry of Echo-Dobutamine [tests]

RIU radioactive iodine uptake

RIVC right inferior vena cava

RIVD ruptured intervertebral disc

RJA regurgitant jet area

RK rabbit kidney; radial keratotomy; reductase kinase; rhodopsin kinase; right kidney

RKG radiocardiogram

RKH Rokitansky-Küster-Hauser [syndrome]

RKM rokitamycin

RKV rabbit kidney vacuolating [virus]

RKY roentgen kymography

RL radial line; radiation laboratory; reduction level; relaxation labeling; renal dysplasia-limb defects [syndrome]; resistive load; reticular lamina; right lateral; right leg; right lung; Ringer's lactate [solution]; run length

R&L right and left

RLA Ranchos de los Amigos [Cognitive Functioning Scale]

RLC residual lung capacity

RLD related living donor; ruptured lumbar disc

RLE right lower extremity

RLF retrolental fibroplasia; right lateral femoral

RLGS restriction landmark genomic scanning

RLL right lobe of liver; right lower limb; right lower lobe; run length limited

RLM right lower medial

RLN recurrent laryngeal nerve; regional lymph node; relaxin

RLNC regional lymph node cell

RLND regional lymph node dissection

RLO residual lymphatic output

RLP radiation leukemia protection; ribosome-like particle

RLPV right lower pulmonary vein

RLQ right lower quadrant

RLR right lateral rectus [muscle]

RLS recursive least square; restless leg syndrome; Ringer lactate solution; Roussy-Levy syndrome; run-length statistics

RLSB right lower scapular border

R-Lsh right-left shunt

RLSL recursive least square lattice

RLT ralitoline

RLV Rauscher leukemia virus

RLWD routine laboratory work done

RLX relaxin

RLXH relaxin H

RLZ right lower zone

RM radical mastectomy; random migration; radon monitor; range of movement; red marrow; reference material; relative magnitude; relative mobility; rehabilitation medicine; reinforced maneuver; resistive movement; respiratory movement; respiratory muscle; restoration-maximization [algorithm]; Riehl melanosis; risk management; routine management; ruptured membranes

Rm relative mobility; remission

R_m membrane resistance

r_m membrane resistance per unit length

rm remission; room

1RM one-repetition maximum

RMA rapid membrane assay; refuses medical advice; Registered Medical Assistant;

relative medullary area; right mentoanterior [fetal position]

RMANOVA repeated measures analysis of variance

RMAT rapid microagglutination test

RMB right mainstem bronchus

RMBF regional myocardial blood flow

RMC reticular magnocellular [nucleus]; right middle cerebral [artery]

RMCA right middle cerebral artery

RMCH rod monochromacy or monochromatism

RMCL right midclavicular line

RMD retromanubrial dullness

RMDP Resource Mothers Development Project

RME rapid maxillary expansion; resting metabolic expenditure; right mediolateral episiotomy

RMEC regional medical education center

RMED rural medical education [program]

RMF recursive median filter; right middle finger

RMI recent myocardial infarction; reticulocyte maturity index

RMK rhesus monkey kidney

RML radiation myeloid leukemia; regional medical library; right mediolateral; right middle lobe

RMLB right middle lobe bronchus

RMLS right middle lobe syndrome

RMLV Rauscher murine leukemia virus

RMM rapid micromedia method

RMN Registered Mental Nurse

RMO Regional Medical Officer; Resident Medical Officer

RMP rapidly miscible pool; Regional Medical Program; regional myocardial infarction; resting membrane potential; ribulose monophosphate pathway; rifampin; right mentoposterior [fetal position]

RMPA Royal Medico-Psychological Association

RMR relative maximum respone; resting metabolic rate; right medial rectus [muscle]

RMRS Regenstrief Medical Record System

RMS rectal morphine sulfate [suppository]; red man syndrome; repetitive motion syndrome; respiratory muscle strength; rhabdomyosarcoma; rheumatic mitral stenosis; rhodomyosarcoma; rigid man syndrome; root-mean-square

rms root-mean-square

RMSA regulator of mitotic spindle assembly; rhabdomyosarcoma, alveolar

RMSa rhabdomyosarcoma

RMSCR rhabdomyosarcoma chromosomal region

RMSD root-mean-square deviation

RMSE root-mean-square error

RMSF Rocky Mountain spotted fever

RMSS Ruvalcaba-Myhre-Smith syndrome

RMT Registered Music Therapist; relative medullary thickness; retromolar trigone; right mentotransverse [fetal position]

RMUI relief medication unit index

RMuLV Rauscher murine leukemia virus

RMV respiratory minute volume

RMZ right midzone

RN radionuclide; red nucleus; Registered Nurse; registry number; residual nitrogen; reticular nucleus

Rn radon

RNA radionuclide angiography; Registered Nurse Anesthetist; ribonucleic acid; rough, noncapsulated, avirulent [bacterial culture]

RNAA radiochemical neutron activation analysis

RNAP ribonucleic acid polymerase

RNAse, RNase ribonuclease

RNase P ribonuclease P

RN-C registered nurse-certification

RNCM registered nurse case manager

RND radical neck dissection; radionuclide dacryography; reactive neurotic depression; respiratory nursing diagnosis

RNFL retinal nerve fiber layer

RNFP Registered Nurse Fellowship Program

RNI reactive nitrogen intermediate

RNIB Royal National Institute for the Blind

RNICU regional neonatal intensive care unit

RNID Royal National Institute for the Deaf

RNINMEGLA rat integral membrane glycoprotein

RNP ribonucleoprotein

RNP-CS ribonucleoprotein consensus sequence

RNR ribonucleotide reductase

RNS reference normal serum; repetitive nerve stimulation; ribonuclease

RNSC radionuclide superior cavography

Rnt roentgenology

RNTMI transfer ribonucleic acid initiator methionine

RNV radionuclide venography; radionuclide ventriculography

rNTP ribonuclease-5;pr-triphosphate

RNVG radionuclide ventriculography

RO radiation oncology; radiation output; ratio of; relative odds; renal osteodystrophy; reverse osmosis; Ritter-Oleson [technique]; routine order; rule out

ro radius of orifice

R/O rule out

ROA regurgitant orifice area; right occipitoanterior [fetal position]

ROAD reversible obstructive airways disease

ROAT repeat open application test

ROATS rabbit ovarian antitumor serum

rob robertsonian translocation

ROBUST Recanalization of Occluded Bypass Graft with Prolonged Urokinase Infusion Site Trial

ROC receiver operating characteristic; receiver operating curve; receptor-operated channels; relative operating characteristic; resident on call; residual organic carbon

ROCF Rey-Osterrieth Complex Figure

ROCKET Regionally Organized Cardiac Key European Trial

RODA rapid opioid detoxification under general anesthesia

rOEF regional oxygen extraction fraction

roent roentgenology

ROESY rotating frame Overhauser effect spectroscopy

ROH rat ovarian hyperemia [test]

ROI reactive oxygen intermediate; region of interest; right occipitolateral [fetal position]

ROIH right oblique inguinal hernia

ROJM range of joint motion

ROLL radioguided occult lesion localization

ROM range of motion; reactive oxygen metabolite; read only memory; reduction of movement; regional office manual; removal of metal [pins or plates in orthopedic surgery]; rupture of membranes

Rom Romberg [sign]

rom reciprocal ohm meter

ROMAS Romanian Multicenter Study

ROM CP range of motion complete and painfree

ROMIO Rule Out Myocardial Infarct Observation [study]

ROOF retro-orbital orbicular fat

ROP removal of pins or plates; removal of plaster [of Paris]; retinopathy of prematurity; right occipitoposterior [fetal position]

RO PACS radiation oncology picture archiving and communication system

ROPE respiratory-ordered phase encoding

ROPS rollover protective structure

Ror Rorschach [test]

ROS reactive oxygen species; reflectance optical shield; relative outcome score; review of systems; rod outer segment

RoS rostral sulcus

ROSC return of spontaneous circulation

ROSETTA Routine vs Selective Exercise Treadmill Test after Angioplasty [trial]

ROSP rod outer segment protein

ROSS review of subjective symptoms

ROSTER Rotational Atherectomy vs Balloon Angioplasty for In-stent Restenosis [trial]

ROT real oxygen transport; remedial occupational therapy; right occipito-transverse [fetal position]

rot rotating, rotation

ROTA rotablator atherectomy

ROTACS rotational angioplasty catheter system

ROTASTENT Rotational Atherectomy with Adjunctive Stenting [trial]

ROU recurrent oral ulcer

ROW Rendu-Osler-Weber [syndrome]; rest of the world

ROXIS Roxithromycin in Ischemic Syndromes [study]

RP radial pulse; radiopharmaceutical; rapid processing [of film]; Raynaud phenomenon; reactive protein; readiness potential; recreation and passtime; rectal prolapse; refractory period; regulatory protein; relapsing polychondritis; reperfusion; replication protein; resident physician; respiratory rate; rest pain; resting potential; resting pressure; retinitis pigmentosa; retrograde pyelogram; retroperitoneal; reverse phase; rheumatoid polyarthritis; ribonucleoprotein; ribose phosphate; ribosomal protein

R5P ribose-5-phosphate
R/P respiratory pulse [rate]
R$_p$ pulmonary resistance
RPA radial photon apsorptiometry; replication protein A; resultant physiologic acceleration; reverse passive anaphylaxis; right pulmonary artery
r-PA reteplase
RPAHPET Royal Prince Albert Hospital Positron Emission Tomography [study]
RPase ribonucleic acid polymerase
RPC reactive perforating collagenosis; relapsing polychondritis; relative proliferative capacity; remote procedure call
RPCF, RPCFT Reiter protein complement fixation [test]
RPCGN rapidly progressive crescenting glomerulonephritis
RPCH rural primary care hospital
RPD removable partial denture
R-PDQ revised prescreening developmental questionnaire
RPE rate of perceived exertion; recurrent pulmonary embolism; retinal pigment epithelium; ribulose 5-phosphate 3-epimerase
RPEP rabies post-exposure prophylaxis
RPET rapid partial exchange transfusion
RPF relaxed pelvic floor; renal plasma flow; retroperitoneal fibrosis
RPG radiation protection guide; Report Program Generator [PC language]; retrograde pyelogram; rheoplethysmography; right paracolic gutter
RPGMEC Regional Postgraduate Medical Education Committee
RPGN rapidly progressive glomerulonephritis
RPGR retinitis pigmentosa guanosine triphosphatase regulator [gene]
RPh Registered Pharmacist
RPHA reversed passive hemagglutination
RPHAMFCA reversed passive hemagglutination by miniature centrifugal fast analysis
RP-HPLC reverse phase-high performance liquid chromatography
RPI regional perfusion index; relative percentage index; reticulocyte production index, ribose 5-phosphate isomerase
RPIPP reverse phase ion-pair partition
RPK ribosephosphate kinase
RPLAD retroperitoneal lymphadenectomy

RPLC reverse phase liquid chromatography
RPLD repair of potentially lethal damage
RPLND retroperitoneal lymph node dissection
RPM, rpm rapid processing mode; revolutions per minute
RPMD rheumatic pain modulation disorder
RPMI Roswell Park Memorial Institute [medium]
RPMS resource and patient management system
RPO right posterior oblique
RPP heart rate-systolic blood pressure product; rate-pressure produce; retropubic prostatectomy
RPPI role perception picture inventory
RPPR red cell precursor production rate
RPR rapid plasmin reagin [test]
RPr retinitis proliferans
RPRC regional primate research center
RPRCT rapid plasma reagin cord test
RPRF rapidly progressive renal failure
Rp:Rs pulmonary to systemic vascular resistance
RPS renal pressor substance; revolutions per second
rps revolutions per second
RPSM residency program in social medicine
RPSP reference preparation for serum proteins
RPS4Y ribosomal protein S4, Y-linked
RPT rapid pull-through; refractory period of transmission; Registered Physical Therapist; renal parenchymal thickness
RPTA renal percutaneous transluminal angioplasty
RPTC regional poisoning treatment center
Rptd ruptured
RPV right portal vein; right pulmonary vein
RPVP right posterior ventricular pre-excitation
RQ recovery quotient; [Hazardous Substance] Reportable Quantities [List]; reportable quantity; respiratory quotient; risk-adjusted quantity
RQDS Revised Quantified Denver Scale of Communication
RQL rejectable quality level

RR radiation reaction; radiation response; rate ratio; rational recovery [group]; recovery room; recurrence risk; regulatory region; relative resistance; relative response; relative risk; renin release; respiratory rate; respiratory reserve; response rate; results reporting [system]; retinal reflex; rheumatoid rosette; ribonucleotide reductase; risk ratio; Riva-Rocci [sphygmomanometer]; Ross River [virus]; ruthenium red

Rr respiratory rate

R&R rate and rhythm; rest and recuperation; rotablator and restenosis

RRA radioreceptor assay; registered record administrator

RRAC Research Realignment Advisory Committee

RRBAT relative rigid body accuracy test

RRC residency review committee; risk reduction component; routine respiratory care; Royal Red Cross; rural referral center

RRC-EM residency review committee for emergency medicine

RRDS radiation-resistant deoxyribonucleic acid [DNA] synthesis

RRE radiation-related eosinophilia; Rev response element

RRE, RR&E round, regular, and equal [pupils]

RRF ragged red fiber; residual renal function

RR-HPO rapid recompression-high pressure oxygen

RRI recurrent respiratory infection; reflex relaxation index; relative response index

RRIS recurrent respiratory infection syndrome

RRL rabbit reticulocyte lysate; Registered Record Librarian

RRM ribonucleic acid [RNA] recognition motif; ribonucleotide reductase M

RRN returning [for advanced studies] registered nurse

rRNA ribosomal ribonucleic acid

rRNP ribosomal ribonucleoprotein

RRP relative refractory period

RRPCE Reduction of Recurrence and Prevention of Cerebral Emboli [study]

RRpm respiratory rate per minute

RRR regular rhythm and rate; relative risk reduction; renin release rate (or ratio)

RR&R regular rate and rhythm

RRS result reporting clinical data repository system; retrorectal space; Richards-Rundle syndrome

RRT random response technique; Registered Respiratory Therapist; relative retention time

RRU respiratory resistance unit

RS radioscaphoid; random sample; rating schedule; Raynaud syndrome; reaction stimulus; recipient's serum; rectal sinus; rectal suppository; rectosigmoid; reducing substance; Reed-Steinberg [cell]; reinforcing stimulus; Reiter syndrome; relative stimulus; remote site; renal specialist; respiratory syncytial [virus]; response to stimulus; resting subject; reticulated siderocyte; retinoschisis; Rett syndrome; review of symptoms; Reye syndrome; right sacrum; Reykjavik Study [coronary diseases in Icelandic males]; ribonucleic acid [RNA] synthetase; right septum; right side; right stellate [ganglion]; Ringer solution; Roberts syndrome; Rous sarcoma

Rs *Rauwolfia serpentina*; systemic resistance

R/s roentgens per second

r$_s$ rank correlation coefficient

RSA rabbit serum albumin; regular spiking activity; relative specific activity; relative standard accuracy; respiratory sinus arrhythmia; reticulum cell sarcoma; right sacroanterior [fetal position]; right subclavian artery; roentgenographic stereogrammetric analysis

Rsa systemic arterial resistance

RSB reticulocyte standard buffer; right sternal border

RSC rat spleen cell; rested state contraction; reversible sickle-cell; right subclavian

RScA right scapuloanterior [fetal position]

RSCN Registered Sick Children's Nurse

RScP right scapuloposterior [fetal position]

RSD reflex sympathetic dystrophy; relative standard deviation

RSDS reflex sympathetic dystrophy syndrome

RSE rapid spin-echo; relative standard error

RSEP right somatosensory evoked potential

RSES Rosenberg Self-Esteem Scale

RSH Royal Society of Health

RSHT regular SNOMED hierarchies table

RSI rapid-sequence induction; rapid sequence intubation; repetition strain injury; repetitive stress injury

RSIC Radiation Shielding Information Center

RSIL respiratory and systemic infection laboratory

R-SIRS Revised Seriousness of Illness Rating Scale

RSIVP rapid-sequence intravenous pyelography

RSL right sacrolateral [fetal position]

RSLD repair of sublethal damage

RSLT test result [UMLS]

RSM risk screening model; Royal Society of Medicine

RSMR relative standard mortality rate

RSN restin; right substantia nigra

RSNA Radiological Society of North America; renal sympathetic nerve activity

RSO radiation safety officer; Resident Surgical Officer; right superior oblique [muscle]

rSO₂ regional oxygen saturation

RSP rapid straight pacing; rat serum protein; recurrent spontaneous pneumothorax; removable silicone plug; ribose-5-phosphatase; right sacroposterior [fetal position]

RSPAC remote sensing public access center

RSPCA Royal Society for the Prevention of Cruelty to Animals

RS₃PE remitting seronegative symmetrical synovitis with pitting edema

RSPH Royal Society for the Promotion of Health

RSPK recurrent spontaneous psychokinesis

RSR rectosphincteric reflex response-stimulus ratio; regular sinus rhythm; relative survival rate; right superior rectus [muscle]

rSr an electrocardiographic complex

RSS rat stomach strip; recombination signal sequence; rectosigmoidoscopy; repetitive stress syndrome; rotary subluxation of the sphenoid; Russell-Silver syndrome; Russian spring-summer [encephalitis]

RSSE Russian spring-summer encephalitis

RSSR relative slow sinus rate

RST radiosensitivity test; rapid surfactant test; reagin screen test; repeated significance test; right sacrotransverse [fetal position]; rubrospinal tract

R$_{st}$ in paper or thin layer chromatography, the distance that a spot of a substance has moved, relative to a reference standard spot

RSTD rectal-skin temperature difference

R-step restoration step

rSTERN recurrent spatiotemporal neuron

RSTI Radiological Service Training Institute

RSTL relaxed skin tension lines

RSTMH Royal Society of Tropical Medicine and Hygiene

RSTS retropharyngeal soft tissue space; Rubinstein-Taybi syndrome

RSU radiological sciences unit

RSV respiratory syncytial virus; right subclavian vein; Rous sarcoma virus

RSVC right superior vena cava

RSVP retired senior volunteer program

RT radiologic technologist; radiotelemetry; radiotherapy; radium therapy; rapid tranquilization; reaction time; reading test; real time; reciprocating tachycardia; recreational therapy; rectal temperature; reduction time; Registered Technician; renal transplantation; resistance transfer; respiratory therapist/therapy; response time; rest tremor; retransformation; retrieved term; reverse transcriptase; reverse transcription; right; right thigh; room temperature; Rubinstein-Taybi [syndrome]

RT3, rT₃ reverse triiodothyronine

Rt right; total resistance

rT ribothymidine

rt right

RTA ray tracing algorithm; renal tubular acidosis; reverse transcriptase assay; road traffic accident

RTAD renal tubular acidification defect

rTag recombinant small T-antigen

rTAP recombinant tick anticoagulant peptide

RT(ARRT) Radiologic Technologist certified by the American Registry of Radiologic Technologists

RTC random control trial; rape treatment center; regional tuberculosis centre; renal tubular cell; residential treatment center; return to clinic; reverse thrust catheter

rtc return to clinic

RT-CT radiotherapy dedicated computed tomography

RTD renal tubular dysplasia or dysgenesis, defect; routine test dilution

Rtd retarded

RTEC Regional Technology and Education Consortium

RTECS Registry of Toxic Effects of Chemical Substances

RTF resistance transfer factor; respiratory tract fluid; rich text format

RTG-2 rainbow trout gonadal tissue cells

RTH resistance to thyroid hormone

rTHF recombinant tumor necrosis factor

RTI reproductive tract infection; respiratory tract infection; reverse transcriptase inhibition

RTK receptor-tyrosine kinase; rhabdoid tumor of the kidney

rtl rectal

rt lat right lateral

RTM registered trademark

RTN renal tubular necrosis

RTn reverse transcription intermediate

RT(N)(ARRT) Radiologic Technologist (Nuclear Medicine) certified by the American Registry of Radiologic Technologists

RTO return to office; right toeoff

RTOG radiation therapy oncology group

RTP radiation treatment planning; renal transplantation patient; reverse transcriptase-producing [agent]

rTPA/rtPA recombinant tissue plasminogen activator

rt-PA recombinant tissue plasminogen activator

RT-PCR reverse transcriptase polymerase chain reaction [PCR]

RTR Recreational Therapist, Registered; red blood cell turnover rate; retention time ratio

RT(R)(ARRT) Registered Technologist, Radiography certified by the American Registry of Radiologic Technologists)

RTRR return to recovery room

RTS real time scan; Rett syndrome; Revised Trauma Score; right toestrike; Rothmund-Thomson syndrome; Rubinstein-Taybi syndrome

RTSS rest technetium-99m sestamibi scan

RT(T)(ARRT) Radiologic Technologist (Radiation Therapy) certified by the American Registry of Radiologic Technologists

RTTP radiation therapy treatment planning

RTU real-time ultrasonography; relative time unit; renal transplantation unit

RT$_3$U resin triiodothyronine uptake

RTUI respiratory therapy utilization index

RTW return to work

RTV room temperature vulcanization

RU radioulnar; rat unit; reading unit; residual urine; resin uptake; resistance unit; retrograde urogram; right upper; roentgen unit

ru radiation unit

RU-1 human embryonic lung fibroblasts

RU-486 mifepristone

RUA reduced under anesthesia

RUC rapid update cycle

RUD recurrent ulcer of the duodenal bulb

RUE right upper extremity

RUG resource utilization group

RUL right upper eyelid; right upper lateral; right upper limb; right upper lobe

RuMP ribulose monophosphate pathway

RUOQ right upper outer quadrant

Ru1,5P ribulose-1,5-biphosphate

Ru5P ribulose-5-phosphate

rupt ruptured

RUP right upper pole

RUPV right upper pulmonary vein

RUQ right upper quadrant

RUR resin-uptake ratio

RURTI recurrent upper respiratory tract infection

RUS radioulnar synostosis; real-time ultrasonography

RUSB right upper sternal border

RUSP right ventricular systolic pressure

RUTH Raloxifene Use for the Heart [study]

RUV residual urine volume

RUX right upper extremity

RUZ right upper zone

RV random variable; rat virus; Rauscher virus; rectovaginal; regurgitant [stroke] volume; reinforcement value; renal vein; residual volume; respiratory volume; retroventral; retroversion; retrovesical; return visit; rheumatoid vasculitis; rhinovirus;

right ventricle, right ventricular; rubella vaccine; rubella virus; Russell viper

R$_V$ radius of view

RVA rabies vaccine activated; re-entrant ventricular arrhythmia; right ventricle activation; right vertebral artery

RVAD right ventricular assist device

RVAW right ventricle anterior wall

RVB red venous blood

RVC reason for visit classification; rectovaginal constriction

RVD relative vertebral density; relative vessel diameter; right ventricular dysplasia

RVDC right ventricular diastolic collapse

RVDO right ventricular diastolic overload

RVDV right ventricular diastolic volume

RVE right ventricular enlargement

RVECP right ventricular endocardial potential

RVED right ventricular end-diastolic [pressure]

RVEDD right ventricular end-diastolic diameter

RVEDP right ventricular end-diastolic pressure

RVEDV right ventricular end-diastolic volume

RVEDVI right ventricular end-diastolic volume index

RVEF right ventricular ejection fraction; right ventricular end-flow

RVESV right ventricular end-systolic volume

RVET right ventricular ejection time

RVF renal vascular failure; residual volume fraction; Rift Valley fever; right ventricular failure; right visual field

RVFP right ventricular filling pressure

RVG right ventral glutens [muscle]; right visceral ganglion

RVH renovascular hypertension; right ventricular hypertrophy

RVHD rheumatic valvular heart disease

RVHR renovascular hypertensive rat

RVI relative value index; right ventricle infarction

RVID ventricular internal dimension

RVIT right ventricular inflow tract

RV-IVRT right ventricular isovolumic relaxation time

RVL right vastus lateralis

RVLG right ventrolateral gluteal

RVLM rostral ventrolateral medulla

RVM right ventricular mean

RVMM rostral ventromedial medulla

RVO Regional Veterinary Officer; relaxed vaginal outlet; right ventricular outflow

RVOT right ventricular outflow tract

RVP red veterinary petrolatum; resting venous pressure; right ventricular pressure

RVPEP right ventricular pre-ejection period

RVPFR right ventricular peak filling rate

RVPRA renal vein plasma renin activity

RVR reduced vascular response; renal vascular resistance; repetitive ventricular response; resistance to venous return

RVRA renal vein rein activity; renal venous renin assay

RVRC renal vein renin concentration

RVS rectovaginal space; relative value scale/study; reported visual sensation; retrovaginal space

RVSO right ventricular stroke output

RVSV right ventricular stroke volume

RVSW right ventricular stroke work

RVSWI right ventricular stroke work index

RVT renal vein thrombosis

RVTE recurring venous thromboembolism

RV/TLC residual volume/total lung capacity

RVU relative value unit

RVV right ventricular volume; rubella vaccine-like virus; Russell viper venom

RVVO right ventricular volume overload

RVVT Russell viper venom time

RVW right ventricular wall

RVWT right ventricle wall thickness

RW radiological warfare; ragweed; respiratory work; Romano-Ward [syndrome]; round window

R-W Rideal-Walker [coefficient]

RWAGE ragweed antigen E

RWC regional weaning center

RWCI right cardiac work index

RWIS restraint and water immersion stress

RWJF Robert Wood Johnson Foundation

RWM regional wall motion

RWMA regional wall motion abnormality

RWP ragweed pollen; R-wave progression

RWS radiology work station; ragweed sensitivity

RWT relative wall thickness

RX reaction
Rx drug; medication; pharmacy; prescribe, prescription, prescription drug; take [Lat. *recipe*]; therapy; treatment
RXLI recessive X-linked ichthyosis
RXN reaction
RXR retinoid X receptor

RXRA retinoid X receptor alpha
RXRE retinoic X response element
RXRG retinoid X receptor gamma
RXT right exotropia
R-Y Roux-en-Y [anastomosis]
RYD ryanodine
RYR ryanodine receptor

S apparent power; in electrocardiography, a negative deflection that follows an R wave [wave]; entropy; exposure time; half [Lat. *semis*]; left [Lat. *sinister*]; mean dose per unit cumulated activity; the midpoint of the sella turcica [point]; sacral; saline; *Salmonella*; saturated; *Schistosoma*; schizophrenia; second; section; sedimentation coefficient; sella [turcica]; semilente [insulin]; senile, senility; sensation; sensitivity; septum; serine; serum; *Shigella*; siderocyte; siemens; sigmoid; signature [prescription]; silicate; single; slow accelerator; small; smooth [colony]; soft [diet]; solid; soluble; solute; sone [unit]; space; spatial; specificity; spherical; *Spirillum*; spleen; standard normal deviation; *Staphylococcus*; stem [cell]; stimulus; *Streptococcus*; streptomycin; subject; subjective findings; substrate; sulfur; sum of an arithmetic series; supravergence; surface; surgery; suture; Svedberg [unit]; swine; Swiss [mouse]; synthesis; systole; without [Lat. *sine*]

S1-S5 first to fifth sacral nerves

S_1-S_4 first to fourth heart sounds

4S Scandinavian Simvastatin Survival Study Group

s atomic orbital with angular momentum quantum number 0; distance; left [Lat. *sinister*]; length of path; sample standard deviation; satellite [chromosome]; scruple; second; section; sedimentation coefficient; sensation; series; signed; suckling

s specific heat capacity; without (Lat. *sine*]

s^{-1} cycles per second

s^2 sample variance

Σ see *sigma*

σ see *sigma*

SA salicylic acid; saline [solution]; salt added; sarcoidosis; sarcoma; scalenus anticus; secondary amenorrhea; secondary anemia; secondary arrest; self-analysis; semen analysis; sensitizing antibody; serum albumin; serum aldolase; sexual abuse; addict; sexual assault; short acting; short axis; sialic acid; simian adenovirus; sinoatrial; sinus arrest; sinus arrhythmia; skeletal age; skin-adipose [unit]; sleep apnea; slightly active; slowly adapting [receptor]; soluble in alkaline medium; specific activity; spectrum analysis; spinal abscess; spinal anesthesia; splenic artery; stable angina; standard accuracy; *Staphylococcus aureas;* status asthmaticus; stimulus artifact; Stokes-Adams [syndrome]; subarachnoid; succinylacetone; suicide attempt; surface antigen; surface area; surgery and anesthesia; surgical assistant; suspended animation; suspicious area; sustained action; sympathetic activity; symptom analysis; synthetic aperture; systemic aspergillosis

S-A sinoatrial; sinoauricular

S&A sickness and accident [insurance]; sugar and acetone

S/A stent-to-artery [ratio]

Sa the most anterior point of the anterior contour of the sella turcica [point]; saline; *Staphylococcus aureus*

sA statampere

SAA serum amyloid Λ; severe aplastic anemia

SAAP selective aortic arch perfusion

SAARD slow-acting antirheumatic drug

SAAS Substance Abuse Attitude Survey

SAAST self-administered alcohol screening test

SAB Scientific Advisory Board; serum albumin; signal above baseline; significant asymptomatic bacteriuria; sinoatrial block; Society of American Bacteriologists; spontaneous abortion; subarachnoid block

SAb spontaneous abortion

SABER Stent-assisted Balloon Angioplasty and Its Effects on Restenosis [study]

SABP spontaneous acute bacterial peritonitis; systolic arterial blood pressure

SAC saccharin; sacrum; screening and acute care; Self-Assessment of Communication [scale]; serum aminoglycoside concentration; short-arm cast; small accessory chromosome; social activity [scale]; splinting for acute closure; stable access cannula; subarea advisory council; substance abuse counselor; symptomatic anomaly complex

sacch saccharin

SACD subacute combined degeneration

SACE serum angiotensin-converting enzyme

SACH small animal care hospital; solid ankle cushioned heel

SACNAS Society for the Advancement of Chicanos and Native Americans in Science

SACS secondary anticoagulation system

SACSF subarachnoid cerebrospinal fluid

SACT sinoatrial conduction time

SAD Scale of Anxiety and Depression; seasonal affective disorder; Self-Assessment Depression [scale]; severe aortic stenosis; sino-aortic denervation; small airway disease; source-to-axis distance; sugar, acetone, and diacetic acid; suppressor-activating determinant

SADD Short-Alcohol Dependence Data [questionnaire]; standardized assessment of depressive disorders; Students Against Drung Driving

SADDAN severe achondroplasia with developmental delay and acanthosis nigricans

SADL simulated activities of daily living

SADR suspected adverse drug reaction

SADS Schedule for Affective Disorders and Schizophrenia; Sudden Adult Death Survey; sudden arrhythmic death syndrome

SADS-C Schedule for Affective Disorders and Schizophrenia-Change

SADS-L Schedule for Affective Disorders and Schizophrenia-Lifetime

SADT Stetson Auditory Discrimination Test

SAE serious adverse event; sexual assault evaluation; short above-elbow [cast]; specific action exercise; subcortical arteriosclerotic encephalopathy; supported arm exercise

SAEB sinoatrial entrance block

SAECG signal averaged electrocardiogram

SAED semiautomatic external defibrillator

SAEM Society for Academic Emergency Medicine

SAEP *Salmonella abortus equi* pyrogen

SAF scrapie-associated fibrils; self-articulating femoral; serum accelerator factor;

simultaneous auditory feedback; standard analytic file [Medicare]

SAFA soluble antigen fluorescent antibody

SAFE Safety After Fifty Evaluation [study]

SAFE-PACE Syncope and Falls in the Elderly–Role of Pacemaker [study]

SAFIRE-D Symptomatic Atrial Fibrillation Investigation and Randomized Evaluation of Dofetilide [study]

SAFTEE-GI systematic assessment for treatment emergent events-general inquiry

SAFTEE-SI systematic assessment for treatment emergent events-systematic inquiry

SAG salicyl acyl glucuronide; sonoangiography; streptavidin-gold; Swiss agammaglobulinemia

sag sagittal

SAGE statistical analysis of genetic epidemiology; Systematic Assessment of Geriatric Drug Use via Epidemiology [study]

SAGES signal-averaged electrocardiographic [ECG] study

SAGM sodium chloride, adenine, glucose, mannitol

SAH S-adenosyl-L-homocysteine; subarachnoid hemorrhage

SAHA seborrhea-hypertrichosis/hirsutism-alopecia [syndrome]

SAHCS Streptokinase-Aspirin-Heparin Collaborative Study

SAHH S-adenosylhomocysteine hydrolase

SAHIGES *Staphylococcus aureus* hyperimmunoglobulinemia E syndrome

SAHS San Antonio Heart Study; sleep apnea-hypersomnolence [syndrome]

SAI Self-Analysis Inventory; Sexual Arousability Inventory; Social Adequacy Index; suppressor of anchorage independence; systemic active immunotherapy

SAICAR sylaminoimidazole carboxylase

SAID specific adaptation to imposed demand [principle]

SAIDS sexually acquired immunodeficiency syndrome; simian acquired immune deficiency syndrome

SAIMS student applicant information management system

SAL sensorineural activity level; sterility assurance level; suction-assisted lipectomy

Sal salicylate, salicylic; *Salmonella*

sAl serum aluminum [level]

sal salicylate, salicylic; saline; saliva

SALAD Surgery vs Angioplasty for Proximal Left Anterior Descending Coronary Artery Stenosis [trial]

Salm *Salmonella*

SALP salpingectomy; salpingography; serum alkaline phosphatase

Salpx salpingectomy

SALT skin-associated lymphoid tissue; Swedish Aspirin in Low Dose Trial

SALTS Strategic Alternatives with Ticlopidine in Stenting [study]

SAM S-adenosyl-L-methionine; scanning acoustic microscope; senescence accelerated mouse; sex arousal mechanism; short-arc motion; staphylococcal absorption method; subject area model; substrate adhesion molecule; sulfated acid mucopolysaccharide; surface active material; system for assembling markers; systolic anterior motion

SAMA schizoaffective mania mainly affective [type]; Student American Medical Association

SAMD S-adenosyl-L-methionine decarboxylase

SAM-DC S-adenosyl-L-methionine decarboxylase

SAMe S-adenosyl-L-methionine

SAMHSA Substance Abuse and Mental Health Services Administration

SAMI Streptokinase and Angioplasty in Myocardial Infarction [trial]; Streptokinase in Acute Myocardial Infarction [study]; Students for Advancement of Medical Instrumentation

SAMII Survey of Acute Myocardial Ischemia and Infarction [study]

SAMIT Streptokinase and Angioplasty Myocardial Infarction Trial

SAMMEC Smoking-Attributable Mortality, Morbidity, and Economic Costs [study]

SAMO Senior Administrative Medical Officer

SAMPLE Study on Ambulatory Monitoring of Pressure and Lisinopril Evaluation

SAMS Society for Advanced Medical Systems

S-AMY serum amylase

SAN sinoatrial node; sinoauricular node; slept all night; solitary autonomous nodule

Sanat sanatorium

SANDR sinoatrial nodal reentry

SANE sexual assault nurse examiner

sang sanguinous

SANGUIS Safe and Good Use of Blood in Surgery [study]

sanit sanitary, sanitation

SANS scale for the assessment of negative symptoms

SANWS sinoatrial node weakness syndrome

SAO small airway obstruction; splanchnic artery occlusion; subvalvular aortic obstruction

S_{AO_2} oxygen saturation in alveolar gas

S_{aO_2} oxygen saturation in arterial blood

SAP sensory action potential; serum acid phosphatase; serum alkaline phosphatase; serum amyloid P; situs ambiguus with polysplenia; sphingolipid activator protein; stable angina pectoris; *Staphylococcus aureus* protease; subjective and physical [findings]; surfactant-associated protein; systemic arterial pressure; systolic arterial pressure

SAPA scan along polygonal approximation

SAPALDIA Swiss Study of Air Pollution and Lung Diseases in Adults

SAPAT Swedish Angina Pectoris Aspirin Trial

SAPD sphingolipid activator protein deficiency

SAPF simultaneous anterior and posterior [spinal] fusion

saph saphenous

SAPHO synovitis-acne-pustulosis hyperostosis-osteomyelitis [syndrome]

SAPK stress-activated protein kinase

SAPPHIRE Stanford Asian Pacific Program in Hypertension and Insulin Resistance

SAPS San Antonio Rotablator Study; simplified acute physiology score; *Staphylococcus aureus* protease sensitivity

SAPX salivary peroxidase

SAQ saquinavir; self-applied questionnaire; short arc quadriceps [muscle]

SAQC statistical analysis of quality control

SAR scatter/air ratio; seasonal allergic rhinitis; sexual attitude reassessment; slowly adapting receptor; specific absorption rate; structure-activity relationship; supra-aortic ridge; supra-aortic ring; synthetic aperture radar

SARA sexually acquired reactive arthritis; Superfund Amendments and Reauthorization

SARB Statistical Application and Research Branch [FDA]

SART simultaneous algebraic reconstruction technique

SAS sarcoma amplified sequence; Scandinavian Angiopeptin Study; self-rating anxiety scale; short arm splint; Sklar Aphasia Scale; sleep apnea syndrome; small animal surgery; small aorta syndrome; social adjustment scale; sodium amylosulfate; space-adaptation syndrome; specific activity scale; statistical analysis system; sterile aqueous solution; sterile aqueous suspension; subaortic stenosis; subarachnoid space; sulfasalazine; supravalvular aortic stenosis; surface-active substance; synchronous atrial stimulation

SASA solvent-accessible surface area

SASMAS skin-adipose superficial musculoaponeurotic system

SASP salicylazosulfapyridine

SASPP syndrome of absence of septum pellucidum with preencephaly

SASS Syngen Acute Stroke Study

SAS-SR social adjustment scale, self-report

SASSY Seniors Active Spirits Staying Young [program]

SAST Self-administered Alcoholism Screening Test; selective arterial secretin injection test; serum aspartate aminotransferase

SAT saliva alcohol test; Saruplase Alteplase Study; satellite; serum antitrypsin; single-agent chemotherapy; slide agglutination test; sodium ammonium thiosulfate; spermatogenic activity test; spontaneous activity test; subacute thyroiditis; subcutaneous adipose tissue; symptomless autoimmune thyroiditis; systematic assertive therapy; systolic acceleration time

Sat, sat saturation, saturated

SATA spatial average, temporal average

SATB special aptitude test battery

satd saturated

SATE Safety Antiarrhythmic Trial Evaluation

SATL surgical Achilles tendon lengthening

SATP spatial average temporal peak

SATS substance, amount ingested, time ingested, symptoms

SATSA Swedish Adoption–Twin Study of Aging

SATT Scottish Adjuvant Tamoxifen Trial

SAU statistical analysis unit

SAUDIS Sudden and Unexpected Death in Sports [study]

SAV sequential atrioventricular [pacing]

SAVD spontaneous assisted vaginal delivery

SAVE saved-young-life equivalent; sudden A-ventilatory event; Survival and Ventricular Enlargement [trial]

SAVED saphenous vein de novo

SAW surface acoustic wave

SAX short axis; surface antigen, X-linked

SAx short axis

SAX-APEX short-axis plane, apical

SAX-MV short-axis, mitral valve

SAX-PM short-axis plane, papillary muscle

SB Bachelor of Science; Schwartz-Bartter [syndrome]; serum bilirubin; shortness of breath; sick bay; sideroblast; single blind [study]; single breath; sinus bradycardia; small bowel; sodium balance; sodium bisulfite; Southern blotting; soybean; spina bifida; spontaneous blastogenesis; spontaneous breathing; standard [hospital] bed; Stanford-Binet [Intelligence Scale]; stereotyped behavior; sternal border; stillbirth; surface binding

S-B Sengstaken-Blakemore [tube]

Sb strabismus

sb stilb

SBA serum bile acid; soybean agglutinin; spina bifida aperta

SBAHC school-based adolescent health care

SBB stimulation-bound behavior

SBBT specialist in blood bank technology

SBC school-based clinic; Schwarz's bayesian criterion; serum bactericidal concentration; strict bed confinement

SBCS Stockholm Breast Cancer Study

SBD selective bowel decontamination; senile brain disease

S-BD seizure-brain damage

SbDH sorbitol dehydrogenase

SBE breast self-examination; short below-elbow [cast]; shortness of breath on exertion; small bowel enema; subacute bacterial endocarditis

SBEH social behavior [UMLS]

SBET Society for Biomedical Engineering Technicians

SBEPI sinusoidal blipped echo-planar imaging

S/ß sickle cell beta-thalassemia

SBF serologic-blocking factor; skin blood flow; specific blocking factor; splanchnic blood flow

SBFT small bowel follow-through

SBG selenite brilliant green

SBH Sabra hypertensive [rat]; sea-blue histiocyte

SBHC school-based health center

SBI soybean trypsin inhibitor

SBIAB secondary bacterial infection acute bronchitis

SBIS Stanford-Binet Intelligence Scale

SBL soybean lecithin

sBL sporadic Burkitt lymphoma

SBLA sarcoma, breast and brain tumors, leukemia, laryngeal and lung cancer, and adrenal cortical carcinoma

SB-LM Stanford-Binet Intelligence Test-Form LM

SBM scientific basis of medicine; sexual intercourse between men; Solomon-Bloembergen-Morgan [equation]

SBMA spinal bulbar muscular atrophy

SBN State Board of Nursing

SBN₂ single-breath nitrogen test]

SBNS Society of British Neurological Surgeons

SBNT single-breath nitrogen test

SBNW single-breath nitrogen washout

SBO small bowel obstruction; spina bifida occulta

SBOM soybean oil meal

SBP schizobipolar; serotonin-binding protein; spontaneous bacterial peritonitis; steroid-binding plasma [protein]; sulfobromophthalein; symmetric biphasic; systemic blood pressure; systolic blood pressure

SBQ Smoking Behavior Questionnaire

SBR small bowel resection; spleen-to-body [weight] ratio; strict bed rest; styrene-butadiene rubber

SBRN sensory branch of radial nerve

SBRT split beam rotation therapy

SBS shaken baby syndrome; short bowel syndrome; sick building syndrome; sinobronchial syndrome; small bowel series; social breakdown syndrome; straight back syndrome; substrate-binding strand

SBSS Seligmann's buffered salt solution

SBT serum bactericidal titer; single-breath test; sulbactam

SBTI soybean trypsin inhibitor

SBTPE State Boards Test Pool Examination

SBTT small bowel transit time

SBV singular binocular vision

SB^V pentavalent antimonial

SC conditioned stimulus; sacrococcygeal; Sanitary Corps; scalenus [muscle]; scapula; Schüller-Christian [disease]; Schwann cell; sciatica; science; sclerosing cholangitis; secondary cleavage; secretory component; self care; semicircular; semilunar valve closure; serum complement; serum creatinine; service-connected; sex chromatin; Sézary cell; short circuit; sick call; sickle cell; sigmoid colon; silicone-coated; single chemical; skin conduction; slow component; Snellen chart; sodium citrate; soluble complex; special care; specialty clinic; spinal canal; spinal cord; squamous carcinoma; start conversion; statistical control; stepped care; sternoclavicular; stratum corneum; subcellular; subclavian; subcorneal; subcortical; subcostal; subcutaneous; subtotal colectomy; succinylcholine; sugar-coated; sulfur-containing; supercoil cruciform [deoxyribonucleic acid, DNA]; supercomputing; superior colliculus; supportive care; supraclavicular; surface colony; surface cooling; switching circuit; systemic candidiasis; systolic click

S/C subcutaneous, sugar-coated [pill]

S-C sickle cell

S&C sclerae and conjunctivae

Sc scandium; scapula; science, scientific; screening

sC statcoulomb

sc subcutaneous

SCA self-care agency; senescent cell antigen; severe congenital anomaly; sickle-cell anemia; single-camera autostereoscopic [imaging]; single-channel analyzer; sperm-coating antigen; spinocerebellar ataxia; starburst calcification; steroidal-cell antibody; subclavian artery; superior cerebellar artery; suppressor cell activity

SCAA Skin Care Association of America; sporadic cerebral amyloid angiopathy

SCABG single coronary artery bypass

SCAD short chain acyl-coenzyme A dehydrogenase

SCAG Sandoz Clinical Assessment-Geriatric [Rating]

SCAI Society for Cardiac Angiography and Interventions

SCAMIA Symposium on Computer Applications in Medical Care

SCAMIN Self-Concept and Motivation Inventory

SCAMP Stanford Coronary Artery Monitoring Project

SCAN Schedules for Clinical Assessment of Neuropsychiatry; suspected child abuse and neglect; systolic coronary artery narrowing

SCAP scapula

SCAR sequence characterized amplified region; severe cutaneous adverse reactions; Society for Computer Application in Radiology

SCARF skeletal abnormalities, cutis laxa, craniostenosis, psychomotor retardation, facial abnormalities [syndrome]

SCARI Spinal Cord Injury Assessment of Risk Index

SCARMD severe childhood autosomal recessive muscular dystrophy

SCAT sheep cell agglutination test; sickle cell anemia test; Simvastatin and Enalapril Coronary Atherosclerosis Trial; Sports Competition Anxiety Test

SCAVF spinal cord arteriovenous fistula

SCAVM spinal cord arteriovenous malformation

SCB strictly confined to bed

SCBA self-contained breathing apparatus

SCBE single contrast barium enema

SCBF spinal cord blood flow

SCBG symmetric calcification of the basal cerebral ganglia

SCBH systemic cutaneous basophil hypersensitivity

SCBP stratum corneum basic protein

SCC self-care center; sequential combination chemotherapy; services for crippled children; short-course chemotherapy; sickle cell disease; small-cell carcinoma; small cleaved cell; spinal cord compression; squamous cell carcinoma; symptom cluster constraint

SC4C subcostal four-chamber [view]

SCCA single-cell cytotoxicity assay; small-cell carcinoma

SCCB small-cell carcinoma of the bronchus

SCCC squamous cell cervical carcinoma

SCCH sternocostoclavicular hyperostosis

SCCHN squamous cell carcinoma of the head and neck

SCCHO sternocostoclavicular hyperostosis

SCCL small cell carcinoma of the lung

SCCM Sertoli cell culture medium; Society of Critical Care Medicine

SCCT severe cerebrocranial trauma

SCD scleroderma; sequential compression device; service-connected disability; sickle-cell disease; spinocerebellar degeneration; subacute combined degeneration; subacute coronary disease; sudden cardiac death; sudden coronary death; support clinical database; systemic carnitine deficiency

ScD Doctor of Science

SCDA situational control of daily activities [scale]

ScDA right scapuloanterior [fetal position] [Lat. *scapulodextra anterior*]

SCDF skin condition data form

SCD-HeFT Sudden Cardiac Death in Heart Failure: Trial of Prophylactic Amiodarone vs Implantable Defibrillator Therapy

SCDMS clinical data management system

SCDNT self-care deficit nursing theory

ScDP right scapuloposterior [fetal position] [Lat. *scapulodextra posterior*]

SCE secretory carcinoma of the endometrium; serious cardiac event; sister chromatid exchange; split hand-cleft lip/palate ectodermal [dysplasia]; subcutaneous emphysema

SCe somatic cell

SCED single case experimental design

SCEP sandwich counterelectrophoresis; spinal cord evoked potential

SCER sister chromatid exchange rate

SCETI Stanford Computer-based Educator Training Intervention

SCF sinusoid containing blood flow; Skin Cancer Foundation; stem cell factor; subcostal frontal [view]

SCFA short-chain fatty acid

SCFE slipped capital femoral epiphysis

SCG serum chemistry graft; serum chemogram; sodium cromoglycate; superior cervical ganglion

SCH student contact hour; succinylcholine

SCh succinylchloride; succinylcholine

SChE serum cholinesterase

schiz schizophrenia

SCHL subcapsular hematoma of the liver

SCI Science Citation Index; spinal cord injury; structured clinical interview

Sci science, scientific

SCID severe combined immunodeficiency [syndrome]; soft copy image display; Structured Clinical Interview for DSM IV [diagnosis]

SCIDS severe combined immunodeficiency syndrome

SCIDX severe combined immunodeficiency disease, X-linked

SCIEH Scottish Centre for Infection and Environmental Health

SCII Strong-Campbell Interest Inventory

SCIM spinal cord injury medicine

SCINT, scint scintigraphy

SCIS spinal cord injury service

SCIU spinal cord injury unit

SCIV subcutaneous intravenous; Subcutaneous vs Intravenous Heparin in Deep Venous Thrombosis [study]

SCIWORA spinal cord injury without radiographic abnormality

SCJ squamocolumnar junction; sternoclavicular joint; sternocostal joint

sCJD sporadic Creutzfeldt-Jakob disease

SCK serum creatine kinase

SCL scleroderma; serum copper level; sinus cycle length; soft contact lens; stromal cell line; subcostal lateral [view]; symptom checklist; syndrome checklist

SCL-90 symptom checklist 90

scl sclerosis, sclerotic, sclerosed

ScLA left scapuloanterior [fetal position] [Lat. *scapulolaeva anterior*]

SCLC small cell lung carcinoma

SCLD sickle-cell chronic lung disease

SCLE subacute cutaneous lupus erythematosus

scler sclerosis, scleroderma

SCLH subcortical laminar heterotopia

ScLP left scapuloposterior [fetal position] [Lat. *scapulolaeva posterior*]

SCL-90-R symptom checklist 90, revised

SCLS systemic capillary leak syndrome

SCM Schwann cell membrane; sensation, circulation, and motion; Society of Computer Medicine; soluble cytotoxic medium; spleen cell-conditioned medium; split cord malformation; spondylitic caudal myelopathy; State Certified Midwife; streptococcal cell membrane; sternocleidomastoid; supernumerary marker chromosome; surface-connecting membrane

SCMC spontaneous cell-mediated cytotoxicity

SCMO Senior Clerical Medical Officer

SCN special care nursing; suprachiasmatic nucleus

SCN1A sodium channel, neuronal alphasubunit type 1

SCNS subcutaneous nerve stimulation

SCNT somatic cell nuclear transfer

SCO sclerocystic ovary; somatic crossing-over; subcommissural organ

SCOP scopolamine; structural classification of proteins

SCOPE Study of Cognition and Prognosis in the Elderly; Surveillance and Control of Pathogens of Epidemiologic Importance [study]

SCOPEG symmetric, centrally-ordered, phase encoded group [imaging]

SCOPME Standing Committee on Postgraduate Medical and Dental Education [UK]

SCOR Specialized Center for Research [NIH]

SCORES Stent Comparative Restenosis [trial]

SCOT subcostal [right ventricle] outflow [view]

SCP single-celled protein; smoking cessation program; sodium cellulose phosphate; soluble cytoplasmic protein; specialty care physician; standard care plan; sterol carrier protein; submucous cleft palate; superior cerebral peduncle

scp spherical candle power

SCPM somatic crossover point mapping

SCPR standard cardiopulmonary resuscitation

SCPS Skin Cancer Prevention Study

SCPK serum creatine phosphokinase

SCPN serum carboxypeptidase N

SCPNT Southern California Postrotary Nystagmus Test

S-CPR standard post-compression remodeling

SCPT schizophrenic chronic paranoid type

SCR Schick conversion rate; short consensus repeat; silicon-controlled rectifier; skin conductance response; slow-cycling rhodopsin; spondylitic caudal radiculopathy

SCr serum creatinine

scr scruple

SCRAM speech-controlled respirometer for ambulation measurement

SCRAS Sheehan clinician-rated anxiety scale

SCRF surface coil rotating frame; Systematized Nomenclature in Medicine Cross-Reference Field

SCRIP Stanford Coronary Risk Intervention Project

SCRIPPS Scripps Coronary Radiation to Inhibit Proliferation Post-stenting [trial]

SCRIPT Smoking Cessation-Reduction in Pregnancy Trial

scRNA small cytoplasmic ribonucleic acid

SCS Saethre-Chotzen syndrome; Seven Country Study; shared computer system; silicon-controlled switch; slow channel syndrome; Society of Clinical Surgery; spinal cord stimulation; splint classification system [American Association of Hand Therapists, ASHT]; systolic click syndrome

SCSA subcostal short axis

SCSB static charge sensitive bed

SCSI enhanced small device interface

SCSIT Southern California Sensory Integration Test

SCSR standard cervical spine radiography

SCT salmon calcitonin; secretin; sex chromatin test; sexual compatibility test; sickle-cell trait; sperm cytotoxicity; spinal computed tomography; spinocervicothalamic; staphylococcal clumping test; sugar-coated tablet

S_{CT} serum creatinine

SCTAT sex cord tumor with annular tubules

SCTN South Carolina Telemedicine Network

SCTR secretin receptor

SCTx spinal cervical traction

SCU self-care unit; special care unit

SCUBA self-contained underwater breathing apparatus

SCUD septicemic cutaneous ulcerative disease

SCUF slow continuous ultrafiltration therapy

SCU-PA single-chain urokinase plasminogen activator

SCUT schizophrenic chronic undifferentiated type

SCV sensory nerve conduction velocity; smooth, capsulated, virulent; subclavian vein; squamous-cell carcinoma of the vulva

SCV-CPR simultaneous compression ventilation-cardiopulmonary resuscitation

SCVIR Society of Cardiovascular and Interventional Radiology

SCWM subcortical white matter

SD Sandhoff disease; selective decontamination; senile dementia; septal defect; serologically defined; serologically detectable; serologically determined; serum defect; Shine-Dalgarno [sequence]; short dialysis; shoulder disarticulation; Shy-Draper [syndrome]; skin destruction; skin dose; solvent/detergent; somatization disorder; speech delay; sphincter dilatation; spontaneous delivery; sporadic depression; Sprague-Dawley [rat]; spreading depression; stable disease; standard deviation; statistical documentation; Stensen duct; Still disease; stone disintegration; straight drainage; strength duration; streptodornase; sudden death; superoxide dismutase; synchronous detector; systolic discharge

S-D sickle-cell hemoglobin D; suicide-depression

S/D sharp/dull; systolic/diastolic

Sd standard; stimulus drive

S^d discriminative stimulus

SDA right sacroanterior [fetal position] [Lat. *sacrodextra anterior*]; serotonin-dopamine antagonist; sialodacryoadenitis; specific dynamic action; strand displacement amplification; structural displacement amplification; succinic dehydrogenase activity

SDAT senile dementia of Alzheimer type; surface digitalization accuracy test

SDAVF spinal dural arteriovenous fistula

SDB shared database; sleep-disordered breathing

SDBP seated (or standing, or supine) diastolic blood pressure

SDC serum digoxin concentration; Smith delay compensator; sodium deoxycholate; subacute combined degeneration; subclavian hemodialysis catheter; succinyldicholine; syndectan; symptomatic developmental complex

SDCL symptom distress check list

SDCN N-syndectan, neural syndectan

SDD selective decontamination of the digestive tract; Skeletal Dysplasia Diagnostician [database]; sporadic depressive disease; sterile dry dressing

SDDS 2-sulfamoyl-4,4;pr-diaminodiphenyl-sulfone

SDE simulation development environment; specific dynamic effect; standard-dose epinephrine; subdural empyema

SDEEG sterotactic depth electroencephalography

SDES symptomatic diffuse esophageal spasm

SDF slow death factor; standard data format; stress distribution factor; stromal derived factor

SDG sucrose density gradient

SDGF schwannoma-derived growth factor

SDH serine dehydratase; sorbitol dehydrogenase; spinal dorsal horn; subdural hematoma; succinate dehydrogenase

SDHD sudden death heart disease

SDI selective dissemination of information; standard deviation interval; survey diagnostic instrument

SDIF standard generalized markup language document interchange format

SDIHD sudden death ischemic heart disease

SDILINE Selective Dissemination of Information Online [data bank]

SDIS Stockholm Diabetes Intervention Study

SDL serum digoxin level; speech discrimination level

sdl sideline; subline

SDM semantic data model; sensory detection method; sparse distributed memory; standard deviation of the mean; system of decision making; Systematized Nomenclature in Medicine [SNOMED] Digital Imaging and Communications in Medicine [DICOM] Microglossary

SDMS Society of Diagnostic Medical Sonographers

SDN sexually dimorphic nucleus

SDNF sliding discrete Fourier transform narrow band filter

SDO sudden dosage onset

SDP right sacroposterior [fetal position] [Lat. *sacrodextra posterior*]; shared decision-making program; signal density plot

SDR Skeletal Dysplasia Registry; spontaneously diabetic rat; surgical dressing room

SDRS social dysfunction rating scale

SDS same day surgery; school dental services; self-rating depression scale; sensory deprivation syndrome; sexual differentiation scale; short depression screen; Shy-Drager syndrome; single-dose suppression; sodium dodecylsulfate; specific diagnosis service; standard deviation score; sudden death syndrome; sulfadiazine silver; sustained depolarizing shift

SDSEM spinocerebellar degeneration-slow eye movements [syndrome]

SD-SK streptodornase-streptokinase

SDSL symmetrical digital single line

SDS/PAGE, SDS-PGE sodium dodecyl-sulfate-polyacrylamide gel electrophoresis

SDT sensory detection theory; right sacrotransverse [fetal position] [Lat. *sacrodextra transversa*]; signal detection theory; single-donor transfusion; speech detection threshold

SD$_t$ standard deviation of total scores

SDU standard deviation unit; step-down unit

SDUB short double upright brace

SDW spin density-weighted

SDYS Simpson dysmorphia syndrome

SE saline enema; sanitary engineering; serum; side effect; smoke exposure; socio-economic; solid extract; sphenoethmoidal; spherical equivalent; spin-echo; spongiform encephalopathy; Spurway-Eddowes [syndrome]; standard error; staphylococcal endotoxin; staphylococcal enterotoxin; starch equivalent; Starr-Edwards [prosthesis]; status epilepticus; subendothelial; subependymal nodule

S&E safety and efficiency

S-E socio-economic; spin-echo [imaging]; substantial equivalence

Se secretion; selenium

S$_e$ external skeleton

$_s$E early systolic wave

SEA sheep erythrocyte agglutination; shock-elicited aggression; soluble egg antigen; spatial envelope area; spinal epidural abscess; spontaneous electrical activity; staphylococcal enterotoxin A

SEARCH Study of the Effectiveness of Additional Reductions of Cholesterol and Homocysteine

SEAT sheep erythrocyte agglutination test

SEB seborrhea; staphylococcal enterotoxin B

SEBA staphylococcal enterotoxin B antiserum

SEBL self-emptying blind loop

SEBM Society of Experimental Biology and Medicine

SEC secretin; Singapore epidemic conjunctivitis; soft elastic capsule; swollen endothelial cell

Sec Seconal; selenocysteine

sec second; secondary; section

sec-Bu sec-butyl

SeCD service for the care of drug addicts

SECG stress electrocardiography

SECORDS South-Eastern Consortium on Racial Differences in Stroke

SECRET stiffness of joint, elderly individuals, constitutional symptoms, arthritis, elevated erythrocyte sedimentation rate, temporal arthritis [in polymyalgia rheumatica]

SECSY spin echo correlated spectroscopy

sect section

SECURE Study to Evaluate Carotid Ultrasound Changes with Ramipril and Vitamin E

SED sedimentation rate; skin erythema dose; spondyloepiphyseal dysplasia; standard error of deviation; staphylococcal enterotoxin D

sed sedimentation; stool [Lat. *sedes*]

SEDL spondyloepiphyseal dysplasia, late

sed rt sedimentation rate

SEDT spondyloepiphyseal dysplasia tarda

SEDT-PA spondyloepiphyseal dysplasia tarda-progressive arthropathy

SEE standard error of estimate

SEEG stereotactic electroencephalography

SEER Surveillance Epidemiology and End Results [Program]

SEF somatically-evoked field; spectral edge frequency; staphylococcal enterotoxin F; structured encounter form; suction effusion fluid

SEG segment; soft elastic gelatin; sonoencephalogram

segm segment, segmented

SEGNE secretory granules of neural and endocrine [cells]

Se-GSH-Px selenium cofactor for glutathione peroxidase

SEH subependymal hemorrhage

SEI Self-Esteem Inventory

SEISMED secure environment for information system in medicine

SE/IVH subependymal/intraventricular hemorrhage

SEL serum ethanol level

SELCA Smooth Excimer Laser Coronary Angioplasty [study]

SELF Self-Evaluation of Life Function [scale]

SEM sample evaluation method; scanning electron microscopy; secondary enrichment medium; standard error of measurement; standard error of the mean; systolic ejection murmur

sem one-half [Lat. *semis*]; semen, seminal

SEMD spondyloepimetaphyseal dysplasia

SEMDIT spondyloepimetaphyseal dysplasia, Irapa type

SEMDJL spondyloepimetaphyseal dysplasia with joint laxity

SEMG semenogelin

sEMG surface electromyography

SEMI subendocardial myocardial infarction

SEMDJL spondyloepimetaphyseal dysplasia with joint laxity

SEN scalp-ear-nipple [syndrome]; State Enrolled Nurse

sen sensitive, sensitivity

SENDCAP St. Mary's Ealing, Northwick Park Diabetes Cardiovascular Prevention [study]

SENIC Study of the Efficacy of Nosocomial Infection Control

SENS sensitivity or sensitization; Stewart evaluation of nursing scale

Sens sensitivity

sens sensation, sensorium, sensory

SENSOR Sentinel Event Notification System for Occupational Risks

SEP self-evaluation process; sensory-evoked potential; septum; somatosensory evoked potential; sperm entry point; spinal evoked potential; standard error of prediction; surface epithelium; systolic ejection period

sEP single evoked potential

separ separation, separation

SEPS Submaximal Exercise Performance Substudy

SEPT septum

SEQ side effects questionnaire

seq sequence; sequel, sequela, sequelae; sequestrum

SEQOL [Bypass Angioplasty Revascularization Investigation] Substudy of Economics and Quality of Life

SER sebum excretion rate; sensitizer enhancement ratio; sensory evoked response; service; smooth endoplasmic reticulum; smooth-surface endoplasmic reticulum; somatosensory evoked response; supination, external rotation [fracture]; surgical emergency room; systolic ejection rate

Ser serine; serology; serous; service

sER smooth endoplasmic reticulum

ser series, serial

SER-IV supination external rotation, type 4 fracture

SerCl serum chloride

SERHOLD National Biomedical Serials Holding Database

SERLINE Serials Online [NLM database]

sero, serol serological, serology

SERPIN serpine protease inhibitor

SERS Stimulus Evaluation/Response Selection [test]

SERT sustained ethanol release tube

serv keep, preserve [Lat. *serva*]; service

SERVHEL Service and Health Records

SES Society of Eye Surgeons; socioeconomic status; spatial emotional stimulus; sphenoethmoidal suture; subendothelial space

SESAM Study in Europe of Saruplase and Alteplase in Myocardial Infarction

SESAP Surgical Educational and Self-Assessment Program

SET surrogate embryo transfer; systolic ejection time

SET-N software evaluation tool for nursing

SETTS subjective experience of therapeutic touch survey

sev severe; severed

SEWHO shoulder-elbow-wrist-hand orthosis

SF Sabin-Feldman [test]; safety factor; salt-free; scarlet fever; scatter factor; screen film; seminal fluid; serosal fluid; serum factor; serum ferritin; serum fibrinogen; sham feeding; shell fragment; shunt flow; sickle cell-hemoglobin F [disease]; simian foam-virus; skin fibroblast; skinfold; soft feces; spinal fluid; spontaneous fibrillation; stable factor; steel factor; sterile female; steroidogenic factor; stress formula; sugar-free; superior facet; suppressor factor; suprasternal fossa; surviving fraction; Svedberg flotation [unit]; swine fever; symptom-free; synovial fluid

S1F Steel factor

SF-36 short-form health survey [36 items]

Sf *Streptococcus faecalis*

S$_f$ Svedberg flotation unit

SFA saturated fatty acid; seminal fluid assay; serum folic acid; skinfold anthropometry; stimulated fibrinolytic activity; superior femoral artery

SFAP single-fiber action potential

SFB Sanfilippo syndrome type B; saphenofemoral bypass; surgical foreign body

SFBL self-filling blind loop

SFC soluble fibrin complex; soluble fibrin-fibrinogen complex; spinal fluid count

SFCP Stanford Five City Project

SFD silo filler's disease; skin-film distance; small for dates; spectral frequency distribution

SFE slipped femoral epiphysis

SFEMG single fiber electromyography

SFFA serum free fatty acid

SFFF sedimentation field flow fractionation

SFFV spleen focus-forming virus

SFG spotted fever group; subglottic foreign body

SFH schizophrenia family history; serum-free hemoglobin; stroma-free hemoglobin

SF/HGF scatter factor/hepatocyte growth factor

SFI Sexual Function Index; Social Function Index

SFIS structural family interaction scale

SFJT saphenofemoral junction thrombophlebitis

SFL synovial fluid lymphocyte

SFM scanning force microscopy; Schimmelpenning-Fuerstein-Mims [syndrome]; self-fitting face mask; serum-free medium; solution-focused management

SFMC soluble fibrin monomer complex

SFMS Smith-Fineman-Myers syndrome

SFNM standard finite normal mixture

SFO subfornical organ

SFP screen filtration pressure; simultaneous foveal perception; spinal fluid pressure; stopped flow pressure

SFR screen filtration resistance; stenosis flow reserve; stroke with full recovery

SFS serial foveal seizures; skin and fascia stapler; social functioning schedule; spatial frequency spectrum; split function study

SFT Sabin-Feldman test; sensory feedback therapy; skinfold thickness

SFU surgical follow-up

SFV Semliki Forest virus; shipping fever virus; Shope fibroma virus; squirrel fibroma virus

SFW sexual function of women; shell fragment wound; slow-filling wave

SG Sachs-Georgi [test]; salivary gland; serum globulin; serum glucose; signs; skin graft; soluble gelatin; specific gravity; subgluteal; substantia gelatinosa; Surgeon General

sg specific gravity; subgenomic

SGA small for gestational age

SG$_{AW}$ specific airway conductance

SGB Simpson-Golabi-Behmel [syndrome]; sparsely granulated basophil

SGBS Simpson-Golabi-Behmel syndrome

SGC spermicide-germicide compound; Swan-Ganz catheter

SGCA subependymal giant cell astrocytoma

SGD specific granule deficiency

SGE secondary generalized epilepsy

SGF sarcoma growth factor; skeletal growth factor

SGH subgluteal hematoma

SGL salivary gland lymphocyte

SGLD spatial gray level dependence

SGLT sodium-glucose transporter

SGM Society for General Microbiology

SGML standard generalized markup language

SGNE secretory granule neuroendocrine [protein]

SGO Surgeon General's Office; surgery, gynecology, and obstetrics

SGOT serum glutamate oxaloacetate transaminase (aspartate aminotransferase)

SGP serine glycerophosphatide; sialoglycoprotein; Society of General Physiologists; soluble glycoprotein; sulfated glycoprotein

SGPA salivary gland pleomorphic adenoma

SGPT serum glutamate pyruvate transaminase (alanine aminotransferase)

SGR Sachs-Georgi reaction; Shwartzman generalized reaction; skin galvanic reflex; submandibular gland renin; substantia gelatinosa Rolandi

sgRNA subgenomic ribonucleic acid [RNA]

SGS Schinzel-Giedion syndrome

SGSG Scandinavian Glioma Study Group

S-Gt Sachs-Georgi test

SGTT standard glucose tolerance test

SGV salivary gland virus; selective gastric vagotomy; short gastric vessel

SGVHD syngeneic graft-versus-host disease

SH Salter-Harris [fracture]; Schönlein-Henoch [purpura]; self-help; serum hepatitis; sexual harassment; sex hormone; Sherman [rat]; sick in hospital; sinus histiocytosis; social history; somatotropic hormone; spontaneously hypertensive [rat]; standard heparin; state hospital; sulfhydryl; surgical history; symptomatic hypoglycemia; syndrome of hyporeninemic hypoaldosteronism; systemic hyperthermia

S/H sample and hold

S&H speech and hearing

Sh sheep; Sherwood number; *Shigella*; shoulder

sh shoulder

SHA simple highest avidity; Southern hybridization analysis; staphylococcal hemagglutinating antibody

sHa suckling hamster

SHAA serum hepatitis associated antigen; Society of Hearing Aid Audiologists

SHAA-Ab serum hepatitis associated antigen antibody

SHAFT sad, hostile, anxious, frustrating, tenacious [patient]

SHAPE Screening Health Assessment and Preventive Education [program]; Stress, Health and Physical Evaluation [program]; Study of Heparin and Actilyse Processed Electronically

SHARE source of help in airing and resolving experiences; Study of Heart Assessment and Risk in Ethnic Groups

SHARK Stroke, Hypertension and Recurrence in Kyushu [study]

SHARP school health additional referral program; Scottish Heart and Arterial Disease Risk Prevention [program]; Subcutaneous Heparin in Angioplasty Restenosis Prevention [trial]

SHAVE Steerable Housing for Atherovascular Excision

SHB sequential hemibody [irradiation]

S-Hb sulfhemoglobin

SHBD serum hydroxybutyric dehydrogenase

SHBG sex hormone binding globulin

SHCC State Health Coordinating Council

SHCO sulfated hydrogenated castor oil

SHD sudden heart death

SHE Syrian hamster embryo

SHEA Society for Hospital Epidemiology of America

SHEENT skin, head, eyes, ears, nose, and throat

SHEP Systolic Hypertension in the Elderly Program

SHF simian hemorrhagic fever

shf super-high frequency

SHFD split hand/foot deformity

SHG synthetic human gastrin

SHH syndrome of hyporeninemic hypoaldosternonism

Shh sonic hedgehog

SHHD Scottish Home and Health Department

SHHH self-help for hard of hearing

SHHS Scottish Heart Health Study; Sleep Heart Health Study

SHHV Society for Health and Human Values

SHI severe head injury

Shig *Shigella*

SHINE Strategic Health Informatics Network in Europe

SHIPS Shiga Pravastatin Study

SHL sensorineural hearing loss

SHLA soluble human lymphocyte antigen

SHLD shoulder

SHMC sinus histiocytosis with massive lymphadenopathy

SHML sinus histiocytosis with massive lymphadenopathy

SHMO, S/HMO social health maintenance organization

SHMP Senior Hospital Medical Officer

SHMT serine-hydroxymethyl transferase

SHN spontaneous hemorrhagic necrosis; subacute hepatic necrosis

SHO secondary hypertrophic osteoarthropathy; Senior House Officer; simple harmonic oscillator

SHOCK Should We Emergently Revascularize Occluded Coronaries for Cardiogenic Shock? [international randomized trial]

SHOP State Hospital Data Project

SHORT, S-H-O-R-T short stature, hyperextensibility of joints or hernia or both, ocular depression, Rieger anomaly, teething delayed

short-FRAME short stature-facial anomalies-Rieger anomaly-midline anomalies-enamel defects [syndrome]

SHOT serious hazards of transfusion; Shunt Occlusion Trial

SHP Schönlein-Henoch purpura; secondary hyperparathyroidism; Skaraborg Hypertension Project; state health plan

SHPDA State Health Planning and Development Agency

sHPT secondary hyperparathyroidism

SHR spontaneously hypertensive rat

SHRED Sedatives and Hemodynamics During Rapid-sequence Intubation in the Emergency Department [trial]

SHRSP stroke-prone spontaneously hypertensive rat

SHS Sayre head sling; sheep hemolysate supernatant; Strong Heart Study; Sutterland-Haan syndrome

SHSF split hand-split foot [malformation]

SHSP spontaneously hypertensive stroke-prone [rat]

SHSS Stanford Hypnotic Susceptibility Scale

SHT simple hypocalcemic tetany; subcutaneous histamine test

SHTTP secure hypertext transport protocol
SHUA system for hospital uniform accounting
SHUR System for Hospital Uniform Reporting
SHV simian herpes virus
SHVRC Shiley Heart Valve Research Center [project]
SI International System of Units [Fr. *le Système International d'Unités*]; sacroiliac; saline infusion; saline injection; saturation index; self-inflicted; sensory integration; septic inflammation; serious illness; serum iron; severity index; sex inventory; shock index; signal intensity; Singh Index; single injection; small intestine; social interaction; soluble insulin; spirochetosis icterohaemorrhagica; stability index; stimulation index; stress incontinence; stroke index; structured interview; sucrase isomaltase; sulfoxidation index; superior-inferior; suppression index; syncytium-inducer
Si the most anterior point on the lower contour of the sella turcica [point]; silicon
S&I suction and irrigation
SIA serum inhibitory activity; stress-induced analgesia; stress-induced anesthesia; subacute infectious arthritis
SIADH syndrome of inappropriate secretion of antidiuretic hormone
SIAM Streptokinase in Acute Myocardial Infarction [study]
SIB self-injurious behavior
sib, sibs sibling, siblings
SIC serum insulin concentration; Standard Industrial Classification
SICCO Stenting in Chronic Coronary Occlusion [study]
SICD serum isocitrate dehydrogenase
SICU spinal intensive care unit; surgical intensive care unit
SID focal spot to imaging-plane distance; single intradermal [test]; Society for Investigative Dermatology; sucrase-isomaltase deficiency; sudden inexplicable death; sudden infant death; suggested indication of diagnosis; systemic inflammatory disease
SIDAM structured interview for the diagnosis of dementia of the Alzheimer type
SIDS sudden infant death syndrome; sulfo-iduronate sulfatase

SIE sis-inducible element; stroke in evolution
SIECUS Sex Information and Education Council of the United States
SIESTA Snooze-induced Excitation of Sympathetically Triggered Activity [study]
SIF serum-inhibition factor
SIFT selector ion flow tube
SIG small inducible gene
SIg, sIg surface immunoglobulin
sig sigmoidoscopy; significant
S-IgA secretory immunoglobulin A
SIGH-D structured interview for the Hamilton Depression Scale
SigInt signal intelligence
Σ Greek capital letter *sigma*; syphilis; summation of series
σ Greek lower case letter *sigma*; conductivity; cross section; millisecond; molecular type or bond; population standard deviation; stress; surface tension; wave number
sigmo sigmoidoscope or sigmoidoscopy
SIGN Scottish Intercollegiate Guideline Network
SIH stimulation-induced hypalgesia; stress-induced hyperthermia; suction-induced hypoxemia
SIHDSPS Stockholm Ischemic Heart Disease Secondary Prevention Study
SIHE spontaneous intramural hematoma of the esophagus
SI-HRDS structured interview Hamilton rating scale for depression
SII self-inflicted injury
SIJ sacroiliac joint
SIL soluble interleukin; speech interference level; squamous intraepithelial lesion
SILD Sequenced Inventory of Language Development
SIM selected ion monitoring; Society of Industrial Microbiology
SIMA single internal mammary artery; Stenting vs Internal Mammary Artery for Single Left Anterior Descending Arterial Lesion [trial]
SIMD single instruction multiple data
SIMP Schmele instrument to measure the process of nursing care; simulation of initial medical problem
SIMP-C Schmele instrument to measure the process of nursing care

SIMP-H Schmele instrument to measure the process of nursing care in home care

SIMPLE symbolic interactive modeling package and learning environment

SIMS secondary ion mass spectroscopy; situational information management system

simul simultaneously

SIMV synchronized intermittent mandatory ventilation; synchronized intermittent mechanical ventilation

SIN salpingitis isthmica nodosa; self-inactivating; Sindbis [virus]

SIN-FM Short Indexed Nomenclature–Family Medicine

SINS Semi-Structured Intelligent Navigation System

SIO sacroiliac orthosis

SIOP International Society of Pediatric Oncology

SIP Short Inventory of Problems; Sickness Impact Profile; slow inhibitory potential; surface inductive plethysmography

SIPS Strategy for Intracoronary Ultrasound-guided Percutaneous Transluminal Coronary Angioplasty and Stenting [trial]

sIPTH serum immunoreactive parathyroid hormone

SIQ Symptom Interpretation Questionnaire

SIQR semi-interquartile range

SIR single isomorphous replacement; specific immune release; standardized incidence ratio; stroke index ratio; syndrome of immediate reactivities

SIRA Scientific Instrument Research Association

SIRE short interspersed repetitive element

SIREF specific immune response enhancing factor

SIRF severely impaired renal function

SIRIS sputter-initiated resonance ionization spectroscopy

SIRS soluble immune response suppressor; Structured Interview of Reported Symptoms; systemic inflammatory response syndrome

SIS semantic indexing system; serotonin irritation syndrome; simian sarcoma; simulator-induced syndrome; social information system; specialized information system; spontaneous interictal spike;

sterile injectable solution; sterile injectable suspension; surgical information system

SISA Stenting in Small Arteries [trial]

SISAMI Silent Ischemia in Survivors of Acute Myocardial Infarction [study]

SISCOM subtraction ictal single proton emission computed tomography coregistered to magnetic resonance imaging [MRI]

SISH Stage I Systolic Hypertension in the Elderly [study]

SISI short increment sensitivity index

SISO single input single output

SISS Sentinel Injury Surveillance System [for Gunshot and Stab Wounds] small inducible secreted substances

SISTEMI Southern Italian Study on Thrombolysis Early in Myocardial Infarction

SISV, SiSV simian sarcoma virus

SIT serum inhibiting titer; Slosson Intelligence Test; sperm immobilization test; suggested immobilization test

SITS supraspinatus, infraspinatus, teres minor, subscapularis [shoulder muscles comprising the rotator cuff]

SIV simian immunodeficiency virus; Sprague-Dawley-Ivanovas [rat]

SIVagm simian immunodeficiency virus from African green monkeys

SIVMAC simian immunodeficiency virus of macaques

SIW self-inflicted wound

SIWIP self-induced water intoxication and psychosis

SIWIS self-induced water intoxication and schizophrenic disorders

S_J Jaccard coefficient

SJA Schwartz-Jampel-Aberfeld [syndrome]

$S_{jb}O_2$ jugular vein oxygen saturation

SjO_2 jugular bulb venous oxygen saturation

SJR Shinowara-Jones-Reinhart [unit]

SJS Schwartz-Jampel syndrome; Stevens-Johnson syndrome; stiff joint syndrome; Swyer-James syndrome

SjS Sjögren syndrome

$SjVO_2$ jugular venous oxygen saturation

SK seborrheic keratosis; senile keratosis; Sloan-Kettering [Institute for Cancer Research]; spontaneous killer [cell]; streptokinase; swine kidney

Sk skin

SKA supracondylar knee-ankle [orthosis]

SKALP skin-derived antileukoproteinase

SKAT Sex Knowledge and Attitude Test

SKDAMI Streptokinase plus Desmopressin in Acute Myocardial Infarction [study]

skel skeleton, skeletal

SKHYDIP Skara Hypertension and Diabetes Project

SKI Sloan-Kettering Institute

SKL serum killing level

SKSD, SK-SD streptokinase-streptodornase

sk trx skeletal traction

SL sarcolemma; scapholunar; sclerosing leukoencephalopathy; secondary leukemia; segment length; sensation level; sensory latency; septal leaflet; short-leg [brace]; Sibley-Lehninger [unit]; signal level; Sinding Larsen [syndrome]; Sjögren-Larsson [syndrome]; slit lamp; small lymphocyte; sodium lactate; solidified liquid; sound level; SPECIALIST Lexicon [UMLS]; Stein-Leventhal [syndrome]; streptolysin; sublingual

S$_L$ systolic wave, latent

S/L sublingual

Sl Steel [mouse]

sl in a broad sense [Lat. *sensu lato*]; stemline; sublingual

SLA left sacroanterior [fetal position] [Lat. *sacrolaeva anterior*]; single-cell liquid cytotoxic assay; slide latex agglutination; soluble liver antigen; superficial linear array; surfactant-like activity

SL$_A$ segment length, anterior

SLAC scapholunate advanced collapse [wrist]

SLAM scanning laser acoustic microscope; systemic lupus erythematosus activity measure

SLAP serum leucine aminopeptidase; superior labrum anterior to posterior

SLAT simultaneous laryngoscopy and abdominal thrusts

SLB short-leg brace

SLC short-leg cast

SLCC short-leg cylinder cast

SLD scapholunar dissociation; sublethal damage

SLD, SLDH serum lactate dehydrogenase

SLDR sublethal damage repair

SLE slit lamp examination; St. Louis encephalitis; systemic lupus erythematosus

SLEA sheep erythrocyte antibody

SLEDAI systemic lupus erythematosus disease activity index

SLEP short latent evoked potential

SLEV St. Louis encephalitis virus

SL-GXT symptom-limited graded exercise test

SLHR sex-linked hypophosphatemic rickets

SLHT straight line Hough transform

SLI selective lymphoid irradiation; somatostatin-like immunoreactivity; specific language impairment; splenic localization index

SL$_I$ segment length, inferior

SLIC scanning liquid ionization chamber

SLIDRC Student Loan Interest Deduction Restoration Coalition

SLIP serial line interface protocol

SLIR somatostatin-like immunoreactivity

SLK superior limbic keratoconjunctivitis

SLKC superior limbic keratoconjunctivitis

SLL small lymphocytic lymphoma

SL$_L$ segment length, lateral

SLM sound level meter

SLMC spontaneous lymphocyte-mediated cytotoxicity

SLN sublentiform nucleus; superior laryngeal nerve

SLNWBC short-leg nonweightbearing cast

SLNWC short-leg nonwalking cast

SLO scanning laser ophthalmoscopy; Smith-Lemli-Opitz syndrome; streptolysin O

SLOS Smith-Lemli-Opitz syndrome

SLP left sacroposterior [fetal position] [Lat. *sacrolaeva posterior*]; segmental limb systolic pressure; sex-limited protein; short luteal phase; subluxation of the patella

SLPI salivary leukocyte protease inhibitor; secretory leukocyte protease inhibitor

SLPP serum lipophosphoprotein

SLR Shwartzman local reaction; single lens reflex; stent-like result; straight leg raising

SLRROM shoulder lateral rotation range of motion

SLRT straight leg raising test

SLS Seattle Longitudinal Study; segment long-spacing; short-leg splint; single leg separation; single limb support; Sjögren-Larsson syndrome; sodium lauryl phosphate; stagnant loop syndrome; Stein-Leventhal syndrome

SL$_S$ segment length, septal

SLT left sacrotransverse [fetal position] [Lat. *sacrolaeva transversa*]; single lung transplantation; smokeless tobacco; solid logic technology

SLTEC/VTEC Shigella-like toxin (verotoxin) producing *Escherichia coli*

SLUD salivation, lacrimation, urination, defecation

SLUDGE salivation, lacrimation, urination, defecation, gastrointestinal upset, emesis

SLVDS San Luis Valley Diabetes Study

SLWC short-leg walking cast

SM Master of Science; sadomasochism; segmental mastectomy; self-monitoring; serum; silicon microphysiometer; simple mastectomy; skim milk; smooth muscle; somatomedin; space medicine; sphingomyelin; splenic macrophage; splenomegaly; sports medicine; streptomycin; Strümpell-Marie [syndrome]; submandibular; submaxillary; submucous; suckling mouse; sucrose medium; suction method; superior mesenteric; surgical microscope; surrogate mother; sustained medication; symptoms; synaptic membrane; synovial membrane; systolic motion; systolic murmur

S/M sadomasochism

Sm samarium; *Serratia marcescens*, Smith [antigen]

sm smear

sM suckling mouse

SMA sequential multichannel autoanalyzer; shape memory alloy; simultaneous multichannel autoanalyzer; smooth muscle antibody; Society for Medical Anthropology; somatomedin A; spinal muscular atrophy; spontaneous motor activity; standard method agar; superior mesenteric artery; supplementary motor area; symptomatic morphologic anomaly

SM-A somatomedin A

SMA-6 Sequential Multiple Analysis-msix different serum tests

SMABF superior mesenteric artery blood flow

SMAC Sequential Multiple Analyzer Computer

SMAE superior mesenteric artery embolism

SMAF smooth muscle activating factor; specific macrophage arming factor

SMAG Special Medical Advisory Group

SMAL serum methyl alcohol level

sm an small animal

SMAO superior mesenteric artery occlusion

SMART Self-measurement for Assessment of the Response to Trandolapril [study]; simultaneous multiple angle reconstruction technique; Study of Medicine vs Angioplasty Reperfusion Trial; Study of Microstent's Ability to Limit Restenosis Trial

SMARTT Serum Markers, Acute Myocardial Infarction, and Rapid Treatment Trial

SMAS submuscular aponeurotic system; superficial musculo-aponeurotic system; superior mesenteric artery syndrome

SMASH Swiss Multicenter Evaluation of Early Angioplasty for Shock [following myocardial infarction]; Sydney Men and Sexual Health [study]

SMAST Short Michigan Alcoholism Screening Test

SMATS Seek Medical Attention in Time Study

SMB selected mucosal biopsy; standard mineral base

sMb suckling mouse brain

SMBFT small bowel follow-through

SMC Scientific Manpower Commission; smooth muscle cell; somatomedin C; succinylmonocholine; supernumerary marker chromosome

SM-C, Sm-C somatomedin C

SMCA smooth muscle contracting agent; suckling mouse cataract agent

SMCD senile macular choroidal degeneration; systemic mast cell disease; systemic meningococcal disease

SM-C/IGF somatomedin C/insulin-like growth factor

SMCR Smith-Magenis chromosome region

SmCS smart classification

SMD senile macular degeneration; spondylometaphyseal dysplasia; submanubrial dullness

SMDA Safe Medical Devices Act [of 1990]; starch methylenedianiline

SMDC sodium-N-methyl dithiocarbamate; standards for medical device communication

SMDM Society for Medical Decision Making

SMDS secondary myelodysplastic syndrome

SME severe myoclonic epilepsy

SMED spondylometaphyseal dysplasia

SMEDI stillbirth-mummification, embryonic death, infertility [syndrome]

SMEI severe myoclonic epilepsy of infancy

SMEM supplemented Eagle minimum essential medium

SMF streptozocin, mitomycin C, and 5-fluorouracil; submembrane region containing thrombosthenin filaments

smf sodium motive force

SMFP state medical facilities plan

SMG specialty medical group; submandibular gland

SmG supramarginal gyrus

SMH state mental hospital; strongyloidiasis with massive hyperinfection

SMHA state mental health agency

SMHC smooth muscle heavy chain myosin

SMI Self-Motivation Inventory; senior medical investigator; severe mental impairment; silent myocardial infarction; small volume infusion; stress myocardial image; Style of Mind Inventory; supplementary medical insurance; sustained maximum inspiration

SmIg surface membrane immunoglobulin

SMILE So Much Improvement with a Little Exercise [program]; Survival of Myocardial Infarction: Long-term Evaluation [study]

SMISS Silent Myocardial Ischemia Stress Study

SMK structured meta knowledge

SML smouldering leukemia

SMM smoldering multiple myeloma

SMMD specimen mass measurement device

SMMHC smooth muscle myosin heavy chain

SMMSE Standardized Mini-Mental State Examination

SMN second malignant neoplasm; stathmin; survival motor neuron

SMN^T telemeric survival motor neuron

SMNB submaximal neuromuscular block

SMO senior medical officer; surveillance medical officer

SMOH Senior Medical Officer of Health; Society of Medical Officers of Health

SMON subacute myeloopticoneuropathy

SMP slow moving protease; standard medical practice; submitochondrial particle; sulfamethoxypyrazine; sympathetically maintained pain

SMPC summary of product characteristics

SMPR small mannose 6-phosphate receptor

SMR senior medical resident; sensorimotor rhythm; severe mental retardation; sexual maturity rating; significantly lower mortality rate; skeletal muscle relaxant; somnolent metabolic rate; standardized mortality ratio; stroke with minimum residuum; submucosal resection

SMRR submucosal resection and rhinoplasty

SMRT silencing mediator of retinoid and thyroid receptors

SMRV squirrel monkey retrovirus

SMS scalable modeling system; senior medical student; serial motor seizures; Shared Medical Systems; Simvastatin Multicenter Study; Smith-Magenis syndrome; somatostatin; stiff-man syndrome; Stockholm Metoprolol Trial; supplemental minimum sodium

SMSA standard metropolitan statistical area

SMSV San Miguel sea lion virus

SMT Spanish Multicentre Study; spontaneous mammary tumor; stereotactic mesencephalic tractomy; Stockholm Metoprolol Trial; surface mouth technology

S-MUAP surface-detected motor unit action potential

SMuLV Scripps murine leukemia virus

SMV superior mesenteric vein

SMX, SMZ sulfamethoxazole

SN school nurse; sclerema neonatorum; scrub nurse; Semantic Network [UMLS]; sensorineural; sensory neuron; serum neutralization; sinus node; spontaneous nystagmus; staff nurse; stromal nodule; student nurse; subnormal; substantia nigra; supernatant; suprasternal notch

S/N signal/noise [ratio]

Sn subnasale

sn small nucleolar
SNA specimen not available; Student Nurses Association; sympathetic nerve activity
SNa serum sodium concentration
SNagg serum normal agglutinator
SNAP Score for Neonatal Acute Physiology [study]; sensory nerve action potential; S-nitroso-N-acetylpenicillamine; Stanford Nutrition Action Program
SNaP Study of Sodium and Blood Pressure
SNAPE Study of Nicorandil in Angina Pectoris in the Elderly
SNB scalene node biopsy
SNC spontaneous neonatal chylothorax
SNCL sinus node cycle length
SNCS sensory nerve conduction studies
SNCV sensory nerve conduction velocity
SND scatterer number density; sinus node dysfunction; striatonigral degeneration; sympathetic nerve discharge
SNDA Student National Dental Association
SNDO Standard Nomenclature of Diseases and Operations
SNE sinus node electrogram; subacute necrotizing encephalomyelography
SNES suprascapular nerve entrapment syndrome
SNF sinus node formation; skilled nursing facility
SNGBF single nephron glomerular blood flow
SNGFR single nephron glomerular filtration rate
SNHL sensorineural hearing loss
SNIPA seronegative inflammatory polyarthritis
SNIVT Society of Non-Invasive Vascular Technology
SNJ nevus sebaceous of Jadassohn
SNK Student-Newman-Keuls [procedure]
SNM Society of Nuclear Medicine; sulfanilamide
SNMP simple network management protocol
SNMA Student National Medical Association
SNMT Society of Nuclear Medical Technologists
sno small nucleolar
SNOBOL String-Oriented Symbolic Language

SNODO Standard Nomenclature of Diseases and Operations
SNOMED Systematized Nomenclature of Medicine
SNOP Systematized Nomenclature of Pathology
snoRNA small nucleolar ribonucleic acid [RNA]
snoRNP small nucleolar ribonucleoprotein [RNP]
SNP school nurse practitioner; sinus node potential; sodium nitroprusside
SNR selective nerve root [block]; signal-to-noise ratio; substantia nigra zona reticulata; supernumerary rib
SNRB selective nerve root block
snRNA small nuclear ribonucleic acid; small nucleolar ribonucleic acid [RNA]
snRNP small nuclear ribonucleoprotein [RNP]; small nuclear ribonucleoprotein particle
snRP small nuclear ribonucleoprotein polypeptide
snRPB small nuclear ribonucleoprotein polypeptide B
snRPN small nuclear ribonucleoprotein polypeptide N
SNRT sinus node recovery time
SNRTd sinus node recovery time, direct measuring
SNRTi sinus node recovery time, indirect measuring
SNS Senior Nursing Sister; Society of Neurological Surgeons; sympathetic nervous system
SNSA seronegative spondyloarthropathy
S-NSE serum neuron-specific enolase
SNST sciatic nerve stretch test
SNT sinuses, nose, and throat; spectral noise threshold
SNU skilled nursing unit
SNuPD single nucleotide primer extension
SNV spleen necrosis virus
SNVDO Standard Nomenclature of Veterinary Diseases
SNW slow negative wave
SO salpingo-oophorectomy; Schlatter-Osgood [test]; second opinion; sex offender; spheno-occipital [synchondrosis]; sphincter of Oddi; standing orders; superior oblique [muscle]; supraoptic; supraorbital
S&O salpingo-oophorectomy

SO₂ oxygen saturation

SOA stimulus onset asynchrony; swelling of ankles

SoA symptoms of asthma

SOAA signed out against advice

SOAMA signed out against medical advice

SOA-MCA superficial occipital artery to middle cerebral artery

SOAP subjective, objective, assessment, and plan [problem-oriented record]

SOAPIE subjective, objective, assessment, plan, implementation, and evaluation [problem-oriented record]

SOAR Safety of Orofiban in Acute Coronary Research [study]

SOB see order blank; shortness of breath; stool occult blood

SOBOE shortness of breath on exertion

SOC sequential oral contraceptive; Standard Occupational Classification; standards of care; synovial osteochondromatosis; syphilitic osteochondritis

SoC state of consciousness

SOCIAIDS Study of Cardiac Involvement in Acquired Immunodeficiency Syndrome [AIDS]

SocSec Social Security

SocServ social services

SOCRATES Study of Coronary Revascularization and Therapeutic Evaluations

S-OCT serum ornithine carbamyl transferase

SOD septo-optic dysplasia; superoxide dismutase

sod sodium

sod bicarb sodium bicarbonate

SODAS spheroidal oral drug absorption system

SODF sperm outer defense fiber

SODH sorbitol dehydrogenase

SOF Study of Osteoporotic Fractures [in association with strokes]; superior orbital fissure

SOFLC self-organizing fuzzy logic control

SOFM self-organization feature map

SOH sympathetic orthostatic hypotension

SOHN supraoptic hypothalamic nucleus

SOHO Solar and Heliospheric Observatory [spacecraft data]

SOI severity of illness

SOL solution; space-occupying lesion

sol soluble, solution

SOLD spatial gray level dependence; Stenting after Optimal Lesion Debulking [trial]

SOLEC stand on one leg eyes closed

Soln, sol'n solution

SOLVD Studies of Left Ventricular Dysfunction

SOM secretory otitis media; sensitivity of method; serous otitis media; somatotropin; state operations manual; superior oblique muscle; suppurative otitis media; sustained outward movement [heart]

SOMA Student Osteopathic Medical Association

somat somatic

SOMI sternal occipital mandibular immobilization

SON superior olivary nucleus; supraoptic nucleus

SONET synchronous optical network transmission

SONH spontaneous osteonecrosis of the hip

SONK spontaneous osteonecrosis of the knee

SOO structured office oral [examination]

SOOF suborbital orbicular fat

SOP service–object pair; standard operating procedure

SoP standard of performance

SOPA Survey of Pain Attitudes; syndrome of primary aldosteronism

SOPCA sporadic olivopontocerebellar ataxia

SOPED Shock Outcome Prediction in the Emergency Department [score]

SOPI service object pair instance

SOQ Suicide Opinion Questionnaire

SOR stimulus-organism response; successive over-relaxation [algorithm in imaging]; superoxide release

SOr supraorbitale

sOR stratified odds ratio

Sorb, sorb sorbitol

SORD sorbitol dehydrogenase

SOREM sleep onset rapid eye movement

SORF spliceable open-reading frame

SOS self-obtained smear; son of sevenless; Southern Oxidant Study; supplemental oxygen system; surgery on site; Swedish Obesity Study

SoS Stent or Surgery [study]
SOSA Student Osteopathic Surgical Association
SOSF single organ system failure
SOT sensory organization test; systemic oxygen transport
SOWS subjective opiate withdrawal scale
SP sacroposterior; sacrum to pubis; salivary progesterone; schizotypal personality; semi-private [room]; senile plaque; sepiaopterin; septum pellucidum; serine/proline [rich protein]; seropositive; serum protein; shunt pressure; shunt procedure; silent period; skin potential; sleep deprivation; smoothed periodogram; soft palate; solid phase; spastic paraplegia; speech pathology; spleen; spontaneous proliferation; standard practice; standard procedure; standardized patient; standardized-patient [assessment]; staphylococcal protease; status post; stool preservative; storage phosphor [radiography]; subliminal perception; substance P; sulfapyridine; suprapatellar; suprapubic; surface polypeptide; surfactant protein; symphysis pubis; systolic pressure
Sp the most posterior point on the posterior contour of the sella turcica; sleep spindle; species; specific; specimen; sphenoid; spine, *Spirillum*; summation potential
S/P, s/p status, post[operative]
S7P sedoheptulose-7-phosphate
sP senile parkinsonism; structural protein
sp space; species; specific; spine, spinal; spirit
SPA salt-poor albumin; sheep pulmonary adenomatosis; spastic ataxia; sperm penetration assay; spinal progressive amyotrophy; spondyloarthropathy; spontaneous platelet aggregation; staphylococcal protein A; student progress assessment; suprapubic aspiration; surface polypeptide, anonymous
SP-A surfactant protein A
SPA-Acad Acadian spastic ataxia
SPACE single potential analysis of cavernous electrical activity
SPACELINE Space Life Science Online
sp act specific activity
SPACTO Stent vs Percutaneous Angioplasty in Chronic Total Occlusion [trial]
SPAD stenosing peripheral arterial disease

SPAF spontaneous paroxysmal atrial fibrillation; Stroke Prevention in Atrial Fibrillation [trial]
SPAF TEE Stroke Prevention in Atrial Fibrillation–Transesophageal Echo [study]
SPAG small particle aerosol generator
SPAI steroid protein activity index
SPAM scanning photoacoustic microscopy
SPAMM spatial modulation of magnetization
sp an spinal anesthesia
sPAP systolic pulmonary artery pressure
SPAR sensitivity prediction by acoustic reflex
SPARC cysteine-rich acidic secreted protein; Stroke Prevention Assessment of Risk and Community [trial]
SPAT slow paroxysmal atrial tachycardia; spatial concept [UMLS]
SPB sinking pre-beta-lipoprotein
SP-B surfactant protein B
SPBI serum protein-bound iodine
SPC salicylamide, phenacetin, and caffeine; scaphopisocapitate, seropositive carrier; single palmar crease; single photoelectron count; soy phosphatidylcholine; spleen cell; statistical process control; synthetizing protein complex
SP-C surfactant protein C
SPCA serum prothrombin conversion accelerator; Society for Prevention of Cruelty to Animals
SPCC Spill Prevention, Control, and Countermeasure [plan]
SPCD syndrome of primary ciliary dyskinesia
Sp Cd, sp cd spinal cord
SPCG spectral phonocardiography
SPD schizotypal personality disorder; sociopathic personality disorder; specific paroxysmal discharge; spermidine; standard peak dilution; sterile processing department; storage pool deficiency
SPDC strio-pallido-dentate calcinosis
SpDur spike duration
SPE septic pulmonary edema; serum protein electrolytes; serum protein electrophoresis; streptococcal pyrogenic exotoxin; sucrose polyester; sustained physical exercise
SPEAK spectral peak [strategy]

SPEAR selective parenteral and enteral anti-sepsis regimen

SPE-C streptococcal pyrogenic exotoxin type C

Spec specialist, specialty; specificity

spec special; specific; specificity; specimen

spec gr specific gravity

SPECT single photon emission computed tomography

SPEED Strategies for Patency Enhancement in the Emergency Department [study]

sPEEP spontaneous peak end-expiratory pressure

SPEG serum protein electrophoretogram

SPEL syndactyly-polydactyly-earlobe [syndrome]

SPEM smooth pursuit eye movement

SPEP serum protein electrophoresis; Structured Patient Education Programme

SPERM spastic paraplegia-epilepsy-mental retardation [syndrome]

SPF skin protection factor; specific-pathogen free; spectrophotofluorometer; S-phase fraction; split products of fibrin; standard perfusion fluid; Stuart-Prower factor; sun protection factor; systemic pulmonary fistula

Sp Fl, sp fl spinal fluid

SPG serine phosphoglyceride; spastic paraplegia; sphenopalatine ganglion; splenoportography; sucrose, phosphate, and glutamate; symmetrical peripheral gangrene

SpG specific gravity

spg sponge

SPGA Bovarnik solution; sucrose

SPGR spoiled gradient [echo]

SpGr, sp gr specific gravity

SPGX spastic paraplegia, X-linked

SPGY spermatogenesis on Y

SPH secondary pulmonary hemosiderosis; severely and profoundly handicapped; spherocyte; spherocytosis; sphingomyelin

Sph sphenoidale; sphingomyelin

sph spherical; spherical lens; spheroid

SPHS Saskatoon Pregnancy and Health Study

sp ht specific heat

SPI Self-Perception Inventory; serum precipitable iodine; serum protein index; Shipley Personal Inventory; standardized-patient instructor; Study of Perioperative Ischemia

SPIA solid-phase immunoabsorption; solid-phase immunoassay

SPICE Simulation Program with Integrated Circuit Emphasis; Study of Patients Intolerant to Converting Enzyme Inhibitors

SPICED TEAS Study of Pacemakers and Implantable Cardioverter Defibrillator Triggering by Electronic Article Surveillance Devices

SPICU surgical pulmonary intensive care unit

SPID summed pain intensity difference

SPIE International Society for Optical Engineering

SPIF solid-phase immunoassay fluorescence

SPIH superimposed pregnancy-induced hypertension

SPIN skeletal plan instantiation

spin spine, spinal

SPINAF Stroke Prevention in Nonrheumatic Atrial Fibrillation [study]

SPIR Study of Perioperative Ischemia Research

spir spiral; spirit

SPIRIT Salvage from Perindopril in Reperfused Infarction Trial; Stroke Prevention in Reversible Ischemia Trial

SPJ saphenopopliteal junction

SPK serum pyruvate kinase; simultaneous pancreas-kidney [transplantation]; superficial punctate keratitis

SPL skin potential level; sound pressure level; splanchnic; spontaneous lesion; staphylococcal phage lysate; superior parietal lobule; surfactant proteolipid

SPLATT split anterior tibial tendon

sPLM sleep-related periodic leg movements

SPLV serum parvovirus-like virus

SPM shocks per minute; spatiotemporal population map; spermine; statistical parametric mapping; subhuman primate model; suspended particulate matter; synaptic plasma membrane

SpM spiriformis medialis [nucleus]

spm spermatogonial metaphase

SPMA spinal progressive muscular atrophy

SPMR standard proportionate mortality ratio (or rate)

SPMSQ Short Portable Mental Status Questionnaire

SPN senior plan network; sialophorin; solitary pulmonary nodule; supplemental parental nutrition; sympathetic preganglionic neuron
SpnCbT spinocerebellar tract
SpO₂ functional oxygen saturation; pulse oximetry
SPOCS surgical planning and orientation computer system
SPOD spouse's perception of disease
spon, spont spontaneous
SPONASTRIME spondylar and nasal alterations with striated metaphyses; spondylar changes–nasal anomaly–associated metaphyses [dysplasia]
SPOOL simultaneous peripheral operation on-line
SPORE Specialized Programs of Research Excellence [study]
SPORT Stent Implantation Postrotational Atherectomy Trial
SPP plural of *species*; Sexuality Preference Profile; skin perfusion pressure; small plaque parapsoriasis; suprapubic prostatectomy
spp plural of *species*
SPPF standard portable patient file
Sp Pn, Sp Pnx spontaneous pneumothorax
SPPP, sppp plural of *subspecies*
SPPS solid phase peptide synthesis; stable plasma protein solution
SPPT superprecipitation response
SPPX X-linked spastic paraplegia
SPR sepiapterin reductase; serial probe recognition; skin potential response; specific pathogen free; Society for Pediatric Radiology; Society for Pediatric Research; solid phase radioimmunoassay; substance P receptor
Spr scan projection radiography
spr sprain
SPRAS Sheehan patient rated anxiety scale
SPRCA solid phase red cell adherence assay
SPRIA solid phase radioimmunoassay
SPRINT Secondary Prevention Reinfarction Israeli Nifedipine Trial
SPROM spontaneous premature rupture of membrane
SPRR small proline-rich protein
SPRRA small proline-rich protein A
SPRRB small proline-rich protein B
SPRRC small proline-rich protein C

SPRS Sixty Plus Reinfarction Study
SPRT sequential probability ratio test; Sixty Plus Reinfarction Trial
SPS scapuloperoneal syndrome; shoulder pain and stiffness; simple partial seizures; slow-progressive schizophrenia; Society of Pelvic Surgeons; sodium polyanethol sulfonate; sodium polystyrene; sound production sample; spermidine synthase; stimulated protein synthesis; Stockholm Prospective Study; Suicide Probability Scale; systemic progressive sclerosis
SpS sphenoid sinus
spSHR stroke-prone spontaneously hypertensive rat
SPST Symonds Picture-Story Test
SPT secretin-pancreazymin [test]; single patch technique; single patient trial; sleep period time; spectrin; station pull-through [technique]
SpT spinal tap
SPTA spectrin alpha
SPTAN spectrin alpha, nonerythroid
Sp tap spinal tap
SPTI systolic pressure time index
SPTS subjective posttraumatic syndrome
SPTx static pelvic traction
SPU short procedure unit; Society of Pediatric Urology; standardized photometric unit
SPV selective proximal vagotomy; Shope papilloma virus; sulfophosphovanillin
SPW subxiphoid pericardial window
SPWVD smooth pseudo-Winger-Ville distribution [heart rate signal]
SPYWS Stroke Prevention in Young Women Study
SPZ sulfinpyrazone
SQ social quotient; status quo; subcutaneous; survey question; symptom questionnaire
Sq subcutaneous
sq square; squamous
SQC statistical quality control
sq cell ca squamous cell carcinoma
SQI signal quality index
SQL standard query language; structured query language
SQP sequential quadratic programming
sq rt square root
SQUID superconducting quantum interference device

SR sample response; sarcoplasmic reticulum; saturation recovery; scanning radiometer; screen; secretion rate; sedimentation rate; seizure resistant; senior resident; sensitivity response; sensitization response; service record; sex ratio; shorthair [guinea pig]; short range; side rails; sigma reaction; sinus rhythm; skin resistance; sleep and rest; slow release; smooth-rough [colony]; specific release; specific response; splenorenal; spontaneous respiration; steroid resistance; stimulus response; stomach rumble; stress related; stretch reflex; sulfonamide-resistant; superior rectus; surface roughness; sustained release; synchronization ratio; systemic resistance; systems research; systems review

S-R smooth-rough [bacteria]

Sr strontium

sr steradian

SRA segmental renal artery; serum renin activity; spleen repopulating activity

SRAM static random access memory

SR$_{AW}$, SR$_{aw}$ specific airway resistance

SRBC sheep red blood cells

SRBD sleep-related breathing disorder

SRC sedimented red cells; sheep red cells; signed reaction center

src Rous sarcoma oncogene

SRCA specific red cell adherence

SRCBC serum reserve cholesterol binding capacity

SR/CP schizophrenic reaction, chronic paranoid

SRD service-related disability; Society for the Relief of Distress; Society for the Right to Die; sodium-restricted diet; specific reading disability

SRDS severe respiratory distress syndrome

SRDT single radial diffusion test

SRE Schedule of Recent Experiences; standard regression effect; sterol regulatory element

SREBP sterol regulatory element binding protein

sREM stage rapid eye movement

SRF severe renal failure; skin reactive factor; somatotropin-releasing factor; split renal function; subretinal fluid

SRFA selective restriction fragment amplification

SRF-A slow-reacting factor-anaphylaxis

SRFS split renal function study

SRG specialty review group

SRH single radial hemolysis; somatotropin-releasing hormone; spontaneously responding hyperthyroidism; stigmata of recent hemorrhage

SRI serotonin reuptake inhibitor; severe renal insufficiency; sorcin; Stanford Research Institute; structured review instrument

SRID single radial immunodiffusion

SRIF somatotropin-release inhibiting factor

SRLE schedule of recent life events

SRM spontaneous rupture of membranes; Standard Reference Material; superior rectus muscle

SMRD stress-related mucosal damage

SRN State Registered Nurse

sRNA soluble ribonucleic acid

SRNG sustained release nitroglycerin

SRNS steroid-responsive nephrotic syndrome

SRO sex-ratio organism; single room occupancy; smallest region of overlap; Steele-Richardson-Olszewski [syndrome]

SROC summary receiver operating characteristic

SROM spontaneous rupture of membrane

SRP scientific review panel; short rib-polydactyly [syndrome]; signal recognition particle; Society for Radiological Protection; State Registered Physiotherapist; synchronized retroperfusion

SRPG simulated respiratory pattern generator

SRPR signal recognition particle receptor

SRPS short rib-polydactyly syndrome

SRQ Self-Reporting Questionnaire

SRR standardized rate ratio; surgery recovery room

SRRS Social Readjustment Rating Scale

SR-RSV Schmidt-Ruppin strain Rous sarcoma virus

SRS schizophrenic residual state; sex reassignment surgery; Silver-Russell syndrome; simple repeat sequence; slow-reacting substance; Snyder-Robinson syndrome; Social and Rehabilitation Service; social relationship scale; spermidine synthase; standard rating scale; suppressor of rad six [locus]; Symptom Rating Scale

SRSA, SRS-A slow-reacting substance of anaphylaxis

SRSCB six random systematic core biopsy

SRSV small round structured virus

SRT sedimentation rate test; simple reaction time; sinus node recovery time; sitting root test; Sorbinil Retinopathy Trial; speech reception test; speech reception threshold; spontaneously resolving thyrotoxicosis; surfactant replacement therapy; sustained-release theophylline; symptom rating test

SRU sample ratio units; side rails up; solitary rectal ulcer; structural repeating unit

SRUS solitary rectal ulcer syndrome

SRV Schmidt-Ruppin virus; simian retrovirus; small round virus; superior radicular vein

SRVT sustained re-entrant ventricular tachyarrhythmia

SRW short ragweed [test]

SRWS super radiology work station

SRY sex-determining region

SS disulfide; sacrosciatic; saline soak; saline solution; saliva sample; saliva substitute; *Salmonella-Shigella* [agar]; salt substitute; saturated solution; Schizophrenia Subscale; Seckel syndrome; seizure-sensitive; selective shunt; serum sickness; Sézary syndrome; short sleep; short stature; siblings; sickle cell; side-to-side; signs and symptoms; single-stranded; Sjögren syndrome; skull series [radiographs]; soap suds; Social Security; social services; somatostatin; Spanish-speaking; sparingly soluble; spatial separation; stainless steel; standard score; statistically significant; steady state; steam sterilization; sterile solution; steroid sensitivity; Stickler syndrome; stimulus separation; stromal sarcoma; subaortic stenosis; subscapular; subspinale; substernal; suction socket; sum of squares; supersaturated; support and stimulation; Sweet syndrome; synchronous sampling; systemic sclerosis

S/S salt substitute; signs/symptoms

S&S signs and symptoms

Ss *Shigella sonnei*; subjects

ss single-stranded

SSA salicylsalicylic acid; sicca syndrome A; single-stranded annealing; skin-sensitizing antibody; skin sympathetic activity; Sjögren syndrome A; Smith surface antigen; Social Security Administration; Social Security Act; social service agency; sperm-specific antiserum; stochastic simulated annealing [imaging]; sulfosalicylic acid

SSA1 Smallest Space Analysis

SSAA sicca syndrome associated antigen A; Sjögren syndrome-associated antigen A; syringomyelia secondary to arachnoid adhesions

SSAV simian sarcoma-associated virus

SSB short spike burst; sicca syndrome B; single-strand break; single-stranded binding [protein]; stereospecific binding

SS-B Sjögren syndrome B

ssb single-strand break

SSBG sex steroid-binding globulin; social services block grant

SSC single-strand conformational [analysis]; sister strand crossover; somatosensory cortex; standard saline citrate; standard sodium citrate; syngeneic spleen cell

SSc systemic scleroderma; systemic sclerosis

SSCA single-strand conformational analysis; spontaneous suppressor cell activity

SSCCS slow spinal cord compression syndrome

ss(c)DNA single-stranded circular deoxyribonucleic acid

SSCF sleep stage change frequency

SSCI Social Science Citation Index

SSCP single-stranded conformational polymorphism

SSCPA single-stranded conformational polymorphism analysis

SSCr stainless steel crown

SSCT stereotactic subcaudate tractotomy

SSD shaded surface display; silver sulfadiazine; single saturating dose; Social Security disability; source-skin distance; source-surface distance; speech-sound discrimination; squared sum of intensity differences; standard deviation score; succinate semialdehyde dehydrogenase; sum of square deviations; syndrome of sudden death

ssD-BP single-stranded D-sequence binding protein

SSDBS symptom schedule for the diagnosis of borderline schizophrenia

SSDD steroid sulfatase deficiency disease

SSDI Social Security Disability Income; Supplemental Security Disability Income
ssDNA single-stranded deoxyribonucleic acid [DNA]
SSE saline solution enema; skin self-examination; soapsuds enema; steady state exercise; subacute spongiform encephalopathy
SSEA stage-specific embryonic antigen
SSEP somatosensory evoked potential; steady-state evoked potential
SSER somatosensory evoked response
SSES Sexual Self-Efficacy Scale
SSF septic scarlet fever; soluble suppressor factor; supplemental sensory feedback
SSFP steady state free procession
SSG side scatter; sublabial salivary gland
SSHL severe sensorineural hearing
SSI segmental sequential irradiation; shoulder subluxation inhibition; small-scale integration; Social Security increment; somatic symptom index; Somatic Symptom Inventory; subshock insulin; supplemental security income; surgical site infection; System Sign Inventory
SSIDS sibling of sudden infant death syndrome [victim]
SSIE Smithsonian Science Information Exchange
SSISS Statewide Sentinel Immunisation Surveillance System
SSKI saturated solution of potassium iodide
SSL secure sockets layer; skin surface lipid; sufficient sleep; suppressor of stem loop
SSLI serum sickness-like illness
SSM solid-state microscopy; subsynaptic membrane; superficial spreading melanoma; system status management
SSMS saturated solution of magnesium iodide
SSN severely subnormal; subacute sensory neuropathy; suprasternal notch
SSNHL sudden sensorineural hearing loss
SSNS steroid-sensitive nephrotic syndrome
SSO sequence-specific oligonucleotide [probe]; Society of Surgical Oncology; special sense organ
SSOP Second Surgical Opinion Program; sequence-specific oligonucleotide probe

SSP Sanarelli-Shwartzman phenomenon; Scottish Society of Physicians; site-specific psoralen; slice sensitivity profile; sporozoite surface protein; subacute sclerosing panencephalitis; subspecies; supersensitivity perception
ssp subspecies
SSPC single-strand conformation polymorphism
SSPCP service-specific practice cost percentage
SSPE subacute sclerosing panencephalitis
SSPG steady state plasma glucose
SSPI steady state plasma insulin
SSPL saturation sound pressure level
SSPP subsynaptic plate perforation
SSPS side-to-side portacaval shunt
SS-PSE Schizophrenic Subscale of the Present State Examination
SSQ Social Support Questionnaire
SSR signal sequence receptor; single sequence repeat; site-specific recombination; solar simulated radiation; somatosensory response; steady state response; surgical supply room; sympathetic skin response
SSr single-strand region
SSrA single-strand region A
SSrB single-strand region B
SSRE shear stress response element
SSRI selective serotonin reuptake inhibitor
ssRNA single-stranded ribonucleic acid
SSS scalded skin syndrome; secondary Sjögren syndrome; sick sinus syndrome; specific soluble substance; Stanford Sleepiness Scale; sterile saline soak; subscapular skinfold; superior sagittal sinus; systemic sicca syndrome
SSSA skin sympathetic sudomotor activity
SSSD Spanish Study on Sudden Death
SSSI Siegel Scale of Support for Innovation
SSSS Scandinavian Simvastatin Survival Study; staphylococcal scalded skin syndrome
SSST superior sagittal sinus thrombosis
SS-STP sum of squares simultaneous test procedure
SSSV superior sagittal sinus velocity
SST skin and soft tissue; sodium sulfite titration; somatostatin
SSTI skin and soft tissue infection

SSTR somatostatin receptor
SSU Sabolt seconds universal; self-service unit; sterile supply unit
SSV Schoolman-Schwartz virus; simian sarcoma virus
SSVEP steady-state visual evoked potential
SSW spike and sharp waves [electroencephalography, EEG]
SSX sulfisoxazole
SSYM sign or symptom [UMLS]
ST esotropia; scala tympani; scaphotrapezoid; sclerotherapy; sedimentation time; semitendinosus; sensory threshold; sharp transients [EEG]; shock therapy; sickle [cell] thalassemia; sincerity test; sinus tachycardia; sinus tympani; skin test; skin thickness; slight trace; slow twitch; soft tissue; solid tumor; spastic torticollis; speech therapist; sphincter tone; stable toxin; standard test; starting time; sternothyroid; stimulus; store; stress test; stria terminalis; striation; string data; subtalar; subtotal; sulfotransferase; surface tension; surgical technologist; surgical treatment; survival time; syndrome of the trephined; systolic time
S&T science and technology
S-T [*segment*] in electrocardiography, the portion of the segment between the end of the S wave and the beginning of the T wave; sickle-cell thalassemia
St, st let it stand [Lat. *stet*]; let them stand [Lat. *stent*]; stage [of disease]; status; stere; sterile; stimulation; stokes; stone [unit]; straight; stroke; stomach; stomion; subtype
STA second trimester abortion; serum thrombotic accelerator; superficial temporal artery
Sta staphylion
stab stabilization; stabnuclear neutrophil
STACK Sequence Tag Alignment Consensus Knowledge-base
STAG slow-target attaching globulin; split-thickness autogenous graft
STAI State Trait Anxiety Inventory
STA-MCA superficial temporal artery to middle cerebral artery
STAMI Stenting for Acute Myocardial Infarction [study]
STAMP Systemic Thrombolysis in Acute Myocardial Infarction with Prourokinase and Urokinase [trial]

STAND sutures to ambulate and discharge
STANDOUT soft thresholding and depth cueing of unspecified techniques
StanPsych standard psychiatric [nomenclature]
Staph, staph *Staphylococcus*, staphylococcal
STAR recombinant streptokinase; Specialty Training and Advanced Research [NIH]; Staphylokinase Recombinant Trial; Study of Tranexamic Acid after Aneurysm Rupture
StAR steroidogenic acute regulatory [protein]
STARNET South Texas Ambulatory Research Network
STARS Standard Treatment with Activase to Reverse Stroke [study]; Stent Anticoagulation Regimen Study; Stent Antithrombolytic Regimen Study; Stent Anticoagulation Restenosis Study; St. Thomas Atherosclerosis Regression Study
START Saruplase and Taprostene Acute Reocclusion Trial; simple triage and rapid treatment; St. Thomas Atherosclerosis Regression Trial; Stent vs Angioplasty Restenosis Trial; Stent vs Directional Coronary Atherectomy Randomized Trial; Study of Thrombolytic Therapy with Additional Response Following Taprostene; Study of Titration and Response to Tiazac
STAR TAP science, technology, and research transit access point
STAS sporadic testicular agenesis syndrome
STAT immediately (Lat. *statim*); signal transducer and activator of transcription; state-trait anxiety inventory; Stent Thrombosis after Ticlopidine [study]; stop teenage addiction to tobacco; Stroke Treatment with Ancrod Trial
Stat statistics, statistical
stat immediately [Lat. *statim*]; radiation emanation unit [German]
STATH statherin
STATRS Stent Antithrombotic Regimen Study
Stb stillborn
STC serum theophylline concentration; soft tissue calcification; stroke treatment center; subtotal colectomy
STD selective T-cell defect; sexually transmitted disease; skin-to-tumor distance;

skin test dose; sodium tetradecyl sulfate; standard test dose; ST segment depression [electrocardiography, ECG]

std saturated; standardized

STDH skin test for delayed hypersensitivity

STE Scholars for Teaching Excellence

STEAM stimulated echo acquisition mode

STEC Shiga toxin-producing *Escherichia coli*

STEL short-term exposure limit

STEM scanning transmission electron microscope; Society of Teachers of Emergency Medicine

STEN staphylococcal toxic epidermal necrolysis

sten stenosis, stenosed

STENT-BY Stent vs Bypass Surgery for Vessels Undergoing Abrupt Closure [trial]

STENTIM Stenting in Acute Myocardial Infarction [study]

STEP Sequential Test of Educational Progress; simultaneous transmission-emission protocol; Study of Taprostene in Elective Percutaneous Transluminal Coronary Angioplasty

STEPHY Starnberg Trial on Epidemiology of Parkinsonism and Hypertension in the Elderly

STEPS Significance of Transesophageal Electrocardiographic Findings in Prevention of Stroke [study]

STEREO Stents and Reopro [trial]

stereo stereogram

STESS self-rating treatment emergent symptom scale

STET submaximal treadmill exercise test

STEV short-term exposure value

STF serum thymus factor; slow-twitch fiber; special tube feeding; specialized treatment center; stefin; Stoffel [buffer]; sudden transient freezing

STFM Society of Teachers of Family Medicine

STFT short-time Fourier transform

STG short-term goal; split-thickness graft; superior temporal gyrus

STH somatotropic hormone; subtotal hysterectomy

STh sickle cell thalassemia

ST/HR ST segment [electrocardiography, ECG] depression with exercise divided by changes in heart rate

STHRF somatotropic hormone releasing factor

STI Scientific and Technical Information; serum trypsin inhibitor; sexually transmitted infection; soybean trypsin inhibitor; structured [cyclic antiretroviral] therapy interruption; systolic time interval

STIC Science and Technology Information Center; serum trypsin inhibition capacity; solid-state transducer intracompartment

STILE Surgery vs Thrombolysis for Ischemic Lower Extremity [trial]

stillb stillborn

STIM state transition information model

stim stimulated, stimulation; stimulus

STIMIS Study of Time Intervals in Myocardial Ischaemic Syndromes

STIMS Swedish Ticlodipine Multicenter Study

STIMULATE Speech, Text, Image, and Multimedia Advanced Technology Effort

STIPAS Safety Study of Tirilazad Mesylate in Patients with Acute Ischemic Stroke

STIR short tau inversion recovery

STJ subtalar joint

STK stem cell tyrosine kinase; streptokinase

STL serum theophylline level; status thymicolymphaticus; stereolithography; swelling, tenderness and limited motion

STLI subtotal lymphoid irradiation

STLOM swelling, tenderness, and limitation of motion

STLS subacute thyroiditis-like syndrome

STLV simian T-lymphotropic virus

STM scanning tunneling microscope; short-term memory; streptomycin

STMS short test of mental status

STMY stromelysin

STN streptozocin; subthalamic nucleus; supratrochlear nucleus

sTNM tumor node metastasis [TNM] staging

STNR symmetric tonic neck reflex

STNV satellite tobacco necrosis virus

STO store

stom stomach

STONE Shanghai Trial of Nifedipine in the Elderly

STOP Shunt Thrombotic Occlusion Prevention by Picotamide [study]; Stenting for Total Occlusion and Restenosis Prevention [study]; Stroke Prevention in Sickle Cell Disease [study]; Study of Hypertension in the Elderly [Sweden] or Swedish Trial in Old Patients with Hypertension; surgical termination of pregnancy; Swedish Trial in Older Patients

STOP 2 Swedish Trial in Old Patients with Hypertension 2

STOP-AF Systematic Trial of Pacing to Prevent Atrial Fibrillation

STOP-Hypertension Swedish Trial in Older Patients with Hypertension

STOP IT Sites Testing Osteoporosis Prevention Intervention Treatment

STOPP Selling Teens on Pregnancy Prevention [study]

STOR summary time-oriented record

STORCH syphilis, toxoplasmosis, rubella, cytomegalovirus, and herpesvirus

STP phenol-preferring sulfotransferase; scientifically treated petroleum; short-term potentiation; sodium thiopental; standard temperature and pressure; standard temperature and pulse; stiripentol; strategic technology planning

STPB skin transient pulse blood

STPS specific thalamic projection system

STQ superior temporal quadrant

STR short tandem repeat; soft tissue relaxation; statherin; stirred tank reactor

Str, str *Streptococcus*, streptococcal

strab strabismus

STRATIFY St Thomas' Risk Assessment Tool in Falling Elderly Patients

STRATUS Study to Determine Rotablator and Transluminal Angioplasty Strategy

Strep *Streptococcus;* streptomycin

STRESS Stent Restenosis Study

STRETCH Symptom Tolerability Response to Exercise Trial of Candesartan Cilexitil in Patients with Heart Failure

STRICU shock, trauma and respiratory intensive care unit

STRIP Special Turku Coronary Risk Factor Intervention Project [for babies]

s-TRSV substrate of tobacco ringspot virus

STRT skin temperature recovery time

struct structure, structural

STRUT stent treatment region assessed by ultrasound tomography

STS sequence tagged site; serologic test for syphilis; sodium tetradecyl sulfate;

sodium thiosulfate; soft tissue sarcoma; standard test for syphilis; steroid sulfatase

STSA Southern Thoracic Surgical Association

STSD Spanish Trial on Sudden Death

STSE split-thickness skin excision

STSG split-thickness skin graft

STSS staphylococcal toxic shock syndrome

STT scaphotrapeziotrapezoid [joint]; serial thrombin time; skin temperature test; space-time toolkit

STU skin test unit

STUR Student Team Utilizing Research [project]

STV spontaneous tidal volume; superior temporal vein

STVA subtotal villose atrophy

STVS short-term visual storage

STX saxitoxin; syntaxin

Stx Shiga toxin

STZ streptozocin; streptozyme

SU salicyluric acid; secretory unit; sensation unit; solar urticaria; sorbent unit; spectrophotometric unit; status uncertain; subunit; sulfonamide; sulfonylurea; supine

Su sulfonamide

SUA serum uric acid; single umbilical artery; single unit activity

subac subacute

subclav subclavian; subclavicular

subcut subcutaneous

subling sublingual

SubN subthalamic nucleus

subq subcutaneous

SUBS substance [UMLS]

subsp subspecies

substd substandard

suc suction

Succ succinate, succinic

SUD skin unit dose; sudden unexpected death

SUDAAN survey data analysis

SUDH succinyldehydrogenase

SUDI sudden unexpected death in infancy

SUFE slipped upper femoral epiphysis

SUI stress urinary incontinence

SUID sudden unexplained infant death

sulf sulfate

sulfa sulfonamide

SULF-PRIM sulfamethoxazole and trimethoprim

SUMA sporadic ulcerating and mutilating acropathy

SUMAA scalable unstructured mesh algorithms and applications

SUMIT streptokinase-urokinase myocardial infarct test

SUMMIT Stanford University Medical Media and Information Technology

SUMSE stroke unit mental status examination

SUN standard unit of nomenclature; serum urea nitrogen

SUO syncope of unknown origin

SUP schizo-unipolar; supination

sup above [Lat. *supra*]; superficial; superior; supinator; supine

supin supination, supine

supp suppository

suppl supplement, supplementary

SUPPORT Study to Understand Prognoses and Preferences for Outcomes and Risks of Treatment

suppos suppository

SUR sulfonylurea receptor

SURE Serial Ultrasound Analysis of Restenosis [study]

SURF surfeit

SURFnet Netherlands Network

SURG, Surg surgery, surgical, or surgeon

SURS solitary ulcer of rectum syndrome; surveillance and utilization review

SUS Saybolt Universal Seconds; solitary ulcer syndrome; stained urinary sediment; suppressor sensitive

SUSHI Stent Use is Superior for Hospitalized Infarction Patients [study]

susp suspension, suspended

SUTAMI Saruplase and Urokinase in the Treatment of Acute Myocardial Infarction [trial]

SUTI symptomatic urinary tract infection

SUUD sudden unexpected unexplained death

SUV small unilamellar vessel

SUVIMAX Supplemental Vitamins, Minerals and Anti-Oxidants [trial]

SUX succinylcholine

SUZI subzonal insemination

SV saphenous vein; sarcoma virus; satellite virus; scattering volume; selective vagotomy; semilunar valve; seminal vesicle; severe; sigmoid volvulus; simian virus;

single ventricle; sinus venosus; snake venom; splenic vein; spontaneous ventilation; stroke volume; subclavian vein; subventricular; supravital; synaptic vesicle

S/V surface/volume ratio

SV2 synaptic vesicle protein 2

SV40, SV$_{40}$ simian vacuolating virus 40

SV40-PML simian vacuolating virus 40 of progressive multifocal leukoencephalopathy

Sv sievert

sv sievert; single vibration

SVA selective vagotomy and antrectomy; selective visceral angiography; sequential ventriculoatrial [pacing]; subtotal villous atrophy

SVAS supravalvular aortic stenosis; supraventricular aortic stenosis

SVAT synaptic vesicle amine transformer

SVB saphenous vein bypass

SVBG saphenous vein bypass grafting

SVC saphenous vein cutdown; segmental venous capacitance; selective venous catheterization; slow vital capacity; spatially varying classification; subclavian vein catheterization; superior vena cava; supraventricular extrasystole

SVCCS superior vena cava compression syndrome

SVCG spatial vectorcardiogram

SVCO superior vena-caval obstruction

SVCP Special Virus Cancer Program

SVCR segmental venous capacitance ratio

SVCS superior vena cava syndrome

SVD single vessel disease; small vessel disease; spontaneous vaginal delivery; spontaneous vertex delivery; swine vesicular disease

SVE slow volume encephalography; soluble viral extract; sterile vaginal examination

SVG saphenous vein graft

SVGA super video graphics array

SVH saphenous vein harvesting

SV-HUC simian virus-human uro-epithelial cell

SVI slow virus infection; stroke volume index; systolic velocity integral

SVL superficial vastus lateralis

SVM seminal vesicle microsome; syncytiovascular membrane

SVMT synaptic vesicle monoamine transformer

SVN selectively vulnerable neurons; sinu-vertebral nerve; small volume nebulizer

SvO₂ venous oxygen saturation

SVOM sequential volitional oral movement

SVP selective vagotomy and pyloroplasty; small volume parenteral [infusion]; standing venous pressure; superior vascular plexus

SVPB supraventricular premature beat

SVPC supraventricular premature complex

SVPD snake venom phosphodiesterase

SVR sequential vascular response; systemic vascular resistance

SVRI systemic vascular resistance index

SVS slit ventricle syndrome; Society for Cardiovascular Surgery

SVT sinoventricular tachycardia; subclavian vein thrombosis; supraventricular tachyarrhythmia; supraventricular tachycardia; sustained ventricular tachycardia

SVTh subvalvular thickening

SVTS Sotalol Ventricular Tachycardia Study

SW seriously wounded; short waves; sine-wave; slow wave; soap and water; social worker; spike wave; spiral wound; stab wound; sterile water; stroke work; Sturge-Weber [syndrome]; Swiss Webster [mouse]

S/W spike wave

Sw swine

SWA seriously wounded in action; slow-wave activity

SWAIDS social workers in acquired immunodeficiency syndrome [AIDS]

SWAP short wavelength automated perimetry

SWAT Stroke Prevention with Warfarin or Aspirin Trial

SWC submaximal working capacity

SWCM social work case manager

SWD short wave diathermy

SWE slow wave encephalography

SWEET Square Wave Endurance Exercise Trial

SWG silkworm gut; standard wire gauge; stimulus waveform generator

SWI sterile water for injection; stroke work index; surgical wound infection

SWIFT Should We Intervene Following Thrombolysis? [study]

SWIM sperm-washing insemination method

SWIORA spinal cord injury without radiologic abnormality

SWISH Swedish Isradipine Study in Hypertension

SWISSI Swiss Interventional Study in Silent Ischemia

SWL shock wave lithotripsy

SWM segmental wall motion

SWMA segmental wall motion analysis

SWMF Semmes-Weinstein monofilament

SWO superficial white onychomycosis

SWOG South West Oncology Group

SWOOP South Wilshire Out of Hours Project

SWORD Survival with Oral D-sotalol [study]; surveillance of work-related and occupational respiratory diseases

SWR serum Wassermann reaction; surgical wound infection rate

SWRF square wave response function

SWS slow-wave sleep; spike-wave stupor; steroid-wasting syndrome; Sturge-Weber syndrome

SWT sine-wave threshold

SWU septic work-up

Sx suction

Sx, Sₓ signs; symptoms

SXCT spiral x-ray computed tomography

SXR skull x-ray [examination]

Sxr sex reversal

Sxs serological sex-specific [antigen]

SXT sulfamethoxazole-trimethoprim [mixture]

SY spectroscopy; syphilis, syphilitic

SYA subacute yellow atrophy

SYB synaptobrevin

SYDS stomach yin deficiency syndrome

sym symmetrical; symptom

sympath sympathetic

symph symphysis

SYMPHONY Sibratiban vs Aspirin to Yield Maximum Protection from Ischemic Heart Events Postacute Coronary Syndromes [trial]

sympt symptom

SYN synapse; synovitis

syn synergistic; synonym; synovial

SYNBIAPACE synchronous biatrial pacing therapy

synd syndrome

SYNDIKATE synthesis of distributed knowledge acquired from text

SynText symbolic text [processor]
SYP synaptophysin
syph syphilis, syphilitic
SYR Syrian [hamster]
syr syrup [Lat. *syrupus*]; syringe
SYREC symmetric recombinant [virus]
SYS stretching-yawning syndrome; systemic
sys system, systemic; systolic
SYS-BP systolic blood pressure

syst system, systole, systolic
SYST-CHINA Systolic Hypertension in Elderly Chinese Trial
SYST-EUR Systolic Hypertension in Europeans Study
SYT synaptotagmin
SZ schizophrenia; streptozocin
Sz seizure; schizophrenia
SZN streptozocin

T absolute temperature; an electrocardiographic wave corresponding to the repolarization of the ventricles [wave]; large T [antigen]; life [time]; period [time]; ribosylthymine; tablespoonful; *Taenia*; tamoxifen; telomere or terminal banding; temperature; temporal electrode placement in electroencephalography; temporary; tenderness; tension [intraocular]; tera-, trillion; tesla; testosterone; tetra; tetracycline; theophylline; therapy; thoracic; thorax; threatened [animal]; threonine; thrombosis; thrombus; thymidine; thymine; thymus [cell]; thymus-derived; thyroid; tidal gas; tidal volume; time; tincture; tocopherol; topical; torque; total; toxicity; training [group]; transition; transducer; transmittance; transverse; treatment; *Treponema*; *Trichophyton*; tritium; tryptamine; *Trypanosoma*; tuberculin; tuberculosis; tumor; turnkey system; type

T₁/₂, t₁/₂ half-life

T1 longitudinal relaxation time

T1-T12 first to twelfth thoracic vertebrae

T₁ spin-lattice or longitudinal relaxation time; tricuspid first sound; tricuspid valve closure sound

T + 1, T + 2, T + 3 first, second, and third stages of increased intraocular tension

T-1, T-2, T-3 first, second, and third stages of decreased intraocular tension

T2 transverse relaxation time

T₂ duudothyronine; spin spin or transverse relaxation time

T2* effective transverse relaxation time

T₂* effective transverse relaxation time

2,4,5-T 2,4,5-trichlorophenoxyacetic acid

T₃ triiodothyronine

T₄ thyroxine

T-7 free thyroxine factor

T₉₀ time required for 90% mortality in a population of microorganisms exposed to a toxic agent

t duration; small T [antigen]; Student t test; teaspoonful; temperature; temporal; terminal; tertiary; test of significance; three times [Lat. *ter*]; time; tissue; tonne; translocation

TA alkaline tuberculin; arterial tension; axillary temperature; tactile afferent; Takayasu arteritis; teichoic acid; temporal abstraction; temporal arteritis; terminal antrum; therapeutic abortion; thermophilic *Actinomyces*; thymocytotoxic autoantibody; thyroarytenoid; thyroglobulin autoprecipitation; thyroid antibody; thyroid autoimmunity; tibialis anterior; tissue adhesive; titratable acid; total alkaloids; total antibody; toxic adenoma; toxin-antitoxin; traffic accident; transactional analysis; transaldolase; transaminase; transantral; transplantation antigen; transposition of aorta; trapped air; triamcinolone acetonide; tricuspid atresia; trophoblast antigen; true anomaly; truncus arteriosus; tryptamine; tryptose agar; tube agglutination; tumor-associated

T/A time and amount

T-A toxin-antitoxin; transfusion-associated

T&A tonsillectomy and adenoidectomy; tonsils and adenoids

Ta tantalum; tarsal

TAA thioacetamide; thoracic aortic aneurysm; total ankle arthroplasty; transverse aortic arch; tumor-associated antigen

TAAF thromboplastic activity of the amniotic fluid

TA-AIDS transfusion-associated acquired immunodeficiency syndrome

TAB total autonomic blockage; typhoid, paratyphoid A, and paratyphoid B [vaccine]

TAb therapeutic abortion

tab tablet

TABC total aerobic bacteria count; typhoid, paratyphoid A, paratyphoid B, and paratyphoid C [vaccine]

TABP type A behavior pattern

Tabs tablets

TABT typhoid, paratyphoid A, paratyphoid B, and tetanus toxoid [vaccine]

TABTD typhoid, paratyphoid A, paratyphoid B, tetanus toxoid, and diphtheria toxoid [vaccine]

TAC tachykinin; terminal antrum contraction; tetracaine, adrenalin, and cocaine; time-activity curve; total abdominal colectomy; total aganglionosis coli; triamcinolone cream; truncus arteriosus communis

TAC-1 tachykinin-1

TAC-2 tachykinin-2

TACE chlorotrianicene; teichoic acid crude extract; tumor-necrosis factor alpha converting enzyme

tachy tachycardia

TACIP Triflusal, Aspirin, Cerebral Infarction Prevention [study]

TACR tachykinin receptor

TACS Thrombolysis and Angioplasty in Cardiogenic Shock [study]

TACT Ticlopidine Angioplasty Coronary Trial; Ticlopidine vs Placebo for Prevention of Acute Closure After Angioplasty Trial

TACTICS Thrombolysis and Counterpulsation to Improve Cardiogenic Shock Survival [trial]

TACTICS-TIMI 18 Treat Angina with Aggrastat and Determine Cost of Therapy with an Invasive or Conservative Strategy–Thrombolysis in Myocardial Infarction [trial]

TAD test of auditory discrimination; thoracic asphyxiant dystrophy; tobacco, alcohol, and drugs; Traffic Accident Deformity [scale]; transient acantholytic dermatosis

TADAC therapeutic abortion, dilatation, aspiration, curettage

TAE transcatheter arterial embolism

TAF albumose-free tuberculin [Ger. *Tuberculin Albumose frei*]; tissue angiogenesis factor; toxin-antitoxin floccules; toxoid-antitoxin floccules; transabdominal hysterectomy; trypsin-aldehyde-fuchsin; tumor angiogenesis factor

TAFU tumor abrasion with focused ultrasound

TAG target attaching globulin; technical advisory group; thymine, adenine, and guanine

TAg large T-antigen

Tag T-antigen

TAGH triiodothyronine, amino acids, glucagon, and heparin

TAGVHD transfusion-associated graft-versus-host disease

TAH total abdominal hysterectomy; total artificial heart

TAH BSO total abdominal hysterectomy and bilateral salpingo-oophorectomy

TAHIV transfusion-acquired human immunodeficiency virus [HIV]

TAI Test Anxiety Inventory

TAIM Trial of Antihypertensive Intervention and Management

TAIS time assessment interview schedule

TAIST Tinzaparin in Acute Stroke Trial

TAL T-cell acute leukemia; tendon of Achilles lengthening; thymic alymphoplasia

talc talcum

TALH thick ascending limb of Henle's loop

TALL theoretical annual loss of life

TALL, T-ALL T-cell acute lymphoblastic leukemia

TALLA T-cell acute lymphoblastic leukemia antigen

TAM tamoxifen; technology acceptance model; technology assessment method; teen-age mother; tele-alarm management; thermoacidurans agar modified; time-averaged mean; total active motion; Total Atherosclerosis Management [study]; toxin-antitoxoid mixture; transient abnormal myelopoiesis

TAME N-alpha-tosyl-1-arginine methyl ester

TAMI Thrombolysis and Angioplasty in Myocardial Infarction [study]; transmural anterior myocardial infarction

TAMIS Telemetric Automated Microbial Identification System

TAMRA tetramethylrhodamine

TAMV temporal average maximal velocity [Doppler]

TAN total adenine nucleotide; total ammonia nitrogen

tan tandem translocation; tangent

TANet Taiwan Network

TANI total axial [lymph] node irradiation

TAO thromboangiitis obliterans; triacetyloleandomycin

TAP technology architecture project; tick anticoagulant peptide; transesophageal atrial pacing; transluminal angioplasty; transmembrane action potential; transporter in antigen processing; trypsinogen-activating peptide

TAPA target of antiproliferative antibody

TAPE temporary atrial pacemaker electrode

TAPIRSS Triflusal vs Aspirin in Preventing Infarction: Randomized Stroke Study

TAPS The Akita Pathology Study; Teenage Attitude and Practices Study; trial assessment procedure scale

TAPVC total anomalous pulmonary venous connection

TAPVD total anomalous pulmonary venous drainage

TAPVR total anomalous pulmonary venous return

Taq *Thermus aquaticus*

taq DNA *Thermus aquaticus* deoxyribonucleic acid [DNA]

TAQW transient abnormal Q wave

TAR thoracic aortic rupture; thrombocytopenia with absent radii [syndrome]; tissue-air ratio; total abortion rate; transactivation response; transanal resection; transaxillary resection; treatment authorization request

TARA total articular replacement arthroplasty; tumor-associated rejection antigen

TAR/PD target nursing hours per patient/day

TARS threonyl transfer ribonucleic acid [RNA] synthetase

TAS tetanus antitoxin serum; therapeutic activities specialist; thoracoabdominal syndrome; transcription-based amplification system; traumatic apallic syndrome

TASA tumor-associated surface antigen

TASC Trial of Angioplasty and Stents in Canada

Tase tryptophan synthetase

TASH Transcoronary Ablation of Septum Hypertrophy [study]

TASMAN Thrombolysis Anticoagulant Study: Mediterranean, Australia, New Zealand

TASO The Acquired Immunodeficiency Syndrome [AIDS] Support Organisation [Australia]

TASS thyrotoxicosis-Addison disease-Sjögren syndrome-sarcoidosis [syndrome]; Ticlopidine Aspirin Stroke Study

TASTE Ticlopidine Aspirin Stent Evaluation

TAT tetanus antitoxin; thematic apperception test; thematic aptitude test; thrombin-antithrombin complex; thromboplastin activation test; total antitryptic activity; toxin-antitoxin; transactivator; transaxial tomography; tray agglutination test; tumor activity test; turnaround time; tyrosine aminotransferase

TATA Pribnow [box]; tumor-associated transplantation antigen

TATD tyrosine aminotransferase deficiency

TATR tyrosine aminotransferase regulator

TATRC Telemedicine and Advanced Technology Research Center

TATST tetanus antitoxin skin test

τ Greek lower case letter *tau*; life [of radioisotope]; relaxation time; shear stress; spectral transmittance; transmission coefficient

TAUSA Thrombolysis and Angioplasty in Unstable Angina [trial]

TAV trapped air volume

TAVB total atrioventricular block

TAX Taxol

TB Taussig-Bind [syndrome]; terabyte; term birth; terminal bronchiole; terminal bronchus; thromboxane B; thymol blue; toluidine blue; total base; total bilirubin; total body; tracheobronchial; tracheal bronchiolar [region]; tracheobronchitis; trapezoid body; tub bath; triple [gene] block; tubercle bacillus; tuberculin; tuberculosis; tumor-bearing

T$_B$ total buffer

Tb Tbilisi [phage]; terabit [trillian bits]; terbium; tubercle bacillus; tuberculosis

T$_b$ biological half-life; body temperature

tb tuberculosis

TBA tertiary butylacetate; testosterone-binding affinity; tetrabutylammonium; thiobarbituric acid; to be absorbed; to be added; total bile acids; trypsin-binding activity; tubercle bacillum; tumor-bearing animal

TBAB tryptose blood agar base

TBAF tetrabutylammonium fluoride

TBAN transbronchial aspiration needle

TBARS thiobarbituric acid reactive substance

TBB transbronchial biopsy

TBBA total body bone ash

TBBM total body bone minerals

TBBx transbronchial biopsy

TBC thyroxine-binding coagulin; total body calcium; total body carbon; total body clearance; tuberculosis

Tbc tubercle bacillus; tuberculosis
TBCa total body calcium
TBCl total body chlorine
TBD total body density; Toxicology Data Base
TBE tick-borne encephalitis; triborate ethylenediamine tetraacetic acid [EDTA]; tuberculin bacillin emulsion
TBEV tick-borne encephalitis virus
TBF total body fat
TBFB tracheobronchial foreign body
TBFM total body fat mass
TBFVL tidal breathing flow-volume loops
TBG beta-thromboglobulin; testosterone-binding globulin; thyroglobulin; thyroid-binding globulin; thyroxine-binding globulin; tracheobronchography; tris-buffered Gey solution
TBGI thyroxine-binding globulin index
TBGP total blood granulocyte pool
TBH total body hematocrit
tBHP terbutyl hydroperoxide
TBHQ tertiary butylhydroquinone
TBHT total-body hyperthermia
TBI thyroid-binding index; thyroxine-binding index; tooth-brushing instruction; total-body irradiation; traumatic brain injury
TBII thyroid-stimulating hormone-binding inhibitory immunoglobulin
T bili total bilirubin
TBIM thoracic bioimpedance monitoring
TBK total body potassium
tbl tablet
TBLB transbronchial lung biopsy
TBLC term birth, living child
TBLI term birth, living infant
TBLTM total body lean tissue mass
TBM total body mass; tracheobronchiomegaly; trophoblastic basement membrane; tuberculous meningitis; tubular basement membrane
TBMC total body mineral content
TBMN thin basement membrane nephropathy
TBN bacillus emulsion; temporal belief network; total body nitrogen
TBNA total body neutron activation; treated but not admitted
TBNa total body sodium
TBNAA total body neutron activation analysis

TBO total blood out
TBP bithionol; testosterone-binding protein; thyroxine-binding protein; total body protein; total bypass; tributyl phosphate; tuberculous peritonitis
TBPA thyroxine-binding prealbumin
TBPr total body protein
Tbps terabits [trillion bits] per second
TBPT total body protein turnover
TBR tumor-bearing rabbit
TB-RD tuberculosis and respiratory disease
TBS total body solids; total body solute; total body surface; total burn size; Townes-Brocks syndrome; tracheobronchial submucosa; tracheobronchoscopy; tribromosalicylanilide; triethanolamine-buffered saline
tbs, tbsp tablespoon
TBSA total body surface area
TBSV tomato bushy stunt virus
TBT tolbutamide test; tracheobronchial toilet; tracheobronchial tree
TBTT tuberculin time test
TBV total blood volume; trabecular bone volume
TBW total body water; total body weight
TBX thromboxane; total body irradiation
TBXA2 thromboxane A2
TBXAS thromboxane A synthase
TBZ tetrabenazine; thiabendazole
TC target cell; taurocholate; temperature compensation; teratocarcinoma; tertiary cleavage; tetracycline; theca cell; therapeutic community; thermal conductivity; thoracic cage; thoracic compression; throat culture; thyrocalcitonin; time constant; tissue culture; to contain; total calcium; total capacity; total cholesterol; total colonoscopy; total correction; transcobalamin; transcutaneous; transplant center; transverse colon; Treacher Collins [syndrome]; true channel; true conjugate; tuberculin contagiosum; tubocurarine; tumor cell; tumor of cerebrum; type and crossmatch
T&C turn and cough; type and crossmatch
$T_4(C)$ serum thyroxine measured by column chromatography
TC_{50} medium toxic concentration
Tc correlation time; technetium; tetracycline; transcobalamin
T_c cytotoxic T-cell; the generation time of a cell cycle; tricuspid closure

t(°C) temperature on the Celsius scale

tc transcutaneous; translational control

TCA T-cell A locus; terminal cancer; tetracyclic antidepressant; total cholic acid; total circulating albumin; total circulatory arrest; total colonic agangliosis; tricalcium aluminate; tricarboxylic acid; trichloroacetic acid; tricyclic antidepressant; thyrocalcitonin

TCAB 3,3',4,4'-tetrachloroazobenzene

TCABG triple coronary artery bypass graft

TCAD tricyclic antidepressant

TCADA Texas Council on Alcohol and Drug Abuse

TCAG triple coronary artery graft

TCAOB 3,3',4,4'-tetrachloroazoxybenzene

TCAP trimethyl-cetyl-ammonium pentachlorophenate

TCB tetrachlorobiphenyl; total cardiopulmonary bypass transcatheter biopsy; transabdominal chorionic biopsy; tumor cell burden

TCAR T-cell antigen receptor

TCBS thiosulfate-citrate-bile salts-sucrose [agar]

TCC terminal complement complex; thromboplastic cell component; transitional-cell carcinoma; trauma center coordination or coordinator; trichlorocarbanilide

Tcc triclocarban

TCCA, TCCAV transitional cell cancer-associated [virus]

TCCD transcranial color-coded Doppler

TCCL T-cell chronic lymphoblastic leukemia

TCCS transcranial color-coded sonography

TCCU&C therapeutic care understanding and control

TCD tapetochoroidal dystrophy; T-cell depletion; thermal conductivity detector; tissue culture dose; transcranial Doppler [sonography]; transverse cardiac diameter; tumoricidal dose

TCD$_{50}$ median tissue culture dose

TCDB turn, cough, deep breathe

TCDC taurochenodeoxycholate

TCDD 2,3,7,8-tetrachlorodibenzo-p-dioxin

TCE T-cell enriched; tetrachlorodiphenyl ethane; trichloroethylene

TCED$_{50}$ 50% tissue effective dose

TCES transcutaneous cranial electrical stimulation

TCESOM trichloroethylene-extracted soybean oil meal

TCET transcerebral electrotherapy

TCF tissue coding factor; total coronary flow; transcription factor; Treacher Collins-Franceschetti [syndrome]

T-CFC T-colony forming cell

TCFU tumor colony-forming unit

TCG therapeutic care–general; time-compensated gain; Thromboprophylaxis Collaborative Group

TCGF T-cell growth factor

TCH tanned-cell hemagglutination; thiophen-2-carboxylic acid hydrazide; total circulating hemoglobin; turn, cough, hyperventilate

TC/HDL total cholesterol/high density lipoproteins [ratio]

TChE total cholinesterase

TCI temporal continuity index; To Come In [open heart surgery program at Cleveland Clinic]; total cerebral ischemia; transcardial catheter therapeutics; transient cerebral ischemia; transcobalamin I

TCi teracurie

TCID tissue culture infective dose; tissue culture inoculated dose

TCID$_{50}$ median tissue culture infective dose; 50% tissue culture infective dose

TCIE transient cerebral ischemic episode

TCII transcobalamin II

TCIII transcobalamin III

TCIMC Trauma Center Information Management Center

TCI$_{pr}$ temporal continuity index for provider

TCI$_{pt}$ temporal continuity index for patients

TCL T-cell leukemia; thermochemiluminescence; total capacity of the lung; transverse carpal ligament

T-CLL T-cell chronic lymphatic leukemia

TC$_{Lo}$ toxic concentration low

TCLP toxicity characteristic leachate procedure [Environmental Protection Agency, EPA]

TCM tissue culture medium; traditional Chinese medicine; transcutaneous monitor

T&CM type and crossmatch

Tc 99m technetium-99m

Tc 99m MDP technetium-99m methylene diphosphonate

TCMA transcortical motor aphasia

TCMI traditional Chinese medicine informatics

TCMP thematic content modification program

TCMZ trichloromethiazide

TCN tetracycline; transcobalamin

T⁻c NM tumor with lymph node metastases

TCNS transcutaneous nerve stimulation/stimulator

TCNV terminal contingent negative variation

TCO transcutaneous oximetry

T$_{CO_2}$ total carbon dioxide

TCP T-complex protein; therapeutic care–psychosocial; therapeutic continuous penicillin; total circulating protein; transcutaneous pacemaker; transcutaneous pacing; transmission control protocol; tranylcypromine; tricalcium phosphate; trichlorophenol; tricresyl phosphate; tumor control probability

TCPA tetrachlorophthalic anhydride

tcPCO₂, tcpCO₂ transcutaneous partial pressure of carbon dioxide

TCPD₅₀ 50% tissue culture protective dose

tcPCO₂, tcPCO₂ transcutaneous carbon dioxide pressure

TCP/IP transmission control protocol/Internet protocol

tcPO₂, tcpO₂ transcutaneous partial pressure of oxygen

tcP₀₂, tcPO₂ transcutaneous oxygen pressure

2,4,5-TCPPA 2-(2,4,5-trichlorophenoxy)-propionic acid

TCPS total cavopulmonary shunt

TCR T-cell reactivity; T-cell receptor; T-cell rosette; thalamocortical relay; total cytoplasmic ribosome; transcriptional control center; transcription-coupled [deoxyribonucleic acid, DNA] repair; trauma center record; true count rate; turn, cough, and rebreathe

TcR T-cell receptor

TCRA T-cell receptor alpha

TCRB T-cell receptor beta

TCRD T-cell receptor delta

TCRG T-cell receptor gamma

tcRNA translational control ribonucleic acid

TCRP total cellular receptor pool

TCRZ T-cell receptor Z

TCRV total red cell volume

TCS T-cell supernatant; tethered cord syndrome; total coronary score; Treacher Collins syndrome

TCSA tetrachlorosalicylanilide

TCSF T-colony-stimulating factor

TCT thrombin clotting time; thyrocalcitonin; trachial cytotoxin; transcardial catheter therapy; transmission computed tomography

Tct tincture

tcTOFA time constrained time-of-flight absorbance

TCU trauma care unit; treatment control unit

TCV thoracic cage volume; three concept view

TCW time coincidence window

TD tabes dorsalis; tardive dyskinesia; T-cell dependent; temporary disability; terminal device; tetanus and diphtheria [toxoid]; tetrodotoxin; thanatophoric dwarfism; thanatophoric dysplasia; therapy discontinued; thermal dilution; thoracic duct; three times per day; threshold of detectability; threshold of discomfort; threshold dose; thymus-dependent; time delay; time dictionary; timed disintegration; tocopherol deficiency; to deliver; tone decay; torsion dystonia; total disability, total discrimination; totally disabled; total dose; Tourette disorder; toxic dose; tracheal diameter; transdermal; transverse diameter; traveler's diarrhea; treatment discontinued; tumor dose; typhoid dysentery

T/D treatment discontinued

T$_D$ the time required to double the number of cells in a given population; thermal death time

Td doubling time; tetanus-diphtheria toxoid

T₄(D) serum thyroxine measured by displacement analysis

TD₅₀ median toxic dose

TDA thyroid-stimulating hormone-displacing antibody

TDB terminologic database; Toxicology Data Bank

T$_{db}$ dry-bulb temperature

TDC taurodeoxycholic acid; total dietary calories

Td-CIA T-cell-derived colony-inhibiting activity

TDCO thermodilution cardiac output [measurement]

TDD telecommunication device for the deaf; tetradecadiene; thoracic duct drainage; total digitalizing dose; toxic doses of drugs; transverse digital deficiency

TDE tetrachlorodiphenylethane; total digestible energy; triethylene glycol diglycidyl

TDF testis-determining factor; thoracic duct fistula; thoracic duct flow; time-dose fractionation; tissue-damaging factor; tumor dose fractionation

TdF thymidine deoxyribose

TDFA testis-determining factor, autosomal

TDFX testis-determining factor X

TDGF teratocarcinoma-derived growth factor

TDH thoracic disc herniation; threonine dehydrogenase

TDI temperature difference integration; three-dimensional interlocking [hip]; time-delay integration; toluene 2,4-diisocyanate; total dose infusion; total dose insulin

TDL tegmental dorsolateral [nucleus]; template definition language; thoracic duct lymph; thymus-dependent lymphocyte; toxic dose level

TDLU terminal ductal lobular unit

TDM therapeutic drug monitoring

TDN total digestible nutrients

tDNA transfer deoxyribonucleic acid

TDNN time-delay neural network

TDO tricho-dento-osseous [syndrome]; tryptophan 2,3-dioxygenase

TDP thermal death point; thoracic duct pressure; thymidine diphosphate; total degradation products

TdP torsades de pointes

TDS temperature, depth, salinity; thiamine disulfide; transduodenal sphincteroplasty

TDSD transient digestive system disorder

TDT terminal deoxynucleotidyltransferase; thermal death time; tone decay test; tumor doubling time

TdT terminal deoxynucleotidyl transferase

TDZ thymus-dependent zone

TE echo-time; expiratory time; tennis elbow; test ear; tetanus; tetracycline; threshold energy; thromboembolism; thymus

epithelium; thyrotoxic exophthalmos; tick-borne encephalitis; time estimation; tissue-equivalent; tonsillectomy; tooth extracted; total estrogen; toxic epidermolysis; *Toxoplasma* encephalitis; trace element; tracheoesophageal; transepithelial; treadmill exercise; trial error

T&E testing and evaluation; trial and error

Te effective half-life; tellurium; tetanic contraction; tetanus

T_E exhalation time; expiratory phase time

TEA temporal external artery; tetraethylammonium; thermal energy analyzer; thromboendarterectomy; total elbow arthroplasty; triethanolamine

TEAB tetraethylammonium bromide

TEAC tetraethylammonium chloride

TEAE triethylammonioethyl

TEAHAT Thrombolysis Early in Acute Heart Attack Trial

TEAM techniques for effective alcohol management; Thrombolytic Trial of Eminase in Acute Myocardial Infarction; Training in Expanded Auxiliary Management; transfemoral endovascular aneurysm management

teasp teaspoon

TEB thoracic electrical bioimpedance

TEBG, TeBG testosterone-estradiol-binding globulin

TEC total electron count; total eosinophil count; total exchange capacity; transient erythroblastopenia of childhood; transluminal extraction catheter; trauma and emergency center

TECBEST Transluminal Extraction Catheter Before Stent [study]

tecMAAP template endonuclear cleavage multiple arbitrary amplicon profiling

TECSAC tele-collaboration for signal analysis in cardiology

TECSS The European Coronary Surgery Study

TECV traumatic epiphyseal coxa vara

TED Tasks of Emotional Development; threshold erythema dose; thromboembolic disease

TEDS anti-embolism stockings

TEE thermic effect of exercise; total energy expenditure; transesophageal echocardiography; tyrosine ethyl ester

TEEP tetraethyl pyrophosphate

TEF thermic effect of food; thyrotroph embryonic factor; tracheoesophageal fistula; transcriptional enhancer factor; trunk extension-flexion [unit]
T$_{eff}$ effective half-life
TEFRA Tax Equity and Fiscal Responsibility Act
TEFS transmural electrical field stimulation
TEG thromboelastogram
TEGDMA tetraethylene glycol dimethacrylate
TEHIP Toxicology and Environmental Health Program
TEIB triethyleneiminobenzoquinone
TEL tetraethyl lead
TEM transmission electron microscope/microscopy; triethylenemelamine
TEMED tetramethylethylenediamine
TEMP temporal concept [UMLS]
temp temperature; temple, temporal
TEMS tactical emergency medical services; Trimetazidine European Multicentre Study
TEN total enteral nutrition; total excretory nitrogen; toxic epidermal necrolysis; transepidermal neurostimulation; Trans-European Network
TENS toxic epidermal necrolysis syndrome; transcutaneous electrical nerve stimulation
TEOAE transient evoked oto-acoustic emissions
TEP tetraethylpyrophosphate; tracheoesophageal puncture; transesophageal pacing
TEPA triethylenephosphamide
TEPP tetraethyl pyrophosphate; triethylene pyrophosphate
TEPR toward an electronic patient record
TER teratogen; total endoplasmic reticulum; transcapillary escape rate
ter rub [Lat. *tere*]; terminal [end of chromosome]; terminal or end; ternary; tertiary; three times; threefold
term terminal
TERT total end range time
tert tertiary
TES thymic epithelial supernatant; toxic epidemic syndrome; *Toxocara canis* excretory/secretory [antigen]; transcutaneous electrical stimulation; transmural electrical stimulation

TeS terminology server
TESA testicular sperm aspiration
TESE testicular sperm extraction
TESPA thiotepa
TESS treatment emergent symptom scale; Tirilazud Efficacy Stroke Study
TEST Timolol, Encainide, Sotalol Trial
TET tetracycline; total ejection time; total exchange thyroxine; treadmill exercise test
Tet tetralogy of Fallot
tet tetanus; tetracycline
tet^r tetracycline resistance
TETD tetraethylthiuram disulfide
TETA triethylenetetramine
tet tox tetanus toxoid
TEV tadpole edema virus; talipes equinovarus
TEWL transepidermal water loss
TEZ transthoracic electric impedance respirogram
TF free thyroxine; tactile fremitus; tail flick [reflex]; temperature factor; term frequency; testicular feminization; tetralogy of Fallot; thymol flocculation; thymus factor; time frequency; tissue-damaging factor; tissue factor; to follow; total flow; transcription factor; transfer factor; transferrin; transformation frequency; transfrontal; tube feeding; tuberculin filtrate; tubular fluid; tuning fork; typhoid fever
t(°F) temperature on the Fahrenheit scale
Tf transferrin
T$_f$ freezing temperature
TFA total fatty acids; transfatty acid; transverse fascicular area; triangular fibrocartilage; trifluoroacetic acid
TFC common form of transferrin; threadable fusion cage
TFCC triangular fibrocartilage complex
TFD time-frequency distribution; Transcriptional Factor Database
TFd dialyzable transfer factor
TFE polytetrafluoroethylene; transcription factor for immunoglobulin heavy chain enhancer
TFF tube-fed food
TFI thoracic fluid index; transient forebrain ischemia
TFIID transcription factor IID
TFJ tibiofemoral joint
TFJA tibiofemoral joint abduction

TFM testicular feminization male; testicular feminization mutation; total fluid movement; transmission electron microscopy

TFMPP 1-(trifluoromethylphenyl)-piperazine

TFN total fecal nitrogen; transferrin

TFO triplex-forming oligonucleotide

TFP tubular fluid plasma

TFPI tissue factor pathway inhibitor

TFPZ trifluoroperazine

TFR time-frequency representation; total fertility rate; total flow resistance; traditional functional retraining; transferrin receptor

TFS testicular feminization syndrome; thyroid function study; tube-fed saline

TFT thin-film transistor; thrombus formation time; thyroid function test; tight filum terminale; trifluorothymidine

TFUN tissue function [UMLS]

TFX toxic effects

TG temperature gradient; tendon graft; testosterone glucuronide; tetraglycine; thioglucose; thioglycolate; thioguanine; thromboglobulin; thyroglobulin; tocogram; total gastrectomy, toxic goiter; transmissible gastroenteritis; treated group; triacylglycerol; trigeminal ganglion; triglyceride; tumor growth

Tg generation time; thyroglobulin; *Toxoplasma gondii;* transglycosylation

T$_g$ glass transition temperature; globe temperature

6-TG thioguanine

tG$_1$ the time required to complete the G$_1$ phase of the cell cycle

tG$_2$ the time required to complete the G$_2$ phase of the cell cycle

TGA taurocholate gelatin agar; thyroglobulin activity; total glycoalkaloids; total gonadotropin activity; transient global amnesia; transposition of great arteries; tumor glycoprotein assay

TgAb thyroglobulin antibody

TGAR total graft area rejected

TGB thromboglobulin beta; tiagabine

tGB triangular Gregory-Bézier [patches]

TGBG dimethylglyoxal bis-guanylhydrazone

TGC time gain compensation

TGD thermal-green dye

TG-DPC temperature gradient deoxyribonucleic acid [DNA] probe chromatography

TGE theoretical growth evaluation; transmissible gastroenteritis; tryptone glucose extract

TGEV transmissible gastroenteritis virus

TGF T-cell growth factor; transforming growth factor; tuboglomerular feedback; tumor growth factor

TG-F transforming growth factor

TGFA transforming growth factor alpha; triglyceride fatty acid

TGFβ transforming growth factor beta

TGG turkey gamma globulin

TGI tracheal gas insufflation

TGL triglyceride; triglyceride lipase

TGN thioguanine nucleotide; trans-Golgi network

TGP tobacco glycoprotein

TGPV total glucose in venous plasma

TgPVR transgenic mice that express human cellular receptor for poliovirus

TGR transgenic rat

6-TGR 6-thioguanine riboside

TGS tincture of green soap

TGs triglycerides

TGT thromboplastin generation test/time; tolbutamide-glucagon test

TGV thoracic gas volume; thoracic great vessel; transposition of great vessels

TGY tryptone glucose yeast [agar]

TGYA tryptone glucose yeast agar

TH tension headache; tetrahydrocortisol; T helper [cell]; theophylline; thorax; thrill; thyrohyoid; thyroid hormone; topical hypothermia; total hysterectomy; triquetrohamate; tyrosine hydrolase; tyrosine hydroxylase

T$_H$, T$_h$, Th T-helper [lymphocyte]; thenar; therapist; therapy; thoracic, thorax; thorium; throat

th thenar; thermie; thoracic; thyroid; transhepatic

THA tacrine; tetrahydroaminoacridine; total hip arthroplasty; total hydroxyapatite; *Treponema* hemagglutination

ThA thoracic aorta

THAL thalassemia

THAM tris(hydroxymethyl)aminomethane

THAMES Tenormin in Hypertension and Myocardial Ischemia Epidemiological Study

THAT Thrombolysis in Myocardial Infarction Trial

THB thrombocyte B; Todd-Hewitt broth; total heart beats

THb total hemoglobin

THBD thrombomodulin

THBI thyroid hormone binding inhibitor

THBP 7,8,9,10-tetrahydrobenzo[a]-pyrene; thyroid hormone binding protein

THBS thrombospondin

THC teen health clinic; tentative human consensus; terpin hydrate and codeine; tetrahydrocannabinol; tetrahydrocortisol; thiocarbanidin; thrombocytopenia; transhepatic cholangiogram; transplantable hepatocellular carcinoma

THCA alpha-trihydroxy-5-beta-cholestannic acid

THD Thomsen disease; transverse heart diameter

Thd ribothymidine

THDOC tetrahydrodeoxycorticosterone

THE tetrahydrocortisone E; tonic hind limb extension; transhepatic embolization; transhiatal esophagectomy; tropical hypereosinophilia

theor theory, theoretical

THER therapeutic procedure [UMLS]

ther therapy, therapeutic; thermometer

therap therapy, therapeutic

Θ Greek capital letter *theta*; thermodynamic temperature

θ Greek lower case letter *theta*; an angular coordinate variable; customary temperature; temperature interval

ther ex therapeutic exercise

therm thermal; thermometer

THF tetrahydrocortisone F; tetrahydrofolate; tetrahydrofolic [acid]; tetrahydrofuran; thymic humoral factor

THFA tetrahydrofolic acid; tetrahydrofurfuryl alcohol

Thg thyroglobulin

THH telangiectasia hereditaria haemorrhagica; trichohyalin

THI transient hypogammaglobulinemia of infancy

Thi thiamine

THIP tetrahydroisoxazolopyridinol

Thio-TEPA thiotriethylenephosphamide

THIS Tissue Plasminogen Activator Heparin Interaction Study

THL trichohyalin

THM total heme mass

thor thorax, thoracic

THO titrated water

Thor thoracic

THORP titanium hollow reconstruction plate

thou thousandth

THP Tamm-Horstall protein; tetrahydropapaveroline; tissue hydrostatic pressure; total hip replacement; total hydroxyproline; transthoracic portography; trihexphenidyl

THPA tetrahydropteric acid

THPP thiamine pyrophosphate; trihydroxy propriophenone

ThPP thiamine pyrophosphate

tHPT tertiary hyperparathyroidism

THPV transhepatic portal vein

THQ tetraquinone

THR targeted heart rate; threonine; thyroid hormone receptor; total hip replacement; transhepatic resistance

Thr thrill; threonine

thr thyroid, thyroidectomy

THRA thyroid hormone receptor alpha

THRF thyrotropic hormone-releasing factor

THRIFT Thromboembolism Risk Factors Study

ThrO thrombotic occlusion

THRM thrombomodulin

throm, thromb thrombosis, thrombus

THS Teebe hypertelorism syndrome; tetrahydro-compound S; thrombohemorrhagic syndrome; Tolosa-Hunt syndrome; Tromsø Heart Study; Turkish Heart Study

THSC totipotent hematopoietic stem cell

THTH thyrotropic hromone

THU tetrahydrouridine

THUG thyroid uptake gradient

THVO terminal hepatic vein obliteration

Thx thromboxane

THY thymosin

Thy thymine

thy thymus, thymectomy

THYB thymosin beta

THz terahertz

TI inversion time; temporal integration; term importance; terminal ileum; thalassemia intermedia; therapeutic index; thoracic index; thymus-independent; time interval; tonic immobility; transischial; translational inhibition; transverse inlet;

tricuspid incompetence; tricuspid insufficiency; tumor induction

T_I inspiration time

Ti titanium; translation imitation

TIA transient ischemic attack; tumor-induced angiogenesis; turbidimetric immunoassay

TIA + CE transient ischemic attack plus carotid endarterectomy

TIAFO toe-inhibiting ankle-foot arthrosis

TIAH total implantation of artificial heart

TIB tibia; time in bed; tumor immunology bank

TIBBS Total Ischaemic Burden Bisoprolol Study

TIBC total iron-binding capacity

TIBET Total Ischemic Burden European Trial

TIBS Trends in Biochemical Sciences

T-IBS T-cell immunoblastic sarcoma

TIC total ion current; Toxicology Information Center; trypsin inhibitory capability; tubulointerstitial cell; tumor-inducing complex

TICC time from cessation of contraception to conception

TICO Thrombolysis in Coronary Occlusion [study]

TICU trauma intensive care unit

TID time interval difference [imaging]; titrated initial dose; trusted image discrimination

TIDA tuberoinfundibular dopaminergic system

TIDE Technology Initiative for Disabled and Elderly People [Europe]

TIDES Transdermal Intermittent Dosing Evaluation Study

TIE transient ischemic episode

TIF tumor-inducing factor; tumor inhibiting factor

TIG Thrombosis Interest Group [study]

TIG, Tig tetanus immunoglobulin

TIGR The Institute for Genome Research

TIH time interval histogram

TIIAP technical information infrastructure assistance program

TIL tumor-infiltrating leukocyte; tumor-infiltrating lymphocyte

TIM transthoracic intracardiac monitoring; Triflusal in Myocardial Infarction [study]; triose phosphate isomerase

TIMAD Ticlodipine in Micro-angiography of Diabetes [study]

TIMC tumor-induced marrow cytotoxicity

TIME Teaching Immunization for Medical Education [study]

TIMED Trials to Investigate Morning vs Evening Dosing [nisoldipine in hypertension]

TIMI thrombolysis in myocardial infarction; transmural inferior myocardial infarction

TIMI IIIA Thrombolysis in Myocardial Ischemia [trial]

TIMI IIIB Thrombolysis in Myocardial Infarction [trial]

TIMI-7 Thrombin Inhibition in Myocardial Ischemia [trial]

TIMI-9 Thrombolysis and Thrombin Inhibition in Myocardial Infarction [trial]

TIMIKO Thrombolysis in Myocardial Infarction in Korea [study]

TIMP tissue inhibitor of metalloproteinases

TIMS Tertatolol International Multicentre Study

TIN tubulointerstitial nephropathy

tinc, tinct tincture

TIOD total iodine organification defect

TINU tubulo-interstitial nephritis-uveitis [syndrome]

TIP telemedicine instrumentation pack; thermal inactivation point; Toxicology Information Program; translation-inhibiting protein; tumor-inhibiting principle

TIPE Thrombolysis in Pulmonary Embolism [study]; Thrombolysis in Peripheral Embolism [study]

TIPI time-insensitive predictive instrument

TIPJ terminal interphalangeal joint

TIPPS tetraiodophenylphthalein sodium

TIPS Transjugular Intrahepatic Portacaval Shunt [study]; transjugular intrahepatic portosystemic shunt

TIPSS transjugular intrahepatic portosystemic stent shunt

TIQ tetrahydroisoquinoline

TIR terminal innervation ratio

TIRES transient infrared emission spectroscopy

TIS tetracycline-induced steatosis; transdermal infusion system; triage illness scale; trypsin-insoluble segment; tumor in situ

TISP total immunoreactive serum pepsinogen

TISS Therapeutic Intervention Scoring System; Ticlodipine Indobufen Stroke Study

TIT *Treponema* immobilization test

TIT, TITh triiodothyronine

TIU trypsin-inhibiting unit

TIUV total intrauterine volume

TIV tomographic image visualization

TIVA total intravenous anesthesia

TIVC thoracic inferior vena cava

TIVT Thrombolysis in Deep Vein Thrombosis [study]

TJ tetrajoule; thigh junction; triceps jerk

TJA total joint arthroplasty

TJR total joint replacement

TK thermokeratoplasty; through knee; thymidine kinase; transketolase; triosekinase; tyrosine kinase

T(°K) absolute temperature on the Kelvin scale

tk thymidine kinase

TKA total knee arthroplasty; transketolase activity; trochanter, knee, ankle

TKase thymidine kinase

TKC torticollis-keloids-cryptorchidism [syndrome]

TKCR torticollis-keloids-cryptorchidism-renal dysplasia [syndrome]

TKD thymidine kinase deficiency; tokodynamometer

TKG tokodynagraph

TKLI tachykinin-like immunoreactivity

TKO to keep open

TKR total knee replacement

TKT transketolase

TL temporal lobe; terminal lumen; thermolabile; thermoluminescence; threat to life; thymus-leukemia [antigen]; thymus lymphocyte; thymus lymphoma; time lapse; time-limited; total lipids; total lung [capacity]; true lumen; tubal ligation

T-L thoracolumbar; thymus-dependent lymphocyte

Tl thallium

TLA thymus leukemia antigen; tissue lactase activity; tongue-to-lip adhesion; translaryngeal aspiration; translumbar aortogram; transluminal angioplasty

TLAA T-lymphocyte-associated antigen

TLam thoracic laminectomy

TLC telephone-linked care; tender loving care; thin-layer chromatography; total L-chain concentration; total lung capacity;

total lung compliance; total lymphocyte count; transverse loop colostomy

TLD thermoluminescent dosimeter; thoracic lymphatic duct; tumor lethal dose

T/LD$_{100}$ minimum dose causing 100% deaths or malformations

TLE temporal lobe epilepsy; thin-layer electrophoresis; total lipid extract

TLI thymidine labeling index; total lymphatic irradiation; trypsin-like immune activity; Tucker-Lewis index

TLL T-cell leukemia or lymphoma; tissue lesion load

TLm median tolerance limit

TLPD thoracolaryngopelvic dysplasia

TLQ total living quotient

TLR tapetal-like reflex; target lesion revascularization; tonic labyrinthine reflex

TLS thoracolumbosacral; Tourette-like syndrome

TLSER theoretical linear solvation energy relationship

TLSO thoracolumboscral orthosis

TLSQL time-line standard query language

TLSSO thoracolumbosacral spinal orthosis

TLT tryptophan load test

TLTP Teaching and Learning Technology Programme [UK]

TLV threshold limit value; tidal liquid ventilation; total lung volume

TLW total lung water

TLX trophoblast-lymphocyte cross-reactivity

TM technology management; tectorial membrane; temperature by mouth; temporalis muscle; temporomandibular; tender midline; tendomyopathy; teres major; thalassemia major; Thayer-Martin [medium]; thrombomodulin; time and materials; time-motion; tobramycin; torus mandibularis; trabecular network; trademark; traditional medicine; transatrial membranotomy; transitional mucosa; transmediastinal; transmembrane; transmetatarsal; transport mechanism; transport medium; transverse myelitis; tropical medicine; tuberculous meningitis; twitch movement; tympanic membrane

T-M Thayer-Martin [medium]

T&M type and crossmatch

Tm temperature; thulium; tubular maximum excretory capacity of kidneys

T$_m$ melting temperature; temperature midpoint; tubular maximum excretory capacity of kidneys

tM the time required to complete the M phase of the cell cycle

tm transport medium; true mean

TMA tetramethylammonium; thrombotic microangiopathy; thyroid microsomal antibody; transcortical mixed aphasia; transcription-mediated amplification; transmetatarsal amputation; trimellitic anhydride; trimethoxyamphetamine; trimethoxyphenyl aminopropane; trimethylamine

TMACl tetramethylammonium chloride

TMAH trimethylphenylammonium (anilinium) hydroxide

TMAI trimethylphenylammonium (anilinium) iodide

TMAO trimethylamine *N*-oxide

TMAS Taylor Manifest Anxiety Scale

T$_{max}$ maximum threshold; time of maximum concentration

TMB transient monocular blindness

TMBA trimethoxybenzaldehyde

TMBF transmural blood flow

TMBJ thermoplastic Minerva body jacket

TMC transmyocardial mechanical channeling; triamcinolone and terramycin capsules

TMD temporomandibular disorder; transient myeloproliferative disease; transmembrane domain; trimethadione

t-MDS therapy-related myelodysplastic syndrome

TME total metabolizable energy; transmissible mink encephalopathy; transmural enteritis

TMEP telangiectasia macularis eruptiva perstans

TMET treadmill exercise test

TMF transformed mink fibroblast; transmitral flow

TM$_g$ maximum tubular reabsorption rate for glucose

TMH tetramethylammonium hydroxide

TM-HSA trimellityl-human serum albumin

TMI testing motor impairment; threatened myocardial infarction; transmural myocardial infarction

TMIC Toxic Materials Information Center

TMIF tumor-cell migratory inhibition factor

TMIS Technicon Medical Information System

TMJ temporomandibular joint; trapeziometacarpal joint

TMJS temporomandibular joint syndrome

TMK thymidylate kinase

TML terminal midline; terminal motor latency; tetramethyl lead

TMLR transmyocardial laser revascularization

TMN thin membrane nephropathy; tumor, metastases and nodes

TMNST tethered median nerve stress test

TMP thiamine monophosphate; thymidine monophosphate; thymidine-5′-monophosphate; thymolphthalein monophosphate; transmembrane potential; transmembrane pressure; trimethaphan; trimethoprim; trimethylpsoralen

TM$_{PAH}$ maximum tubular excretory capacity for para-aminohippuric acid

TMPD tetramethyl-p-phenylinediamine

TMPDS temporomandibular pain and dysfunction syndrome; thiamine monophosphate disulfide

TMP-SMX trimethoprim-sulfamethoxazole

TMR the medical record; tissue maximum ratio; topical magnetic resonance; trainable mentally retarded; transmyocardial revascularization

TMRM tetramethylrhodamine

TMS thalium myocardial scintigraphy; The Muscatine Study; thread mate system; thymidilate synthase; total morbidity score; trapezoidocephaly-multiple synostosis [syndrome]; trimethylsilane

TMST treadmill stem test

TMT tarsometatarsal; thiol methyltransferase; Trail-Making Test; trimethyllin

TMTD tetramethylthiuram disulfide

TMTJ tarsometatarsal joint

TMTX trimetrexate

TMU tetramethyl urea

TMV tobacco mosaic virus

TMX tamoxifen

TMZ transformation zone

TN talonavicular; tarsonavicular; team nursing; temperature normal; tenascin; test negative; trigeminal nucleus; total negatives; trigeminal neuralgia; trochlear nucleus; true negative

T/N tar and nicotine
T₄N normal serum thyroxine
Tn normal intraocular tension; transposon
TNA total nutrient admixture
TNB transnasal butorphanol
TNBP tri-n-butyl phosphate
TND term normal delivery
t-NE total norepinephrine
TNEE titrated norepinephrine excretion
TNF true negative fraction; tumor necrosis factor
TNFA tumor necrosis factor alpha
TNFAIP tumor necrosis factor, alpha-induced protein
TNFAR tumor necrosis factor alpha receptor
TNFB tumor necrosis factor beta
TNFBR tumor necrosis factor beta receptor
TNFR1 tumor necrosis factor type 1 receptor
TNG trinitroglycerin
tng tongue
tNGF truncated nerve growth factor
TNH teaching nursing home; transient neonatal hyperammonemia
T-NHL T-cell-derived non-Hodgkin leukemia
TNHP teaching nursing home program
TNI total nodal irradiation
TNM primary tumor, regional nodes, metastasis [tumor staging]; thyroid node metastases; tumor node metastasis
TNMR tritium nuclear magnetic resonance
TNP total net positive; trinitrophenyl
TNPACK truncated Newton program package
TNR tonic neck reflex; true negative rate
TNS total nuclear score; transcutaneous nerve stimulation; tumor necrosis serum
TNT tetranitroblue tetrazolium; Transderm-Nitro Trial; 2,4,6-trinitrotoluene
TnT troponin T
TNTC too numerous to count
TNV tobacco necrosis virus
TO old tuberculin; oral temperature; original tuberculin; target organ; telephone order; thoracic orthosis; thromboangiitis obliterans; thrombotic occlusion; tincture of opium; total obstruction; tracheoesophageal; treatment object; tubo-ovarian; turnover
T(O) oral temperature

TO₂ oxygen transport
T₀ tricuspid opening
to tincture of opium
TOA total quality assessment; tubo-ovarian abscess
TOAP thioguanine, oncovin, cytosine arabinoside, and prednisone
TOAST Treatment of Acute Stroke Trial; Trial of Org 10172 in Acute Stroke Trial
TOAT The Open Artery Trial
TOB tobramycin
TOBEC total body electrical conductivity [test]
TobRV tobacco ringspot virus
TOC total organic carbon
TOCC Total Occlusion of Coronary Arteries, Chronic [study]
TOCP tri-o-cresyl phosphate
TOCSY total correlation spectroscopy
TOD right eye tension [Lat. *oculus dexter*]; target organ disease; Time-Oriented Data [Bank]; titanium optimized design [plate]
TOD/CCD target organ disease/clinical cardiovascular disease
TODS toxic organic dust syndrome
TOE tender on examination; tracheoesophageal; transesophageal echography; transferred nuclear Overhauser effect
TOEFL Test of English as a Foreign Language [for foreign medical graduates]
TOES toxic oil epidemic syndrome
TOF tetralogy of Fallot; time-of-flight; train of four [monitor]; tracheo[o]esophageal fistula
TOFA time-of-flight absorbance; time-of-flight and abstinence [imaging]
T of F tetralogy of Fallot
TOFHLA test of functional health literacy in adults
TOFMS time-of-flight mass spectrometry
TOFS total organ failure score
TOH transient osteoporosis of hip; tower of Hanoi [neurophysiological test]
TOHP Trial of Hypertension Prevention
TOL trial of labor
tol tolerance, tolerated
TOLB, tolb tolbutamine
TOLC Treatment of Low-density Lipoprotein-bound Cholesterol [study]
TOLD top-level driver
TOM toxic oxygen metabolite
TOMA tri-octylmethylammonium chloride

TOMAS torsional ocular movement analysis system

TOMHS Treatment of Mild Hypertension Study

TOMIIS Total Occlusion Postmyocardial Infarction Intervention Study

Tomo tomography, tomogram

tomos tomograms

TOMS The Oklahoma Marker Study

TON traumatic optic neuropathy

TONE tilted optimized nonsaturating excitation; Trial of Nonpharmacologic Interventions in the Elderly

tonoc tonight

TOP termination of pregnancy; Thrombolysis in Old Patients [study]; topoisomerase

top topical

TOPAS Thrombolysis or Peripheral Arterial Surgery [study]

TOPCAD topical prevention or conception and disease

TOPLIT Transluminal Extraction Catheter or Percutaneous Transluminal Coronary Angioplasty in Thrombus [study]

TOPS Take Off Pounds Sensibly [program]; Thrombolysis in Old Patients Study; Treatment of Post-thrombolytic Stenosis [study]

TOPV trivalent oral poliovaccine

TORCH toxoplasmosis, other [congenital syphilis and viruses], rubella, cytomegalovirus, and herpes simplex virus

TORCHS toxoplasmosis and other diseases: rubella, cytomegalovirus infections, herpes simplex, syphilis

TORP total ossicular replacement prosthesis

torr mm Hg pressure

TOS thoracic outlet syndrome; toxic oil syndrome

TOSCA Total Occlusion Study in Canada

TOT The Oslo Trial; total operating time

TOTAL Total Occlusion Trial with Angioplasty by Using Laser Guidewire

TOV trial of voiding

TOVA trigger of ventricular arrhythmia

TOWARD Toyama Warfarin Rational Dosage [study]

tox toxicity, toxic

TOXICON Toxicology Conversational Online Network [NLM database]

TOXLINE Toxicology Information On-Line [NLM database]

TOXLIT Toxicology Literature [NLM database]

TOXNET Toxicology Data Network [NLM database]

TP temperature and pressure; temperature probe; template; temporal peak; temporoparietal; tension pneumothorax; terminal phalanx; terminal protein; testosterone propionate; thick padding; thin-plate; threshold potential; thrombocytopenic purpura; thrombophlebitis; thromboxane prostaglandin; thymopentin; thymopoietin; thymus polypeptide; thymus protein; torsades de pointes; torus palatinus; total positives; total protein; transaction processing; transforming principle; transition point; transverse polarization; transverse process; treatment progress; *Treponema pallidum*; triazolophthalazine; trigger point; triphosphate; true positive; tryptophan; tryptophan pyrrolase; tube precipitin; tuberculin precipitate; tumor protein

6-TP 6-thiopurine

T&P temperature and pressure; temperature and pulse

T+P temperature and pulse

Tp primary transmission; time of preparation; *Treponema pallidum;* tryptophan

T$_p$ physical half-life

TPA tannic acid, polyphosphomolybdic acid, and amino acid; 12-0-tetradecanoylphorbol-13-acetate; third-party adnistrator; tissue plasminogen activator; total parenteral alimentation; *Treponema pallidum* agglutination; tumor polypeptide antigen

t-PA tissue plasminogen activator

TPAI tissue plasminogen activator inhibitor

TPase thymidine phosphorylase

TPASK Tissue Plasminogen Activator vs Streptokinase [trial]

TPAT Tissue Plasminogen Activator, Toronto Trial

TPB tetraphenyl borate; tryptone phosphate broth

TPBF total pulmonary blood flow

TPBG trophoblast glycoprotein

TPBS three-phase radionuclide bone scanning

TPC thromboplastic plasma component; thyroid papillary carcinoma; total patient care; total plasma catecholamines; total plasma cholesterol; *Treponema pallidum* complement

TPCF *Treponema pallidum* complement fixation

TPCV total packed cell volume

TPD temporary partial disability; thiamine propyl disulfide; tripotassium phenolphthalein disulfate; tumor-producing dose

TP-DNA template deoxyribonucleic acid [DNA]

TPDS tropical pancreatic diabetes syndrome

TPE therapeutic plasma exchange; totally protected environment; typhoid-parathyroid enteritis

T^{Pe} expiratory pause time

T$_{peak}$ time-to-peak

TPEY tellurite polymyxin egg yolk [agar]

TPF thymus permeability factor; thymus to peak flow; true positive fraction

TPG transmembrane potential gradient; transplacental gradient; transpulmonary gradient; tryptophan peptone glucose [broth]

TPGS E-alpha-tocopheryl polyethylene glycol succinate; Talairach Proportional Grid System

TPGYT trypticase-peptone-glucose-yeast extract-trypsin [medium]

TPH transplacental hemorrhage; tryptophan hydroxylase

TpH tryptophane hydroxylase

TPHA *Treponema pallidum* hemagglutination

TPHU Tropical Public Health Unit [Australia]

TPI Thrombolytic Predictive Instrument [project]; time period integrator; treponemal immobilization test; *Treponema pallidum* immobilization; triose phosphate isomerase

T^{Pi} inspiratory pause time

TPIA *Treponema pallidum* immune adherence

TPIIA time of postexpiratory inspiratory activity

TPK tyrosine protein kinase

TPL third party liability; titanium proximal loading; tumor progression locus; tyrosine phenol-lyase

tpl transplantation, transplanted

TPLV transient pulmonary vascular lability

TPM temporary pacemaker; thrombophlebitis migrans; topiramate; total particulate matter; total passive motion; triphenylmethane; tropomyosin

TPMT thiopurine methyltransferase

TPN thalamic projection neuron; total parenteral nutrition; transition protein; triphosphopyridine nucleotide

TPNH reduced triphosphopyridine nucleotide

TPO thrombopoietin; thyroid peroxidase; tryptophan peroxidase

Tpo thrombopoietin

TPP tetraphenylporphyrin; thiamine pyrophosphate; transpulmonary pressure; treadmill performance test; tripeptidyl peptidase; triphenyl phosphite

TPPase thiamine pyrophosphatase

TPPD thoracic-pelvic-phalangeal dystrophy

TPPI time proportional phase incrementation

TPPN total peripheral parenteral nutrition

TPQ Threshold Planning Quantity

TPR temperature, pulse, and respiration; testosterone production rate; tetraricopeptide repeat; third party reimbursement; total peripheral resistance; total pulmonary resistance; true positive rate; tumor potentiating region; true positive rate

TPRI total peripheral resistance index

TPS time to peak shortening; trypsin; tryptase; tumor polysaccharide substance

TPSE 2-(p-triphenyl)sulfonylethanol

TPST true positive stress test; tyrosyl protein sulfotransferase

TPT tetraphenyl tetrazolium; Thrombosis Prevention Trial; topotecan; total protein tuberculin; triphalangeal thumb; typhoid-paratyphoid [vaccine]

TPTE 2-(p-triphenyl)thioethanol

TPTX thyro-parathyroidectomized

TPTZ tripyridyltriazine

TPV tetanus-pertussis vaccine; tipranavir

TPVR total peripheral vascular resistance; total pulmonary vascular resistance

TPVS transhepatic portal venous sampling

TPX testis-specific protein

TPZ thioproperazine

TQ tocopherolquinone; tourniquet

TQFCOSY triple-quantum filtered correlated spectroscopy

TQM total quality management

TR recovery time; rectal temperature; repetition time; residual tuberculin; terminal repeat; tetrazolium reduction; therapeutic radiology; therapeutic ratio; therapeutic recreation; thrombin receptor; thyroid [hormone] receptor; time release; time to relengthening; total resistance; total response; trachea; transfusion reaction; transmission rate; transrectal; tricuspid regurgitation; Trinder reagent; tuberculin R [new tuberculin]; tuberculin residue; turbidity-reducing; turnover ratio

T&R treated and released

T(°R) absolute temperature on the Rankine scale

TR_{90} time to 90 percent relengthening

Tr trace; tragion; transferrin; trypsin

T_r radiologic half-life; retention time

tr tincture; trace; traction; transaldolase; trauma, traumatic; tremor; triradial

TRA total renin activity; tumor-resistant antigen

tra transfer

TRAb thyrotoxin receptor antibody

TRABS thiobarbituric reactive substance

TRAC tool for referral assessment of continuity [of health]

trac traction

TRACE Trandolapril Cardiac Evaluation [trial]

trach trachea, tracheal, tracheostomy

TRAJ time repetitive ankle jerk

TRALT transfusion-related acute lung injury

TRAM transport remote acquisition monitor; transverse rectus abdominis muscle; Treatment Rating Assessment Matrix; Treatment Response Assessment Method; trisaminomethane

TRAMPE tricho-rhino-auriculophalangeal multiple exostoses

TRANDA Trandolapril Andalusian Study

trans transfer; transference; transverse

trans D transverse diameter

TRANSFAIR Transfatty Acids in Food in Europe [study]

transm transmitted, transmission

transpl transplantation, transplanted

TRAP carpal tunnel syndrome, Raynaud phenomenon, aching muscles, proximal muscle weakness [rheumatic disorders associated with hypothyroidism]; tartrate-resistant acid phosphatase; transport and rapid accessioning for additional procedures; triiodothyronine receptor auxiliary protein; Twin Reversed Arterial Perfusion [study]

trap trapezius

TRAPIST Trapadil vs Placebo to Prevent In-Stent Intimal Hyperplasia [study]

TRAS transplanted renal artery stenosis

TRASHES tuberculosis, radiotherapy, ankylosing spondylitis, histoplasmosis, extrinsic allergic alveolitis, silicosis [chest x-ray findings]

traum trauma, traumatic

TRB terbutalone; tropanyl benzylate

TRBF total renal blood flow

TRC tanned red cell; therapeutic residential center; total renin concentration; total respiratory conductance; total ridge count

TRCA tanned red cell agglutination

TRCF transcription repair coupling factor

TRCH tanned red cell hemagglutination

TRCHI tanned red cell hemagglutination inhibition

TRCV total red cell volume

TRD tongue-retaining device

TRDN transient respiratory distress of the newborn

TRE target registration error; thymic reticuloendothelial; thyroid hormone response; triplet rapid expansion; true radiation emission

TREA triethanolamine

TREAT Tranilast Restenosis Following Angioplasty Trial

treat treatment

TREND Trial on Reversing Endothelial Dysfunction

Trend Trendelenburg [position]

TRENT Trial of Early Nifedipine Treatment of Acute Myocardial Infarction

Trep Treponema

TRF targeted ribonucleic acid [RNA] fingerprinting; T-cell replacing factor; thyrotropin-releasing factor; tubular rejection fraction

TRFC total rosette-forming cell

TRG T-cell rearranging gene; transfer ribonucleic acid glycine

TRH tension-reducing hypothesis; thyrotropin-releasing hormone

TRHR thyrotropin-releasing hormone receptor

TRH-ST thyrotropin-releasing hormone stimulation test

TRI tetrazolium reduction inhibition; Thyroid Research Institute; total response index; Toxic Chemical Release Inventory (NLM database); tubuloreticular inclusion

tri tricentric

T$_3$RIA, T$_3$(RIA) triiodothyronine radioimmunoassay

T$_4$RIA, T$_4$(RIA) thyroxine radioimmunoassay

TRIAC 3,5,3'-triiodothyroacetic acid

TRIC Thrombolysis with Recombinant Tissue Plasminogen Activator During Instability in Coronary Artery Disease [trial]; trachoma inclusion conjunctivitis [organism]

TRICB trichlorobiphenyl

Trich Trichomonas

TRIFACTS Toxic Chemical Release Inventory Facts

trig trigger; triglycerides; trigonum

TRIM Thrombin Inhibition in Myocardial Ischemia [study]

TRIMIS Tri-Service Medical Information Systems [Department of Defense]

TRIMM Triggers and Mechanisms of Myocardial Infarction [study]

TRINS totally reversible ischemic neurological symptoms

TRIS tris-(hydroxymethyl)-aminomethane

TRISS trauma and injury severity score

TRIT triiodothyronine

trit triturate

TRITC tetrahodamine isothiocyanate

TRK transketolase; throsine kinase

TRL transfer ribonucleic acid leucine

TRLP triglyceride-rich lipoprotein

TRM traditional medicines

TRMA thiamine-responsive megaloblastic anemia

TRMC trimethylrhodamino-isothiocyanate

TRMI transfer ribonucleic acid initiator methionine

TRML, Trml terminal

TRM-SMX trimethoprim-sulfamethoxazole

TRN tegmental reticular nucleus

tRNA transfer ribonucleic acid

tRNA GLU transfer ribonucleic acid glutamic acid

tRNA-i(met) transfer ribonucleic acid initiator methionine

tRNA-SER transfer ribonucleic acid serine

TRNG tetracycline-resistant *Neisseria gonorrhoae*

TRNOE transfer nuclear Overhauser effect

TRNS transfer ribonucleic acid serine

TRO tissue reflectance oximetry

Troch trochanter

TROM torque range of motion

Trop tropical

TROPCAB total revascularization off pump by coronary artery bypass

TROPHY Treatment Effects of Lisinopril vs Hydrochlorothiazide in Obese Patients with Hypertension [trial]; Treatment of Obese Patients with Hypertension [trial]; Trial of Preventing Hypertension

TRP total refractory period; transfer ribonucleic acid proline; trichorhinophalangeal [syndrome]; tubular reabsorption of phosphate; tyrosine-related protein

Trp tryptophan

TRPA tryptophan-rich prealbumin

TrPl treatment plan

TRPM testosterone-repressed prostate message

TRPO tryptophan oxygenase

TRPS trichorhinophalangeal syndrome

TRPT theoretical renal phosphorus threshold

TRR temporal representation and reasoning; total respiratory resistance

TRS testicular regression syndrome; total reducing sugars; tubuloreticular structure

TrS trauma surgery

TRST triage risk screening tool

TRSV tobacco ringspot virus

TRT thoracic radiotherapy; transfer ribonucleic acid threonine

TR/TE repetition time/echo time

T-RTS triage-revised trauma score

TRU task-related unit; turbidity-reducing unit

T$_3$RU triiodothyronine resin uptake

TRUS transrectal ultrasonography

TRUSP transrectal ultrasonography of prostate

TRUST Trial in United Kingdom for Stroke Treatment

TRV tobacco rattle virus

TRVV total right ventricular volume

Tryp tryptophan
TRX thioredoxin
trx traction
TS Takayasu syndrome; Tay-Sachs; temperature sensitivity; temperature sensor; temperature, skin; temporal stem; tensile strength; test solution; thermal stability; thoracic surgery; thymidylate synthetase; tissue space; total solids [in urine]; Tourette syndrome; toxic substance; toxic syndrome; tracheal sound; transferrin saturation; transitional sleep; transsexual; transverse section; transverse sinus; trauma score; treadmill score; triceps surae; tricuspid stenosis; triple strength; tropical sprue; Troyer syndrome; trypticase soy [plate]; T suppressor [cell]; tuberous sclerosis; tumor-specific; Turner syndrome; type-specific
T/S transverse section
T+S type and screen
Ts skin temperature; tosylate
T$_s$ T-cell suppressor; T suppressor [cell]
tS time required to complete the S phase of the cell cycle
ts temperature sensitivity
ts, tsp teaspoon
TSA technical surgical assistance; time series analysis; toluene sulfonic acid; total shoulder arthroplasty; total solute absorption; toxic shock antigen; transcortical sensory aphasia; trypticase-soy agar; tumor-specific antigen; tumor surface antigen; type-specific antibody
T$_4$SA thyroxine-specific activity
TSAb thyroid-stimulating antibody
TSAP toxic-shock-associated protein
TSAS total severity assessment score
TSAT tube slide agglutination test
TSB total serum bilirubin; trypticase soy broth; tryptone soy broth
TSBA total serum bile acids
TSBB transtracheal selective bronchial brushing
TSC technetium sulfur colloid; thiosemicarbazide; transient spontaneous circulation; transverse spinal sclerosis; tuberous sclerosis complex
TSCA Toxic Substances Control Act
TSCOHS Tri-Service Comprehensive Oral Health Survey
TSCS Tennessee Self-Concept Scale

TSD target-skin distance; Tay-Sachs disease; theory of signal detectability
TSE testicular self-examination; tissue-specific extinguisher; total skin examination; transmissible spongiform encephalopathy; trisodium edetate
TSEB total skin electron beam
T sect transverse section
TSEM transmission scanning electron microscopy
TSES Target Symptom Evaluation Scale
T-set tracheotomy set
TSF testicular feminization syndrome; thrombopoiesis-stimulating factor; total systemic flow; triceps skinfold
TSG tumor suppressor gene
TSG, TSGP tumor-specific glycoprotein
TSGE temperature sweep gel electrophoresis
TSH thyroid-stimulating hormone; transient synovitis of the hip
TSHA thyroid-stimulating hormone, alpha chain
TSHB thyroid-stimulating hormone, beta chain
TSHR thyroid-stimulating hormone receptor
TSH-RF thyroid-stimulating hormone-releasing factor
TSH-RH thyroid-stimulating hormone-releasing hormone
TSHW Thyroid Study in Healthy Women
TSI thyroid stimulating immunoglobulin; triple sugar iron [agar]
TSIA total small intestine allotransplantation; triple sugar iron agar
tSIDS totally unexplained sudden infant death syndrome
TSL task specification language; terminal sensory latency
TSM type-specific M protein
TSMDB Tuberous Sclerosis Mutation Database
TSO transient spastic occlusion; trans-stilbene oxide
TSOP time from symptom onset to presentation
TSP testis-specific protein; thrombin-sensitive protein; thrombospondin; total serum protein; total suspended particulate; trisodium phosphate; tropical spastic paraparesis
tsp teaspoon

TSPA thiotepa

TSPAP total serum prostatic acid phosphatase

TSPL transplant

TSPP tetrasodium pyrophosphate

TSR theophylline sustained release; thyroid to serum ratio; total systemic resistance

TSS toxic shock syndrome; tropical splenomegaly syndrome

TSSA tumor-specific cell surface antigen

TSSE toxic shock syndrome exotoxin

TSST toxic shock syndrome toxin

TST thiosulfate sulfur-transferase; thromboplastin screening test; total sleep time; transforming sequence, thyroid; treadmill stress test; triceps skinfold thickness; tricipital skinfold thickness; tumor skin test

TSTA toxoplasmin skin test antigen; tumor-specific tissue antigen; tumor-specific transplantation antigen

TSU triple sugar urea [agar]

TSV total stomach volume

TSVR total systemic vascular resistance

TSWT tree-structured wavelet transform

TSY trypticase soy yeast

TT tablet triturate; tactile tension; tendon transfer; test tube; testicular torsion; tetanus toxin; tetanus toxoid; tetrathionate; tetrazol; therapeutic touch; thrombin time; thrombolytic therapy; thymol turbidity; tibial tubercle; tick typhus; tilt table; tiny T [antigen]; tolerance test; total thyroxine; total time; transient tachypnea; transferred to; transit time; transthoracic; transtracheal; treadmill test; tuberculin test; tuberculoid [in Ridley-Jopling Hansen disease classification]; tube thoracostomy; tumor thrombus; turnover time

T&T time and temperature; touch and tone

TT₂ total diiodothyronine

TT₃ total triiodothyronine

TT₄ total thyroxine

TTA tetanus toxoid antibody; timed therapeutic absence; total toe arthroplasty; transtracheal aspiration

TTAP threaded titanium acetabular prosthesis

TTATTS Thrombolytic Therapy in Acute Thrombotic/Thromboembolic Stroke [study]

TTB third trimester bleeding

TTC triphenyltetrazolium chloride; T-tube cholangiogram

TTD temporary total disability; tissue tolerance dose; transfusion-transmitted disease; transient tic disorder; transverse thoracic diameter; trichothiodystrophy

TTE transthoracic echocardiography

TTF thyroid transcription factor

TTFD tetrahydrofurfuryldisulfide

TTG T-cell translocation gene; telethermography; tellurite, taurocholate, and gelatin

TTGA tellurite, taurocholate, and gelatin agar

TTH thyrotropic hormone; tritiated thymidine

TTI tension-time index; time-temperature indicator; time-tension index; time-to-intubation; torque-time interval; transtracheal insufflation

TTIdi tension time index diaphragm

TTIM T-cell tumor invasion and metastasis

T-TIME tourniquet time

TTL total thymus lymphocytes; training test lung; transistor-transistor logic

TTLC true total lung capacity

TTLD terminal transverse limb defect

TTN titin; transient tachypnea of the newborn

TTNA transthoracic needle aspiration

TTNB transthoracic needle biopsy

TTO time trade-off [method]

TTOPP Thrombolytic Therapy in Older Patient Population [study]

TTP thiamine triphosphate; thrombotic thrombocytopenic purpura; thymidine triphosphate; time to peak; tocopherol transfer protein; tristetraprolin

TTPA triethylene thiophosphoramide

TTR transthoracic resistance; transthyretin; triceps tendon reflex

TTS tarsal tunnel syndrome; temporary threshold shift; The Tromsø Study; through the scope; through the skin; tilt table standing; transdermal therapeutic system; twin transfusion syndrome

TTT thymol turbidity test; tolbutamide tolerance test; total twitch time; tuberculin tine test

TTTT test tube turbidity test; Tokyo Trop-T Trial

TTV tracheal transport velocity; transfusion-transmitted virus

TTVS Transfusion Transmitted Viruses Study

TTWB toe touch weightbearing

TTX tetrodotoxin

TU thiouracil; thyroid uptake; Todd unit; toxin unit; transmission unit; transurethral; tuberculin unit; turbidity unit

T$_3$U triiodothyronine uptake

TUB tubulin

TUBA tubulin alpha

TUBAL tubulin alpha-like

TUBB tubulin beta

tuberc tuberculosis

TUBG tubulin gamma

TUBS traumatic unidirectional Bankart surgical

TUCC Tissue Plasminogen Activator/Urokinase Comparison in China [study]

TUD total urethral discharge

TUG total urinary gonadotropin

TUGMI Tsukuba University Group for Myocardial Infarction

TUGSE traumatic ulcerative granuloma with stromal eosinophilia

TUI transurethral incision

TUL tumescent ultrasound liposculpture

TULIP transurethral ultrasound-guided laser-induced prostatectomy

TUN total urinary nitrogen

TUR transurethral resection

TURB, TURBT transurethral resection of bladder [tumor]

turb turbidity, turbid

truboFLASH turbo fast low angle shot

TURP transurethral resection of the prostate

TURS transurethral resection syndrome

TURV transurethral resection of valves

TUS trauma ultrasound

TUTase terminal urydilate transferase

TV talipes varus; television; tetrazolium violet; thoracic vertebra; tickborne virus; tidal volume; total volume; toxic vertigo; transvaginal; transvenous; transverse; trial visit; *Trichomonas vaginalis*; tricuspid valve; trivalent; true vertebra; truncal vagotomy; tuberculin volutin; tubovesicular typhoid vaccine

Tv Trichomonas vaginalis

TVA truncal vagotomy and antrectomy

TVC timed vital capacity; total viable cells; total volume capacity; transvaginal cone; triple voiding cystogram; true vocal cords

TVCV transvenous cardioversion

TVD transmissible virus dementia; triple vessel disease

TVF tactile vocal fremitus

TVFD time-varying frequency dependence

TVG time-varied gain

TVH total vaginal hysterectomy; turkey virus hepatitis

TVI time-velocity integral

TVL tenth value layer; tunica vasculosa lentis

TVMF time varying magnetic field

TVP tensor veli palatini [muscle]; textured vegetable protein; transvenous pacemaker; tricuspid valve prolapse; truncal vagotomy and pyloroplasty

TVR target vessel revascularization; tonic vibratory reflex; total vascular resistance; tricuspid valve replacement

TVRE transvaginal resection or endometrium

TVS transvesical sonography

TVSS transient voltage surge suppressor

TVT tension-free vaginal tape; transmissible venereal tumor; tunica vaginalis testis

TVU total volume of the urine

TW tap water; terminal web; test weight; thyroid weight; total body water; travelling wave

Tw twist

TWA time weighted average

T$_{wb}$ wet-bulb temperature

TWBC total white blood cells; total white blood count

TWD total white and differential [cell count]; travelling-wave dielectrophoresis

TWE tap water enema; tepid water enema

TWIST time without symptoms of disease and subjective toxic effects of treatment

TWISTER Trial of Within Stent Treatment of Endoluminal Restenosis

TWL transepidermal water loss

TWS tranquilizer withdrawal syndrome

TWs triphasic waves

TWT total waiting time

TWWD tap water wet dressing

TX a derivative of contagious tuberculin; tamoxifen; thromboxane; thyroidectomized; transplantation; treatment

T&X type and crossmatch

6TX 6-thioxanthine

Tx transplant or transplantation
Tx, T$_x$ treatment; therapy, traction
tx traction
TXA, TxA thromboxane A
TXA2, TXA$_2$ thromboxane A2 (A$_2$)
TXB2, TXB$_2$ thromboxane B2 (B$_2$)
TXDS qualifying toxic dose
TXN thioredoxin
Ty type, typhoid; tyrosine
TYH tyrosine hydrolase
Tymp tympanum, tympanic

TYMS thymidylate synthetase
TYMV turnip yellow mosaic virus
Ty-neg tyrosinase negative
Ty-pos tyrosinase positive
Tyr tyrosine
TyRIA thyroid radioisotope assay
TYRL tyrosinase-like
TYRP tyrosine-related protein
TZ zymoplastic tuberculin [the dried residue which is soluble in alcohol] [Ger. *Tuberculin zymoplastische*]

U congenital limb absence; in electrocardiography, an undulating deflection that follows the T wave; internal energy; International Unit of enzyme activity; Mann-Whitney rank sum statistic; potential difference (in volts); ulcer; ulna; ultralente [insulin]; umbilicus; uncertain; unerupted; unit; universial application [residency]; unknown; unsharpness; upper; uracil; uranium; urea; urethra; uridine; uridylic acid; urinary concentration; urine; urology; uterus; uvula; volume velocity

u unified atomic mass unit; velocity

U/2 upper half

U/3 upper third

UA absorption unsharpness; ultra-audible; ultrasonic arteriography; umbilical artery; unauthorized absence; unicystic ameloblastoma, unit of analysis; unstable angina; upper airways; upper arm; uric acid; uridylic acid; urinalysis; urinary aldosterone; uronic acid; uterine activity; uterine aspiration

U/A urinalysis; uric acid

ua urinalysis

UAC umbilical artery catheter; unusual-appearing child

UA/C uric acid/creatinine [ratio]

U-AMY urinary amylase

UAE unilateral absence of excretion; urine albumin excretion

UAEM University Association for Emergency Medicine

UAGA Uniform Anatomical Gift Act

UAI uterine activity interval

UAI-C unprotected anal intercourse with casual partners

UAL ultrasound-assisted liposuction

UAN uric acid nitrogen

UAO upper airway obstruction

UAP unlicensed assistive personnel; unstable angina pectoris; urinary acid phosphatase; urinary alkaline phosphatase

UAPA unilateral absence of pulmonary artery

UAR upper airway resistance; uric acid riboside

UAS upper abdomen surgery; upstream activating sequence; upstream activation site

UAU uterine activity unit

UB ultimobranchial body; Unna boot; upper back; urinary bladder

UB 82 universal billing document [1982]

UBA undenatured bacterial antigen; ureidoisobutyric acid

UBB ubiquitin B

UBBC unsaturated vitamin B12 binding capacity

UBC ubuquitin C; University of British Columbia [brace]

UBE ubiquitin-activating enzyme

UBF uterine blood flow

UBG, Ubg urobilinogen

UBI ultraviolet blood irradiation

UBL undifferentiated B-cell lymphoma

UBM ultrasound biomicroscopy

UBN urobilin

UBO unidentified bright object

UBP ureteral back pressure

UBS unidentified bright signal

UBW usual body weight

UC ulcerative colitis; ultracentrifugal; umbilical cord; unchanged; unclassifiable; unconscious; undifferentiated cells; unit clerk; unsatisfactory condition; untreated cells; urea clearance; urethral catheterization; urinary catheter; urinary catheterization; urine concentrate; urine culture; uterine contractions

U&C urethral and cervical; usual and customary

UCAID University Corporation for Advanced Internet Development

UCARE, U-CARE Unexplained Cardiac Arrest Registry of Europe

UCB unconjugated bilirubin

UCBC umbilical cord blood culture

UCD urine collection device; usual childhood diseases

UCDS uniform clinical data set

UCE urea cycle enzymopathy

UCG ultrasonic cardiography; urinary chorionic gonadotropin

UCHD usual childhood diseases

UCI unusual childhood illness; urethral catheter in; urinary catheter in

UCL ulnar collateral ligament; upper collateral ligament; upper confidence limit; upper control limit; urea clearance

UCLP unilateral cleft of lip and palate

UCO ultrasonic cardiac output; urethral catheter out; urinary catheter out

UCOD underlying cause of death

UCP uncoupling protein; urinary coproporphyrin; urinary C-peptide

UCPT urinary coproporphyrin test

UCR unconditioned response; usual, customary, and reasonable [fees]

U$_{Cr}$ urinary creatinine

UCS unconditioned stimulus; unconscious; uterine compression syndrome

ucs unconscious

UCT urological care table

UCTD undifferentiated (unclassifiable) connective tissue disease

uCTD undifferentiated connective tissue disease

UCV uncontrolled variable; unconventional viral [disease]

UCVA uncorrected visual acuity

UD ulcerative dermatosis; ulnar deviation; undetermined; underdeveloped; unit dose; urethral dilatation; urethral discharge; uridine diphosphate; uroporphyrinogen decarboxylase; uterine delivery

UD-AHF UD-CG 115 BS in Acute Heart Failure [study]

UDB universal database

UDC usual diseases of childhood

UDCA ursodeoxycholic acid

UDKase uridine diphosphate kinase

UDN ulcerative dermal necrosis

UDO undetermined origin

UDP uridine diphosphate; user datagram protocol

UDPG uridine diphosphate glucose; urine diphosphoglucose

UDPGA uridine diphosphate-glucuronic acid

UDPGT uridine diphosphate glucuronosyl transferase

UDR-BMD ultradistal radius bone mineral density

UDRP urine diribose phosphate

UDS ultrasound Doppler sonography; uniform data system; unscheduled deoxynucleic acid synthesis; unscheduled deoxyribonucleic acid [DNA] synthesis

UE uncertain etiology; under elbow; uninvolved epidermis; upper esophagus; upper extremity

uE$_s$ unconjugated estriol

UEA *Ulex europaeus* agglutinin

UEFFDE upper extremity fitness for duty evaluation

UEG ultrasonic encephalography; unifocal eosinophilic granuloma

UEHB uniform effective health benefits

UEL upper explosive limit

UEM universal electron microscope

UEMC unidentified endosteal marrow cell

UES upper esophageal sphincter

u/ext upper extremity

UF film unsharpness; ultrafiltrate; ultrafiltration; ultrafine; ultrasonic frequency; unaffected female; universal feeder; unknown factor; urinary formaldehyde

UFA unesterified fatty acid

UFB urinary fat bodies

UFC urinary free cortisol

UFCT ultrafast computed tomography

UFD ultrasonic flow detector; unilateral facet dislocation

UFFI urea formaldehyde foam insulation

UFH unfractionated heparin

UFL upper flammable limit

UFN unreamed femoral nail

UFP ultrafiltration pressure

UFR ultrafiltration rate; urine filtration rate

uFSH urinary follicle-stimulating hormone

UG geometric unsharpness; urogastrone; urogenital

μg microgram

Ug uracyl glycol

UGD urogenital diaphragm

UGDP University Group Diabetes Project

UGF unidentified growth factor

UGH uveitis-glaucoma-hyphema [syndrome]

UGH+ uveitis-glaucoma-hyphema plus vitreous hemorrhage [syndrome]

UGI upper gastrointestinal [tract]

UGIH upper gastrointestinal hemorrhage

UGIS upper gastrointestinal series

UGME undergraduate medical education

UGP uridyl diphosphate glucose pyrophosphorylase

UGPA undergraduate grade-point average

UGPP uridyl diphosphate glucose pyrophosphorylase

UGS urogenital sinus

UGT uridine diphosphate-glucuronosyltransferase; urogenital tract; urogenital tuberculosis

UH umbilical hernia; uncontrolled hemorrhage; unfavorable histology; upper half

UHC university hospital consortium

UHD unstable hemoglobin disease

UHDDS uniform hospital discharge data set

UHF ultrahigh frequency

UHID universal healthcare identifier

UHIS universal healthcare information system; university hospital information system

UHL universal hypertrichosis lanuginosa

UHMW ultrahigh molecular weight

UHMWPE ultrahigh molecular weight polyethylene

UHR underlying heart rhythm

UHS uncontrolled hemorrhagic shock

UHSC university health services clinic

UHT ultrahigh temperature

UI urinary incontinence; uroporphyrin isomerase; user interface

U/I unidentified

UIBC unsaturated iron-binding capacity

UICAO unilateral internal carotid artery occlusion

UICC Union Internationale Contre Cancre

UID unique image identifier

UIF undegraded insulin factor

UIL user interface language

UIP usual interstitial pneumonia

UIQ upper inner quadrant

UIR unsolicited information retrieval

UIS Utilization Information Service

UJT unijunction transistor

UK unknown; uridine kinase; urinary kallikrein

UKa urinary kallikrein

UKAEA United Kingdom Atomic Energy Authority

UKase uridine kinase

UKCCSG United Kingdom Children's Cancer Study Group

UK-COMA United Kingdom Committee on Medical Aspects [food and nutrition]

UKCSG United Kingdom Collaborative Study Group [timolol trial]

UKEGNS United Kingdom Epidemiology Group for the Nutrition Society

UKHAS United Kingdom Heart Attack Study

UKHEART United Kingdom Heart Failure Evaluation and Assessment of Risk Trial

UK in USA Urokinase in Unstable Angina [study]

UKM urea kinetic modeling

ukn unknown

UKNCSPAIVS United Kingdom National Collaborative Study of Pulmonary Atresia with Intact Ventricular Septum

UKPACE United Kingdom Pacing and Cardiovascular Events [study]; United Kingdom Pacing and Clinical Events [study]

UKPDS United Kingdom Prospective Diabetes Study

UKSAT United Kingdom Small Aneurysm Trial

UK-TIA United Kingdom Transient Ischemic Attack [aspirin trial]

UKTSSA United Kingdom Transplant Support Service Authority

UL ultrasonic; Underwriters Laboratories; undifferentiated lymphoma; upper limb; upper limit; upper lobe

U&L upper and lower

U/l units per liter

ULAM United Network for Organ Sharing Liver Allocation Model

ULBW ultralow birth weight

ULD Unverricht-Lundborg disease

ULDH urinary lactate dehydrogenase

ULLE upper lid of left eye

ULN upper limits of normal

uln ulna, ulnar

ULP ultra low profile

ULPA ultra low penetration air filter

ULPE upper lobe pulmonary edema

ULQ upper left quadrant

ULRE upper lid of right eye

ULT ultrahigh temperature

ult ultimate

ULTC urban level trauma center

ULTIMA Unprotected Left Main Trunk Intervention Multicenter Assessment

ULTRA utilizing GFX 2.5 stent in small diameter arteries

UltraSTAR ultrasound structured attribute reporting

ULV ultralow volume

UM movement unsharpness; unaffected male; upper motor [neuron]; uracil mustard; utilization management

uM, μM micromole, micromolar

UMA ulcerative mutilating acropathy; upright membrane assay; urinary muramidase activity

Umax maximum urinary osmolality

umb umbilicus, umbilical

UMC unidimensional chromatography; university medical center

UMCV-TO ulnar motor conduction velocity across thoracic outlet

UMDNS Universal Medical Device Nomenclature System

UME undergraduate medical education

UMHDS uniform minimum health data set

UMI urinary meconium index

UMIN university medical information network

UMKase uridine monophosphate kinase

UMLS Unified Medical Language System

UMN upper motor neuron

UMNL upper motor neuron lesion

UMNS upper motor neuron syndrome

UMP uridine monophosphate

UMPH uridine 5′-monophosphate phosphohydrolase

UMPK uridine monophosphate kinase

UMPS uridine monophosphate synthase

UMS urethral manipulation syndrome

UMT units of medical time

UN ulnar nerve; undernourished; unilateral neglect; updraft nebulizer; urea nitrogen; urinary nitrogen

UNa, U$_{Na}$ urinary sodium

UNAI uniform needs assessment for posthospital care

UNAIDS United Nations Acquired Immunodeficiency Syndrome [AIDS] [program]

UNASEM Unstable Angina Study Using Eminase

uncomp uncompensated

uncond unconditioned

UNCV ulnar nerve conduction velocity

undet undetermined

UNDRO United Nations Disaster Relief Organization

UNE urinary norepinephrine

UNFPA United Nations Population Fund

UNG uracil deoxyribonucleic acid glycosylase

UNHCR United Nations High Commission on Refugees

unilat unilateral

UNIS Urological Nursing Information System

univ universal

unk, unkn unknown

UNL upper normal limit

UNLS Unified Nursing Language System

UNOS United Network for Organ Sharing

UNRPCA Use of Nicardipine to Retard the Progression of Coronary Atherosclerosis [trial]

UNSA Unstable Angina Study

unsat unsatisfactory; unsaturated

UNT untreated

UNTS unilateral nevoid telangiectasia syndrome

UNX uninephrectomy

UO under observation; undetermined origin; urethral orifice; urinary output

U/O urinary output

u/o under observation

UOP urinary output

UOQ upper outer quadrant

UOsm urinary osmolality

UOV units of variance

UOX urate oxidase

UP parallax unsharpness; ulcerative proctitis; ultrahigh purity; unipolar; upright posture; ureteropelvic; uridine phosphorylase; uroporphyrin

U/P urine to plasma [ratio]

UPase uridine phosphorylase

UPC usual provider continuity

UPD ulcerative periodontal disease; uniparental disomy; urinary production

UPDIC Uppsala Prospective Diabetes Control [study]

UPDRS unified Parkinson disease rating scale

UPF universal proximal femur [prosthesis]

UPEP urinary protein electrophoresis; urine protein electrophoresis

UPET Urokinase Pulmonary Embolism Trial

UPG uroporphyrinogen

UPGMA unweighted pair group method with averages

UPI uteroplacental insufficiency; uteroplacental ischemia

UPID uniparental isodisomy

UPIN universal physician identifier number [Health Care Financing Administration, HCFA]

UPJ ureteropelvic junction

UPJO ureteropelvic junction obstruction

UPL unusual position of limbs

UPP urethral pressure profile

UPPP uvulopalatopharyngoplasty

UPPRA upright peripheral plasma renin activity

UPS ultraviolet photoelectron spectroscopy; uninterruptible power supply; uroporphyrinogen synthetase; uterine progesterone system

Υ Greek capital letter *upsilon*

υ Greek lower case letter *upsilon*

UPSIT University of Pennsylvania Smell Identification Test

UPSIZE Ultrasound-controlled Percutaneous Transluminal Coronary Angioplasty with Optional Balloon Size [study]

UpU uridyl (3′-5′)uridine

UQ ubiquinone; upper quadrant

UQAC unit quality assurance committee

UQCRC ubiquinol-cytochrome C reductase core

UQL unacceptable quality level

UQS upper quadrant syndrome

UR unconditioned reflex; upper respiratory; uridine; urinal; urology; utilization review

Ur urea; urine; urinary

URA unilateral renal agenesis

URA, Ura uracil

URAC Utilization Review Accreditation Commission

URALMI Urokinase and Alteplase in Myocardial Infarction [study]

URC upper rib cage; utilization review committee

URD unrelated donor; unspecified respiratory disease; upper respiratory disease

Urd uridine

ureth urethra

URF unidentified reading frame; uterine relaxing factor

URG urogastrone

URI uniform resource identifier; upper respiratory illness; upper respiratory infection

URK urokinase

URL uniform resource locator

URN uniform resource name

U-RNA uridylic acid ribonucleic acid

URO urology; uroporphyrin; uroporphyrinogen; utilization review organization

UROD uroporphyrinogen decarboxylase

URO-GEN urogenital

Urol urology, urologist

UROS uroporphyrinogen synthase

URQ upper right quadrant

URS ultrasonic renal scanning; upstream repressing sequence

URT upper respiratory tract

URTI upper respiratory tract infection

URVD unilateral renovascular disease

US screen unsharpness ultrasonic, ultrasound; ultrasonography; unconditioned stimulus; unique sequence; unit separator; upper segment; upper strength; urinary sugar; Usher syndrome

u/s ultrasonic or ultrasound

US1 Usher syndrome type I

US1A Usher syndrome type IA

US1B Usher syndrome type IB

US1C Usher syndrome type IC

US2 Usher syndrome type II

US2A Usher syndrome type IIA

US2B Usher syndrome type IIB

US3 Usher syndrome type III

US4 Usher syndrome type IV

USAFH United States Air Force Hospital

USAFRHL United States Air Force Radiological Health Laboratory

USAH United States Army Hospital

USAHC United States Army Health Clinic

USAIDR United States Army Institute of Dental Research

USAMEDS United States Army Medical Service

USAMRMC US Army Medical Research and Materiel Command

USAMRIID United States Army Medical Research Institute for Infectious Diseases

USAN United States Adopted Names

USAR urban search and rescue

USASI United States of America Standards Institute

USAT ultrasmall aperture terminal

USB upper sternal border

USBS United States Bureau of Standards

USCG ultrasonic cardiography

USCR universal self-care requisites

USD United States Dispensary

USDA United States Department of Agriculture

USDHEW United States Department of Health, Education, and Welfare

USDHHS United States Department of Health and Human Services

USE ultrasonic echography; ultrasonography

USEIR United States Eye Injury Registry

USF upstream stimulatory factor

USFA United States Fire Administration

USFMG United States foreign medical graduate

USFMS United States foreign medical student

USG ultrasonography

USH Usher syndrome

USH1 Usher syndrome type I

USH1A Usher syndrome type IA

USH1B Usher syndrome type IB

USH1C Usher syndrome type IC

USH2 Usher syndrome type II

USH2A Usher syndrome type IIA

USH2B Usher syndrome type IIB

USH3 Usher syndrome type III

USH4 Usher syndrome type IV

US+HC ultrasound-driven hydrocortisone

USHL United States Hygienic Laboratory

USHMAC United States Health Manpower Advisory Council

USI universal serial interface; urinary stress incontinence

USIA United States Information Agency

USIMG United States citizen international medical school graduate

US/LS upper strength/lower strength [ratio]

USMG United States or Canada medical school graduate

USMH United States Marine Hospital

USMLE United States Medical Licensing Examination

USN ultrasonic nebulizer; unilateral spatial neglect

USNCHS United States National Center for Health Statistics

USNH United States Naval Hospital

USO unilateral salpingo-oophorectomy

USP United States Pharmacopeia

US+P ultrasound and placebo

USPC United States Pharmacopeia Convention

USPDI United States Pharmacopeia Drug Information

USPET Urokinase Streptokinase Pulmonary Embolism Trial

USPHS United States Public Health Service; United States Physicians' Health Study

USPSTF United States Preventive Services Task Force

USPTA United States Phyical Therapy Association

USR unheated serum reagin

USRDS United States Renal Data System

USS ultrasound scanning; user support system

USUHS Uniformed Services University of the Health Services

USVH United States Veterans Hospital

USVMD urine specimen volume measuring device

USW ultrashort waves

UT total unsharpness; Ullrich-Turner [syndrome]; Unna-Thost [syndrome]; untested; untreated; urinary tract; urticaria

uT unbound testosterone

UTBG unbound thyroxine-binding globulin

UTC upper thoracic compression

UTD up to date

UT-ETT ultrathin endotracheal tube

UTI urinary tract infection; urinary trypsin inhibitor

util rev utilization review

UTO upper tibial osteotomy; urinary tract obstruction

UTOPIA Utilization of Platelet Inhibition in Angina [trial]

UTP unilateral tension pneumothorax; unshielded twisted pair; uridine triphosphate

UTR untranslated region

UTS Ullrich-Turner syndrome; ulnar tunnel syndrome; ultimate tensile strength

UTTS-ETT two-stage ultrathin-walled endotracheal tube

UTZ ultrasound

UU urinary urea; urine urobilinogen

UUID universal unique identifier

UUN urinary urea nitrogen

UUO unilateral urethral obstruction

UUP urinary uroporphyrin

UV ultraviolet; umbilical vein; ureterovesical; Uppsala virus; urinary volume

UVA ultraviolet A; ultraviolet germicidal irradiation; ureterovesical angle

UVAL-MED universal visual associative language for medicine

UVB ultraviolet B
UVC umbilical venous catheter
UVEB unifocal ventricular ectopic beat
UVER ultraviolet-enhanced reactivation
UVGI ultraviolet germicidal irradiation
UVI ultraviolet irradiation
UVJ ureterovesical junction
UVL ultraviolet light
UVO uvomorulin

UVP ultraviolet photometry
UVR ultraviolet radiation
UW unilateral weakness
UWB unit of whole blood
UWD Urbach-Wiethe disease
UWSC unstimulated whole saliva collection
UWW underwater weight
UX uranium X, proactinium
UYP upper yield point

V in cardiography, unipolar chest lead; coefficient of variation; electrical potential (in volts); in electroencephalography, vertex sharp transient; five; a logical binary relation that is true if any argument is true, and false otherwise; luminous efficiency; potential; potential energy (joules); vaccinated, vaccine; vagina; valine; valve; vanadium; variable, variation, varnish; vector; vegetarian; vein [Lat. *vena*]; velocity; ventilation; ventricular [fibrillation]; verbal comprehension [factor]; vertebra; vertex; vestibular; *Vibrio*; vincristine; violet; viral [antigen]; virulence; virus; vision; visual acuity; voice; volt; voltage; volume; vomiting

V1 to V6 ventral 1 to ventral 6 [chest leads in ECG]

V$_O$ rest volume

V$_1$ mean flow velocity

v or [Lat. *vel*]; rate of reaction catalyzed by an enzyme; see [Lat. *vide*]; specific volume; valve; vein [Lat. *vena*]; velocity; venous; ventricular; versus; very; virus; vision; volt; volume

VA vacuum aspiration; valproic acid; vasodilator agent; ventricular aneurysm; ventricular arrhythmia; ventriculoatrial; ventroanterior; Veterans Administration; Veterans Affairs; vincristine, adriamycin; viral antigen; visual acuity; visual aid; visual axis; volt-ampere; volume-average

V$_A$ alveolar ventilation

V/A volt/ampere

V-A veno-arterial

Va activated factor V

V$_a$ alveolar ventilation

VAAE vaccine-associated adverse events

VAB vincristine, actinomycin D, and bleomycin; violent antisocial behavior

VABS Vineland adaptive behavior scales

VAB-6 vincristine, actinomycin, bleomycin, cis-platinum, Cytoxan

VABP venoarterial bypass pumping

VAC ventriculoatrial conduction; vincristine, doxorubicin, and cyclophosphamide; virus capsid antigen

vac vacuum

VACA Valvuloplasty and Angioplasty in Congenital Anomalies [registry]

VAcc visual acuity with correction

vacc vaccination

VACO Veterans Affairs Central Office

VACS Veterans Administration Cooperative Study

VACSDM Veterans Affairs Cooperative Study on Glycemic Control and Complications in Non-Insulin Dependent Diabetes Mellitus

VACT Veterans Administration Cooperative Trial

VACTERL vertebral abnormalities, anal atresia, cardiac abnormalities, tracheoesophageal fistula and/or esophageal atresia, renal agenesis and dysplasia, and limb defects [association]

VAD venous access device; ventricular assist device; vinblastine and dexamethasone; vitamin A deficiency; virus-adjusting diluent

VAE venous air emboli

VA-ECMO venoarterial extracorporeal membrane oxygenation

VAERS Vaccine Adverse Events Reporting System [UK]

VAF viral-free antigen

VAG vibroarthrography

vag vagina, vaginal, vaginitis

VAG HYST vaginal hysterectomy

VAH vertebral ankylosing hyperostosis; Veterans Affairs Hospital; virilizing adrenal hyperplasia

VA-HIT Veterans Affairs High-density Lipoprotein Intervention Trial

VAHS virus-associated hemophagocytic syndrome

VAIN vaginal intraepithelial neoplasm

V$_{ak}$ atrial volume constant

Val valine

val valve

VALE visual acuity, left eye

Val-HeFT Valsartan–Heart Failure Trial

VALIANT Valsartan in Acute Myocardial Infarction [study]

VALID Velocity Assessment for Lesions of Intermediate Severity [trial]

VALID II Velocity Assessment for Lesions of Indeterminate Severity [trial]

ValRS valyl ribonucleic acid [RNA] synthetase

VALUE Valsartan Antihypertensive Long-term Use Evaluation

VAN value-added network

VANQWISH Veterans Affairs Non–Q-wave Infarction Strategies in Hospital [study]

VAM ventricular arrhythmia monitor

VAMC Veterans Affairs Medical Center

VAMP venous arterial blood management protection system; vincristine, amethopterine, 6-mercaptopurine, and prednisone

VAP vaginal acid phosphatase; variant angina pectoris; ventilator-associated pneumonia

vap vapor

VAPP vaccine-associated paralytic poliomyelitis

VAPS visual analog pain score

VAPSHCS Veterans Affairs Puget Sound Health Care System

V_a/Q alveolar ventilation/perfusion

V_A/Q_C ventilation-perfusion [ratio]

VAR visual-auditory range

Var, var variable; variant, variation, variety

var varicose

VARE visual acuity, right eye

VA RNA virus-associated ribonucleic acid [RNA]

VARS valyl-transfer ribonucleic acid synthetase

VAS vagal afferents; vascular; vascular access service; ventriculo-atrial shunt; Verapamil Angioplasty Study; vesicle attachment site; viral arthritis syndrome; Visual Analogue Scale

VASC vascular; Verbal Auditory Screen for Children; visual-auditory screening

VAsc visual acuity without correction

vasc vascular

VASD Vascular Access Service Database

VASPNAF Veterans Administration Stroke Prevention in Nonrheumatic Atrial Fibrillation [study]

VAS RAD vascular radiology

VAST visual analysis systems technology

VAST/STT visual analysis systems technology/space-time toolkit

VAT variable antigen type; ventricular accommodation test; ventricular activation time; vesicular amine transformer; video-assisted thoracoscopy; visceral adipose tissue; visual action therapy; visual action time; visual apperception test; vocational apperception test

VATER vertebral defects, imperforate anus, tracheoesophageal fistula, and radial and renal dysplasia

VATS Veterans Administration medical center transference syndrome; video-assisted thoracic surgery

VATs surface variable antigen

VATT vascular anatomy teaching tool

VB vaginal bulb; valence bond; venous blood; ventrobasal; Veronal buffer; vertebrobasilar; viable birth; vinblastine; virus buffer; voided bladder

Vb vinblastine

VBAC vaginal birth after cesarean section

VBAIN vertebrobasilar artery insufficiency nystagmus

VBC vincristine, bleomycin, and cisplatin; visualization in biomedical computing; volumetric based capnometry

VBD vanishing bile duct; Veronal-buffered diluent

VBG vagotomy and Billroth gastroenterostomy; venous blood gases; venous bypass graft; vertical-banded gastroplasty

VBI ventral blood island; vertebrobasilar insufficiency; vertebrobasilar ischemia

VBL vinblastine

VbMF vinblastine, methotrexate, 5-fluorouracil

vBNS very high-performance backbone network services

VBOS Veronal-buffered oxalated saline

VBP vagal body paraganglia; venous blood pressure; ventricular premature beat

VBR ventricular brain ratio; vertebral body repositioning

VBS Veronal-buffered saline; vertebrobasilar system

VBS:FBS Veronal-buffered saline-fetal bovine serum

VBWG Vascular Biology Working Group

VBX visual basic controls

VC color vision; variance cardiography; variation coefficient; vascular changes;

vasoconstriction; vena cava; venereal case; venous capacitance; ventilatory capacity; ventral column; ventricular contraction; vertebral caval; Veterinary Corps; video-casette; vincristine; vinyl chloride; visual capacity; visual cortex; vital capacity; vocal cord

V/C ventilation/circulation [ratio]

VCA vancomycin, colistin, and anisomycin; viral capsid antigen

VCAM vascular cell adhesion molecule

VCAP vincristine, cyclophosphamide, Adriamycin, and prednisone

vCBF venous cerebral blood flow

VCC vasoconstrictor center; ventral cell column

VCD Van Capelle-Durrer [model of cardiac cell depolarization-repolarization]; vibrational circular dichroism

VCE vagina, ectocervix, and endocervix

VCF velocardiofacial [syndrome]; velocity of circumferential fiber [lengthening]

VCFG volume-cycled flow generator

VCF$_{min}$ minimum velocity of circumferential fiber [lengthening]

VCFS velo-cardio-facial syndrome

VCG vectorcardiogram, vectorcardiography; voiding cystography, voiding cystourethrography

VCL vinculin

VCM vinyl chloride monomer

VCMP vincristine, cyclophosphamide, melphalan, and prednisone

VCN vancomycin, colistomethane, and nystatin; *Vibrio chloreae* neuraminidase

VCO voltage-controlled oscillator

VCO, V$_{CO}$ endogenous production of carbon monoxide

VCO$_2$, V$_{CO2}$ carbon dioxide output

VCP vincristine, cyclophosphamide, and prednisone

VCR vasoconstriction rate; vincristine; volume clearance rate

VCS vasoconstrictor substance; vesicocervical space; virtual chart system

VCSA viral cell surface antigen

VCSF ventricular cerebrospinal fluid

VCT venous clotting time; voluntary counselling and testing

VCU videocystourethrography; voiding cystourethrogram, voiding cystourethrography

VCUG vesicoureterogram; voiding cystourethrogram

VD vapor density; vascular disease; vasodilation, vasodilator; venereal disease; venous dilatation; ventricular dilator; ventrodorsal; verbal dysphasia; vertical deviation; vertical divergence; video-disk; viral diarrhea; voided; volume of dead space; volume of distribution

V&D vomiting and diarrhea

V$_D$ dead space; volume of distribution

Vd voided, voiding; volume dead space; volume of distribution

V$_d$ apparent volume of distribution

VDA visual discriminatory acuity

VDAC voltage-dependent anion channel

VDB virtual database

VdB van der Bergh [test]

VDBR volume of distribution of bilirubin

VDC vasodilator center

VDD atrial synchronous ventricular inhibited [pacemaker]; vitamin D-dependent

VDDR vitamin D-dependent rickets

VDEL Venereal Disease Experimental Laboratory

VDEM vasodepressor material

VDF ventricular diastolic fragmentation

VDG, VD-G venereal disease-gonorrhea

vdg voiding

VDH valvular disease of the heart

VDI virus defective interfering [particle]

V$_{dia}$ diastolic potential

VDL vasodepressor lipid; visual detection level

VDM vasodepressor material

vDOC virtual distributed online clinic

VDP ventricular premature depolarization

VDR venous diameter ratio; vitamin D receptor

VDRG vitamin D-binding alpha-globulin

VDRL Venereal Disease Research Laboratory [test for syphilis]

VDRR vitamin D-resistant rickets

VDRS Verdun Depression Rating Scale

VDRT venereal disease reference test

VDS vasodilator substance; vindesine

VDS, VD-S venereal disease-syphilis

VDT vector distance transform; vibration disappearance threshold; visual display terminal; visual distortion test

V$_D$V$_T$ dead space to tidal volume [ratio]

VDU video display unit

VDV ventricular end-diastolic volume

Vd/Vt dead space ventilation/total ventilation [ratio]

VDWS van der Woude syndrome

VE vaginal examination; Venezuelan encephalitis; venous emptying; venous extension; ventilation; ventilatory equivalent; ventricular elasticity; ventricular extrasystole; vertex; vesicular exanthema; viral encephalitis; virtual endoscopy; visual efficiency; vitamin E; volume ejection; voluntary effort

V_E environmental variance; respiratory minute volume

Ve ventilation

V&E Vinethine and ether

VEA ventricular ectopic activity; ventricular ectopic arrhythmia; viral envelope antigen

VEB ventricular ectopic beat

VECG vector electrocardiogram

VEC-MR velocity encoded cine-magnetic resonance

VECP visually evoked cortical potential

VED vacuum erection device; ventricular ectopic depolarization; vital exhaustion and depression

VEE vagina, ectocervix, endocervix; Venezuelan equine encephalomyelitis

VEF ventricular ejection fraction; visually evoked field

VEG vegetation; von Egner gland [protein]

VEGAS Vein Graft Angiojet Study; ventricular enlargement with gait apraxia syndrome

VEGP von Ebner gland protein

vehic vehicle

VEI volume [lung] at the end of inspiration

VEINES Venous Insufficiency Epidemiologic and Economic Study

vel, veloc velocity

VEM vasoexcitor material

VEMR virtual electronic medical record

VENC velocity encoding

vent ventilation; ventral; ventricle, ventricular

vent fib ventricular fibrillation

ventric ventricle

VENUS Very Early Nimopidine Use in Stroke [trial]

VEP visual evoked potential

VEPID video-based electronic portal imaging device

VEPT volume of electrically participating thoracic tissue

VER visual evoked response

Verc vervet (African green monkey) kidney cells

VERDI Verapamil vs Diuretics [trial]

VERDICT Verapamil Digoxin Cardioversion Trial

vert vertebra, vertebral

VES virtual endoscope system; viscoelastic substance

ves bladder [Lat. *vesica*]; vesicular; vessel

VESA virtual endoscopy software application

vesic a blister [Lat. *vesicula*]

VEST Vesnarinone Trial

vest vestibular

ves ur urinary bladder [Lat. *vesica urinaria*]

VET ventricular ejection time; vestigial testis

Vet veteran; veterinarian, veterinary

VetMB Bachelor of Veterinary Medicine

Vet Med veterinary medicine

VETS Veterinary Expert Technology System; Veterans Adjustment Scale

Vet Sci veterinary science

VEUD virtual emergency and urgency department

VF left leg [electrode]; ventricular fibrillation; ventricular fluid; ventricular flutter; ventricular function; videofluorography; visual field; vitreous fluorophotometry; vocal fremitus

Vf visual frequency

V_f variant frequency

vf visual field

VFA volatile fatty acid

VFC ventricular function curve

VFD visual feedback display

VFDP variant familial developmental pattern

VFI venous filling index; visual field intact

V fib ventricular fibrillation

VFID virtual focus-isocenter-distance

VFL ventricular flutter

VFP ventricular filling pressure; ventricular fluid pressure; vocal fold pathology

VFR voiding flow rate

VFS vascular fragility syndrome; very fast sedimentation

VFT venous filling time; ventricular fibrillation threshold

VF/VT ventricular fibrillation/ventricular tachycardia

VG van Gieson [stain]; ventricular gallop; volume of gas

V$_G$ genetic variance

VGA video graphics array

VGB vigabatrin

VGCC voltage-gated calcium channels

VGH very good health

vGI ventral giant interneuron

VGM venous graft myringoplasty

VGP viral glycoprotein

VGPO volume-guaranteed pressure options [ventilation]

VH vaginal hysterectomy; venous hematocrit; ventral hippocampus; ventricular hypertrophy; veterans hospital; viral hepatitis; virtual hospital; Visible Human [project]

V$_H$ variable domain of heavy chain; variable heavy chain

VHA Veterans Health Administration; Voluntary Hospital Association

V/Hallu visual hallucinations

VHAS Verapamil in Hypertension Atherosclerosis Study

VHCD virtual health care databank

VHD valvular heart disease; viral hematodepressive disease; Visible Human Dataset

VHDL very high density lipoprotein

V-HeFT Vasodilator Heart Failure Trial; Veterans Administration Heart Failure Trial

VHF very high frequency; viral hemorrhagic fever; visual half-field

VHL von Hippel-Lindau [syndrome]

VHN Vickers hardness number

VHP vaporized hydrogen peroxide; Visible Human Project

VHR ventricular heart rate

VHS veterans health study

VHS&RA Veterans Health Service and Research Administration

VI Roman numeral six; vaginal irrigation; variable interval; vastus intermedius; ventilation index; virgo intacta; virulence, virulent; viscosity index; visual impairment; visual inspection; vitality index; volume index

Vi virulence, virulent

VIA virus inactivating agent; virus infection-associated antigen

vib vibration

vib & perc vibration and percussion

VIC vasoinhibitory center; verbal intelligence quotient; virtual information center; visual communication therapy; voice intensity control

VICP Vaccine Injury Compensation Program

VI-CTS vibration-induced carpal tunnel syndrome

VID visible iris diameter

VIDA viability identification with dipyridamole-dobutamine administration

VIF variance inflation factor; virus-induced interferon

VIG, VIg vaccinia immunoglobulin

VIGOUR Virtual Coordinating Center for Global Collaborative Cardiovascular Research

VIGRE velocity imaging with gradient-recalled echos

VIIag factor VII antigen

VIIIc factor VIII clotting activity

VIII$_{vwf}$ von Willebrand factor

VIL villin

VIM video-intensification microscopy; vimentin

VIN vulvar intraepithelial neoplasm

vin vinyl

VINDICATE **v**ascular, **i**nflammatory/infectious, **n**eoplastic/neurologic/psychiatric, **d**egenerative/dietary, **i**ntoxication/idiopathic/iatrogenic, **c**ongenital, **a**llergic/autoimmune, **t**rauma, **e**ndocrine/metabolic

VIP vaccine information pamphlet; vasoactive intestinal peptide; vasoinhibitory peptide; venous impedance plethysmography; ventricular inotropic parameter; Viability Impact on Prognosis [study]; voluntary interruption of pregnancy

VIPERS Virtual Intelligent Patient Electronic Record System

VIPoma vasoactive intestinal polypeptide-secreting tumor

VIPOR Vermont Integrated Problem-Oriented Record

VIQ Verbal Intelligence Quotient

VIR virology

Vir virus, viral

vir virulent

VIS vaginal irrigation smear; value-intensity-strength; venous insufficiency syndrome; vertebral irritation syndrome; visible; visual information storage

vis vision, visual

VISC vitreous infusion suction cutter

visc viscera, visceral; viscosity

VISI volar intercalated segment instability

VISN veterans integrated service network

VISP Vitamin Intervention for Stroke Prevention [trial]

Vit vitamin

vit vital

VITA Vicenza Thrombophilia and Atherosclerosis Project

VITALS vital indicators of teaching and learning success

vit cap vital capacity

VIVAS Vaccination Information Vaccination Administration System

VIVIAN virtual intracranial visualization and navigation

VJ ventriculojugular

VJC ventriculojugularcardiac

VK vervet (African green monkey) kidney cells

VKC vernal keratoconjunctivitis

VKH, VKHS Vogt-Koyanagi-Harada [syndrome]

VL left arm [electrode]; vastus lateralis [muscle]; ventralis lateratis [nucleus]; ventrolateral; viral load; visceral leishmaniasis; vision, left [eye]

V_L lung volume; variable domain of the light chain; variable light chain

VLA very late activation [antigen or protein]; virus-like agent

VLAB, VLA-BETA very late activation protein beta

V LACT venous lactate

VLAN virtual online area network

VLB vinblastine; vincaleukoblastine

VLBR very low birth rate

VLBW very low birth weight

VLCAD very long chain acyl-coenzyme A dehydrogenase

VLCD very low calorie diet

VLCFA very long chain fatty acid

VLD very low density; volume limiter disk

VLDL, VLDLP very low density lipoprotein

VLDLR very low density lipoprotein receptor

VLDL-TG very-low-density lipoprotein–triglyceride complex

VLF very low frequency

VLG ventral nucleus of the lateral geniculate body

VLH ventrolateral nucleus of the hypothalamus

VLM ventrolateral medulla; visceral larva migrans

VLO vastus lateralis obliquus

VLP vincristine, L-asparaginase, and prednisone; virus-like particle

VLPA ventrolateral pressure area

VLR vinleurosine

VLS vascular leak syndrome

VLSI very large scale integration

VM vasomotor; ventilator management; ventralis medialus; ventricular mass; ventriculomegaly; ventriculometry; ventromedial; vestibular membrane; viomycin; viral myocarditis; voltmeter

V/m volts per meter

V_m membrane potential; muscle volume; peak velocity

VMA vanillylmandelic acid; ventilator management advisor

VMAP, Vmap velocity mapping

VMAT vesicular monoamine transformer

Vmax maximum velocity

VMC vasomotor center

VMCG vector magnetocardiogram

VMCHN Victorian Maternal and Child Health Nurses

VMD Doctor of Veterinary Medicine; virtual medical device; vitelliform macular dystrophy

vMDV virulent Marek disease virus

VME Volunteers for Medical Engineering

VMF vasomotor flushing

VMGT Visual Motor Gestalt Test

VMH ventromedial hypothalamus

VMI, VMIT visual-motor integration [test]

VML ventriculomegaly

VMLS virtual medical library system

VMN ventromedial nucleus

VMO vastus medialis obliquus [muscle]; visiting medical officer

VMR vasomotor rhinitis

VMRS Vermont Medical Record System

VMS visual memory span

VMST visual motor sequencing test

VMT vasomotor tonus; ventilatory muscle training; ventromedial tegmentum

$V_m(t)$ time-averaged membrane potential

$V_m(x,t)$ absolute transmembrane potential

VN vesical neck; vestibular nucleus; virus neutralization; visceral nucleus; visiting nurse; vitronectin; vocational nurse; vomeronasal

VNA Visiting Nurse Association

VNDPT visual numerical discrimination pre-test

VNO vomeronasal organ

VNR vitronectin receptor

VNRA vitronectin receptor alpha

VNS virtual notebook system; visiting nursing service

VNTR variable number of tandem repeats; variable copy number tandem repeats

VO verbal order; volume overload; voluntary opening

Vo standard volume

VO$_2$, V$_{o2}$ volume of oxygen utilization

VOC volatile organic compound

VOCC voltage-operated calcium channel

VOD veno-occlusive disease

VOI volume of interest

VO$_2$I volume of oxygen utilization index

V̇O$_2$ Max, V̇O$_2$max maximum volume of oxygen utilization

vol volar; volatile; volume; voluntary, volunteer

VOM volt-ohm-milliammeter

VON Victorian Order of Nurses

V-ONC viral oncogene

VOO ventricular asynchronous (competitive, fixed-rate) [pacemaker]

VOP vaso-occlusive pain; venous occlusion plethysmography

VOR vestibulo-ocular reflex; volume of regret

VOS videothoracoscopic operator staging; vision, left eye [Lat. *visio, oculus sinister*]

VOT voice onset time

VOTE Value of Transesophageal Echocardiography [study]

VP physiological volume; vapor pressure; Varadi-Papp [orofaciodigital syndrome]; variegate porphyria; vascular permeability; vasopressin; velopharyngeal; venipuncture; venous pressure; ventricular pacing; ventricular pericardium; ventricular premature [beat]; ventroposterior; VePepsid; verbal paraphrasia; vertex potential; vincristine and prednisone; viral protein; Voges-Proskauer [medium or test]; volume-pressure; vulnerable period

V/P ventilation/perfusion [ratio]

V&P vagotomy and pyloroplasty

Vp peak velocity; peak voltage; phenotype variance; plasma volume; ventricular premature [beat]

vp vapor pressure

VPA valproic acid

VPB ventricular premature beat

VPC vapor-phase chromatography; ventricular premature complex; ventricular premature contraction; volume-packed cells; volume percent

VPCT ventricular premature contraction threshold

VPD vaccine-preventable disease; ventricular premature depolarization

VPF vascular permeability factor

VPG velopharyngeal gap

VPGSS venous pressure gradient support stockings

VPI vapor phase inhibitor; velopharyngeal insufficiency

VPL ventroposterolateral

VPM ventilator pressure manometer; ventroposteromedial

vpm vibrations per minute

VPN ventral pontine nucleus

VPO velopharyngeal opening; vertical pendular oscillation

VPP vacuolar proton pump; viral porcine pneumonia

VPR ventricular paced rhythm; virtual patient record; Voges-Proskauer reaction; volume/pressure ratio

VPRBC volume of packed red blood cells

VPRC volume of packed red cells

VPRS variable precision rough set [model]

VPS Vasovagal Pacemaker Study; ventriculoperitoneal shunt; verbal pain scale; virtual point source; visual pleural space; volume performance standard

vps vibrations per second

VPT vibratory perception threshold

VQ vector quantization

V/Q ventilation-perfusion; ventilation perfusion [ratio]; voice quality

VQE visa qualifying examination [for foreign medical graduates]

VQI ventilation perfusion index

VR right arm [electrode]; valve replacement; variable ratio; variable region; vascular resistance; vasopressin receptor; venous flow reversal; venous reflux; venous return; ventilation rate; ventilation ratio; ventral root; ventricular rale; ventricular rhythm; vesicular rosette; virtual reality; vision, right [eye]; vital records; vocal resonance; vocational rehabilitation

Vr relaxation volume

V2R vasopressin 2 receptor [gene]

VRA visual reinforcement audiometry

VRBC red blood cell volume

VRC venous renin concentration

VRCP vitreoretinochoroidopathy

VRD ventricular radial dysplasia; viral reference division

VRE vancomycin-resistant enterococcus

VR&E vocational rehabilitation and education

VREF vancomycin-resistant *Enterococcus faecium*

V_rest resting potential

VRI viral respiratory infection; virtual reality imaging

VRL Virus Reference Laboratory

VRML Virtual Reality Modeling Language

VRNA viral ribonucleic acid

VRNI neovascular inflammatory vitreoretinopathy

VROM voluntary range of motion

VRP ventral root potential

VRR ventral root reflex

VRS verbal rating scale; Virchow-Robin space

VRSA vancomycin-resistant *Staphylococcus aureus*

VRT vehicle rescue technician; volume-rendering technique

VRV ventricular residual volume; viper retrovirus

VS vaccination scar; vaccine serotype; vagal stimulation; vasospasm; venesection; ventricular septum; verapamil shock; vesicular stomatitis; veterinary surgeon; vibration syndrome; visual storage; vital sign; Vogt-Spielmeyer [syndrome]; volatile solid; volume support; volumetric solution; voluntary sterilization

Vs venesection

V·s vibration second; volt-second

V_s system tissue volume

V x s volts by seconds

vs see above [Lat. *vide supra*]; single vibration; versus; vibration seconds; vital signs

VSA variant-specific surface antigen

VSAT very small aperture terminal

VSBE very short below-elbow [cast]

VSC voluntary surgical contraception

VSD ventricular septal defect; vesicular stomatitis virus; virtually safe dose

VSFP venous stop flow pressure

VSG variant surface glycoprotein; Vesnarinone Study Group

VSHD ventricular septal heart defect

VSIE volume surface integral equation [method]

VSINC Virus Subcommittee of the International Nomenclature Committee

VSM vascular smooth muscle

VSMC vascular smooth muscle cell

VSMS Vineland Social Maturity Scale

vsn vision

VSO vertical supranuclear ophthalmoplegia

VSOK vital signs normal

VSP variable spine plating; very short patch [deoxyribonucleic acid, DNA, repair]

VSR venous stasis retinopathy; visceral/subcutaneous adipose tissue ratio

VSRA variable speech rate audiometry

VSS vital signs stable

VST ventral spinothalamic tract; video-see-through; volume-selective excitation

VSV vesicular stomatitis virus

VSV-G G protein of Gibbon ape leukemia virus

VSW ventricular stroke work

VT tetrazolium violet; tidal volume; total ventilation; vacuum tube; vacuum tuberculin; vasotonin; venous thrombosis; ventricular tachyarrhythmia; ventricular tachycardia; verocytotoxin; verotoxin; vibration threshold

V_T tidal volume; total ventilation

V&T volume and tension

VTA ventral tegmental area

V tach ventricular tachycardia

VTE venous thromboembolism; ventricular tachycardia event

VTEC verotoxin-producing *Escherichia coli*

VTEU Vaccine and Treatment Evaluation Unit

VTG volume thoracic gas

VTI velocity-time integral; volume thickness index

VTK visualization toolkit

VTM mechanical tidal volume; virus transport medium

VT-MASS Metoprolol and Sotalol for Sustained Ventricular Tachycardia [study]

VTN vitronectin

VTOP vaginal termination of pregnancy

VTR variable tandem repeats; videotape recording; vesicular transport system

VTSRS Verdun Target Symptom Rating Scale

VTVM vacuum tube voltmeter

VTX, vtx vertex

VU varicose ulcer; volume unit

vu volume unit

VUC voided urinary cytology

VUJ vesico-ureteral junction

UVO vesico-ureteral orifice

VUR vesico-ureteral reflux

VUV vacuum ultraviolet

VV vaccinia virus; variable volume; varicose veins; venous volume; veno-venous; vertical vein; viper venom; vulva and vagina

V&V verification and validation

V-V veno-venous [bypass]

vv varicose veins; veins

v/v percent volume in volume

VVAS vertical visual analog scale

VVD vaginal vertex delivery

VVDL venovenous double-lumen [catheter]

VVFR vesicovaginal fistula repair

VVGF vaccinia virus growth factor

VVI ventricular inhibited [pacemaker]; vocal velocity index

v$_{vk}$ ventricular volume constant

VVLBW very very low birth weight

vvMDV very virulent Marek disease virus

VVol venous volume

VVS vesicovaginal space; vesicovaginal space; vestibulo-vegetative syndrome

VVT ventricular triggered [pacemaker]

VW van der Woude [syndrome]; vascular wall; vessel wall; Volterra-Wiener [approach]; von Willebrand [disease]

v/w volume per weight

VWD ventral wall defect

vWD von Willebrand disease

VWDFAg, vWDFAg von Willebrand factor antigen

VWF velocity waveform; vibration-induced white finger; von Willebrand Factor Database

vWF, vWf von Willebrand factor

VWM ventricular wall motion; verbal working memory

vWS van der Woude syndrome; viewing work station; von Willebrand syndrome

Vx vertex

VYS visceral yolk sac

VZ varicella-zoster

VZIG, VZIg varicella zoster immunoglobulin

VZV varicella-zoster virus

W dominant spotting [mouse]; energy; section modulus; a series of small triangular incisions in plastic surgery [plasty]; tryptophan; tungsten [Ger. *Wolfram*]; wakefulness; ward; water; watt; Weber [test]; week; wehnelt; weight; white; widowed; width; wife; Wilcoxson rank sum statistic; Wistar [rat]; with; word fluency; work; wound
W3 World Wide Web
w water; watt; while; with; velocity (m/s)
Wt weakly positive
WA when awake; white adult; Wiskott-Aldrich [syndrome]
W/A watt/ampere
W&A weakness and atrophy
WAAT Warfarin Plus Aspirin vs Aspirin Trial
WAB Western Aphasia Battery
WACS Women's Atherosclerosis Cardiovascular Study
WAF weakness, atrophy and fasciculation; white adult female
WAFUS Warfarin Anticoagulation Follow-up Study
WAGR Wilms tumor, aniridia, genitourinary abnormalities, and mental retardation
WAI Web Accessibility Initiative
WAIS Wechsler Adult Intelligence Scale; Western Angiographic and Interventional Society; wide area information server
WAIS-R revised Wechsler Adult Intelligence Scale
WAK wearable artificial kidney
WALK Walking with Angina–Learning is the Key [program]
WAM white adult male; work area model; worksheet for ambulatory medicine
WAN wide area network
WANTO WEB-Aided Nursing the Old Information System
WAP wandering atrial pacemaker; whey acid protein

WAR Wasserman antigen reaction; without additional reagents
WARCRY Wegener and Related Diseases Compassionate Regimen Yield [study]
WARDS Welfare of Animals Used for Research in Drugs and Therapy
WARF warfarin [Wisconsin Alumni Research Foundation]
WARIS Warfarin Reinfarction Study
WARIS II Warfarin-Aspirin Reinfarction Study–Norwegian
WARSS Warfarin-Aspirin Recurrent Stroke Study
WAS weekly activities summary; Wiskott-Aldrich syndrome
WASH Warfarin-Aspirin Study of Heart Failure
WASID Warfarin-Aspirin Symptomatic Intracranial Disease [study]
WASP Weber Advanced Spatial Perception [test]; Wiskott-Aldrich syndrome protein
Wass Wasserman [reaction]
WAT word association test
WATCH Warfarin Antiplatelet Trial in Chronic Heart Failure; Worcester-area Trial for Counseling in Hyperlipidemia
WATSMART Waterloo Spatial Motion Analysis and Recording Technique
WAVE Women's Angiographic Vitamin and Estrogen [trial]
WB waist belt; washable base; washed bladder; water bottle; Wechsler-Bellevue [Scale]; weight-bearing; well baby; Western blot [assay]; wet bulb; whole blood; whole body; Willowbrook [virus]; Wilson-Blair [agar]
Wb weber; well-being
WBA wax bean agglutinin; Western blot assay; whole body activity
Wb/A webers/ampere
WBAPTT whole blood activated partial thromboplastin time
WBC well baby care/clinic; white blood cell; white blood cell count; whole blood cell count
WBCT wet-bulb globe temperature; whole-blood clotting time
WBDC whole-body digital scanner
WBE whole-body extract
WBF whole-blood folate**

WBGT wet bulb global temperature

WBH whole-blood hematocrit; whole-body hyperthermia

WBLT Watson-Barker Listening Test

Wb/m² weber per square meter

WBN whole-blood nitrogen

WBPTT whole-blood partial thromboplastin time

WBR whole-body radiation

WBRT whole-blood recalcification time

WBS Wechsler-Bellevue Scale; whole-blood serum; whole-body scan; Wiedemann-Beckwith syndrome; Williams-Beuren syndrome; withdrawal body shakes

WBT wet bulb temperature

WC ward clerk; water closet; Weber-Christian [syndrome]; wheel chair; white cell; white cell casts; white cell count; white child; whooping cough; wild caught [animal]; work capacity; workers' compensation; writer's cramp

WC' whole complement

W/C watch carefully; wheel chair

W3C World Wide Web Consortium

wc wheel chair

WCC Walker carcinosarcoma cells; white cell count; windowed cross correlation

WCD Weber-Christian disease

WCE whole cell extract; work capacity evaluation

WCGS Western Collaborative Group Study

WCL Wenckebach cycle length; whole cell lysate

w/cm² watts per square centimeter

WCPs whole chromosome paints

WCS white clot syndrome; Wisconsin Card Sort [test]

WCST Wisconsin Card Sorting Test

WCT word categorization test

WCTU Women's Christian Temperance Union

WCUS Wiktor Stent and Cutting Balloon Angioplasty Study

WD wallerian degeneration; well developed; well differentiated; wet dressing; Whitney Damon [dextrose]; Winger distribution; Wilson disease; with disease; withdraw or withdrawn; without dyskinesia; Wolman disease; wrist disarticulation

W/D warm and dry

Wd ward

wd well developed; wound, wounded

WDCC well-developed collateral circulation

WDHA watery diarrhea, hypokalemia, achlorhydria [syndrome]

WDHH watery diarrhea, hypokalemia, and hypochlorhydria

WDI warfarin dose index

WDL well-differentiated lymphocytic

WDLL well-differentiated lymphatic lymphoma

WDMF wall-defective microbial forms

WDR wide dynamic range

WDS watery diarrhea syndrome; wet dog shakes [syndrome]

WDSCC well-differentiated squamous cell carcinoma

WDWN, wdwn well developed and well nourished

WE wax ester; Wernicke encephalopathy; western encephalitis; western encephalomyelitis; wound of entry

We weber

WEB Women's Experience with Battering [scale]

WECN Wisconsin Ethics Committee Network

WEDI Workshop for Electronic Data Interchange

WEE western equine encephalitis/ encephalomyelitis

WELL-HART Women's Estrogen/Progestin and Lipid-lowering Hormone Atherosclerosis Regression Trial

WELLSTENT-CABG Wellstent European Study on Stenting for Coronary Artery Bypass Grafts

WER wheal erythema reaction

WERN Workgroup of European Nurse Researchers

WES wall echo sign; work environment scale; wound evaluation scale

WESDR Wisconsin Epidemiologic Study of Diabetic Retinopathy

WESH West European Study of Health

WEST Western European Stent Trial; Women's Estrogen for Stroke Trial

WF Weil-Felix reaction; white female; Wistar-Furth [rat]

W/F, wf white female

WFC workflow cycle

WFD word-finding difficulty

WFE Williams flexion exercise

WFI water for injection
WFL within function limits
WfMS workflow management system
WFOT World Federation of Occupational Therapists
WFR Weil-Felix reaction; wheal-and-flare reaction
WFS Waterhouse-Friederichsen syndrome
WFSL workflow specification language
WFT windowed Fourier transform
WG water gauge; Wegener granulomatosis; Wright-Giemsa [stain]
WGA wheat germ agglutinin
WGE wheat germ extract
WG-RH whole genome radiation hybrid task
wgt weight
WH well hydrated; Werdnig-Hoffmann [syndrome]; whole homogenate; wound healing
Wh, wh white
w·h watt-hour
WHA warm and humid air; World Health Assembly
WHAP Women's Health Australian Project
WHAS Women's Health and Aging Study; Women's Heart Attack Study
WHAT Worcester Heart Attack Trial
wh ch wheel chair; white child
WHCOA White House Conference on Aging
WHCR Wolf-Hirschhorn chromosome region
WHD Werdnig-Hoffmann disease
WHEASE What Happens Eventually to Asthmatics Sociologically and Epidemiologically? [study]
WHHHIMP Wernicke encephalopathy/withdrawal, hypertensive encephalopathy, hypoglycemia, hypoxemia, intracranial bleeding/infection, meningitis/encephalitis, poison/medication
WHHL Watanaby heritable hyperlipidemia; Watanaby heritable hyperlipidemic [rabbit]
WHI Women's Health Initiative
WHIMS Women's Health Initiative Memory Study
WHIN Wisconsin Health Information Network
WHML Wellcome Historical Medical Library

WHO World Health Organization; wrist-hand orthosis
WHO/ISH World Health Organization/International Society of Hypertension [survey]
whp whirlpool
WHR waist:hips girth ratio
whr watt-hour
WHRC World Health Research Centre
WHS Werdnig-Hoffmann syndrome; Wolf-Hirschhorn syndrome; Women's Health Study
WHT Warm Heart Trial
WHTVS Women's Health Trial Vanguard Study
WHV woodchuck hepatic virus
WHVP wedged hepatic venous pressure
WHYMPI West Haven–Yale Multidimensional Pain Inventory
WI human embryonic lung cell line; walk-in [patient]; water ingestion; weaning index; Wistar [rat]
WIA wounded in action
WIBC Wiggins Interpersonal Behavior Circle
WIC walk-in clinic; women, infants, and children
WICHEN Western Interstate Commission for Higher Education in Nursing
WIHS Women's Interagency Human Immunodeficiency Virus [HIV] Study
WIL workflow intermediate language
WIMP windows, icons, menus, pointing
WIN Wallstent in Native Vessel [study]; Weight Control Information Network
WINS Wallstent in Saphenous Vein Grafts [study]
WIPI Word Intelligibility Picture Identification
WIS Wechsler Intelligence Scale
WISC Wechsler Intelligence Scale for Children
WISCR Wisconsin clinical record
WISC-R Wechsler Intelligence Scale for Children-Revised
WISE Women's Ischemic Syndrome Evaluation
WIST Whitaker Index of Schizophrenic Thinking
WITS Women and Infants Transmission Study
WITT Wittenborn [Psychiatric Rating Scale]

W-J Woodcock-Johnson [Psychoeducational Battery]

WJG Wilders-Jongsma-van Ginneken [pacemaker model]

WK week; Wernicke-Korsakoff [syndrome]; Wilson-Kimmelstiel [syndrome]

wk weak; week; work

WKD Wilson-Kimmelstiel disease

W/kg watts per kilogram

WKS Wernicke-Korsakoff syndrome

WKY Wistar-Kyoto [rat]

WL waiting list; waterload; wavelength; weight loss; withdrawal; Wood's lamp; working level; workload

wl wavelength

WLE wide local excision

WLF whole lymphocytic fraction

WLI weight-length index

WLM white light microscopy; working level month [radon]

WLS wet lung syndrome

WLT whole lung tomography

WM Waldenström macroglobulinemia; wall motion; ward manager; warm and moist; Wernicke-Mann [hemiplegia]; wet mount; white male; white matter; whole milk; Wilson-Mikity [syndrome]; working memory

W-M Weil-Marchesani [syndrome]

W/M white male

wm white male; whole milk; whole mount

w/m² watts per square meter

WMA wall motion abnormality; wall motion analysis; World Medical Association

WMC weight-matched control

WME Williams' medium E

WMH white matter hyperintensities

WMHP Women's Medical Health Page

WML white matter lesion

WMO ward medical officer

WMP weight management program

WMR work metabolic rate; World Medical Relief

WMS Wechsler Memory Scale; Weill-Marchesani syndrome; Williams syndrome

WMS-R Wechsler memory scale–revised

WMX whirlpool, massage, exercise

WN, wn well nourished

WNE West Nile encephalitis

WNF well-nourished female

WNL within normal limits

WNM well-nourished male

WNPW wide, notched P wave

WNV West Nile virus

WO wash out; will order; written order

W/O water in oil [emulsion]

w/o without

wo weeks old

WOB work of breathing

WOB$_I$ imposed work of breathing

WOB$_P$ physiologic work of breathing

WOB$_T$ total work of breathing (WOB$_P$ plus WOB$_I$

WOB$_V$ work of breathing performed by ventilator

WOE wound of entry

WOLF Work, Lipids, Fibrinogen [study]

WONCA World Organization of Family Doctors

WOOFS Warfarin Optimized Outpatient Follow-up Study

WOP without pain

WOSCOPS West of Scotland Coronary Prevention Study

WOU women's outpatient unit

WOWS weak opiate withdrawal scale

WOX wound of exit

WP weak-plate; weakly positive; wedge pressure; wet pack; wettable powder; whirlpool; white pulp; word processor; working point

W/P water/powder ratio

wp wettable powder

WPAI work productivity and activity impairment [questionnaire]

WP-ANAT weak-plate with anatomic information

WPB whirlpool bath

WPCU weighted patient care unit

WPDL workflow process definition language

Wpf wave at a pilot frequency

WPFM Wright peak flow meter

WPk Ward's pack; wet pack

WPPSI Wechsler Preschool and Primary Scale of Intelligence

WPR written progress report

WPRS Wittenborn Psychiatric Rating Scale

WPS wasting pig syndrome

WPW Wolff-Parkinson-White [syndrome]

WQAC ward quality assurance committee

W-QLI Wisconsin quality of life index

WR Wassermann reaction; water retention; weakly reactive; weak response; whole response; Wiedemann-Rautenstrauch [syndrome]; wiping reaction; work rate

Wr wrist; writhe

WRAIN Walter Reed Army Medical Center Institute of Nursing

WRAMC Walter Reed Army Medical Center

WRAML Wide Range Assessment of Memory and Learning

WRAT Wide Range Achievement Test

WRBC washed red blood cells

WRE wahole ragweed extract

WRC washed red cells; water retention coefficient

WRISS Weapons Related Injury Surveillance System

WRIST Washington Radiation for In-stent Restenosis Trial

WRK Woodward reagent K

WRMD work-related musculoskeletal disorder

WRMT Woodcock Reading Mastery Test

WRN Werner [syndrome]

WRS Ward-Romano syndrome; Wiedemann-Rautenstrauch syndrome

WRSI Work-related Strain Inventory

WRVP wedged renal vein pressure

WS Waardenburg syndrome; ward secretary; Warkany syndrome; warning stimulus; Warthin-Starry [stain]; water soluble; water swallow; Wollens' syndrome; Werner syndrome; West syndrome; Wilder silver [stain]; Williams syndrome; Wolfram syndrome; workstation

W·s watt-second

ws water-soluble

WSB wheat-soy blend

WSDRN Western Satellite Data Relay System

w-sec watt-second

WSI Waardenburg syndrome type I

WSA water-soluble antibiotic

WSC water-soluble contrast [medium]

WSL Wesselsbron [virus]

WSP withdrawal seizure prone

WSPHU Western Sector Public Health Unit [Australia]

WSR Westergren sedimentation rate; withdrawal seizure resistant

W/sr watts per steradian

WSS Weaver-Smith syndrome; wrinkly skin syndrome

WT wall thickness; water temperature; wavelet transform; wild type [strain]; Wilms tumor; wisdom teeth; work therapy

wt weight; white; wild type [virus]

WT-1 Wilms tumor gene-1

wtAAV wild type adeno-associated virus

wtAd wild type adenovirus

WTCC wavelet transform cross correlation

WTE whole time equivalent

WTF weight transferral frequency

WTH Women Take Heart [project]

WTP willingness to pay

WTR waist/thigh circumference ratio

WTS Wilson-Turner syndrome

W/U workup

WV walking ventilation

W/V, w/v percent weight in volume, weight/volume

W^v variable dominant spotting [mouse]

WVD wavelet-vaguelette decomposition; Winger-Ville distribution

WW Weight Watchers; wet weight; whisker weaving

W/W, w/w weight; percent weight

WWICT Western Washington Intracoronary Streptokinase Trial

WWISK Western Washington Intracoronary Streptokinase Trial

WWIST Western Washington Intravenous Streptokinase Trial

WWIV Western Washington Intravascular Streptokinase Trial

WWIVSK Western Washington Intravenous Streptokinase Trial

WWM world wide microscope

W/wo with or without

WWS Walker-Warburg syndrome; Wieacker Wolff syndrome; Working Well Study

WWSIMIT Western Washington Streptokinase in Myocardial Infarction Trials

WWU weighted working unit

WWW World Wide Web

WX wound of exit

WxB wax bite

WxP wax pattern

WY women years

WYSIWYG what you see is what you get

WZa wide zone alpha

WZS Weissenbacher-Zweymuller syndrome

X androgenic [zone]; cross; crossbite; exophoria distance; exposure; extra; female sex chromosome; ionization exposure; Kienböck's unit of x-ray exposure; magnification; multiplication times; reactance; removal of; respirations [anesthesia chart]; Roman numeral ten; start of anesthesia; "times"; translocation between two X chromosomes; transverse; unknown quantity; X unit; xylene

X̄ sample mean

Ẋ ionization exposure rate

x except; extremity; horizontal axis of a rectangular coordinate system; mole fraction; multiplication times; position; roentgen [rays]; sample mean; times; unknown factor; xanthine

X², χ² chi-square

X3 orientation as to time, place, and person

XA xanthurenic acid; x-ray analysis

X-A xylene and alcohol

Xa activated factor X; chiasma

Xaa unknown amino acid

XAD External Atrial Defibrillation [trial]

Xam examination

Xan xanthine

Xanth xanthomatosis

Xao xanthosine

XBP X-box binding protein

XBSN X-linked bulbospinal neuropathy

XC, Xc excretory cystogram

X-CAR cross-relational computer-based retention

XCE X-chromosome controlling element

X-CGD X-linked chronic granulomatous disease

XCMD external [computer] command

XD x-ray diffraction

XDH xanthine dehydrogenase

XDP xanthine diphosphate; xeroderma pigmentosum

XDR transducer

Xe electric susceptibility; xenon

XECT xenon-enhanced computed tomography

XEF excess ejection fraction

XES x-ray energy spectrometry

Xfb cross-linked fibrin

XGP xanthogranulomatous pyelonephritis

XGPT xylosylprotein-4-beta-galactosyltransferase

Ξ Greek capital letter *xi*

ξ Greek lower case letter *xi*

XIC X-inactivation center

XIP x-ray-induced polypeptide

XISHF Xamoterol in Severe Heart Failure [study]

XIST X-inactivation specific transcript

XL excess lactate; X-linked [inheritance]; xylose-lysine [agar base]

XLA, X-LA X-linked agammaglobulinemia

XLAS X-linked aqueductal stenosis

XLCM X-linked dilated cardiomyopathy

XLD X-linked dominant; xylose-lysine-deoxycholate [agar]

XLH X-linked hydrocephalus; X-linked hypophosphatemia

XLHED X-linked hypohidrotic ectodermal dysplasia

XLI X-linked ichthyosis

XLM extended markup language

XLMR X-linked mental retardation

XLMTM, XLMTm X-linked myotubular myopathy

XLOS X-linked Opitz syndrome

XLP X-linked lymphoproliferative [syndrome]

XLPD X-linked lymphoproliferative disease

XLR X-linked recessive

XLRP X-linked retinitis pigmentosa

XLS X-linked recessive lymphoproliferative syndrome

XLSP X-linked spastic paraplegia

XM crossmatch

Xm maternal chromosome X

xma chiasma

X-mas Christmas [factor]

x-mat crossmatch [blood]

X-match crossmatch

XML extensible markup language

XMP xanthine monophosphate
XMMR Xenopus molecular marker resource
XMR X-linked mental retardation
XN night blindness
XO presence of only one sex chromosome; xanthine oxidase
XOAD X-linked ocular albinism with deafness
XOAN X-linked ocular albinism of Nettleship-Fall
XOM extraocular movements
XOR exclusive operating room
XP xanthogranulomatous pyelonephritis; xeroderma pigmentosum
Xp paternal chromosome X; short arm of chromosome X
XPA xeroderma pigmentosum group A
XPC xeroderma pigmentosum group C
XPN xanthogranulomatous pyelonephritis
XPS x-ray photoemission spectroscopy
Xq long arm of chromosome X
XR xeroradiography; X-linked recessive [inheritance]; x-ray
x-rays roentgen rays
XRD x-ray diffraction
XRF x-ray fluorescence
XRII X-ray image intensifier
XRMR X-linked recessive mental retardation
XRN X-linked recessive nephrolithiasis
XRS x-ray sensitivity
XRT x-ray therapy
XS cross-section; excessive; xiphisternum

X/S cross-section
xs excess
XSA cross-section area
XSCID X-linked severe combined immunodeficiency [syndrome]
XSCLH X-linked subcortical laminar heterotopia
X-sect cross-section
XSP xanthoma striatum palmare
XT exotropia
Xt extra toe
Xta chiasmata
Xtab cross-tabulating
XTE xeroderma, talipes, and enamel defect [syndrome]
X-TEP crossed immunoelectrophoresis
XTM xanthoma tuberosum multiplex
XTP xanthosine triphosphate
X-TUL external tumescent ultrasound liposculpture
XU excretory urogram; X unit
Xu X-unit
XuMP xylulose monophosphate
Xu5P, Xu5p xylulose-5-phosphate
XX double strength; female chromosome type
46, XX 46 chromosomes, 2 X chromosomes (normal female)
XXL xylocaine
XX/XY sex karyotypes
XY male chromosome type
46, XY 46 chromosomes, 1 X and 1 Y chromosome (normal male)
Xyl xylose

Y a coordinate axis in a plane; male sex chromosome; tyrosine; year; yellow; yield; yttrium; *Yersinia*

y the vertical axis of a rectangular coordinate system

Y see *upsilon*

ʋ see *upsilon*

YA *Yersinia* arthritis

Y/A years of age

YAC yeast artificial chromosome

YACP young adult chronic patient

YADH yeast alcohol dehydrogenase

YAG yttrium aluminum garnet [laser]

Yahoo Yet Another Hierarchically Officious Oracle [hierarchical subject index to Web sites]

Yb ytterbium

YBOCS Yale-Brown Obsessive Compulsive Scale

YCB yeast carbon base

YCMI Yale Center for Medical Informatics

YCT YMCA Cardiac Therapy [program]

yd yard

YDV yeast-derived hepatitis B vaccine

YCVDS Yugoslavia Cardiovascular Disease Study

YDYES yin deficiency yang excess syndrome

YE yeast extract; yellow enzyme

YEH₂ reduced yellow enzyme

YEI *Yersinia enterocolitica* infection

Yel yellow

YF yellow fever

YFI yellow fever immunization

YFMD yellow fever membrane disease

YFV yellow fever virus

YHAP Yale Health and Aging Project

YLC youngest living child

YLD year lived with disability

YLS years of life saved

YM yeast and mannitol; Young's modulus

Y$_{max}$ maximum yield

YMB yeast malt broth

YNB yeast nitrogen base

YNS yellow nail syndrome

y/o years old

YOB year of birth

YOS Yale Observation Scale

YP yeast phase; yield pressure

YPA yeast, peptone, and adenine sulfate

YPLL years of potential life lost

yr year

YRBS Youth Risk Behavior Survey

YRD Yangtze River disease

YRRM Y ribonucleic acid [RNA] recognition motif

YS yellow spot; yolk sac

ys yellow spot; yolk sac

YSHR younger spontaneously hypertensive rat

YST yolk sac tumor

YT, yt yttrium

Y2K year 2000

yWACC younger woman with aggressive cervical cancer

YWKY younger Wistar-Kyoto rat

Z acoustic impedance; atomic number; complex impedance; contraction [Ger. *Zuckung*]; the disk that separates sarcomeres [Ger. *Zwischenscheibe*]; glutamine; impedance; ionic charge number; no effect; point formed by a line perpendicular to the nasion-menton line through the anterior nasal spine; proton number; section modulus; standard score; standardized deviate; zero; zone; a Z-shaped incision in plastic surgery

Z′,Z″ increasing degrees of contraction

z algebraic unknown or space coordinate; axis of a three-dimensional rectangular coordinate system; catalytic amount; standard normal deviate; zero

ZAG, ZA2G zinc-alpha-2-glycoprotein

ZAP zeta-associated protein zymosan-activated plasma [rabbit]

ZAPF zinc adequate pair-fed

ZAS zymosan-activated autologous serum

ZB zebra body

ZBG zinc-binding group

ZCP zinc chloride poisoning

ZD zero defects; zero discharge; zinc deficiency

Z-D Zamorano-Duchovny [digitizer]

ZDDP zinc dialkyldithiophosphate

ZES Zutphen Elderly Study

ZEST Zocor Early Start Trial

Z-DNA zig-zag (left-handed helical) deoxyribonucleic acid

ZDO zero differential overlap

ZDS zinc depletion syndrome

ZDV zidovudine

ZE Zollinger-Ellison [syndrome]

ZEBRA zero blanaced reimbursement account

ZEC Zinsser-Engman-Cole [syndrome]

ZEEP zero end-expiratory pressure

ZEPI zonal echo planar imaging

Z-ERS zeta erythrocyte sedimentation rate

ZES Zollinger-Ellison syndrome; Zutphen Elderly Study

ZEST Zocor Early Start Trial

Z Greek capital letter *zeta*

ζ Greek lower case letter *zeta*

ZF zero frequency; zinc finger [protein]; zona fasciculata

ZFF zinc fume fever

ZFP zinc finger protein

ZFX X-linked zinc finger protein

ZG zona glomerulosa

ZGM zinc glycinate marker

ZIFT zygote intrafallopian tube transfer

ZIG, ZIg zoster immunoglobulin

ZIP zoster immune plasma

ZK Zuelzer-Kaplan [syndrome]

ZLS Zimmerman-Laband syndrome

Zm zygomaxillare

ZMA zinc meta-arsenite

ZNF zinc finger [protein]

ZnOE zinc oxide and eugenol

ZNS zonisamide

ZO Zichen-Oppenheim [syndrome]; Zuelzer-Ogden [syndrome]

Zo impedance; thoracic fluid

ZOE zinc oxide-eugenol

ZOL zoladex

Zool zoology

ZP zona pellucida

ZPA zone of polarizing activity

ZPC zero point of change

ZPG zero population growth

ZPO zinc peroxide

ZPP zinc protoporphyrin

ZR zona reticularis

Zr zirconium

ZS Zellweger syndrome; Zutphen Study

ZSR zeta sedimentation ratio

ZT Zwolle Trial

ZTS zymosan-treated serum

Z-TSP zephiran-trisodium phosphate

ZTT zinc turbidity test

ZVD zidovudine

ZVT Zehlenverbindungstest

ZW Zellweger [syndrome]

ZWCHRS Zellweger cerebrohepatorenal syndrome

ZWOLLE Primary Coronary Angioplasty Compared with Intravenous Streptokinase [trial from Zwolle, The Netherlands]

ZWS Zellweger syndrome
ZXF zero crossing frequency
Zy zygion

ZyC zymosan complement
zyg zygotene
Zz ginger [Lat. *zingibar*]